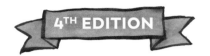

4TH EDITION

Cooking à la Heart

500 Easy and Delicious Recipes to Help Make Every Meal Healthy

**Linda Hachfeld, MPH, RDN, and
Amy Myrdal Miller, MS, RDN, FAND**

Foreword by James M. Rippe, MD

THE EXPERIMENT

NEW YORK

COOKING À LA HEART, FOURTH EDITION:
500 Easy and Delicious Recipes to Help Make Every Meal Heart Healthy
Text copyright © 2023 by Linda Hachfeld, MPH, RDN, and Amy Myrdal Miller, MS, RDN, FAND
Photographs copyright © 2023 by Sarah Hone
Foreword copyright © 2023 by James M. Rippe, MD

STRAWBERRY, PINEAPPLE & MINT SALAD (PAGE 145)

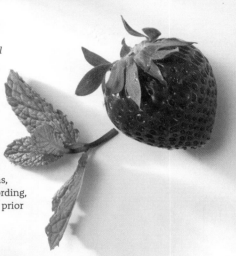

The Experiment, LLC
220 East 23rd Street, Suite 600
New York, NY 10010-4658
theexperimentpublishing.com

This book contains the opinions and ideas of its authors. It is intended to provide helpful and informative material on the subjects addressed in the book. It is sold with the understanding that the authors and publisher are not engaged in rendering medical, health, or any other kind of personal professional services in the book. The authors and publisher specifically disclaim all responsibility for any liability, loss, or risk—personal or otherwise—that is incurred as a consequence, directly or indirectly, of the use and application of any of the contents of this book.

THE EXPERIMENT and its colophon are registered trademarks of The Experiment, LLC. Many of the designations used by manufacturers and sellers to distinguish their products are claimed as trademarks. Where those designations appear in this book and The Experiment was aware of a trademark claim, the designations have been capitalized.

The Experiment's books are available at special discounts when purchased in bulk for premiums and sales promotions as well as for fundraising or educational use. For details, contact us at info@theexperimentpublishing.com.

Library of Congress Cataloging-in-Publication Data

Names: Hachfeld, Linda, author. | Myrdal Miller, Amy, author.
Title: Cooking à la heart : 500 easy and delicious recipes to help make every meal heart healthy / Linda Hachfeld, MPH, RDN, and Amy Myrdal Miller, MS, RDN, FAND.
Description: 4th edition. | New York : The Experiment, [2023] | Includes bibliographical references and index.
Identifiers: LCCN 2022029884 | ISBN 9781615197583 | ISBN 9781615197590 (ebook)
Subjects: LCSH: Low-fat diet--Recipes. | Low-cholesterol diet--Recipes. | Salt-free diet--Recipes. | Cooking. | LCGFT: Cookbooks.
Classification: LCC RM237.7 .H325 2023 | DDC 641.5/6384--dc23/eng/20220802
LC record available at https://lccn.loc.gov/2022029884

ISBN 978-1-61519-758-3
Ebook ISBN 978-1-61519-759-0

Cover and text design by Beth Bugler
Food styling by Melissa Mileto
Illustrations by Adobe Stock

Manufactured in China

First printing February 2023
10 9 8 7 6 5 4 3 2 1

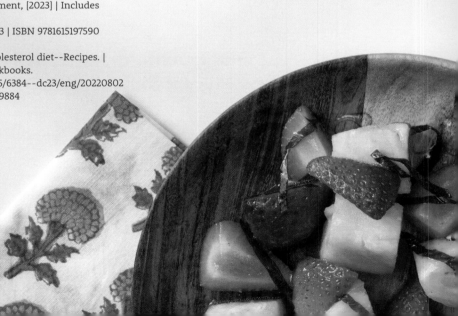

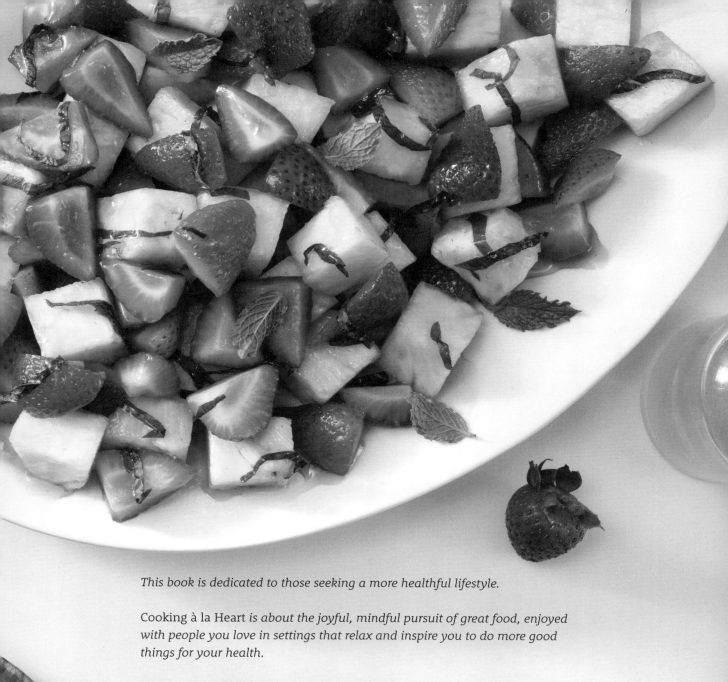

This book is dedicated to those seeking a more healthful lifestyle.

Cooking à la Heart is about the joyful, mindful pursuit of great food, enjoyed with people you love in settings that relax and inspire you to do more good things for your health.

We've honored plant-forward eating patterns inspired by cultural traditions and referenced the science that supports these eating patterns to produce a book we hope will build confidence and competence in your home kitchen.

We support and encourage you to do the best you can every day in pursuit of better health.

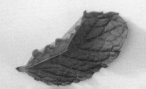

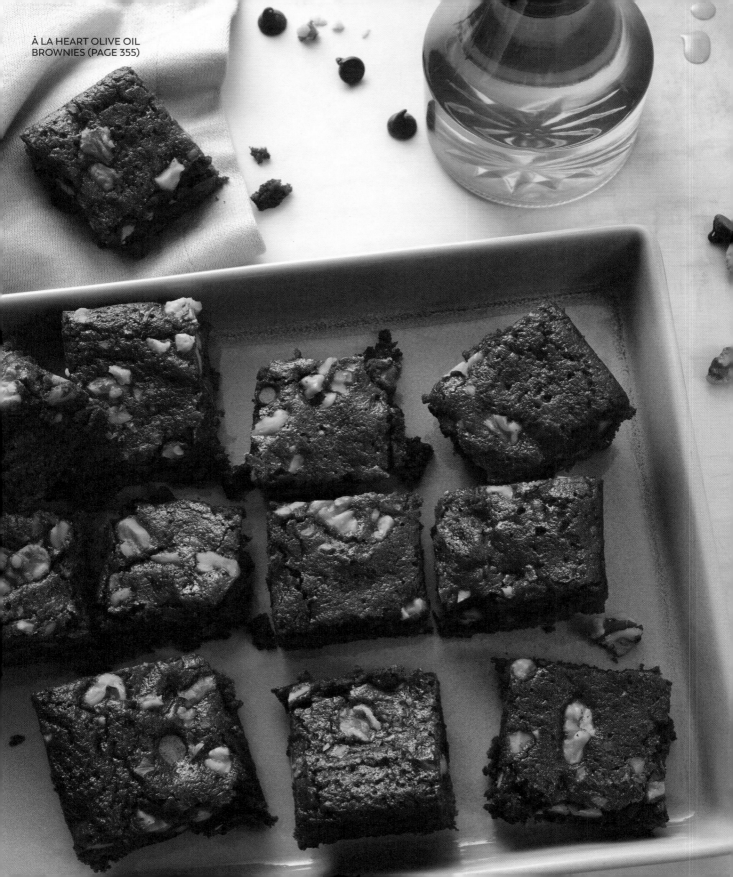

À LA HEART OLIVE OIL
BROWNIES (PAGE 355)

Contents

Foreword by James M. Rippe, MD 1

Introduction 3

1 The Science & Cultures Behind Heart-Healthy
   Eating Patterns 5

2 The Principles & Practices of *Cooking à la Heart* 11

3 Seasonings 28

4 Sauces, Salsas, Dressings & More 42

5 Stocks, Soups & Stews 68

6 Quick Breads & Yeast Breads 92

7 Breakfast & Brunch 118

8 Fruit & Vegetable Side Salads 142

9 Entrée Salads 158

10 Burgers, Sandwiches, Tacos & More 176

11 Pizzas, Piadine & Flatbreads 192

12 Pasta 204

13 Whole Grains 220

14 Legumes 238

15 Vegetables 254

16 Fish & Shellfish 282

17 Chicken & Turkey 302

18 Beef, Pork & Lamb 322

19 Appetizers, Snacks & Nibbles 338

20 Desserts & Sweet Treats 350

References 364

Acknowledgments 367

Index 369

About the Authors 378

Foreword

By James M. Rippe, MD

What a pleasure to write a foreword to this wonderful and important book! As a cardiologist and researcher studying how daily habits impact both short- and long-term health, I have been inextricably drawn to both nutrition and physical activity for many years. These two modalities—together with healthy sleep, stress reduction, and positive interpersonal relationships—form the cornerstones of lifestyle medicine, an academic discipline that originated with the textbook I edit carrying this very title, initially published in 1999.

Over the past twenty-five years, an enormous literature has emerged concerning how nutrition impacts chronic diseases in general and heart disease in particular. Not surprisingly, this literature underpins evidence-based guidelines from prestigious organizations like the US Department of Agriculture, American Heart Association, and World Health Organization: namely that to prevent obesity, people should eat more fruits, vegetables, whole grains, and fish (particularly oily fish) while not over-consuming calories. These nutrition recommendations, along with other lifestyle-related factors such as regular physical activity, reduce the risk of heart disease by over eighty percent and that of diabetes by more than ninety-one percent.

In addition, emerging literature suggests that inflammation represents a significant link connecting chronic disease conditions including cardiovascular disease, diabetes, obesity, and even cancer and Alzheimer's. Some investigators have even suggested that we coin the phrase "cardiodiabesity" to underscore their common underlying etiology. Of note, the standard American diet has also been shown to significantly provoke inflammation. (Ironically, the acronym for this diet is "SAD.")

The strategies recommended by these prestigious international bodies may seem simple, but how are we really doing as individuals? Sadly, not very well! Only twelve percent of adults in the United States eat the recommended servings of fruits, and just seven percent consume the recommended servings of vegetables. The standard American diet contains only half the fiber recommended by the Centers for Disease Control, and over seventy percent of the US adult population is overweight or obese.

Unfortunately, the medical community has largely stood on the sidelines while these problems have continued to accelerate. Just twenty-five percent of individuals with diabetes receive nutritional counseling from their physician, and only fifteen percent of the rest of the patient population receives any nutrition counseling. This is a tragic, wasted opportunity, since over seventy percent of adults see their primary care physician at least once a year.

Why aren't we doing better? The simple answer is that change is hard and many of the processed food items in the standard American diet are convenient and tasty. The more complex answer is that nutrition is complicated, and individuals often have difficulty carrying out changes to make their eating patterns more heart healthy.

One thing I have learned from my work in nutrition is that knowledge alone is typically not enough to promote change. We need to find ways to effectively communicate to the public and motivate them to change. Furthermore, we must make heart-healthy nutrition *easy and enjoyable*.

All this brings me back to this important book: a motivational, science-based compendium of information that is both practical and user-friendly. *Cooking à la Heart* will be enjoyable for beginning and advanced chefs alike who are looking to improve their personal and family nutrition.

I was particularly pleased to see that three of the book's core principles are evidence-based and practical: focus on flavor (lower salt), prioritize plants, and embrace enjoyment. The fourth core principle about finding good sources of protein is also important since it combats the common misperception that plants cannot be a major source of protein.

I am also pleased that the authors emphasized the Mediterranean, MIND, and DASH diets. These diets are loaded with fruits and vegetables and are proven to decrease the risk of heart disease and other chronic illnesses. (They even improve mental health and lower the risk of dementia!)

One of my early mentors in cooking and nutrition was my friend Julia Child. (I met Julia at the Harvard Radcliffe Pottery Studio, which I built and ran for five years before going to medical school; Julia used to come by and purchase or commission various pots I made. In fact, if you look at the cover of her classic *The Way to Cook*, you will see a covered casserole pot that I made for her in the upper right-hand corner of the picture.) One of many important things Julia often said was, "As we think about health and nutrition, don't forget the 'pleasure of the table.'" The authors of *Cooking à la Heart* clearly embrace this significant concept!

These authors are also highly qualified and very skilled at developing recipes. Linda Hachfeld has been a guiding light in all four editions of this book, which began with her work with the Minnesota Heart Health Program in the 1980s, an important research endeavor that sought to improve public health and reduce risk of heart disease through individual and community interventions. I have known Amy Myrdal Miller for over twenty-five years, as I initially hired her for her first job in nutrition research: Amy consulted on hundreds of patients in our Cardiac Research Program, and she and I coauthored two books on heart-healthy nutrition. She subsequently enhanced her culinary knowledge by working for The Culinary Institute of America, where she organized more than fifty conferences on nutrition, health, world cuisines, and sustainability over seven years. I'd like to think that I launched Amy into her book-writing career, but even from her earliest days, her nutrition knowledge far surpassed mine!

This extraordinary book comes at an auspicious time. Even as the scientific links between nutrition and heart health have exploded, we still face the daunting challenge of motivating people to use this knowledge to lower their risk of heart disease and other chronic illnesses. Books like *Cooking à la Heart* will play a substantial role in this important mission. I applaud the authors and am grateful for the effort that they have made to help reduce the risk of heart disease, the number-one killer in the United States and around the world, with delicious and healthy recipes. As Julia Child often said, "Bon appétit!"

James M. Rippe, MD, is the founder and director of the Rippe Lifestyle Institute, the largest research organization in the world exploring how daily habits impact health. He is also a professor of medicine focusing on cardiology at the University of Massachusetts Chan Medical School.

Introduction

Thank you for choosing this book to explore heart-healthy eating patterns! We created and curated recipes for *Cooking à la Heart* with busy home cooks in mind, people like us who are juggling many roles and responsibilities. We focused on foods and flavors that both are delicious and offer nutrition and health benefits. Finally, we've included both quick and easy recipes and recipes that take more time and effort. Like life, this book is all about balance.

Rest assured, this is not a book about diets and deprivation. Instead, it focuses on foods and flavor development strategies that promote good health and enjoyment of food. We want to help you find a way of eating that is enjoyable and doable for the long haul, one that helps promote and protect your cardiovascular health.

Why is this so important? Your heart is the primary organ that pumps blood throughout your body. The arteries and veins through which blood flows to all of our organs, including the brain, can be negatively impacted by high blood pressure, high blood cholesterol, smoking, inactivity, stress, genetics, and more. When arteries leading to the heart are damaged, it can cause a heart attack.

Plaques in the brain can lead to dementia and Alzheimer's. A complete blockage in an artery in the brain can cause a stroke, possibly resulting in loss of vision, movement on one side of the body, or the ability to speak. Protecting your heart and the rest of your cardiovascular system is essential for overall wellness and quality of life. Our goal is to provide you with information, insights, strategies, and recipes that can protect your cardiovascular system, keeping it as healthy as possible, so you can live your very best life!

We also want to help you develop new attitudes and habits that motivate you to make the best possible choices, recognizing that "perfect is the enemy of good" when it comes to food, fitness, and health. Life is too short to waste time on guilt. *Cooking à la Heart* is about the joyful, mindful pursuit of great food enjoyed with people you love.

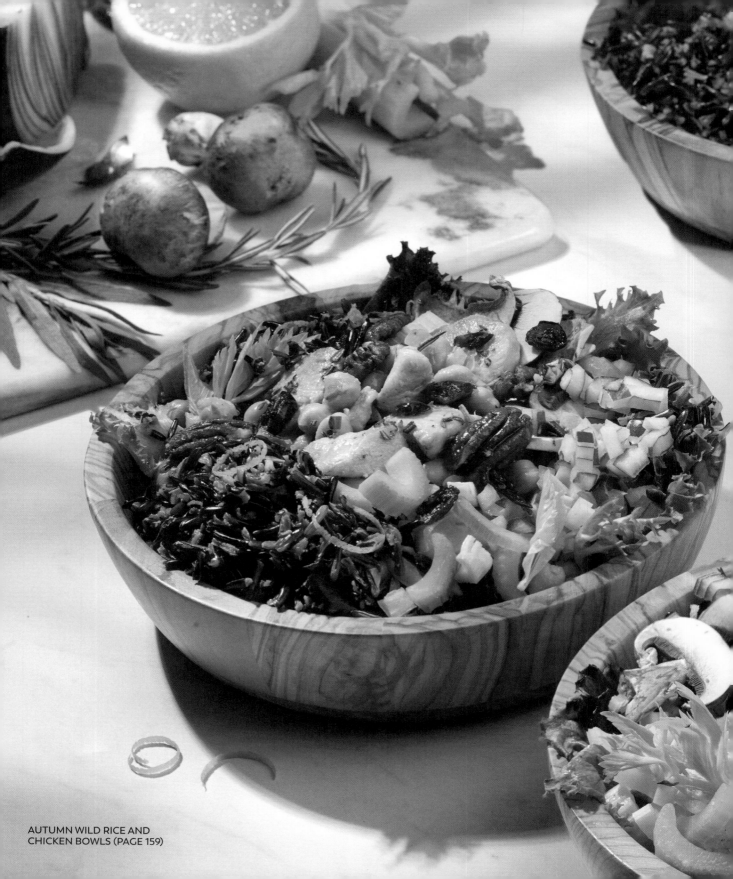

AUTUMN WILD RICE AND
CHICKEN BOWLS (PAGE 159)

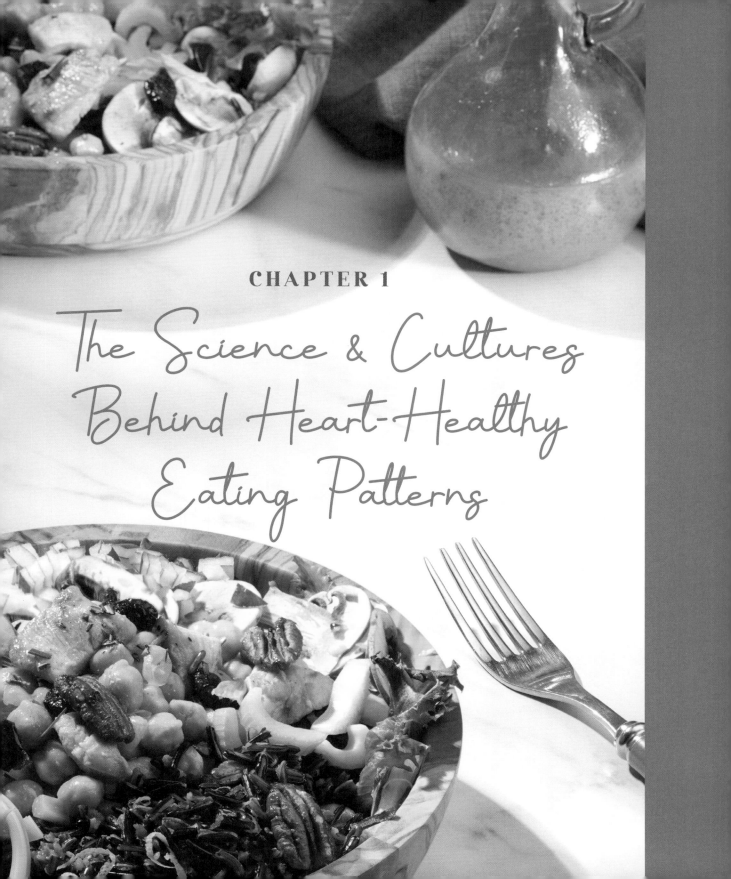

CHAPTER 1

The Science & Cultures Behind Heart-Healthy Eating Patterns

There are five principles to keep in mind as you read through this book.

1 There is no single dietary pattern best suited to every person, but there are traits common among eating patterns from around the world that predict better health outcomes, including greater consumption of fruits, vegetables, and other minimally processed plant-based foods.

2 Healthful dietary patterns do not have to be low in total fat—the traditional Mediterranean eating pattern, perhaps the most studied, contains more than 40 percent calories from fat, of which most is unsaturated fats from plant-based sources like olive oil.

3 Health-promoting eating patterns never need to eliminate entire food groups; in fact, eating a broad variety of foods across all food groups promotes greater nutrient intake, which can in turn promote better health outcomes.

4 If you want to focus on limiting a single nutrient to promote better health, focus on limiting your sodium intake, as this can reduce your risk of developing high blood pressure. According to the World Health Organization, high blood pressure (hypertension) is a major cause of premature death around the world. Hypertension increases risk of heart disease, kidney disease, and other diseases. It can also cause headaches, vision changes, and even anxiety.

5 Just like there's no single consummate dietary pattern, there's no single ideal food that will lead to perfect health. We'll say it again: There are no superfoods, only super eating patterns. Healthful eating patterns should be filled with a wide variety of foods from all food groups, some enjoyed in great abundance every day, like fruits and vegetables, and others enjoyed less often in smaller amounts, like alcohol and sugar-sweetened desserts.

Mediterranean-Style Eating Patterns and Health Outcomes

Nutrition researchers have been evaluating the impact of eating habits and other lifestyle factors on health outcomes since the mid-1950s, beginning with the Seven Countries Study by Dr. Ancel Keys and his colleagues at the University of Minnesota. Researchers looked at the diets of people in Finland, Yugoslavia (now Bosnia and Herzegovina, Croatia, Macedonia, Montenegro, Serbia, and Slovenia), Greece, Italy, Japan, the Netherlands, and the United States. Despite many socioeconomic and cultural differences among these countries, the data showed that people who ate the most saturated fat had higher blood cholesterol levels and higher risk of cardiovascular disease.

One interesting finding, which led to more research focused on traditional Mediterranean eating patterns, was that people living on the Greek island of Crete ate the most vegetables, had the highest fat intake (mostly unsaturated fat from sources like olives and olive oil), and had the lowest rates of cardiovascular disease compared to people in the other six countries.

The Seven Countries Study was an epidemiological study: People filled out forms about their diet and lifestyle factors, had certain diagnostic tests run occasionally, and were followed over many years to determine associations between diet and lifestyle factors, like exercise levels or smoking habits, and health outcomes, like heart attacks and stroke. Epidemiological studies show associations, not cause and effect. Think about umbrellas—people are more likely to carry them when rain is predicted, but carrying an umbrella doesn't cause it to rain.

While many people think there is one Mediterranean diet, there are actually distinct differences in eating patterns among Mediterranean countries and within regions. Think about Italy: The foods and cultural eating patterns on the island of Sicily are very

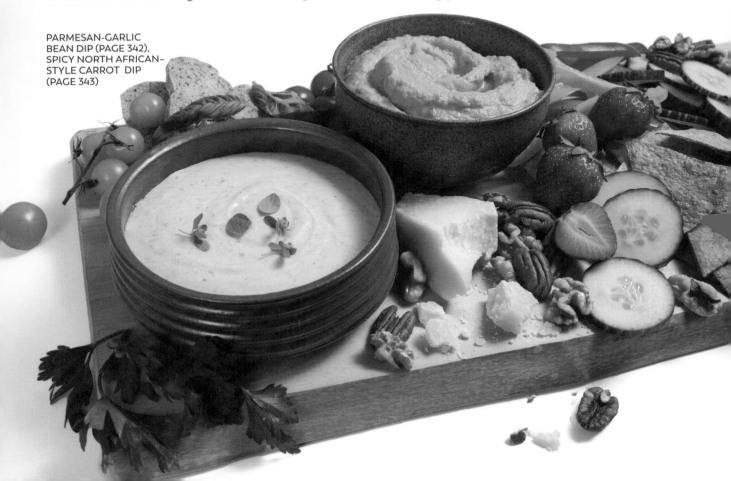

PARMESAN-GARLIC BEAN DIP (PAGE 342), SPICY NORTH AFRICAN-STYLE CARROT DIP (PAGE 343)

different from those of Northern Italy, for example, where dairy products play a much larger role in traditional diets. Likewise, coastal regions of Spain eat much more seafood than inland areas where meat—often in the form of sausage—is a more common source of protein. The one trait all regions of the Mediterranean have in common is abundant use of plant-based foods: fruits, vegetables, legumes, whole grains, nuts, seeds, and plant-based oils like olive oil.

In the early 2000s, a group of researchers in Spain wanted to design and conduct a randomized controlled trial (RCT) to see if following a Mediterranean diet could truly reduce the risk of cardiovascular disease among adults living in Spain who were at high risk of having a heart attack or stroke. The researchers enrolled nearly 7,500 people with multiple risk factors for cardiovascular disease, including having type 2 diabetes, high blood pressure, and high cholesterol, and being overweight. Participants were randomly assigned to one of three groups: a control group asked to eat a low-fat diet, a group asked to follow a Mediterranean-style eating pattern and consume a liter (a little more than a quart) of olive oil per week, or a group asked to follow a Mediterranean-style eating pattern and consume an ounce (28 g) of nuts (almonds, hazelnuts, and walnuts) every day.

Called the PREDIMED study, it was halted early due to ethical concerns about the significant cardiovascular risk reduction for participants in the two Mediterranean diet groups. Participants in both groups had a decreased risk of a heart attack, stroke, or death from a cardiovascular incident. It wasn't fair to keep the participants in the control group on a diet that didn't help reduce their risk, especially since all the study participants were at increased risk.

What was most astounding about this study is that participants in the group that ate a Mediterranean diet with olive oil didn't gain weight. The average household size was 1.6 persons, and study participants were encouraged to share their olive oil with their household. A liter of olive oil contains more than 8,000 calories, which meant that study participants could have consumed, on average, an additional 720 calories per day. An ounce (28 g) of nuts, which the other Mediterranean diet group was directed to eat each day, contains 190 calories. In theory, participants in both groups should have gained some weight, but researchers believe they made other subtle changes to their eating patterns to accommodate for the additional calories. If those changes included eating fewer foods containing refined carbohydrates, they got significant benefits. Researchers at Harvard have shown that replacing highly processed carbohydrates with saturated fat reduces risk of heart disease, likely because this decreases the

A Closer Look at Triglycerides and Cholesterol

Triglycerides are a type of fat found in the blood; they travel through our blood stream. They rise after meals and drop after a few hours. Triglycerides can come from food, but most are made by the liver. The same is true for cholesterol. Most of the cholesterol in our bodies comes from what our livers make; very little comes from the foods we eat. Lipoproteins carry cholesterol through the blood. Very-low-density lipoproteins (VLDL) are likely the most dangerous lipoprotein; they are more likely to cause plaques to build up in arteries throughout the body.

Choosing more fiber-rich plant-based foods encourages your liver to make less low-density lipoproteins (LDL), while choosing more healthful sources of fat, like extra virgin olive oil and nuts, encourages your liver to make more high-density lipoproteins (HDL). HDL is a good type of lipoprotein that clears cholesterol—from the foods we eat as well as the cholesterol our livers create—from our blood.

inflammation associated with consuming these processed carbohydrates. We share more information about saturated fat in chapter 2 (see pages 15–17).

The PREDIMED study conclusively showed that the type of fat you consume is much more important than the total amount; that limiting fat is not necessary if you are choosing foods with mostly unsaturated fat, like extra virgin olive oil and nuts; and that you can maintain your weight and protect your cardiovascular health while eating more fat if you reduce your intake of highly processed carbohydrates, such as sugar-sweetened beverages, sugar-sweetened cereals and coffee creamers, refined breads, cookies, cakes, donuts, and other desserts made with refined flours and sweeteners.

Dietary Approaches to Stop Hypertension: The DASH Diet

The DASH Diet was created by researchers at the U.S. National Institutes of Health (NIH) to see if a specific dietary pattern could be as powerful as prescription medications in reducing blood pressure. Results from controlled feeding studies showed that a low-fat dietary pattern rich in fruits, vegetables, and low-fat dairy products—all foods that contribute potassium—could significantly reduce blood pressure. Follow-up studies with higher fat levels in the DASH diet have shown that this pattern can significantly reduce blood pressure while also reducing triglyceride and very low-density lipoprotein (VLDL) levels without increasing low-density lipoprotein (LDL) cholesterol levels. Additional follow-up studies have shown that in people over age 50, the most important factor in reducing blood pressure is reducing dietary sodium as well as saturated fat. These findings form the basis for the development of many of the recipes in this book, which contain lower quantities of sodium and use limited amounts of foods that contribute saturated fat.

The Mediterranean-DASH Intervention for Neurodegenerative Delay: The MIND Diet

Since 1997, when the original DASH research results were published, there has been a steady stream of peer-reviewed studies of the potential benefits of adopting a Mediterranean-style eating pattern that closely matches the DASH diet. (Keep in mind that the Mediterranean diet was created by people living in certain cultures, while the DASH diet was created by researchers.) The latest researcher-developed diet is called the MIND diet, which was designed to determine if food choices have an impact on brain health. While the MIND diet is very similar to a Mediterranean-style eating pattern and to the DASH diet, it emphasizes certain foods, such as extra virgin olive oil, nuts, dark leafy greens, and berries, that contain nutrients associated with reducing the risk of dementia (when consumed as part of a healthful dietary pattern). Results show that following the MIND diet can slow the cognitive declines associated with aging.

To reduce the risk of dementia and Alzheimer's, embrace these findings and focus on incorporating more extra virgin olive oil (versus other plant-based oils), nuts, dark leafy greens, and berries in your diet, knowing that the cognitive benefits, along with the cardiovascular benefits, are significant. You'll see these foods used throughout the recipes in this book, with extra virgin olive oil taking the largest role. It's the oil we call for most often in recipes; we'll share more about why in the next chapter.

In the next chapter, we present our ten principles and practices for Cooking à la Heart, share tips about how to shop for and select ingredients from various categories, offer recommendations for making your home-cooked meals more flavorful and delicious, clear up confusion about the most common myths we hear (e.g., sea salt is a better than regular table salt), and much more.

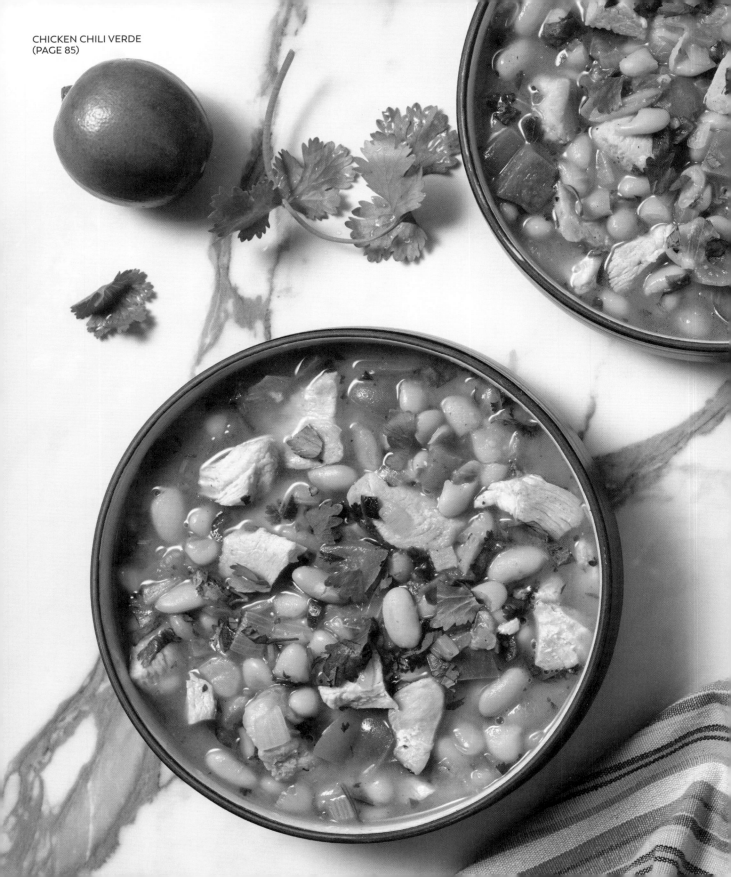

CHICKEN CHILI VERDE
(PAGE 85)

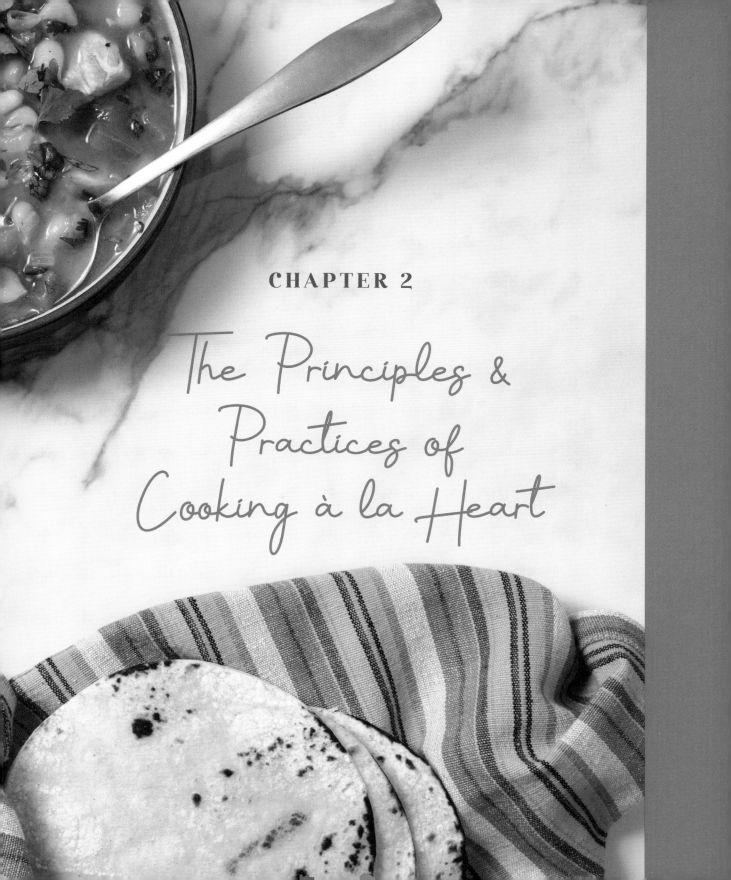

CHAPTER 2

*The Principles &
Practices of
Cooking à la Heart*

Our aim with *Cooking à la Heart* is to help you gain a greater understanding of the importance of developing a healthful eating pattern. The healthiest eating patterns focus on fruits, vegetables, legumes, whole grains, nuts, seeds, healthy sources of protein, and plant-based oils, and are lower in sodium and saturated fat. To make your cooking a bit easier and your food more delicious and enjoyable, we'd like to introduce you to our favorite strategies.

Here are ten principles and practices to guide you as you fully embrace *Cooking à la Heart*.

PRINCIPLES & PRACTICES OF COOKING À LA HEART
Inspired by the Mediterranean, DASH, and MIND Diets

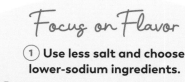

Focus on Flavor
1. Use less salt and choose lower-sodium ingredients.
2. Use more spice blends that don't rely on added salt for flavor.
3. Choose the best-quality oils for your cooking.
4. Make sauces, salsas, and dressings to add additional flavors and textures to your food.

Embrace Enjoyment

10. Enjoy desserts made more thoughtfully with better-for-you ingredients.

Prioritize Plants
5. Use more whole grain flours in your baking, and add more intact whole grains to your meals.
6. Use more fruits and vegetables in all their glorious forms in your cooking.

Pick Powerful Proteins
7. Choose healthy sources of protein from plants and animals.
8. Eat more seafood!
9. Snack on nuts and other nourishing nibbles.

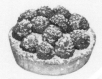

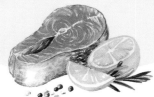

Use Less Salt and Choose Lower-Sodium Ingredients

Reducing the amount of sodium in your diet is one way to reduce blood pressure. Sodium comes from many sources, but the two biggest contributors for most people are processed and restaurant foods. If you start to cook more and you focus on using unprocessed or minimally processed ingredients, you can quickly start to reduce your sodium intake. Here are some specific tips.

> • **Choose a salt that contains less sodium per measure.** We recommend Diamond Crystal kosher salt, which is available in many grocery stores as well as online. Standard table salt contains approximately 2,300 milligrams per teaspoon. Diamond Crystal contains 1,120 milligrams per teaspoon. The Diamond Crystal salt crystals are larger and fluffier than the crystals in other sodium chloride salts. Diamond Crystal works just like any other salt in cooking.

• **Choose processed foods with less sodium.** Compare nutrition labels among brands, including store-brand products. The sodium in foods like canned tomato paste can vary greatly. And if you can buy a lower-sodium, low-sodium, or no-added-sodium version of a product, go with that. This will help you control the amount of sodium you're adding to your recipes.

• **If you're cooking with and eating fewer processed and restaurant foods, you can add salt at the table.** Our recipes focus on developing flavor without relying too much on salt, and when you start cooking with lower-sodium ingredients and recipes, it can take time to adjust. Adding salt at the table, especially if you're using a lower-sodium salt like Diamond Crystal, allows you to have control and adjust more easily to lower-sodium foods and cooking styles. Allowing people to add a sprinkle of salt to their food also encourages them to enjoy new foods and flavors. Food only offers nutrition if it's eaten; if adding a little salt at the table gets people to eat more vegetables, whole grains, and other healthful foods, then you've achieved your goal.

Use Seasonings and Spice Blends That Don't Rely on Added Salt for Flavor

We devoted an entire chapter to recipes for seasonings and spice blends. Of the twenty-eight recipes in chapter 3, there are only six that include a small amount of added salt to heighten the flavor impact of the other ingredients. The Italian Seasoning (page 34) and Seafood Seasoning (page 37) are two versatile salt-free seasonings we keep on hand for everyday use.

One of the keys to maximizing the flavor you get from herbs, spices, and seasoning blends is the freshness of the ingredients. Buying spices in their whole forms and grinding just what you need for a recipe is one way to maximize freshness and flavor impact. Storing spice blends in ways that limit exposure to air is another way to protect the flavor. We like to store ours in small zipper bags, with as much air pressed out as possible, or in small resealable, airtight jars. Many people worry about the effort that goes into

What About Sea Salt?

Many people believe sea salt is somehow better for their health than regular table salt, but that's just not true. Sea salt is just like table salt in that it's mostly sodium chloride. The color of certain sea salts, like pink Himalayan salt, comes from trace amounts of minerals like copper. While sea salts can take on different crystalline shapes (and be used as elegant finishing salts), they are still contributing sodium to the diet and should be used sparingly.

grinding their own spices. You can use a mortar and pestle to grind some spices, but a small coffee or spice grinder is a great tool for grinding spices quickly. Clean the grinder by grinding a few grains of rice after grinding the spices.

We also recommend using freshly ground black pepper. In fact, every time we call for black pepper in our recipes, it's listed as "freshly ground." Preground black pepper typically provides very little flavor, whereas grinding pepper during cooking or at the table is a very effective way to add bursts of bright flavor to your dishes. If you don't have a pepper grinder, consider buying one—it makes a huge difference.

There are two other strategies for enhancing flavor without relying on sodium. One is the use of spicy ingredients. Our taste buds are able to perceive salt in food at lower levels when accompanied by spicy ingredients. Our Habanero Spice Rub (page 33) is an example of a seasoning that can be used in foods like chicken wings, which typically rely on high levels of sodium in Buffalo sauce for flavor. But not everyone loves spicy foods. Thankfully, there's another strategy: the use of umami-rich ingredients like dashi broth, mushrooms, and aged cheeses. Umami, or savoriness, is one of the five basic tastes (the others are sweet, sour, salty, and bitter). Ingredients with umami compounds help enhance our perception of sodium in food. You'll notice we use mushrooms in many ways—sometimes as the star of a dish and other times as a supporting ingredient, to aid in developing flavor. We also use aged umami-rich cheeses, such as Parmesan, Manchego, Gruyère, and Gouda, to boost the perception of sodium in many recipes. To learn more about umami and umami-rich ingredients, visit the Umami Information Center's website at www.umamiinfo.com.

Choose the Best-Quality Oils for Your Cooking

Is there one perfect oil to use for all types of recipes and cooking applications? No. But the one we recommend and prefer most often is a good-quality extra virgin olive oil. In addition to contributing excellent flavor to dishes, good-quality extra virgin olive oil contains mostly unsaturated fatty acids and beneficial phenols.

Quality in extra virgin olive oil depends on many factors, but the most important is freshness. Olives are fruit, and olive oil is essentially fruit juice, which can deteriorate if not handled and stored properly. To buy a fresh oil with the best flavor, look for one with a harvest date (typically found on the back label) within one year of the current day's date. Next, look for oils in dark brown or dark green bottles. Exposure to light as well as heat and air will cause the oil to go rancid. Buying oils that are certified extra virgin is another smart move; many oils that state "extra virgin" on the label are actually adulterated with other oils or have defects that negatively affect their flavor. Good-quality olive oil is never cheap; we believe a good oil is worth the price.

There are three sensory attributes related to extra virgin olive oil quality: fruitiness, bitterness, and pungency. (Sensory defects include fustiness, mustiness, and rancidity.) Fruitiness refers to the aroma of fresh olive fruit in an oil. Bitterness and pungency are correlated with certain naturally occurring compounds in olives, like phenols, that have very powerful health benefits. The phenol content of an oil depends on several factors, such as the type of olive used to make the oil, where the olives were grown, and the growing conditions (e.g., stress under drought conditions will produce more phenolic compounds). Many experts in olive oil sensory evaluation talk about "one cough, two cough, and three cough" oils: A more pungent oil with more phenols will make someone cough more than a less pungent oil.

The benefits of extra virgin olive oil extend far beyond its fatty acid profile. For example, it contains oleuropein, a potent antioxidant that reduces inflammation and thereby reduces blood pressure. Antioxidant phenols like oleuropein also work to protect the integrity of extra virgin olive oil's fatty acids when the oil is heated, making sure you still get all the benefits.

If you're wondering what the difference is between olive oil and extra virgin olive oil, the biggest difference is the amount of phenols. Extra virgin olive oils contain far higher levels of phenols compared to olive oil and virgin olive oil, which are more processed. You'll still get some nutrition benefits from non–extra virgin olive oil, but if you can afford to buy good-quality extra virgin olive oil, we encourage you to do so.

A final note on cooking with extra virgin olive oil: uncooked and cooked oils provide different benefits. For example, when vegetables like carrots, sweet potatoes, and dark green leafy vegetables like broccoli and spinach are sautéed in extra virgin olive oil, the vegetables absorb beneficial phenols from the oil and the bioavailability of the carotenoids in the vegetables increases.

When selecting fats and oils for cooking, there are many factors to consider: saturated fat content, other potential nutrition and health benefits, cost, flavor profile, and stability when exposed to heat (i.e., smoke point). It's also important to consider the best way to store fats and oils to maintain the integrity of the fatty acids and the flavor of the oil. Cooking with rancid or oxidized oil is never a good idea.

The following tables can help guide your decisions when selecting, storing, and using fats and oils in your cooking and baking.

Table 1: Factors to Consider for Fats and Oils

INGREDIENT	COST	SATURATED FAT (% TOTAL FAT)	CULINARY APPLICATION	OTHER TIPS & INSIGHTS
Butter & Lard				
Butter, salted, stick	$$	63%	Great for special occasion baking, but there are better fats to use for everyday cooking.	
Butter, unsalted, stick	$$	63%	If a dessert or pastry recipe calls for unsalted butter and you don't have any, you can use salted butter—just cut back on added salt. On average, one stick of butter contains 730 mg sodium, the amount found in a generous ¼ teaspoon of fine grain table salt.	Salt helps preserve the shelf life of butter. If you buy unsalted butter and don't use all of it, store the extra in the freezer to preserve the flavor.
Butter, soft, whipped	$$	58%	Convenient for spreading on breads, muffins, and scones.	If you like the flavor of butter but want a lower saturated fat content, look for products that blend butter with vegetable oils.
Ghee (clarified butter)	$$$$	63%	Best known for its use in Indian cooking. It provides a rich, nutty flavor that, when used sparingly, can add great flavor to dishes, but there are better options with lower saturated fat content to use for everyday cooking.	Expensive, but you can make your own by melting butter and allowing it to simmer over low heat until all the water has evaporated. Spoon off the milk solids and voilà!
Lard	$	39%	Can create very flaky pie doughs, biscuits, and pastries.	May contribute unwanted flavor; if you want a neutral fat with less saturated fat, choose vegetable shortening instead.

INGREDIENT	COST	SATURATED FAT (% TOTAL FAT)	CULINARY APPLICATION	OTHER TIPS & INSIGHTS
Plant-Based Alternatives to Butter				
Margarine, stick	$	25%		We don't recommend using stick margarines; their firmness is created by chemically converting the fatty acids in the plant oils in a process called "hydrogenation" that creates harmful trans fats.
Margarine, soft	$$	17%	Great for spreading on toast or quick breads, or for sauteing vegetables.	
Vegetable shortening	$$	25%	Like lard, can create very flaky pie doughs, biscuits, and pastries.	Store in the refrigerator to maintain the integrity of plant-based fatty acids.
Everyday Cooking Oils				
Canola oil	$	7%	A good everyday cooking oil that has a neutral flavor and high smoke point. Can be used for baking, sauteing, stir-frying, marinades, vinaigrettes, and frying.	The heart healthy omega-3s in canola oil break down when exposed to heat, causing rancid, off flavors to develop. It's best to store canola oil in the refrigerator.
Corn oil	$	13%	A good everyday cooking oil that has a neutral flavor and high smoke point. Can be used for baking, sauteing, stir-frying, marinades, vinaigrettes, and frying.	Can be stored at room temperature.
Extra virgin olive oil (imported)	$$	14%	Contributes delicious flavor to foods. Can be used for baking, sauteing, stir-frying, marinades, vinaigrettes, and frying.	Research from UC Davis indicates that many imported EVOO are not high quality and may be blended with other oils. The price will tell you a bit about quality; poorer quality oils, especially blended oils, are much less expensive than high-quality EVOO. EVOO can be stored at room temperature, away from heat sources like your stove or oven.
Extra virgin olive oil (domestic)	$$$	14%	Great quality EVOO contributes flavor to foods ranging from fresh, green vegetal tastes to peppery bitterness. Can be used for baking, sauteing, stir-frying, marinades, and vinaigrettes. Has a lower smoke point compared to other oils; its ability to hold up to high temperatures depends on the oil's phenol content.	Great quality EVOO contains not only beneficial fatty acids but also natural plant compounds called phenols that contribute flavor and potential health benefits. Look for bottles that have olive harvest dates listed on the label; choose those harvested within the past 12 months.
Olive oil (may also be called light olive oil, which refers to color, not fat content)	$$	14%	Has a higher smoke point compared to extra virgin olive oil, which means it can be used for frying at higher temperatures.	Pure olive oil is refined and does not offer the potential nutrition and health benefits of extra virgin olive oil.
Peanut oil	$	18%	A good everyday cooking oil that has a neutral flavor and high smoke point. Can be used for baking, sauteing, stir-frying, marinades, vinaigrettes, and frying.	Can be stored at room temperature.

INGREDIENT	COST	SATURATED FAT (% TOTAL FAT)	CULINARY APPLICATION	OTHER TIPS & INSIGHTS
Safflower oil	$$	6%	A good everyday cooking oil that has a neutral flavor and high smoke point. Can be used for baking, sauteing, stir-frying, marinades, vinaigrettes, and frying.	Like canola oil, the heart healthy omega-3s in safflower oil break down when exposed to heat, causing rancid, off flavors to develop. It's best to store safflower oil in the refrigerator.
Soybean oil	$	16%	A good everyday cooking oil that has a neutral flavor and high smoke point. Can be used for baking, sauteing, stir-frying, marinades, vinaigrettes, and frying.	It's difficult to find 100% soybean oil, but it's nearly always found in vegetable oil blends. Can be stored at room temperature.
Sunflower oil	$	10%	A good everyday cooking oil that has a neutral flavor and high smoke point. Can be used for baking, sauteing, stir-frying, marinades, vinaigrettes, and frying.	Can be stored at room temperature.
Vegetable oil blends	$	14%	A good everyday cooking oil that has a neutral flavor and high smoke point. Can be used for baking, sauteing, stir-frying, marinades, vinaigrettes, and frying.	Can be stored at room temperature.
Specialty Oils				
Avocado oil	$$$	12%	Has a very high smoke point, higher than the everyday oils listed above. The flavor profile will depend on the ripeness of the fruit and the oil extraction method.	There is very little research on potential health benefits of avocado oil. If you want the nutrition and health benefits from avocadoes, eat the fruit.
Coconut oil	$$	82%	Can contribute flavor and functional benefits in cooking and baking. Due to its high saturated fat content and impact on LDL cholesterol, should be used infrequently if at all.	"Coconut oil may be viewed as one of the most deleterious cooking oils that increases risk for cardiovascular disease."—Frank Sacks, MD, Harvard School of Public Health, Department of Nutrition
Flaxseed oil	$$$$	8%	More than 50% of this oil is alpha-linolenic acid, the plant form of omega-3s.	This oil goes rancid easily. It's wise to store it in the refrigerator.
Grapeseed oil	$	10%	Grapeseed oil has a neutral flavor, high smoke point, and low price point, which makes it a great everyday oil.	This oil is typically made from the seeds of wine grapes.
Hempseed oil	$$$$	10%	Hempseed oil has a mild nutty flavor but a high price point.	
Sesame seed oil	$$$$	14%	Due to its strong flavor, this is best used in small amounts.	Sesame seed oil goes rancid easily. It's best stored in the refrigerator.
Walnut oil	$$$	9%	Walnut oil is great for adding flavor to baked goods like banana bread and vinaigrettes for salads, especially ones that include walnuts!	More than 10% of this oil is alpha-linolenic acid, the plant form of omega-3s. This oil goes rancid easily. It's wise to store it in the refrigerator.

Cost per Tablespoon
Pricing data based on store brands, when available, and smaller size bottles.

$ = $0.05–$0.10 per tablespoon
$$ = $0.11–$0.20 per tablespoon
$$$ = $0.21–$0.30 per tablespoon
$$$$ = $0.31+ per tablespoon

Make Sauces, Salsas, and Dressings to Add Additional Flavors and Textures to Your Food

Many chefs will talk about the importance of layering flavors to increase deliciousness in foods. This is just one of the many reasons we love to add sauces like aïolis, chutneys, dressings, pestos, salsas, and vinaigrettes to food. A great sauce can add not only appealing flavors, textures, and even temperature contrast, but also nutrition from extra virgin olive oil or other sources of unsaturated fat, as well as fruits, vegetables, nuts, seeds, herbs, and spices. Sauces can also add playful aspects to food. Seriously, who doesn't love dunking and dipping something crunchy into something creamy? So try adding some new sauces to your repertoire!

Use More Whole Grain Flours in Your Baking and Add More Intact Whole Grains to Your Meals

Many people think the biggest benefit of eating more whole grains is that you'll get more fiber. While that is true, it tells only part of the story about the health benefits of whole grains. Like extra virgin olive oil, fruits, vegetables, legumes, and other plant-based foods, whole grains provide beneficial phenols, many of which are metabolized by good bacteria in our lower intestines. Whole grains can also slow down the speed at which our bodies absorb the carbohydrates; the more refined the grain, the more quickly the carbohydrate enters our bloodstream as blood glucose.

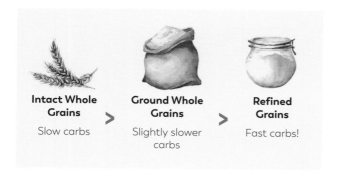

Intact Whole Grains		Ground Whole Grains		Refined Grains
Slow carbs	>	Slightly slower carbs	>	Fast carbs!

Choosing more "slow carbs" helps reduce the inflammation caused by quick increases in blood sugar levels, even in people without diabetes. Slowly digested carbohydrate sources also have the benefit of keeping hunger at bay longer, which in turn can affect our mood. We all know how being hungry can make us "hangry," grumpy, and anxious, right?

One of the many reasons we love cooking with whole grains is the abundant and exciting variety. We've included recipes for common whole grains like oatmeal and popcorn and those that may be less familiar, like farro, millet, and sorghum. And though we provide many options, we've barely scratched the surface of the whole grain options available today, including whole grain flours for baking. If you love baking with whole grains, we recommend *Flavor Flours: A New Way to Bake with Teff, Buckwheat, Sorghum, Other Whole & Ancient Grains, Nuts & Non-Wheat Flours* by famed chocolatier and baker Alice Medrich.

We used whole wheat pastry flour in many of our dessert recipes, and none of our taste testers could tell a difference between an item made with all-purpose flour and one made with whole wheat pastry flour. The biggest discernible difference for us was cost: Specialty flours, including whole wheat pastry flour, are more expensive.

To get more whole grains into your diet in place of their refined counterparts, consider trying a "half & half" approach. If you currently serve only white rice with meals, try mixing white and brown rice in varying proportions, starting with one-quarter brown rice one week and moving to half brown rice the next week, until you can transition to 100 percent brown rice. In certain applications, like in fried rice, you may not even need this technique, since there's no visual difference between white and brown rice when they're mixed with other ingredients.

As you're striving to eat more whole grains, keep in mind that perfect is the enemy of good. Try to make more of your grain choices whole grain, but don't stress about choosing refined grain products for certain purposes. Amy is a big fan of eating hamburgers or ahi tuna burgers on bakery-fresh brioche buns!

Use More Fruits and Vegetables in All Their Glorious Forms in Your Cooking

Did you know that only one out of ten Americans eats the recommended *minimum* five cups of fruits and vegetables every day? The same is true in many developed countries around the world. People are simply not buying and eating enough fruits and vegetables and therefore not gaining all the potential nutrition and health benefits.

There are many reasons for this, but if time and effort are a few of your reasons, consider this: Research shows that people who eat the most fruits and vegetables—regardless of how they were grown, processed, or packaged—have the lowest risk of cardiovascular disease. That's right—you don't have to eat fresh, whole fruits and vegetables to reap the benefits. You can buy fruits and vegetables fresh-cut, frozen, canned, dried, and even in the form of 100% juice products. These options not only save precious prep time, but they can also reduce food waste, especially frozen options.

Processing fruits and vegetables can also make vitamins and phytonutrients more bioavailable to our bodies. One of the best-known examples of this is the bioavailability of lycopene from tomatoes. Lycopene, a carotenoid that gives tomatoes and watermelon, for example, their red color, is stored between tomato cell walls; processing the tomatoes breaks the cell walls open, releasing the lycopene and making it easier for our bodies to absorb it. Lycopene is most often associated with promoting breast and prostate cell health. Another example is frozen spinach, which is a concentrated source of the bioavailable carotenoids lutein and zeaxanthin, which help protect eyes, thereby decreasing risk of macular degeneration, the leading cause of vision loss in people over age fifty. Lutein and zeaxanthin are also found in eggs. If macular degeneration runs in your family, consider adding our Spinach Scramble Pita Pockets (page 127) to your weekly breakfast routine.

One strategy you can use to add more fruits and vegetables to your cooking is to buy the largest items

The Produce for Better Health Foundation (PBH), a nonprofit organization based in the United States, leads the Have A Plant movement, designed to help more people enjoy the benefits of all fruits and vegetables. They commission research to evaluate the emotions, intentions, habits, and behaviors that lead people to eat more fruits and vegetables. The PBH website, www.fruitsandveggies.org, offers tips and tools for everyone who is striving to eat more fruits and vegetables.

possible. Many of our savory recipes that use market amounts (e.g., 1 carrot or 1 cucumber) can accommodate larger pieces of produce. Buying larger sizes can also save time prep time. Why peel two smaller onions when you can save time by peeling and dicing one larger one?

We're also proponents of using the whole item. Nearly all our recipes call for using whole pieces of fresh produce. (We do have one smoothie that calls for half a banana to add sweetness. But it's frozen, so the other half won't go to waste!) If other recipe sources call for "½ apple," throw caution to the wind and use the whole apple. This may seem like a small victory, but when you're trying to eat more fruits and vegetables, we encourage you to use every strategy possible.

We're also big fans of using kitchen tools to make prepping produce easier. If you have a food processor, use it to process onions, celery, and carrots for soup and stew bases or to shred cabbage for coleslaw. (Or just buy shredded cabbage!) A handheld citrus zester or Microplane is a wonderful tool for gently removing the outermost peel from citrus fruit, and for grating fresh ginger or garlic.

Speaking of garlic, this is one ingredient we recommend you buy whole, peel, and prep. The flavor of garlic changes quickly depending on its form. When garlic is trimmed, chopped, or minced, it releases enzymes that start to change its flavor. We also prefer the flavor of whole garlic, processed just before cooking, to garlic powder. With that said, if you prefer the convenience and flavor of garlic powder, use it! If this gets you in the kitchen cooking vegetables more often, do what works for you.

You'll notice that we specify the use of many convenience products like canned beans, canned tomato products, and canned fruits in 100% juice in our recipes. You can still make recipes like Greek-Inspired Baked Chickpeas with Tomatoes & Feta (page 246) if you haven't taken the time to cook chickpeas from dry or grow, harvest, and can your own tomatoes. Buy the canned versions, keep them on hand, and embrace the joy of making a delicious, nutrient-rich meal in minutes.

We're serious about this! Too many people think that cooking and eating more healthfully takes extensive effort. The biggest challenge is the mental effort, convincing yourself this is something you want to do for your health and well-being. After that, finding strategies to make the process easier is the biggest trick to building habits that lead to better health.

Are Potatoes a Vegetable?

Yes, they are! While many people think of potatoes as simply starch, they are actually nutrient dense and a top source of many nutrients that contribute to cardiovascular health, including potassium, a mineral that helps maintain healthy blood pressure levels. Cooked and cooled potatoes (used in recipes like potato salad) offer resistant starch, a form of carbohydrate that is harder for our bodies to digest, lessening its impact on blood sugar. It's also important to recognize that potatoes are a very diverse family. Different varieties offer differences in calories, carbohydrates, fiber, vitamin C, potassium, and other nutrients. And different types of potatoes are suitable for various cooking methods; some are great for frying while others are naturally creamy, making them perfect for mashing. Potatoes pair well with so many other vegetables as well as other health-promoting ingredients like extra virgin olive oil.

Choose Healthy Sources of Protein from Plants and Animals

Protein is found in many foods, including animal sources like dairy products, beef, chicken, pork, fish, and shellfish; grains like wheat, barley, and oats; vegetables like dark leafy greens and potatoes; and legumes like chickpeas, black beans, and pinto beans.

But not all protein is created equal. Proteins are made up of amino acids, and foods that contain protein vary in their amino acid composition and the bioavailability of those amino acids. Today, the gold standard for assessing protein quality is a measurement called DIAAS (Digestible Indispensable Amino Acid Score), which determines the digestibility of amino acids. In general, animal sources have higher DIAAS scores than plant sources and are thereby considered higher-quality sources of protein. They typically provide more essential amino acids, including ones the human body can't produce.

With that said, it's important to look at the full package of nutrients a food provides as well as the context of that food within an overall dietary pattern. Protein sources like legumes, for example, provide much more than protein; they contain fiber and potassium, nutrients many people need more of in their diets. It's also important to note that no single food can meet all nutrient needs. Eating a wide variety of foods, including foods that contain protein, is the best way to ensure your nutrient needs are met.

The following table compares the protein quality of various foods and notes why including protein sources with low protein-quality scores is still important for meeting other nutrient needs.

When it comes to choosing animal proteins, we have three specific recommendations.

1. **Choose lean sources of animal protein that contain less saturated fat.** One trick for identifying leaner sources of beef and pork is to look for the term "loin" on the label. Cuts like tenderloin and sirloin qualify for the United States Department of Agriculture standards for lean if they contain less than 10 grams of total fat, 4.5 grams or less of saturated fat, and less than 95 milligrams of cholesterol per 3-ounce (85 g) serving. Ground beef, pork, and lamb are often labeled with the percent lean on the package; look for packages with the highest percentage of lean available, which can be as high as 97%. Research has shown that lean, unprocessed cuts of beef and pork can be part of a healthful Mediterranean-style eating pattern that reduces risk of cardiovascular disease by decreasing blood pressure, blood cholesterol, blood glucose, and inflammation.

2. **Choose less-processed sources of protein that contain little or no added sodium.** Choosing lean ground meat and whole muscle cuts of meat ensures no sodium is added. You'll notice as that we rarely call for a processed meat product like bacon or sausage. While they can be convenient options, we limit their use due to their sodium content. When it comes to processed products like canned beans, draining and rinsing the beans prior to adding to a recipe can reduce sodium levels by up to 35 percent. It's also important to compare processed products while shopping, since levels of added sodium can vary greatly among brands.

3. **Eat more seafood.** We'll cover this recommendation in greater detail in the next section.

Eat More Seafood!

We've had many people tell us they want to eat more seafood, but they either don't know how to cook it, don't like how it makes their house smell, or find it too expensive. We're here to help, with options to address these concerns and more in chapter 16. But first, let us explain why we believe it is so important to eat more seafood. People who eat more seafood have a lower risk of cardiovascular disease. All seafood, including fish and shellfish, can provide beneficial omega-3s. Seafood with higher levels of fat, like salmon, tuna, mackerel, anchovies, and herring, have corresponding higher levels of omega-3 fats. High omega-3 intake is also associated with reduced risk of depression, dementia, and arthritis.

There are many convenience products that can make cooking with and eating fish and shellfish easier, including canned products like salmon, tuna, clams, and oysters, which work well in soups, stews, and chowders. There are also many frozen products like cooked peeled and deveined shrimp, cooked frozen scallops and mussels, or portioned, individually packed fish fillets that allow you to thaw and heat or cook just what you need without having to do any prep work other than opening a package. We include several recipes like Hearty Clam Chowder (page 88) and Mini Crab Cakes (page 289) that feature the use of these convenience products.

One of the biggest benefits of cooking with seafood is how quickly much of it cooks. Broiling or grilling a piece of fish can put dinner on the table in a matter of minutes. Cooking en papillote (in paper; see page 283) is an easy way to cook fish without worrying about overcooking it; this cooking method retains moisture and also seals in flavor and aromas, which is a bonus if you're worried about how cooking fish makes your home smell. Chapter 16 includes three en papillote recipes.

While we hope you'll cook more fish and shellfish at home, if you'd prefer to get your seafood in restaurants, go for it. Order the wood-grilled salmon for dinner one night and enjoy a tuna burger for lunch a few days later. But speaking of tuna burgers, do try one of our seafood recipes in Chapter 10—we offer five handheld recipes, including an awesome Ahi Burgers with Wasabi-Ginger Slaw (page 177) and light, refreshing, and beautiful Salmon Spring Rolls (page 188). And if you're a fan of Taco Tuesdays, put Fish Tacos (page 184) or Shrimp Tacos (page 185) on the menu!

Table 2: Comparing the Protein Quality of Various Foods

The Food and Agriculture Organization of the United Nations uses DIAAS (digestible indispensable amino acid scores) to assess protein quality. Foods that score 100 or greater are considered high-quality sources of protein; foods that score 75 to 99 are considered good sources, and foods that score less than 75 are considered low quality-protein foods.

FOOD	DIAAS (%)	PROTEIN QUALITY	NOTES
Almonds	40	Low	A good source of magnesium and dietary fiber; a top food source of vitamin E for many people
Barley	47	Low	Contains beta-glucans, a form of soluble fiber that binds to dietary cholesterol in the gut. Instead of being absorbed into your blood stream, the cholesterol is excreted from your body.
Beef	112	High	All beef offers high-quality protein; choose lean cuts to reduce saturated fat intake, and unprocessed beef to reduce sodium intake.
Black beans	63	Low	Like other legumes, a good source of fiber and iron
Chicken	108	High	Both white and dark meat are high-quality protein sources.
Chickpeas	83	Good	Whether whole or processed in foods such as hummus, a good source of protein
Eggs	113	High	Not only a high-quality protein source, but also very affordable
Milk	114	High	Dairy milk only. Plant-based alternatives, other than soy milk, do not offer high-quality protein, and protein content can vary greatly.
Oatmeal	54	Low	Like barley, contains beta-glucan fibers that bind cholesterol in the gut
Peas	58	Low	Like other vegetables in the legume family, a good source of fiber
Pork	114	High	Like beef, all pork offers high-quality protein; choose lean cuts to reduce saturated fat intake, and unprocessed pork to reduce sodium intake.
Potatoes	100	High	While the protein quality of potatoes is high, potatoes contain very little protein and should not be relied upon for adequate protein intake.
Rice	57	Low	Rice is culturally important for many people. Choose whole grain rice, which contains all the goodness of the entire rice kernel (i.e., fibrous bran, starchy endosperm, and protein-, vitamin-, and mineral-packed germ) when possible.
Sorghum	29	Low	Whole grain; provides fiber and slowly digested carbohydrates
Tilapia	100	High	All fish and shellfish contain high-quality protein.
Tofu	52	Low	Protein quality is low, but offers many other benefits. Studies suggest tofu may help protect the lining of our arteries, reduce LDL cholesterol levels, and promote bone health.
Wheat	92	Good	Includes gluten proteins; anyone diagnosed with celiac disease should avoid products containing gluten from wheat and other cereal grains.

What About Grass-Fed Beef?

Many people mistakenly believe grass-fed or grass-finished beef is leaner than grain-fed beef. This may or may not be true depending on many factors like where the cattle are raised, how they are fed (i.e., exclusively grass and hay or majority grass/hay and supplemental feed, if needed) and the climate. One important thing to note is that while grass-fed beef often contains higher levels of omega-3 fatty acids, the total amount is so small that it's not considered a good source of omega-3s. Eating seafood regularly is a much better way to ensure you're getting adequate omega-3s in your diet. It's important to note that grain-fed beef typically costs less per pound than grass-fed when comparing the same grades. Finally, there's the issue of flavor. Many people think grass-fed beef has a more "beefy" flavor than grain-fed beef. From our point of view, the best beef choice is lean beef of whatever grade or production system you prefer at a price you can afford.

Is It Okay to Eat Eggs?

Eggs are a convenient, versatile, affordable, and high-quality source of protein and many nutrients that support cardiovascular health, including choline. For many years, people worried that the cholesterol in egg yolks had a negative impact on blood cholesterol levels, but research has shown that eggs can be eaten on a regular basis without increasing risk of cardiovascular disease, if they're eaten as part of an overall healthful dietary pattern. Eggs are often thought of as a breakfast food, and when used as a gateway to greater vegetable consumption at breakfast, they can be especially powerful in improving the quality and healthfulness of a person's eating pattern. It's important to recognize that egg yolks contain significant amounts of essential nutrients and phytonutrients like choline, lutein, and zeaxanthin, while egg whites contain mostly protein. For this reason we encourage you to eat whole eggs.

Should I Eat Less Cheese?

Many types of cheese offer appealing flavors and some types offer unctuous creaminess, but all offer essential nutrients like high-quality protein. While cheese is a top source of saturated fat in the diets of many people, this saturated fat is not associated with an increased risk of cardiovascular disease. The saturated fat in dairy products does increase LDL ("bad") cholesterol, but it also increases HDL ("good") cholesterol. And there are other beneficial nutrients in full-fat dairy products that are potentially protective against cardiovascular disease. Moreover, the way saturated fat from butter affects cardiovascular disease risk markers differs from saturated fat from cheese or cream; emerging evidence suggests that the way the fatty acids are packaged in the food matrix of fat, protein, and water affects how our bodies use them to make cholesterol. Saturated fatty acids that are packaged in a food matrix with protein are less likely to prompt our livers to use the saturated fat to make cholesterol. There is also emerging research on how our bodies react to fermented versus nonfermented dairy foods, with some studies suggesting that fermented full-fat dairy products, like whole milk Greek yogurt, are more supportive of cardiovascular health than low-fat dairy products. Our biggest concern with cheese is the sodium content; for this reason, we limit its use in our recipes. When we do use cheese, we either use smaller amounts of good-quality cheese (like Parmesan) or use fresh cheeses (like part-skim ricotta or fresh mozzarella) that contain far less sodium than hard cheeses.

Snack on Nuts and Other Nourishing Nibbles

Snacking is a habit that can make significant contributions to meeting our daily nutrient needs, particularly if we choose our snacks thoughtfully. Consider snacking on nutrient-dense foods that you don't eat enough of, like fruits and vegetables, or that can have an impact on reducing your risk of chronic disease, like nuts.

Research shows that people who eat the most nuts, averaging about 5 ounces (150 g) per week, have the lowest risk of cardiovascular disease. People with type 2 diabetes can reduce their risk of cardiovascular disease by eating nuts in place of refined carbohydrates, and women who eat walnuts can significantly reduce their risk of developing type 2 diabetes.

We've included many recipes for spiced and lightly candied nuts, and you can almost always swap one nut for another if you have a preference. Nuts can be great as crunchy toppings for salads and bowls that feature vegetables, legumes, whole grains, and healthy sources of protein. They can be incorporated into recipes as nut butters and nut flours.

Chapter 19 includes recipes for dips and spreads that include nuts, providing a way to add delicious flavors and creamy textures to crunchy vegetables and whole grain crackers or crisps. Do we seem a wee bit obsessed with nuts? Or a bit nuts, pun intended? Well, we are. We love nuts for all their amazing culinary, nutrition, and health benefits!

Enjoy Desserts . . . Made More Thoughtfully with Better-For-You Ingredients

Ah . . . we saved room to talk about dessert. Yes, desserts can be part of heart-healthy eating patterns! The key is to be thoughtful about how much and how often you eat them, and how they're made. We focused on including more plant-based ingredients like fruit, vegetables, whole grains, nuts, seeds, dark chocolate, plant-based oils, and sweeteners like honey in our recipes. We also focused on "right sizing" portions to keep the calorie, added sugars, and saturated fat contributions of desserts lower than what is typical. We are not fans of messages like "If you eat all your vegetables, then you can have dessert." Dessert shouldn't be a reward; it should be part of healthful, balanced, delicious meals enjoyed in the company of people you love and who bring you joy. We've also included recipes for dairy-based toppings that bring added creaminess or a bit of contrasting tanginess to a sweeter dessert. If you haven't tried Buttermilk Crème Fraîche (page 361) on a piece of galette or a fruit crisp, be prepared to be delighted!

We've also included butter in some recipes—and granulated sugar—to show you how to make room for these ingredients in certain recipes. In many cases, we found we could replace all the butter with an alternative like extra virgin olive oil, but sometimes the best approach was to just replace half the butter with oil. We also demonstrate how to balance the use of whole wheat pastry flour with all-purpose flour to achieve a great texture. But what we most want to show you is that you can still enjoy desserts and sweet treats once in a while when striving to eat a more health-promoting diet.

A Final Note About Sustainability

We know that many readers are interested in making more sustainable food choices. We also know that sustainable food production is a complex issue. A sustainable production practice on one farm, in one region, or in one part of the world may not work well in another part of the world. Similarly, an important consideration in sustainable food production is financial sustainability. One of the biggest ways every reader of this book can contribute to sustainable food production is by reducing food waste. Food waste occurs all across our food system, from agriculture and food processing to retail and food-service establishments, as well as in our homes.

Globally, experts estimate that more than 35 percent of all food that is grown and produced using precious natural resources is wasted—from crop losses due to climate change, shortage of labor for hand-harvested crops, large portions served in restaurants, or food spoiling and being thrown away in homes. In the United States, food wasted in the home represents the largest portion of waste. Food waste not only wastes natural and financial resources, but also contributes to global warming, because food in landfills produces methane, a greenhouse gas. Making a commitment to reducing food waste in your home is one of the best ways you can help mitigate climate change. We provide tips throughout the book for reducing food waste, but here are a few to help get you started.

1. **Plan to plan.** Take inventory of the perishable foods you have on hand and plan your meals accordingly. Prepare a shopping list before ordering groceries or going to a store.

2. **Transport and store food properly.** Some foods, like dairy products, can spoil more quickly if not stored at proper temperatures during transport or in the home. Using insulated cooler bags when bringing dairy products, meat, and seafood from the grocery store to your home can help maintain quality and freshness.

3. **Embrace canned and frozen products.** Many people think fresh is best, but fresh foods like fruits and vegetables spoil with age, while their canned and frozen counterparts last much longer and maintain their quality.

4. **Embrace leftovers.** Leftovers are a joy for busy people because you cook only once and can eat twice or more. We've created many recipes that show you how to plan to use leftovers in future meals. Sometimes this means a meal the next day, but it can also mean freezing extras and using them in the future. (See Table 3 for details.)

Table 3: Recipes That Allow You to Cook Once, Eat Twice

RECIPE	EAT TWICE STRATEGY
Chicken Stock (page 70)	Use the richly flavored chicken meat to make Chicken & Bean Burritos (page 186).
Vegetable Broth (page 72)	Use the vegetables from the stock to make Mirepoix Soupe (page 77), a recipe specifically designed to reduce food waste.
Any Simply Cooked whole grain in chapter 13	Serve part at the first meal, then freeze the rest to use in other recipes, like many of the bowl recipes in chapter 9, or as an accompaniment to future meals.
Any Simply Cooked legume in chapter 14	Serve part at the first meal, then freeze the rest to use in other recipes, like our soup recipes in chapter 5, or as an accompaniment to future meals.
Roast Chicken with Lemon & Thyme (page 313)	Use leftovers to make Chicken Fried Rice (page 306); Chicken Enchiladas (page 306); or Chicken & Bean Burritos (page 186).
Simply Cooked Pork Tenderloin (page 332)	Use leftovers to make Pork Fried Rice (page 332).
Sheet Pan Tri-Tip Roast (page 328)	Use leftovers to make Beef & Lentil Salad Bowls (page 160).

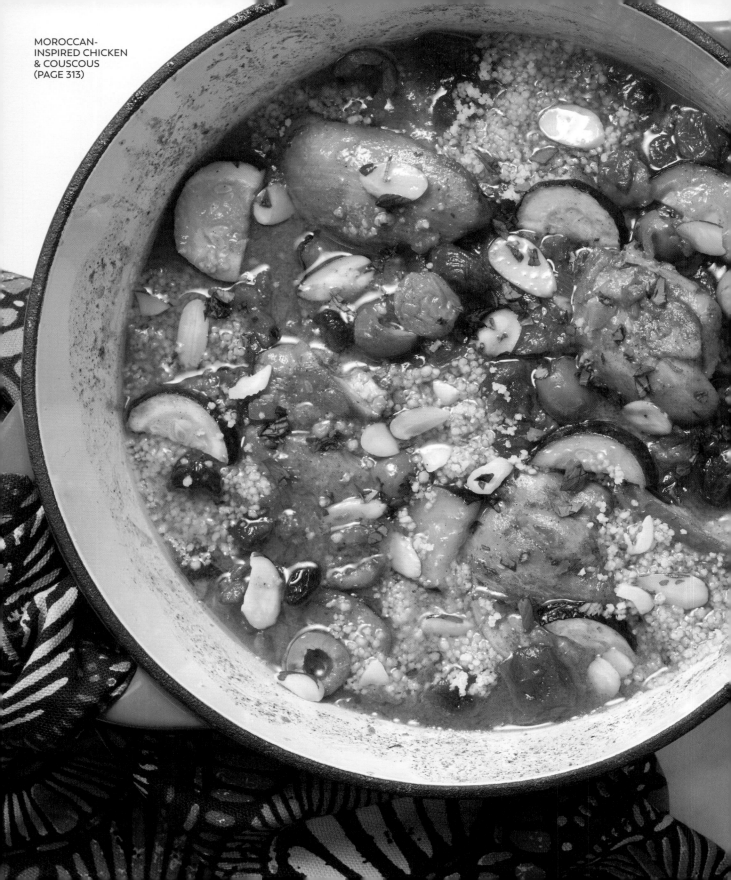

MOROCCAN-
INSPIRED CHICKEN
& COUSCOUS
(PAGE 313)

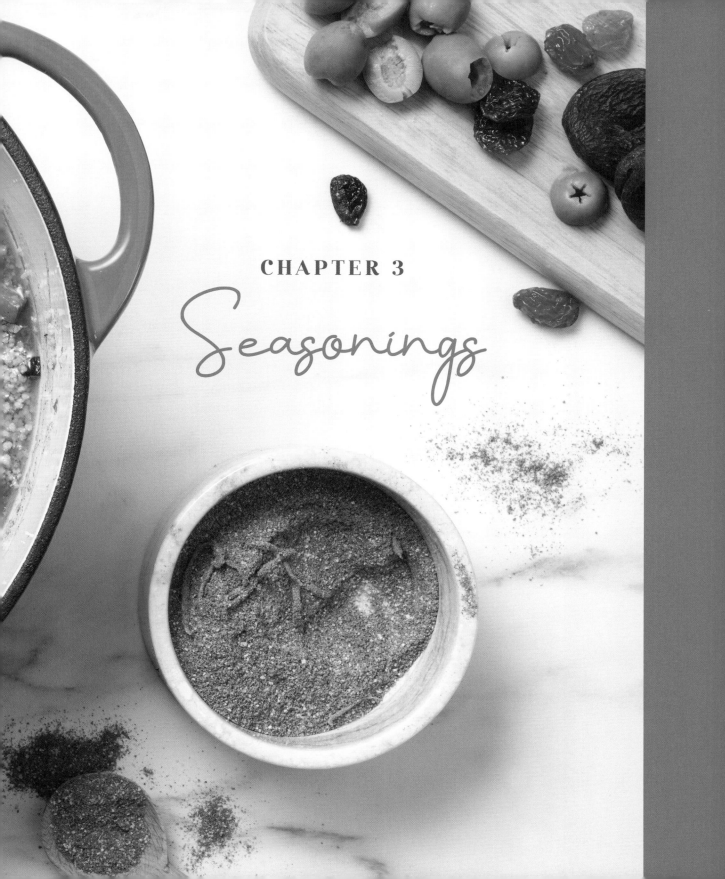

CHAPTER 3

Seasonings

Seasonings

Helpful Hints for
Cooking with Herbs 29

Adobo Seasoning 30

Bouquet Garni. 30

Cajun Seasoning 30

Chinese Five-Spice Blend 31

Cinnamon Spice Mix. 31

Coffee & Fennel Rub 31

Cumin, Sage & Turmeric Seasoning 32

Curry Powder 32

East Indian–Inspired Spice Blend 32

Garlic & Herb Bread Crumbs 33

Habanero Spice Rub 33

Herb Blend for Beef 34

Herb Blend for Pork 34

Herb Blend for Poultry. 34

Italian Seasoning 34

Jamaican Jerk Rub 35

Moroccan-Style Seasoning. 35

Persian Fresh Herb Mix 35

Rustic Herb Seasoning 36

Salmon Rub 36

Savory Nut Crumb Topping 36

Seafood Seasoning. 37

Smoke & Pepper Ginger Rub 37

Smoky Workaday Seasoning 37

Southwest Seasoning 37

Taco Seasoning 38

Tofu Seasoning 38

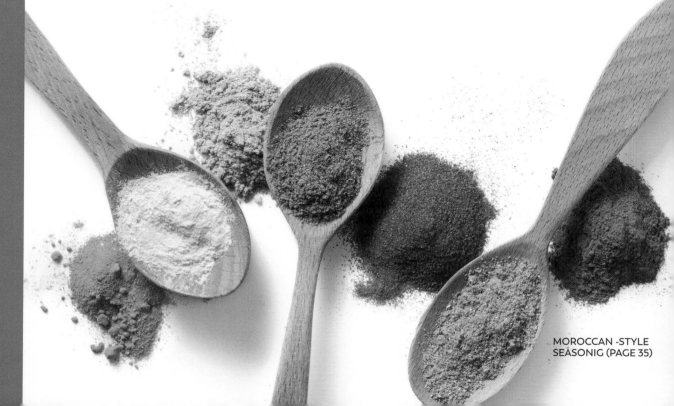

MOROCCAN -STYLE
SEASONIG (PAGE 35)

Flavor is the top reason we choose our most frequently consumed foods and beverages. Learning how to use spices, herbs, aromatics, and other ingredients in your cooking can enhance the flavor—and therefore your enjoyment—of food. But that's not all: Many ingredients that enhance flavor also contain natural health-promoting compounds or increase the health-promoting properties of plant-based foods. Something as simple as adding freshly ground black pepper to a dish can increase your body's absorption of carotenoids (compounds that may decrease inflammation or boost immune function) in vegetables like spinach, carrots, corn, and tomatoes.

Using spices, herbs, and aromatics has the additional benefit of reducing the need for added sodium to add flavor to foods. Yes, we need some sodium in our diets, but most adults consume too much. Using fewer processed foods in cooking and choosing lower-sodium versions of processed foods can make a significant impact on your diet's overall sodium content. We share more information on this important topic in chapter 2.

Some of these recipes you'll use less frequently than others, and you may wish to make some of the recipes in larger batches to always have on hand. (Amy uses our Italian Seasoning, on page 34, in her home kitchen nearly every day!) Our goal is to help you explore more flavor profiles you can use to make crave-worthy meals and snacks. Speaking of crave-worthy, be sure to check out the spiced nuts in the Appetizers, Snacks & Nibbles chapter!

Helpful Hints for Cooking with Herbs

Fresh herbs can add freshness and fantastic flavor to foods. Many fresh herbs are available at supermarkets across the country, but home gardeners know hearty herbs can grow year-round in many climates or, if potted, can be transitioned indoors when temperatures drop. And herbs can be successfully dried for later use. We recommend using fresh herbs when they're available and dried or ground herbs when you don't have access to fresh. A general rule of thumb is that one tablespoon of a fresh herb is equal to 1 teaspoon dried or ½ teaspoon ground dried herbs.

When buying spices, buy whole spices when possible and grind them fresh to get the maximum flavor benefit. If you buy ground spices, buy them in small quantities and try to use them within a year of purchase. Labeling spice containers can help you keep track of their age. Be sure to store spices and herbs in cool, dry, and dark environments in airtight containers.

Aside from pepper grinders, few people have grinders for specific spices. Small coffee grinders can be used to grind whole spices, and grinding a few grains of rice after grinding spices is an easy way to clean the grinder. But you may find that grinding certain spices, like cardamom, and then immediately grinding coffee beans may impart a very pleasant aroma and flavor to your coffee! A mortar and pestle works well for some spices, but you may struggle with very hard spices like cloves; for those, we recommend the coffee grinder.

There are many schools of thought on when to add spices and herbs during the cooking process. A general rule of thumb is to add spices early and herbs later. Spices can stand up to higher temperatures and longer cooking times without losing their flavor impact better than herbs.

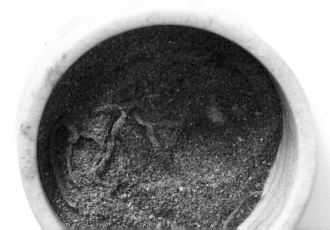

ADOBO SEASONING

Makes ½ cup (65 g)

Food historians place the origins of adobo seasoning in Spanish colonial times, during which it traveled to Latin America and the Caribbean. It's an all-purpose savory seasoning that provides a smoky, garlicky flavor when used as a rub to season or marinate tofu, fish, chicken, beef, or pork. Apply 2 tablespoons per pound (454 g) of meat, rubbing and massaging it into all sides. Let rest for 5 minutes before cooking. Adobo seasoning's versatile flavor profile makes it perfect for Simply Roasted Cauliflower (page 258) and Spicy Black Bean Chili (page 244).

- 2 tablespoons garlic powder
- 2 tablespoons onion powder
- 2 tablespoons smoked paprika
- 1 tablespoon dried oregano
- 2 teaspoons chili powder
- 2 teaspoons ground cumin
- 2 teaspoons freshly ground black pepper

Whisk together the garlic powder, onion powder, paprika, oregano, chili powder, cumin, and pepper in a small bowl. Use immediately or store in an airtight container in a cool, dark place for up to 3 months.

BOUQUET GARNI

French for "garnished bouquet," a bouquet garni is a bundle of fresh and/or dried herbs used to add flavor and depth to stocks and soups. Try this in the Beef Stock (page 70) or the Vegetable Broth (page 72), then experiment with any herb combinations that intrigue you or speak to your taste preferences.

- 4 parsley sprigs
- 2 thyme sprigs
- 1 marjoram sprig
- ¼ cup (25 g) fresh tarragon leaves
- 2 bay leaves
- 2 garlic cloves, halved
- 8 black peppercorns
- Cheesecloth or large, flat-bottomed coffee filter
- Kitchen string

Place the parsley, thyme, marjoram, tarragon, bay leaves, garlic, and peppercorns in the center of a 6-inch (15 cm) square of double-layered cheesecloth or coffee filter. Bring the corners of the cheesecloth together in the middle and tuck in the sides; if using a coffee filter, bring the sides together in a bundle. Tie securely with kitchen string, with a large bow to help retrieve the bouquet garni when it's time to remove it from the dish.

TIP: If you don't have cheesecloth or a coffee filter on hand, you can simply tie the herbs together with string. Strain the stock or broth through a fine-mesh sieve to remove the peppercorns, any leaves from the herbs that have come off their stems, and the garlic cloves.

CAJUN SEASONING

Makes about ½ cup (60 g)

This Cajun seasoning blend is smoky, savory, and spicy. Try it in our Cajun-Spiced Peanuts (page 345) and Turkey Jambalaya (page 318).

- 2 tablespoons garlic powder
- 2 tablespoons smoked paprika
- 1 tablespoon cayenne
- 1 tablespoon onion powder
- 1 tablespoon ground oregano
- 1 tablespoon ground thyme
- 1 teaspoon white pepper
- ½ teaspoon kosher salt

Whisk together the garlic powder, paprika, cayenne, onion powder, oregano, thyme, white pepper, and salt in a small bowl. Use immediately or store in an airtight container in a cool, dark place for up to 1 year.

SODIUM TIP: Using Diamond Crystal Kosher Salt will dramatically reduce the sodium in any recipe that uses kosher salt. This salt contains 50% less sodium per measure than regular kosher salt and 60% less than fine grain table salt.

CHINESE FIVE-SPICE BLEND

Makes ⅓ cup (30 g)

There are two theories about how this spice blend came to be: One says it represents the five elements (earth, fire, metal, wood, and water), and the other says it represents the five tastes (sweet, sour, salty, bitter, and umami). Regardless, this seasoning offers amazingly complex flavors for dishes like fried rice.

- 5 whole star anise
- 2 tablespoons ground cinnamon
- 2 tablespoons fennel seeds
- 2 tablespoons Sichuan peppercorns
- 1 tablespoon whole cloves

Combine the star anise, cinnamon, fennel seeds, peppercorns, and cloves in a spice grinder. Grind to a relatively smooth powder. Use immediately or store in an airtight container in a cool, dark place for up to 3 months.

NOTE: *Sichuan peppercorns not only provide flavor, but also offer some interesting benefits. They contain oleoresin, a compound that can enhance our perception of sodium in food, and hydroxy-alpha sanshool, a compound that interacts with taste buds to create a tingling, numbing sensation on the tongue.*

CINNAMON SPICE MIX

Makes about 2½ tablespoons

If you're striving to eat more fruit for dessert (we encourage you to do so!), make it more fun—and flavorful—by adding a teaspoon or so of this blend to Creme Fraiche (page 361) for topping a bowl of mixed fruit, berries, diced mango, or sliced bananas. You can also add a pinch or two to vanilla yogurt for dipping apple or pear slices.

- 2 teaspoons ground cinnamon
- 2 teaspoons ground nutmeg
- 1 teaspoon ground ginger
- 1 teaspoon dried granulated orange peel
- ½ teaspoon ground allspice
- ½ teaspoon ground cardamom
- ¼ teaspoon ground cloves

Whisk together the cinnamon, nutmeg, ginger, orange peel, allspice, cardamom, and cloves in a small bowl.

Use immediately or store in an airtight container in a cool, dark place for up to 6 months.

COFFEE & FENNEL RUB

Makes ½ cup (60 g)

Coffee works both as a meat tenderizer and as a spice, enhancing the flavor of whatever cut of meat you choose. Here, coffee is teamed with other spices to develop a sweet and savory outer crust on your finished roast or steak. Apply 2 tablespoons per pound (454 g) of meat, rubbing and massaging it into all sides. Let rest for 5 minutes before cooking. This rub also works well as a dry marinade; just coat your meat, place in a covered container in the fridge, and allow to marinate overnight.

- ¼ cup (30 g) ground coffee (origin and roast of choice)
- 1 tablespoon crushed fennel seeds
- 1 tablespoon garlic powder
- 2 teaspoons ground mustard
- 2 teaspoons smoked paprika
- 1 teaspoon lemon pepper
- 1 teaspoon ground star anise
- ⅛ teaspoon kosher salt

Whisk together the coffee, fennel seeds, garlic powder, mustard, paprika, lemon pepper, star anise, and salt in small bowl. Use immediately or store in an airtight container in a cool, dark place for up to 1 year.

CUMIN, SAGE & TURMERIC SEASONING
Makes about ½ cup (30 g)

Turmeric is a popular Indian spice that gives many curry powders their intense yellow color. It has an earthy flavor, while cumin, a much-used ingredient in Mexican and Indian cooking, provides a spicy, nutty flavor with lemony undertones. Use this seasoning as a spice rub to enhance the flavor of fish, poultry, or meat, or mix into rice or a casserole to boost and infuse flavors while adding a gorgeous golden color.

- 1 tablespoon celery seed
- 2 tablespoons dried basil
- 2 teaspoons ground cumin
- 1 tablespoon dried lemon thyme or thyme
- 1 tablespoon dried marjoram
- 1 tablespoon ground sage
- 1 tablespoon ground turmeric

Use a mortar and pestle or spice grinder to grind the celery seed to powder. Whisk together the celery seed, basil, cumin, lemon thyme, marjoram, sage, and turmeric in a small bowl. Use immediately or store in an airtight container in a cool, dark place for up to 6 months.

CURRY POWDER
Makes about 1 cup (100 g)

Curry can refer to three things in Indian cuisine: any dish with a sauce; curry leaves, which are used similarly to bay leaves; and curry spice blend, for which every family has their secret recipe. What most Americans think of as curry powder was invented by the British to mimic the flavors of Indian dishes "discovered" during seafaring voyages to the Far East. Our curry blend has a combination of savory and sweet spices that offer a deep, earthy flavor with pleasantly sweet undertones. The cumin, ginger, cayenne, and turmeric provide heat, but if you prefer less heat, use paprika in place of the cayenne. We use this to prepare Curry-Glazed Chicken (page 311).

- ¼ cup (15 g) ground coriander
- 3 tablespoons ground turmeric
- 2 tablespoons ground cumin

- 1 tablespoon freshly ground black pepper
- 1 tablespoon ground fenugreek seeds
- 1 tablespoon ground ginger
- 2 teaspoons ground cardamom
- 2 teaspoons cayenne or paprika
- 2 teaspoons ground cinnamon
- 2 teaspoons ground nutmeg
- 1 teaspoon ground cloves
- 1 teaspoon ground mustard

Whisk together the coriander, turmeric, cumin, pepper, fenugreek, ginger, cardamom, cayenne, cinnamon, nutmeg, cloves, and mustard in a small bowl. Use immediately or store in an airtight container in a cool, dark place for up to 6 months.

EAST INDIAN–INSPIRED SPICE BLEND
Makes about ⅔ cup (65 g)

East Indian cuisine is usually savory because it uses a number of warm spices like black pepper, cinnamon, and cumin. This mild, versatile blend can be used as a rub for firm white fish, shrimp, chicken wings, or even steak before grilling, baking, or roasting.

- 2 tablespoons chili powder
- 2 tablespoons ground cumin
- 2 tablespoons Curry Powder (page 32)
- 1 tablespoon plus 2 teaspoons ground allspice
- 1 tablespoon ground cinnamon
- 1 tablespoon freshly ground black pepper
- 1 teaspoon cayenne

Whisk together the chili powder, cumin, curry powder, allspice, cinnamon, pepper, and cayenne in a small bowl. Use immediately or store in an airtight container in a cool, dark place for up to 3 months.

GARLIC & HERB BREAD CRUMBS

Makes 1 cup (220 g)

If no one in your home is a fan of the crusty end pieces of a loaf of bread, you can use them to make the most delicious bread crumb topping to coat fish or chicken pieces, sprinkle on top of casseroles or soups, or give a finishing touch to grains or greens bowls. We use it as a crispy topping to our Mushroom & Spinach–Stuffed Tomatoes (page 275), and alternate it with the Savory Nut Crumb Topping (page 36) when we make Cauliflower-Walnut Casserole (page 276).

- 4 slices whole grain bread (whole wheat, oat, rye, or multigrain)
- 1 tablespoon extra virgin olive oil
- 2 garlic cloves, minced
- 3 tablespoons chopped fresh parsley
- 1 tablespoon chopped fresh thyme
- 3 tablespoons freshly grated Parmesan
- Freshly ground black pepper

1. Adjust an oven rack to the middle position. Preheat the oven to 250°F (120°C).

2. Place the bread slices in a single layer on a large baking sheet. Bake for 15 minutes or until completely dry, flipping the slices after 8 minutes. Remove from the oven and let cool about 20 minutes.

3. Break the bread into pieces and place in a heavy zipper bag. Squeeze all the air out of the bag and seal. Crush the bread into crumbs by rocking a rolling pin back and forth across the bag until you reach the size needed for your dish (smaller to use as a coating; larger for a topping).

4. Heat the oil in a medium skillet over medium heat. When the oil is shimmering, add the garlic; cook until fragrant, about 2 minutes. Stir in the bread crumbs and cook about 1 minute. Add the parsley and thyme, stirring constantly. When the crumbs are crispy and the herbs fragrant, about 1 minute, remove from the heat.

5. If using immediately, transfer the crumbs to a medium bowl and add the cheese and 2 or 3 grinds of pepper. For later use, add the cheese after the crumbs have completely cooled, then pour into a resealable container with 2 or 3 grinds of pepper. Refrigerate until ready to use. Store in an airtight container in the refrigerator for up to 5 days or in the freezer for up to 3 months.

TIP: *You can also prepare the bread crumbs by pulsing the dried bread in a food processor until they reach the desired crumb size.*

HABANERO SPICE RUB

Makes ¾ cup (85 g)

If you love lingering heat in your food, this is the rub for you! We use it on our Habanero Chicken Wings (page 311). It's also fantastic as a wet rub for grilled or roasted chicken: Blend ¼ cup (30 g) with 1 tablespoon extra virgin olive oil for a wet rub for a whole chicken.

- ¼ cup plus 2 tablespoons (45 g) onion powder
- 2 tablespoons dried oregano
- 1 tablespoon plus 2 teaspoons ground mustard
- 1 tablespoon garlic powder
- 1 tablespoon sugar
- 2 teaspoons ground habanero chiles

Whisk together the onion powder, oregano, mustard, garlic powder, sugar, and habanero in a small bowl. Use immediately or store in an airtight container in a cool, dark place for up to 3 months.

TIPS: *To use as a dry rub, apply 2 tablespoons per pound (454 g) of meat, rubbing and massaging it into all sides. Let rest for 5 minutes.*

Make a wet rub for meat by combining 2 tablespoons with 2 tablespoons extra virgin olive oil; rub into all sides before roasting or grilling.

HERB BLEND FOR BEEF

Makes ¼ cup (15 g)

We use this use this rub for Sheet Pan Tri-Tip Roast (page 328). You can also use it to season the braising liquid for a beef or pork roast, or add it to a simple beef and vegetable soup.

- 2 teaspoons dried basil
- 2 teaspoons celery seed
- 2 teaspoons dried marjoram
- 2 teaspoons dried oregano
- 2 teaspoons dried parsley
- 2 teaspoons dried thyme

Combine the basil, celery seed, marjoram, oregano, parsley, and thyme in a small bowl. Use immediately or store in an airtight container in a cool, dark place for up to 6 months.

HERB BLEND FOR PORK

Makes ¼ cup (10 g)

Add subtle flavor to pork chops or a pork roast, or try it as a dry rub on our Simply Cooked Pork Tenderloin (page 332).

- 1 tablespoon dried basil
- 1 tablespoon dried marjoram
- 1 tablespoon dried sage
- 1 tablespoon dried thyme

Whisk together the basil, marjoram, sage, and thyme in a small bowl. Use immediately or store in an airtight container in a cool, dark place for up to 6 months.

HERB BLEND FOR POULTRY

Makes 6 tablespoons

This flavorful blend of spices enhances the flavor of baked, roasted, or grilled chicken and turkey, and will help retain their moisture. To use, pat the poultry dry; brush with 1 to 2 teaspoons olive or vegetable oil, then sprinkle with the herb rub and massage it in with your hands. If you have fresh basil, marjoram, or thyme, add a sprig or two under the breast flap or skin of the chicken or turkey after applying. This rub is excellent in our Herb-Roasted Turkey Breast with Vegetables (page 317).

- 1 tablespoon plus 1 teaspoon dried marjoram
- 1 tablespoon dried basil
- 1 tablespoon dried parsley
- 1 tablespoon dried rosemary
- 1 tablespoon dried thyme
- 2 teaspoons rubbed sage

Whisk the marjoram, basil, parsley, rosemary, thyme, and sage together in a small bowl. Use immediately or store in an airtight container in a cool, dark place for up to 6 months.

ITALIAN SEASONING

Makes ½ cup (25 g)

We use this versatile seasoning in many recipes throughout the book, such as Spaghetti with Meat Sauce (page 215) and Italian-Inspired Beef & Farro Bowls (page 327). It's also great for seasoning oven-roasted vegetables prior to roasting.

- 2 tablespoons dried basil
- 2 tablespoons dried marjoram
- 1 tablespoon dried rosemary
- 2 teaspoons dried oregano
- 2 teaspoons dried sage
- 2 teaspoons dried savory
- 2 teaspoons dried thyme
- 1 teaspoon freshly ground black pepper

Whisk together the basil, marjoram, rosemary, oregano, sage, savory, thyme, and pepper in a small bowl. Use immediately or store in an airtight container in a cool, dark place for up to 6 months.

JAMAICAN JERK RUB

Makes about ½ cup (50 g)

One of the most popular flavors in Caribbean food is the legendary jerk seasoning, a delicious marinade or rub for meat, poultry, and fish. The spicy kick comes from indigenous red peppers grown on the island. Apply 1 to 2 tablespoons per pound (454 g) of meat, rubbing it into all sides. Let rest for 5 minutes before cooking.

1 tablespoon brown sugar

1 tablespoon cayenne

1 tablespoon garlic powder

1 tablespoon lemon pepper

1 tablespoon onion powder

1 teaspoon smoked paprika

1 tablespoon dried thyme

2 teaspoons ground allspice

⅛ teaspoon kosher salt

Whisk together the sugar, cayenne, garlic powder, lemon pepper, onion powder, paprika, thyme, allspice, and salt in a small bowl. Use immediately or store in an airtight container in a cool, dark place for up to 3 months.

MOROCCAN-STYLE SEASONING

Makes ½ cup (55 g)

Here we present a blend of spices and aromatics that create a harmony of hot and sweet flavors prevalent in North African cuisine. This seasoning can be added to extra virgin olive oil and lemon juice and used as a marinade or to coat chicken or fish. It's also delicious added to couscous and rice dishes. We use it in the Moroccan-Spiced Almonds (page 346) and the Moroccan-Inspired Chicken & Couscous (page 313).

1 tablespoon cayenne

1 tablespoon ground coriander

1 tablespoon ground cumin

1 tablespoon ground ginger

1 tablespoon grated lemon zest

1 tablespoon onion powder

2 teaspoons ground turmeric

1 teaspoon ground cinnamon

1 teaspoon sugar

½ teaspoon ground cloves

½ teaspoon freshly ground black pepper

2 saffron threads, crumbled

⅛ teaspoon kosher salt

Whisk together the cayenne, coriander, cumin, ginger, lemon zest, onion powder, turmeric, cinnamon, sugar, cloves, pepper, saffron, and salt in a small bowl. Use immediately or store in an airtight container in a cool, dark place for up to 6 months.

PERSIAN FRESH HERB MIX

Makes about 3 cups (100 g)

This fresh herb mix is inspired by Persian sabzi—an assortment of herbs, radishes, and green onions—that often accompanies meals. We suggest serving this with our Simply Broiled Salmon (page 298) or Moroccan-Inspired Chicken & Couscous (page 313).

1 cup (20 g) chopped fresh arugula

1 cup (8 g) finely chopped fresh dill

½ cup (8 g) finely chopped fresh cilantro

½ cup (15 g) finely chopped fresh mint

2 tablespoons finely chopped fresh tarragon

Grated zest of 1 lemon

Combine the arugula, dill, cilantro, mint, tarragon, and lemon zest in a bowl. Use immediately or store in an airtight container in the refrigerator, covered with a lightly damp paper towel to preserve freshness, for up to 3 days.

NOTE: *First wash and fully dry your herbs on a clean absorbent kitchen or paper towel before chopping. Wet herbs will turn to mush. Use a sharp knife to chop herbs by bunching the herbs together, and chop up and down in a circular motion. Then, placing your free hand on the top of the knife, rock the blade of the knife up and down and back and forth through the herbs until they are chopped as fine as you'd like. Avoid handling herbs too much, as overchopping causes them to bruise and lose their vitality.*

RUSTIC HERB SEASONING

Makes ½ cup (35 g)

Add this seasoning to any tomato-based dish like lasagna, spaghetti sauce, or tomato soup to deepen and intensify as well as brighten flavors. It's also good stirred into mashed or scalloped potatoes.

2 tablespoons dried chives

1 tablespoon ground aniseed

1 tablespoon ground basil

1 tablespoon garlic powder

1 tablespoon dried (granulated) lemon peel

1 tablespoon ground oregano

1 tablespoon dried rosemary

Whisk together the chives, aniseed, basil, garlic powder, lemon peel, oregano, and rosemary in a small bowl. Use immediately or store in an airtight container in a cool, dark place for up to 6 months.

TIP: *Mix 1 tablespoon seasoning with 2 tablespoons olive oil and drizzle over roasted carrots, cauliflower, or potatoes hot from the oven.*

SALMON RUB

Makes 6 tablespoons

This sweet, smoky rub is an easy way to add fantastic flavor to salmon fillet. Simply rub a tablespoon on each fillet, sear the skin side in an oven-safe skillet (start with a cold pan so the skin doesn't stick), and place in the oven to finish cooking the salmon. We use this rub in our Smoky Seared Salmon for One (page 298).

2 tablespoons brown sugar

1 tablespoon chili powder

1 tablespoon grated lemon zest

2 teaspoons smoked paprika

1 teaspoon garlic powder

1 teaspoon onion powder

1 teaspoon freshly ground black pepper

½ teaspoon ground coriander

½ teaspoon kosher salt

½ teaspoon ground mustard

Whisk together the brown sugar, chili powder, lemon zest, paprika, garlic powder, onion powder, pepper, coriander, salt, and mustard in a small bowl. Use immediately or store in an airtight container at room temperature for up to 1 month.

TIP: *After 1 month, the spices will lose some of their strength and you may need to use more of the blend to get the same flavor impact.*

SAVORY NUT CRUMB TOPPING

Makes 1 cup (235 g)

This topping can be made from any kind of nut you have on hand. Consider almonds, walnuts, pistachios, peanuts, cashews, or leftover mixed nuts. This mixture can be used to bread chicken tenders, top a casserole, or sprinkle on a gratin. We use it in our Mushroom & Spinach–Stuffed Tomatoes (page 275) and Potato-Turnip Gratin (page 278). It forms the crust for the Shiitake & Spinach Quiche with Rosemary & Sage (page 125) and, when made with almonds, it's a star ingredient in our Almond-Crusted Chicken Strips (page 303).

½ cup (70 g) unsalted nuts

½ cup (40 g) panko bread crumbs

⅓ cup (20 g) chopped fresh flat-leaf parsley

2 tablespoons chopped fresh thyme or lemon thyme

1 tablespoon grated lemon, lime, or orange zest

½ teaspoon freshly ground black pepper

¼ teaspoon kosher salt

1. Preheat oven to 200°F (95°C). Line a rimmed baking sheet with parchment paper.

2. Place the nuts, bread crumbs, parsley, thyme, zest, pepper, and salt in a blender or food processor. Pulse to form fine crumbs, about 1 minute. Spread the mixture on the baking sheet and bake for 12 to 15 minutes, until completely dry.

3. Cool completely. Use immediately or store in an airtight container in a cool, dark place for up to 1 month or in the refrigerator for up to 3 months.

SEAFOOD SEASONING

Makes ½ cup (15 g)

This very versatile seasoning blend can be used with a wide variety of fish and shellfish, during cooking or offered as a seasoning to add at the table. We use it extensively in our fish and shellfish recipes, including our delicious Seafood Trio Rolls (page 294), which include fish, shrimp, and crab to create a very elegant yet easy entrée.

3 tablespoons dried tarragon

2 tablespoons dried parsley

1 tablespoon dried basil

1 tablespoon dried (granulated) lemon peel

1 tablespoon dried marjoram

Whisk together the tarragon, parsley, basil, lemon peel, and marjoram in a small bowl. Use immediately or store in an airtight container in a cool, dark place for up to 6 months.

SMOKE & PEPPER GINGER RUB

Makes ½ cup (65 g)

This can be used dry or as a wet rub: Combine 1 tablespoon with 2 tablespoons olive oil and 2 tablespoons apple cider vinegar to marinate lean cuts of pork or beef, such as a blade chop or flank steak, before grilling or roasting.

2 tablespoons onion powder

2 tablespoons smoked paprika

1 tablespoon chili powder

1 tablespoon garlic powder

1 tablespoon ground ginger

1 tablespoon freshly ground black pepper

Whisk together the onion powder, paprika, chili powder, garlic powder, ginger, and pepper in a small bowl. Use immediately or store in an airtight container in a cool, dark place for up to 6 months.

SMOKY WORKADAY SEASONING

Makes about ¾ cup (70 g)

This alluring blend combines onion, parsley, and garlic with a hint of smoke. Stir into bean soups or white sauces for casseroles. You can also add 1 tablespoon to 1 pound (454 g) lean ground beef for hamburgers. It's the hero ingredient in our Smoky Workaday Sweet Corn & Pepper Sauté (page 268) and Smoky Workaday Pork Tenderloin (page 333).

¼ cup (30 g) onion powder

¼ cup (4 g) dried parsley

3 tablespoons smoked paprika

1 tablespoons garlic powder

Whisk together the onion powder, parsley, paprika, and garlic powder in a small bowl. Use immediately or store in an airtight container in a cool, dark place for up to 6 months.

SOUTHWEST SEASONING

Makes ½ cup (45 g)

This is the perfect seasoning to add to poultry, meat, vegetables, or beans that need a flavor boost from the earthy nuttiness of cumin and the subtle heat from cayenne. We feature this in our Southwest Pita Chips (page 340) and Southwestern Beef & Bean Burgers (page 180).

2 tablespoons cayenne

2 tablespoons ground cumin

2 tablespoons sweet paprika

2 teaspoons onion powder

2 teaspoons ground thyme

1 teaspoon garlic powder

1 teaspoon freshly ground black pepper

Whisk together the cumin, paprika, cayenne, onion powder, thyme, garlic powder, and pepper in a small bowl. Use immediately or store in an airtight container in a cool, dark place for up to 3 months.

TACO SEASONING

Makes ½ cup (55 g)

Most commercial taco seasoning mixes contain high amounts of sodium. Our version contains no sodium, allowing you to enjoy other taco ingredients (like hard shells, tortillas, and cheese) without worrying about the total sodium content of your meal. You can use ¼ cup (25 g) of this blend in place of a 1-ounce (28 g) packet of taco seasoning mix. We use it in our Fish Tacos (page 184) and Beef & Mushroom Taco Filling (page 183).

- 3 tablespoons chili powder
- 1 tablespoon cornstarch
- 1 tablespoon ground cumin
- 1 tablespoon dried minced onion
- 1 tablespoon dried oregano
- 2 teaspoons garlic powder
- 1 teaspoon cayenne

Whisk together the chili powder, cornstarch, cumin, onion, oregano, garlic powder, and cayenne in a small bowl. Use immediately or store in an airtight container in a cool, dark place for up to 6 months.

TOFU SEASONING

Makes ½ cup (70 g)

There are so many layers of flavor in this seasoning. You can use it as a dry rub on tofu, or combine 1 tablespoon with 1 tablespoon extra virgin olive oil or canola oil and brush it on tofu steaks before grilling, sautéing, or baking.

- 2 tablespoons ground mustard
- 2 tablespoons paprika or smoked paprika
- 1 tablespoon dried thyme
- 1 tablespoon dried basil
- 1 tablespoon garlic powder
- 1 tablespoon white pepper

Whisk together the mustard, paprika, thyme, basil, garlic powder, and pepper in a small bowl. Use immediately or store in an airtight container in a cool, dark place for up to 6 months.

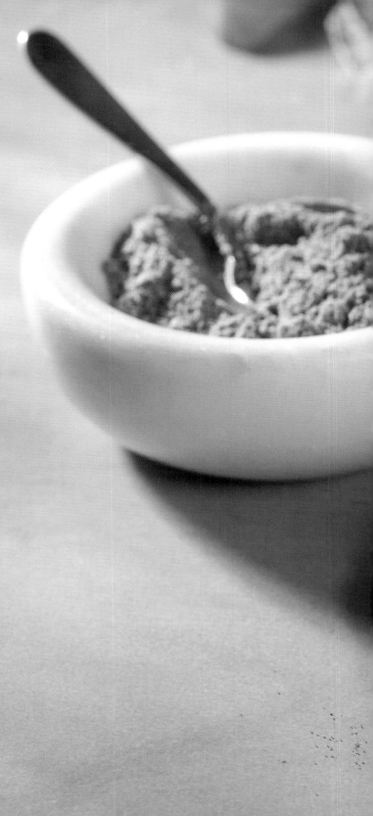

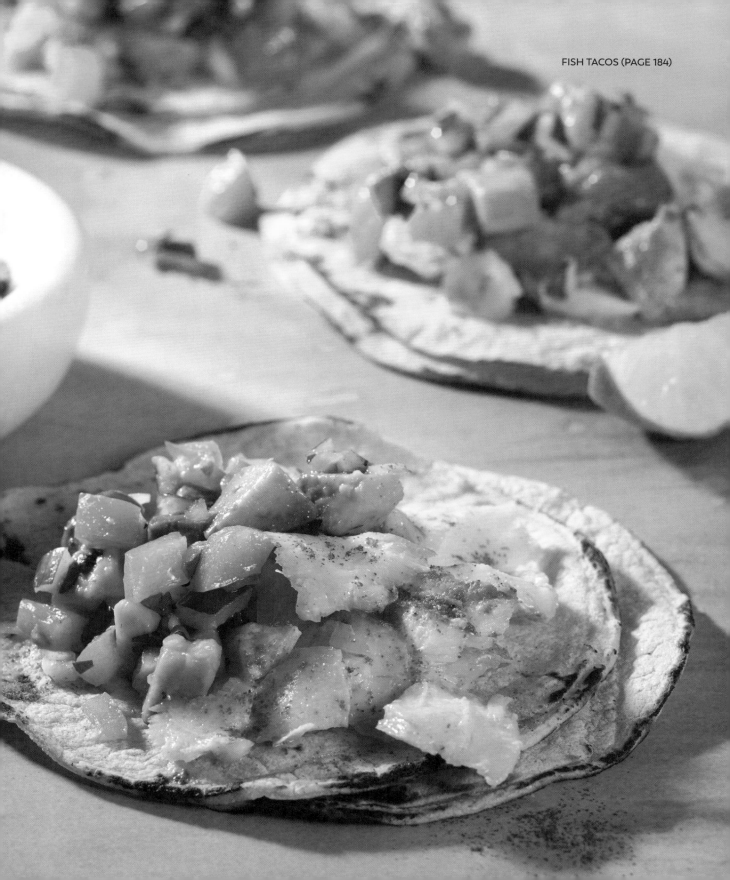

FISH TACOS (PAGE 184)

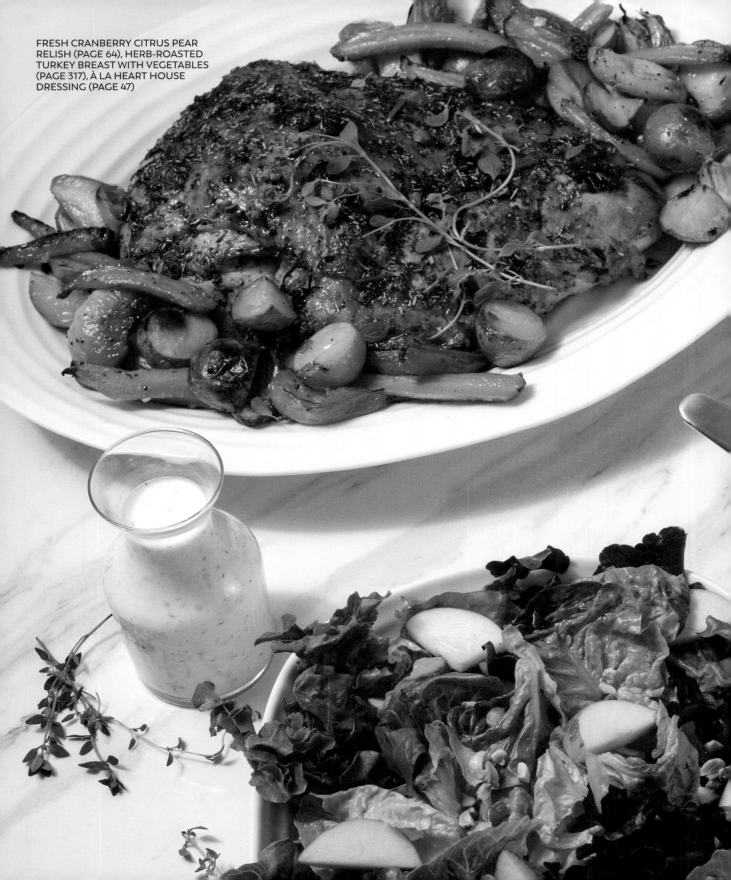

FRESH CRANBERRY CITRUS PEAR RELISH (PAGE 64), HERB-ROASTED TURKEY BREAST WITH VEGETABLES (PAGE 317), À LA HEART HOUSE DRESSING (PAGE 47)

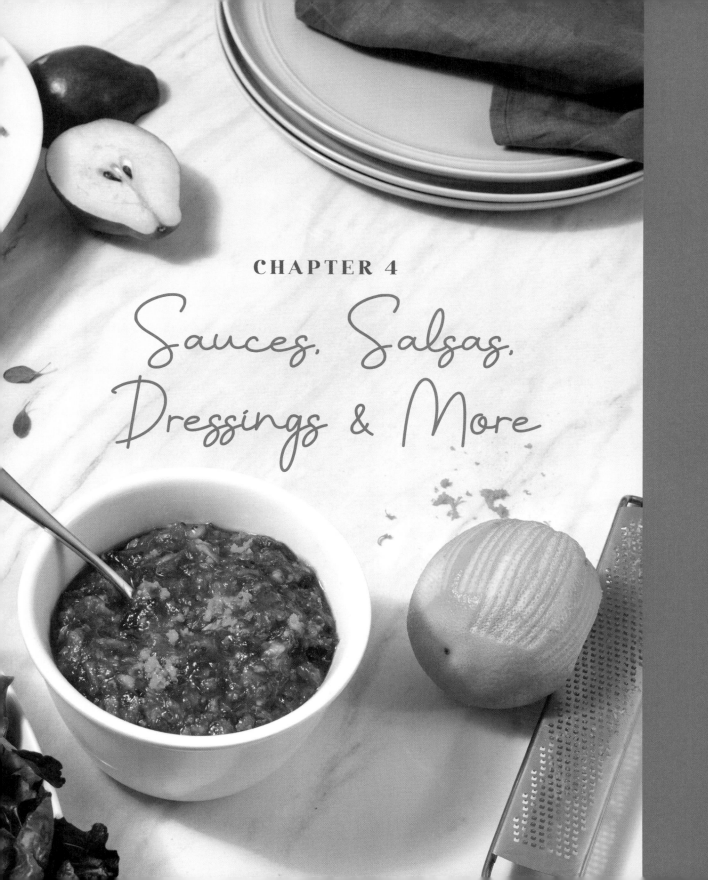

CHAPTER 4

Sauces, Salsas, Dressings & More

Sauces, Salsas, Dressings & More

Aïolis

Avocado Lemon Dill Aïoli 43

Avocado Lime Cilantro Aïoli 44

Chipotle Aïoli 44

Horseradish-Dijon Aïoli 44

Roasted Garlic Aïoli 45

Pestos

Basil Pesto 45

Cilantro Pesto 46

Cilantro-Mint Pesto 46

Spinach Pesto 46

Dressings & Vinaigrettes

À la Heart Caesar Dressing 47

À la Heart House Dressing 47

Blue Cheese Vinaigrette 48

Creamy Cucumber Dressing 48

Creamy Dijon Dressing 48

Creamy Dill Dressing 49

Creamy Feta & Mint Dressing 49

Dill Vinaigrette 49

Herbed Red Wine Vinaigrette 50

Herb-Infused Vinegar 50

Honey-Ginger Dressing 50

Lime & Thyme Vinaigrette 50

Sweet & Sour Sesame Dressing 51

Tarragon & Thyme Vinaigrette 51

Yogurt-Cardamom Dressing 52

Sauces

À la Heart Velouté Sauce 52

Alfredo Sauce 52

Béchamel 53

Caramelized Garlic Sauce 53

Chimichurri 54

Cranberry Sauce with Lime &
Crystallized Ginger 54

Cucumber-Dill Sauce 54

Homestyle Barbecue Sauce 55

Honey Mustard Sauce 55

Jalapeño-Peach Barbecue Sauce 56

Peanut Sauce 56

Plum Sauce 57

Raspberry-Chipotle Sauce 57

Rhubarbecue Sauce 58

Romesco Sauce 58

Simply Cooked Fresh Tomato Sauce . . . 59

Skordalia 59

Sweet & Sour Sauce 60

Sweet & Tangy Red Pepper Sauce 60

Tzatziki 60

Salsas

Avocado Salsa 61

Pico de Gallo 61

Pineapple Salsa with Tomato & Lemon . . 62

Stone Fruit Salsa 62

Strawberry Salsa 62

Tomato-Corn Salsa 62

Tropical Fruit Salsa 63

And More

Citrusy Walnut Gremolata 63

Cucumber Raita 63

Fresh Cranberry Citrus Pear Relish 64

Garlic-Tomato Confit 64

Honey Balsamic Onion Jam 64

Hot Mango Chutney 65

Rosemary-Sage Gremolata 65

There's a saying in the restaurant industry: "Sauce is boss." That's because most people love the additional flavor, richness, or creaminess a great sauce offers. In this chapter, we offer you a wide variety of sauces—from aïolis and pestos to dressings, vinaigrettes, salsas, barbecue sauces, and more—that can contribute to your greater enjoyment of a wide variety of health-promoting foods.

We're particularly proud of how many of the sauces use fruits and vegetables in all their glorious forms—fresh, frozen, canned, dried, and 100% juice. Enjoying these sauces helps contribute to increased fruit and vegetable consumption, which is an important part of heart-healthy eating. Many of the recipes feature sources of unsaturated, heart-healthy fats from plant-based oils, nuts, nut butters, and seeds.

When a recipe calls for a sweetener, we most often choose honey. From a metabolic point of view, honey is just like sugar, but honey also has flavor, antioxidants, and small amounts of minerals and B vitamins. Finally, our recipes limit added salt as well as other ingredients that contribute sodium. Most of the recipes in this chapter contain much less sodium than comparable products you'll find in your local grocery store.

Some of the recipes can be made in a matter of minutes, while others take more time to prepare. But nearly every recipe in this chapter can be made ahead of time and refrigerated until needed, or re-warmed to serve. In fact, many of the sauces get better if they have some time to settle and allow the flavors of the ingredients to "marry."

You may notice that serving sizes for fruit- and vegetable-based sauces, especially the salsas, are generous (typically ¼ to ½ cup/50 to 160 g), while sauces that include more fat—and therefore more calories—are conservative (typically 2 to 4 tablespoons). Keep in mind that heart-healthy eating isn't about limiting total fat, just saturated fat, but we do encourage you to think about portion sizes and the impact they can have on total calorie intake.

We hope you'll use these sauces as the gateway to greater consumption of foods with proven heart health benefits, including fruits, vegetables, legumes, whole grains, and healthy proteins.

AVOCADO LEMON DILL AÏOLI
Makes 2 cups (440 g)

This aïoli is wonderful accompaniment for fish or shellfish. Need a fast yet elegant lunch option? Toss it with cooked crab for a quick and easy crab salad.

- 2 garlic cloves, sliced
- 1 avocado, halved, pitted, flesh scooped out
- One 5.3-ounce (150 g) container plain Greek yogurt (about ⅔ cup)
- ¼ cup (55 g) mayonnaise
- 2 tablespoons chopped fresh flat-leaf parsley
- Grated zest of 1 lemon
- 1 tablespoon fresh lemon juice
- 1 tablespoon chopped fresh dill

Crush the garlic with a mortar and pestle to a creamy paste. Combine the garlic with the avocado in a small bowl. Mash the avocado and mix to combine. Add the yogurt, mayonnaise, parsley, lemon and juice, and dill. Whisk until well blended. Store in an airtight container in the refrigerator for up to 1 week. Do not freeze.

Serving Size 2 tablespoons; Calories 51; Protein 1 g; Carbs 1 g; Dietary Fiber 1 g; Added Sugars 0 g; Total Fat 5 g; Sat Fat 1 g; Omega-3s 0 mg; Sodium 24 mg; Potassium 83 mg

AVOCADO LIME CILANTRO AÏOLI

Makes 2 cups (440 g)

This smooth and intensely flavorful sauce pairs well with eggs, fish, poultry, roasted vegetables, and pasta dishes. Serve the aïoli in an avocado shell with a lime twist and cilantro sprig as garnish. Consider serving as a dipping sauce with Kale Chips (page 340) or Cumin Garlic Tortilla Chips (page 340).

2 garlic cloves, sliced

1 avocado, halved, pitted, flesh scooped out

One 5.3-ounce (150 g) container plain
  Greek yogurt (about ⅔ cup)

¼ cup (55 g) mayonnaise

2 tablespoons chopped fresh cilantro

Grated zest of 1 lime

1 tablespoon fresh lime juice

1 tablespoon chopped fresh tarragon or thyme

Crush the garlic with a mortar and pestle to form a creamy paste. Combine the garlic with the avocado in a small bowl. Mash the avocado and mix to combine. Add the yogurt, mayonnaise, cilantro, lime zest and juice, and tarragon. Whisk until well blended. Store in an airtight container in the refrigerator for up to 1 week. Do not freeze.

Serving Size 2 tablespoons; Calories 51; Protein 1 g; Carbs 1 g; Dietary Fiber 1 g; Added Sugars 0 g; Total Fat 5 g; Sat Fat 1 g; Omega-3s 0 mg; Sodium 23 mg; Potassium 80 mg

CHIPOTLE AÏOLI

Makes 1 cup (275 g)

This recipe is a must-try. You can buy a small can of chipotle chiles in adobo at most any supermarket. For a milder sauce, use just the adobo sauce from the can. If you prefer more heat, add one or more chiles from the can, diced. We use this to top off the Portobello Street Tacos (page 184) or use as a dipping sauce with the Wonton Crisps (page 341).

One 5.3-ounce (150 g) container plain
  Greek yogurt (about ⅔ cup)

⅓ cup (75 g) mayonnaise

2 tablespoons adobo sauce (from canned
  chipotles in adobo)

1 tablespoon fresh lime juice

½ teaspoon Adobo Seasoning (page 30) or
  ground chipotle chiles

½ teaspoon sugar

Whisk the yogurt, mayonnaise, adobo sauce, lime juice, adobo seasoning, and sugar together in a small bowl. Refrigerate until ready to use. Store in an airtight container in the refrigerator for up to 2 weeks. Do not freeze.

Serving Size 2 tablespoons; Calories 90; Protein 2 g; Carbs 2 g; Dietary Fiber 0 g; Added Sugars 0 g; Total Fat 9 g; Sat Fat 2 g; Omega-3s 500 mg; Sodium 90 mg; Potassium 5 mg

HORSERADISH-DIJON AÏOLI

Makes 1 cup (275 g)

Use this zesty aïoli as a spread for any of our sandwiches, as a dipping sauce with our Crispy Chicken Nuggets (page 310), or served on the side with the Sheet Pan Tri-Tip Roast (page 328).

⅔ cup (145 g) mayonnaise

⅓ cup (75 g) plain Greek yogurt

2 tablespoons prepared horseradish, well
  drained

1 tablespoon fresh lemon juice

1 teaspoon Dijon mustard

1 garlic clove, minced or grated

Whisk the mayonnaise, yogurt, horseradish, lemon juice, mustard, and garlic together in a small bowl. Refrigerate until ready to use. Store in an airtight container in the refrigerator for up to 2 weeks. Do not freeze.

NOTE: *Did you know that most of the oil used to make mayonnaise is unsaturated fat? Like extra virgin olive oil, the fatty acids in regular mayonnaise are 85 percent unsaturated. Enjoy the creaminess and heart-healthy fats it adds to other health-promoting foods.*

Serving Size 2 tablespoons; Calories 135; Protein 1 g; Carbs 1 g; Dietary Fiber 0 g; Added Sugars 0 g; Total Fat 14 g; Sat Fat 3 g; Omega-3s 0 mg; Sodium 127 mg; Potassium 14 mg

ROASTED GARLIC AÏOLI

Makes ½ cup (130 g)

A small drizzle of this French aïoli is a wonderful way to add a bit of mellow garlic flavor and creamy richness—compliments of heart-healthy fats from the extra virgin olive oil—to Simply Roasted Potatoes (page 260) or a piece of lean grilled beef. It's also very good tossed with Simply Cooked White Beans (page 241).

1 large egg yolk

3 or 4 Simply Roasted Garlic cloves (page 258)

1 tablespoon fresh lemon juice

1 teaspoon Dijon mustard

¼ teaspoon kosher salt

⅓ cup (80 ml) extra virgin olive oil

Combine the egg yolk, garlic, lemon juice, mustard, and salt in a food processor. Blend until smooth, then slowly drizzle in the oil while the motor is running, until emulsified. Refrigerate until ready to use. Store in an airtight container in the refrigerator for up to 5 days.

TIP: You can make a quick roasted garlic aïoli by combining ½ cup (110 g) mayonnaise with 3 or 4 roasted garlic cloves. Add 1 tablespoon lemon juice to brighten the flavor and thin the consistency.

Serving Size 2 tablespoons; Calories 180; Protein 1 g; Carbs 1 g; Dietary Fiber 0 g; Added Sugars 0 g; Total Fat 20 g; Sat Fat 3 g; Omega-3s 10 mg; Sodium 127 mg; Potassium 20 mg

BASIL PESTO

Makes 1 cup (245 g)

Pesto is a very versatile sauce that can be used to dress warm whole grains or beans, or as a base for lively dressings for pasta or vegetable salads. It can also be spread on mild white fish prior to baking or mixed with mayonnaise for an aromatic sandwich spread. We use it as a topping for our Italian-Inspired Beef & Farro Bowls (page 327).

3 cups (70 g) firmly packed fresh basil leaves

¼ cup (30 g) walnuts, toasted

3 garlic cloves, crushed

1 tablespoon fresh lemon juice

1 tablespoon chopped fresh thyme

⅓ cup (80 ml) extra virgin olive oil

¼ teaspoon freshly ground black pepper

¼ teaspoon kosher salt

½ cup (40 g) freshly grated Parmesan

1. Combine the basil, walnuts, garlic, lemon juice, and thyme in a food processor or blender. Pulse until coarsely chopped.

2. Slowly drizzle the oil into the food processor while the motor is running, or add in 2-tablespoon increments if using a blender. Add the pepper and salt. Stop blending when the pesto is a little chunkier than your desired consistency.

3. Add the Parmesan and pulse until as smooth as desired.

4. Store in an airtight container in the refrigerator for up to 5 days or in the freezer for up to 3 months.

TIP: If storing pesto to use later (in a pasta, salad, grain bowl, or fish recipe, for example), add the cheese just before serving. If freezing, drizzle a teaspoon or two of extra virgin olive oil over the top of the pesto in the container. To freeze the pesto in ice cube trays, measure 1 to 2 tablespoons into each compartment. Freeze for 4 hours or until solid. Remove the cubes from the tray and store in an airtight container.

Serving Size 2 tablespoons; Calories 127; Protein 3 g; Carbs 2 g; Dietary Fiber 1 g; Added Sugars 0 g; Total Fat 13 g; Sat Fat 2 g; Omega-3s 370 mg; Sodium 93 mg; Potassium 66 mg

CILANTRO PESTO

Makes 1 cup (235 g)

This pesto pairs beautifully with chicken, including our Roast Chicken with Lemon & Thyme (page 313). Use left-over chicken to fill warmed tortillas spread with some of this pesto for a quick and easy lunch.

- 2 cups (30 g) packed fresh cilantro leaves
- ½ cup (30 g) packed fresh flat-leaf parsley leaves
- ¼ cup (35 g) unsalted roasted cashews
- 3 garlic cloves, crushed
- 1 tablespoon fresh lime juice
- ⅓ cup (80 ml) extra virgin olive oil
- ¼ teaspoon freshly ground black pepper
- ¼ teaspoon kosher salt
- ½ cup (40 g) freshly grated Parmesan

1. Combine the cilantro, parsley, cashews, garlic, and lime juice in a food processor or blender. Pulse until coarsely chopped.

2. Slowly drizzle the oil into the food processor while the motor is running or add in 2-tablespoon increments if using a blender. Add the pepper and salt. Stop blending when the pesto is a little chunkier than your desired consistency.

3. Add the Parmesan and pulse it until it is as smooth as desired.

4. Store in an airtight container in the refrigerator for up to 5 days or in the freezer for up to 3 months (see Tip on page 45).

Serving Size 2 tablespoons; Calories 128; Protein 3 g; Carbs 2 g; Dietary Fiber 0 g; Added Sugars 0 g; Total Fat 13 g; Sat Fat 2 g; Omega-3s 360 mg; Sodium 97 mg; Potassium 70 mg

CILANTRO-MINT PESTO

Makes 1 cup (200 g)

This pesto is a perfect pairing with lamb. It's featured in our Lamb Chops with Cilantro-Mint Pesto (page 333).

- 1 cup (15 g) packed fresh cilantro leaves and stems
- ½ cup (15 g) packed fresh mint leaves
- ½ cup (60 g) walnuts, toasted
- 1 teaspoon minced garlic
- 1 teaspoon fresh lemon juice
- ¼ teaspoon kosher salt
- ⅓ cup extra virgin olive oil

1. Combine the cilantro, mint, walnuts, garlic, lemon juice, and salt in a food processor or blender. Pulse until coarsely chopped.

2. Slowly drizzle the oil into the food processor while the motor is running or add in 2-tablespoon increments if using a blender. Stop blending when the pesto is your desired consistency. For a thinner consistency, add a tablespoon or two of water.

3. Store in an airtight container in the refrigerator for up to 5 days or in the freezer for up to 3 months (see Tip on page 45).

Serving Size 2 tablespoons; Calories 131; Protein 1 g; Carbs 2 g; Dietary Fiber 1 g; Added Sugars 0 g; Total Fat 14 g; Sat Fat 2 g; Omega-3s 680 mg; Sodium 60 mg; Potassium 56 mg

SPINACH PESTO

Makes 1 cup (260 g)

Tossing pasta with this sauce is an easy way to get people to eat more vegetables. It also works well as a sandwich spread. This pesto is featured in our Turkey Tenderloins with Spinach Pesto & Pistachios (page 319) and Portobello-Pesto Pizza with Leeks (page 198).

- 3 cups (90 g) packed fresh baby spinach leaves
- ¼ cup (35 g) pine nuts or walnuts, toasted
- 3 garlic cloves, crushed
- 1 tablespoon chopped fresh basil
- 1 tablespoon fresh lemon juice
- ⅓ cup (80 ml) extra virgin olive oil
- ¼ teaspoon freshly ground black pepper
- ¼ teaspoon kosher salt
- ½ cup (40 g) freshly grated Parmesan

1. Combine the spinach, pine nuts, garlic, basil, and lemon juice in a food processor or blender. Pulse until coarsely chopped.

2. Slowly drizzle the oil into the food processor while

the motor is running or add in 2-tablespoon increments if using a blender. Add the black pepper and salt. Add the Parmesan and pulse until as smooth as desired.

3. Store in an airtight container in the refrigerator for up to 5 days or in the freezer for up to 3 months (see Tip on page 45).

Serving Size 2 tablespoons; Calories 126; Protein 3 g; Carbs 1 g; Dietary Fiber 1 g; Added Sugars 0 g; Total Fat 13 g; Sat Fat 2 g; Omega-3s 40 mg; Sodium 101 mg; Potassium 93 mg

À LA HEART CAESAR DRESSING

Makes 2 cups (475 g)

If you love Caesar salads with lots of creamy dressing, you'll love this version, which offers all the creamy goodness but fewer calories and less cholesterol and sodium than traditional Caesar dressings. This version has an added nutrition bonus from the yogurt and beans. We feature it in our Chicken Caesar Salad (page 161).

- 1 cup (175 g) Simply Cooked White Beans (page 241) or drained and rinsed canned cannellini beans
- 1 cup (230 g) plain Greek yogurt
- ¼ cup (60 ml) extra virgin olive oil
- ¼ cup (20 g) freshly grated Parmesan
- 3 garlic cloves, minced
- 2 tablespoons fresh lemon juice
- 1½ teaspoons Dijon mustard
- 1 teaspoon anchovy paste or 1 anchovy fillet
- 1 teaspoon freshly ground black pepper
- ½ teaspoon kosher salt

Combine the beans, yogurt, oil, Parmesan, garlic, lemon juice, mustard, anchovy paste, pepper, and salt in a blender or food processor. Blend or process until smooth. Store in an airtight container in the refrigerator for up to 2 weeks or until the yogurt's use by date.

Serving Size 2 tablespoons; Calories 68; Protein 2 g; Carbs 3 g; Dietary Fiber 1 g; Added Sugars 0 g; Total Fat 5 g; Sat Fat 2 g; Omega-3s 75 mg; Sodium 125 mg; Potassium 65 mg

À LA HEART HOUSE DRESSING

Makes 2 cups (535 g)

If only one dressing could be selected to be Cooking à la Heart's house dressing, this is it! A trio of familiar herbs— oregano, basil, and tarragon—adds a balanced finish to mixed greens. We serve it with our Crab, Asparagus & Avocado Salad (page 163) and as a dipping sauce for Savory Sweet Potato Fries (page 272) and Crispy Chicken Nuggets (page 310).

- 1 cup (240 ml) cultured buttermilk
- ½ cup (110 g) mayonnaise
- ½ cup (115 g) plain Greek yogurt
- ¼ cup (40 g) minced sweet onion (such as Vidalia or Walla Walla) or shallots
- 2 garlic cloves, minced
- 2 teaspoons fresh lemon or lime juice
- 1 tablespoon chopped fresh chives
- 1 tablespoon chopped fresh parsley
- 1 teaspoon chopped fresh basil
- 1 teaspoon chopped fresh oregano
- 1 teaspoon chopped fresh tarragon

Whisk together the buttermilk, mayonnaise, and yogurt in a medium bowl. Add the onion, garlic, lemon juice, chives, parsley, basil, oregano, and tarragon. Mix gently, then whisk vigorously until well blended. Pour the dressing into an airtight bottle or glass jar and refrigerate for at least 1 hour before serving. Store in the refrigerator for up to 1 week.

TIP: *This dressing can also be made in your blender.*

NOTE: *We like to add lemon juice to recipes that call for fresh garlic and/or onion, as the lemon juice mellows their intensity, keeping them from becoming too overpowering.*

Serving Size 2 tablespoons; Calories 60; Protein 1 g; Carbs 2 g; Dietary Fiber 0 g; Added Sugars 1 g; Total Fat 6 g; Sat Fat 1 g; Omega-3s 380 mg; Sodium 71 mg; Potassium 38 mg

BLUE CHEESE VINAIGRETTE

Makes 1½ cups (340 g)

Our blue cheese vinaigrette provides all the rich flavors you love in a traditional blue cheese dressing, but with less saturated fat and sodium. You can use it on our very simple Wedge Salad (page 155).

- ¼ cup (60 ml) vinegar (champagne or white wine)
- 1 tablespoon Dijon mustard
- 1 tablespoon honey
- ¾ cup (180 ml) extra virgin olive oil
- 2 tablespoons minced shallot
- 2 ounces (57 g) blue cheese, finely crumbled
- ½ teaspoon freshly ground black pepper

Combine the vinegar, mustard, and honey in a bowl. Whisk to combine. Slowly drizzle in the oil while whisking to emulsify and thicken the vinaigrette. Stir in the shallot, blue cheese, and pepper. Use immediately or store in an airtight container in the refrigerator for up to 1 week.

TIP: *To get the best flavor from this vinaigrette, use the best-quality blue cheese you can find. Buying a wedge in the cheese section will likely provide better quality than buying a tub of the crumbled version.*

Serving Size 2 tablespoons; Calories 153; Protein 1 g; Carbs 2 g; Dietary Fiber 0 g; Added Sugars 2 g; Total Fat 15 g; Sat Fat 3 g; Omega-3s 110 mg; Sodium 85 mg; Potassium 24 mg

CREAMY CUCUMBER DRESSING

Makes 2 cups (570 g)

This versatile dressing can be paired with sliced tomatoes or used to dress a simple salad of shaved carrots and tender baby greens.

- 1 cup (230 g) plain Greek yogurt
- ¾ cup (165 g) mayonnaise
- ½ cup (65 g) chopped English cucumber
- 1 teaspoon Dijon mustard
- 4 green onions, sliced
- ¼ cup (15 g) minced fresh parsley
- 1 garlic clove, peeled

Combine the yogurt, mayonnaise, cucumber, mustard, green onions, parsley, and garlic in a blender. Blend until smooth. Refrigerate until ready to use. Store in an airtight container in the refrigerator for up to 1 week.

TIP: *You can use a regular slicing cucumber instead of an English cucumber, but be sure to peel it, as the peel on a regular cucumber is much thicker. English cucumbers are often sold wrapped in plastic because their thin skin makes them dry out easily.*

Serving Size 2 tablespoons; Calories 93; Protein 1 g; Carbs 1 g; Dietary Fiber 0 g; Added Sugars 0 g; Total Fat 9 g; Sat Fat 2 g; Omega-3s 560 mg; Sodium 82 mg; Potassium 24 mg

CREAMY DIJON DRESSING

Makes 2 cups (500 g)

This versatile and simple dressing whips up super fast to dress a last-minute mixed greens salad, top roasted vegetables, coat the inside of a pita pocket, or drizzle on roasted meat like our Sheet Pan Tri-Tip Roast (page 328).

- 1 cup (230 g) plain Greek yogurt
- ¾ cup (165 g) mayonnaise
- 1 teaspoon Dijon mustard
- 4 green onions, sliced
- ¼ cup (15 g) minced fresh parsley
- 1 garlic clove, peeled

Combine the yogurt, mayonnaise, mustard, green onions, parsley, and garlic in a blender. Blend until smooth. Refrigerate until ready to use. Store in an airtight container in the refrigerator for up to 1 week.

Serving Size 2 tablespoons; Calories 93; Protein 1 g; Carbs 1 g; Dietary Fiber 0 g; Added Sugars 0 g; Total Fat 9 g; Sat Fat 2 g; Omega-3s 560 mg; Sodium 82 mg; Potassium 18 mg

CREAMY DILL DRESSING

Makes 2 cups (505 g)

We love pairing this dressing with seafood like shrimp, salmon, or canned tuna. It's also great served with our Mini Crab Cakes (page 289).

- 1 cup (230 g) plain Greek yogurt
- ¾ cup (165 g) mayonnaise
- 1 teaspoon Dijon mustard
- 4 green onions, sliced
- ¼ cup (5 g) chopped fresh dill or 2 teaspoons dried dill
- ¼ cup (15 g) minced fresh parsley
- 1 garlic clove, chopped

Combine the yogurt, mayonnaise, mustard, green onions, dill, parsley, and garlic in a blender. Blend until smooth. Refrigerate until ready to use. Store in an airtight container in the refrigerator for up to 1 week.

Serving Size 2 tablespoons; Calories 93; Protein 1 g; Carbs 1 g; Dietary Fiber 0 g; Added Sugars 0 g; Total Fat 9 g; Sat Fat 2 g; Omega-3s 560 mg; Sodium 82 mg; Potassium 19 mg

CREAMY FETA & MINT DRESSING

Makes 1½ cups (315 g)

This dressing works well on any Mediterranean dish, especially with chickpeas or grains. It's a good mix-in, adding flavor and a creamy texture when used as a sauce for the Simply Cooked Bulgur (page 224) or Simply Steamed Couscous (page 205).

- 1 cup (230 g) plain Greek yogurt
- 2 ounces (57 g) feta, crumbled (about ½ cup)
- 2 garlic cloves, minced
- 2 tablespoons chopped fresh parsley
- 1 tablespoon chopped fresh mint

Whisk together the yogurt, feta, garlic, parsley, and mint in a small bowl. Cover and refrigerate for at least 30 minutes before using. Store in an airtight container in the refrigerator for up to 1 week.

Serving Size 2 tablespoons; Calories 42; Protein 2 g; Carbs 2 g; Dietary Fiber 0 g; Added Sugars 0 g; Total Fat 3 g; Sat Fat 2 g; Omega-3s 10 mg; Sodium 54 mg; Potassium 11 mg

DILL VINAIGRETTE

Makes ½ cup (120 ml)

This dressing can be used in the Dilly Cucumber Salad (page 152) or to make pickled vegetables.

- ½ cup (120 ml) extra virgin olive oil
- 2 tablespoons sherry vinegar
- 1 tablespoon fresh lemon juice
- 2 garlic cloves, minced
- 1 tablespoon chopped fresh dill
- 1 tablespoon chopped fresh oregano
- ¼ teaspoon freshly ground black pepper

In a jar with a tight-fitting lid, combine the oil, vinegar, lemon juice, garlic, dill, oregano, and pepper. Cover and shake vigorously. Refrigerate until ready to use. Shake again just before using. Store in an airtight container in the refrigerator for up to 2 weeks.

Serving Size 2 tablespoons; Calories 88; Protein 0 g; Carbs 1 g; Dietary Fiber 0 g; Added Sugars 0 g; Total Fat 9 g; Sat Fat 1 g; Omega-3s 100 mg; Sodium 15 mg; Potassium 8 mg

HERBED RED WINE VINAIGRETTE

Makes 1 cup (240 ml)

This bright, vibrant herb-infused vinaigrette is our preferred dressing for the Salad Niçoise (page 166). It can also be used as a dressing for a simple potato salad, made with steamed halved baby red potatoes.

- ½ cup (120 ml) extra virgin olive oil
- ¼ cup (60 ml) red wine vinegar
- 2 tablespoons fresh lemon juice
- 1 tablespoon honey
- 1 teaspoon Dijon mustard
- 1 tablespoon chopped fresh rosemary
- 1 tablespoon chopped fresh tarragon
- ½ teaspoon freshly ground black pepper

Combine the oil, vinegar, lemon juice, honey, mustard, rosemary, tarragon, and pepper in a jar with a tight-fitting lid. Cover and shake vigorously. Store in an airtight container in the refrigerator for up to 2 weeks. Shake again just before using.

Serving Size 2 tablespoons; Calories 131; Protein 0 g; Carbs 3 g; Dietary Fiber 0 g; Added Sugars 2 g; Total Fat 14 g; Sat Fat 2 g; Omega-3s 100 mg; Sodium 17 mg; Potassium 16 mg

HERB-INFUSED VINEGAR

Makes 1¼ cups (300 ml)

To make your own herbed vinegar, start with a very good-quality vinegar. Add your choice of garden-fresh herb; experiment to find favorites. Then use this vinegar in vinaigrettes, marinades, and sauces. You can also use herb-infused vinegar on roasted vegetables or salad greens along with extra virgin olive oil.

- 1 cup (240 ml) vinegar (champagne or white balsamic)
- 1 tablespoon chopped fresh herbs (such as dill, oregano, thyme, tarragon, or mint), plus 1 sprig
- 2 fresh chives, minced
- 1 garlic clove, halved

Whisk together the vinegar, chopped herbs, chives, and garlic in a small bowl. Transfer to a glass jar or bottle with a lid and add the herb sprig. Refrigerate for at least 4 days to allow flavors to blend. Strain before using. Store in a clean jar or bottle in the refrigerator for up to 3 months.

Serving Size 2 tablespoons; Calories 9; Protein 0 g; Carbs 2 g; Dietary Fiber 0 g; Added Sugars 0 g; Total Fat 0 g; Sat Fat 0 g; Omega-3s 0 mg; Sodium 1 mg; Potassium 37 mg

HONEY-GINGER DRESSING

Makes 1 cup (265 g)

This dressing pairs beautifully with lettuce salads that include apples and walnuts. We love using it on salads made with butter lettuce, Honeycrisp apples, diced celery, and toasted walnuts for a crunchy hit of omega-3s!

- ½ cup (115 g) mayonnaise
- ½ cup (115 g) plain Greek yogurt
- 1 tablespoon honey
- 2 teaspoons fresh lemon juice
- 1 teaspoon grated fresh ginger
- ½ teaspoon smoked paprika

Whisk together the mayonnaise, yogurt, honey, lemon juice, ginger, and paprika in a small bowl. Refrigerate until ready to use. Store in an airtight container in the refrigerator for up to 1 week.

Serving Size 2 tablespoons; Calories 123; Protein 1 g; Carbs 3 g; Dietary Fiber 0 g; Added Sugars 2 g; Total Fat 12 g; Sat Fat 3 g; Omega-3s 750 mg; Sodium 95 mg; Potassium 10 mg

LIME & THYME VINAIGRETTE

Makes ½ cup (115 g)

This dressing is perfect on our Citrus, Spinach & Mushroom Salad (page 147). It's also wonderful paired with mixed greens and added to rice bowls; it brightens and heightens the flavors of the greens and rice while also adding moisture.

- ¼ cup (60 ml) extra virgin olive oil
- Grated zest of 1 lime
- 2 tablespoons fresh lime juice
- 1 tablespoon finely chopped fresh thyme
- 1 tablespoon sherry vinegar
- 1 garlic clove, minced

Mix the oil, lime zest, lime juice, thyme, vinegar, and garlic in a jar with a tight-fitting lid. Shake well. Use immediately or store in an airtight container in the refrigerator for up to 2 weeks. Shake again just before using.

Serving Size 2 tablespoons; Calories 131; Protein 0 g; Carbs 1 g; Dietary Fiber 0 g; Added Sugars 0 g; Total Fat 14 g; Sat Fat 2 g; Omega-3s 100 mg; Sodium 25 mg; Potassium 11 mg

SWEET & SOUR SESAME DRESSING

Makes ½ cup (120 ml)

This light, sweet-sour dressing, enhanced by the nutty flavor of toasted sesame, is excellent splashed on the Simply Stir-Fried Vegetables (page 262).

¼ cup (35 g) sesame seeds

⅓ cup (80 ml) rice vinegar

½ teaspoon freshly ground black pepper

½ teaspoon sugar

⅛ teaspoon kosher salt

1. Toast the sesame seeds in a dry skillet over medium heat until fragrant, 1 to 2 minutes. Shake or stir and watch carefully! They can go from toasted to burned in the blink of an eye. Transfer to a plate to cool.

2. Combine the vinegar, pepper, sugar, and salt in a small bowl. Add the sesame seeds, stir to combine, cover, and refrigerate until ready to use. Store in an airtight container in the refrigerator for up to 2 weeks.

Serving Size 2 tablespoons; Calories 42; Protein 1 g; Carbs 2 g; Dietary Fiber 1 g; Added Sugars 0 g; Total Fat 3 g; Sat Fat 0 g; Omega-3s 0 mg; Sodium 73 mg; Potassium 18 mg

TARRAGON & THYME VINAIGRETTE

Makes 1 cup (240 ml)

This all-purpose dressing doubles as a marinade—and is Linda's workhorse classic to splash on fresh greens, brush on grilled fish hot from the oven, or use to make quick-pickling vegetables, as in the Marinated Vegetable Salad (page 152). It also tenderizes and infuses flavor into beef or pork (omit the water) when used as a marinade.

¼ cup (60 ml) white wine vinegar

¼ cup (60 ml) cold water

3 tablespoons extra virgin olive oil

2 garlic cloves, crushed

2 tablespoons fresh lemon juice

2 tablespoons minced shallot

1 tablespoon honey

1 tablespoon chopped fresh tarragon

1 tablespoon chopped fresh thyme

1 teaspoon Dijon mustard

½ teaspoon paprika

¼ teaspoon freshly ground black pepper

Whisk together the vinegar, water, oil, garlic, lemon juice, shallot, honey, tarragon, thyme, mustard, paprika, and pepper in a small bowl. Use immediately or store in an airtight container in the refrigerator for up to 2 weeks.

Serving Size 2 tablespoons; Calories 66; Protein 0 g; Carbs 4 g; Dietary Fiber 0 g; Added Sugars 2 g; Total Fat 5 g; Sat Fat 1 g; Omega-3s 40 mg; Sodium 61 mg; Potassium 33 mg

YOGURT-CARDAMOM DRESSING
Makes 1 cup (245 g)

This mellow, creamy dressing filled with warming spices pairs well with many fruits, from citrus and apples to berries, cherries, and plums. We use it on our Mixed Fruit with Yogurt-Cardamom Dressing (page 144).

- 1 cup (230 g) vanilla Greek yogurt
- 1 teaspoon grated lemon zest
- ½ teaspoon ground cinnamon
- ¼ teaspoon ground cardamom
- ¼ teaspoon ground nutmeg

Whisk together the yogurt, lemon zest, cinnamon, cardamom, and nutmeg in a small bowl. Use immediately or store in an airtight container in the refrigerator for up to 1 week.

Serving Size 2 tablespoons; Calories 31; Protein 2 g; Carbs 4 g; Dietary Fiber 0 g; Added Sugars 2 g; Total Fat 1 g; Sat Fat 1 g; Omega-3s 0 mg; Sodium 16 mg; Potassium 49 mg

À LA HEART VELOUTÉ SAUCE
Makes 1 cup (240 ml)

We created this lighter version of a traditional velouté, which pairs well with roasted or grilled chicken breasts or served as a sauce with our Roast Chicken with Lemon & Thyme (page 313). If serving this sauce with fish and vegetables, consider using our Fish Broth (page 71) in place of chicken. In either recipe, you can also add 2 tablespoons of chopped fresh herbs or 2 teaspoons of lemon juice during the last minute of cooking to brighten the flavor.

- 1 tablespoon butter
- 1 tablespoon all-purpose flour
- 1 cup (240 ml) Chicken Stock (page 70) or reduced-sodium chicken broth
- ⅛ teaspoon white pepper

1. Melt the butter in a small saucepan. Add the flour, stirring constantly, until the mixture bubbles, 2 to 3 minutes. Cook and stir for 1 additional minute. Do not let it brown.

2. Add the broth and continue stirring until the mixture comes to a boil and thickens, 2 to 3 minutes. Add

the pepper, stir again, and serve. Store in an airtight container in the refrigerator for up to 5 days. Gently reheat prior to use.

Serving Size 2 tablespoons; Calories 19; Protein 0 g; Carbs 1 g; Dietary Fiber 0 g; Added Sugars 0 g; Total Fat 2 g; Sat Fat 1 g; Omega-3s 20 mg; Sodium 27 mg; Potassium 2 mg

ALFREDO SAUCE
Makes 2½ cups (680 g)

Alfredo sauce is typically made with heavy cream, but ours is made with milk, half-and-half, and a roux made with extra virgin olive oil and whole grain flour, for a thick, rich consistency. Italian seasoning and this recipe make enough to generously coat 1 pound (454 g) of fettuccine or other cooked whole grain pasta with vegetables.

- 2 tablespoons extra virgin olive oil
- 2 tablespoons whole wheat pastry flour
- 1 cup (240 ml) milk (of choice)
- 1 cup (240 ml) half-and-half
- 3 garlic cloves, minced
- 1 tablespoon Italian Seasoning (page 34)
- 1½ cups (120 g) freshly grated Parmigiano-Reggiano (see Tip)
- 1 tablespoon fresh lemon juice
- ½ teaspoon ground nutmeg
- ⅛ teaspoon kosher salt
- ¼ teaspoon freshly ground black pepper

1. Heat the oil in a medium skillet or saucepan over medium heat. Whisk in the flour 1 tablespoon at a time, until smooth. Slowly whisk in ½ cup (120 ml) of the milk until smooth. Slowly add the remaining ½ cup of milk and the half-and-half, whisking continuously.

2. Add the garlic and Italian seasoning, and bring to a gentle simmer for 4 to 5 minutes. Do not boil. Whisk to keep the sauce smooth, then cook until thickened, 3 to 4 minutes. Reduce the heat to medium-low if it the sauce starts to boil.

3. Add the cheese and whisk to combine. Add the lemon juice, nutmeg, salt, and pepper. Cook, whisking, until the cheese is melted and the sauce is smooth, about 1 minute.

4. Serve immediately. Store in an airtight container in the refrigerator for up to 5 days. Do not freeze. Gently reheat prior to use.

TIP: *Use freshly grated Parmigiano-Reggiano cheese, which melts smoothly and differentiates Alfredo sauce from any other cheese sauce.*

Serving Size 2 tablespoons; Calories 64; Protein 3 g; Carbs 3 g; Dietary Fiber 0 g; Added Sugars 0 g; Total Fat 5 g; Sat Fat 2 g; Omega-3s 20 mg; Sodium 133 mg; Potassium 55 mg

BÉCHAMEL
Makes 1 cup (240 ml); eight 2-tablespoon servings

Béchamel is one of the five "mother sauces" of classic French cuisine, which are the foundation for creating derivative "daughter" sauces. We use it in our À la Heart Mexican-Inspired Mac & Cheese (page 206).

- 1 tablespoon butter
- 1 tablespoon all-purpose flour
- 1 cup (240 ml) milk
- ⅛ teaspoon white pepper

1. Melt the butter in a small saucepan. Add the flour, stirring constantly, until the mixture bubbles. Cook and stir for 1 minute. Do not let it brown.

2. Add the milk and continue stirring until the mixture comes to a boil and thickens, 2 to 3 minutes. Add the pepper. Use immediately or store in an airtight container in the refrigerator for up to 5 days. Gently reheat prior to use.

TIP: *You can turn this sauce into an Alfredo sauce by stirring in ¼ cup (20 g) grated Parmigiano-Reggiano when you add the pepper.*

Serving Size 2 tablespoons; Calories 32; Protein 1 g; Carbs 2 g; Dietary Fiber 0 g; Added Sugars 0 g; Total Fat 2 g; Sat Fat 1 g; Omega-3s 10 mg; Sodium 23 mg; Potassium 48 mg

CARAMELIZED GARLIC SAUCE
Makes ½ cup (530 g)

Caramelizing garlic produces a mild, faintly sweet sauce similar to onion butter. This sauce is excellent served with beef, pork, veal, or lamb chops, or used as a spread inside wraps and pocket breads.

- 10 garlic cloves, peeled
- 1 cup (240 ml) water
- 3 teaspoons extra virgin olive oil
- ¾ cup (180 ml) reduced-sodium vegetable or chicken broth
- 3 white or cremini mushrooms, finely sliced
- 1 bay leaf
- 1 tablespoon chopped fresh parsley

1. Place the garlic cloves in small saucepan. Add the water, 1 teaspoon of the oil, and bring to a boil. Cover loosely and simmer until most of the water has evaporated and the garlic has softened, 15 to 20 minutes.

2. Mash the garlic with the back of a fork and return it to the saucepan. Add the remaining 2 teaspoons oil, the broth, mushrooms, and bay leaf. Cook over medium heat, stirring and simmering until the sauce is reduced and thickened, 4 to 5 minutes.

3. Discard the bay leaf, add the parsley, and mix well. Use immediately or store in an airtight container in the refrigerator for up to 1 week.

Serving Size 2 tablespoons; Calories 49; Protein 1 g; Carbs 3 g; Dietary Fiber 0 g; Added Sugars 0 g; Total Fat 4 g; Sat Fat 1 g; Omega-3s 0 mg; Sodium 20 mg; Potassium 85 mg

CHIMICHURRI

Makes 1½ cups (340 g)

Chimichurri is a fresh herb–based sauce most often associated with Argentinian cuisine. It's vibrant and aromatic, and you can make it quickly to serve with grilled seafood and meat. We love to serve it with grilled shrimp or our Smoked Tri-Tip (page 329). Chimichurri can also be mixed with mayonnaise or our Roasted Garlic Aïoli (page 45) to make a delicious spread for sandwiches.

- 1 bunch cilantro, ends trimmed, roughly chopped
- 1 bunch flat-leaf parsley, ends trimmed, roughly chopped
- 1 garlic clove, crushed
- ½ cup (120 ml) red wine vinegar
- ¼ cup (60 ml) extra virgin olive oil
- ½ teaspoon red pepper flakes
- ½ teaspoon kosher salt
- ½ teaspoon freshly ground black pepper

Combine the cilantro, parsley, garlic, vinegar, olive oil, red pepper flakes, salt, and pepper in a blender or food processor. Blend or pulse briefly, just long enough to combine the ingredients. Use immediately or store in an airtight container in the refrigerator for up to 1 week. The herbs will darken in color, but the vibrant flavor will remain.

TIP: *Use both the leaves and stems of the parsley and cilantro—the stems offer great flavor, and using them helps reduce food waste.*

Serving Size 2 tablespoons; Calories 44; Protein 0 g; Carbs 1 g; Dietary Fiber 0 g; Added Sugars 0 g; Total Fat 5 g; Sat Fat 1 g; Omega-3s 0 mg; Sodium 82 mg; Potassium 43 mg

CRANBERRY SAUCE WITH LIME & CRYSTALLIZED GINGER

Makes 2 cups (665 g)

Making homemade cranberry sauce is a family tradition for Linda. Maple syrup, lime, and crystallized ginger brings out the best flavor qualities of the cranberries, reducing their tartness with sweetness and warmth.

- ½ cup (120 ml) real maple syrup
- ½ cup (120 ml) water
- Grated zest and juice of 1 lime
- 1 tablespoon finely chopped crystallized ginger (see Notes)
- One 12-ounce (340 g) bag fresh or frozen cranberries, rinsed

1. Place the maple syrup, water, lime zest and juice, and ginger in a medium saucepan over medium-high heat. Bring to a simmer, add the cranberries, stir, and reduce the heat to a simmer.

2. Cook, stirring occasionally, until most of the berries have popped and the mixture has thickened, 5 to 6 minutes. Allow to cool before serving. Store in an airtight container in the refrigerator for up to 1 week.

NOTES: *Cranberries eaten straight from the bag are hard, sharp, and sour; they need a little sweetening to make them palatable. Like all berries, they have many health-promoting properties. Due to their seasonal availability as a fresh product, we like to freeze fresh berries so we can cook and bake with them throughout the year.*

Store your crystallized ginger in the freezer and use kitchen shears to handily chop the gummy pieces. Ginger packs a powerful punch in a small amount and can overpower; always taste before adding more.

Serving Size 2 tablespoons; Calories 38; Protein 0 g; Carbs 10 g; Dietary Fiber 1 g; Added Sugars 21 g; Total Fat 0 g; Sat Fat 0 g; Omega-3s 10 mg; Sodium 1 mg; Potassium 15 mg

CUCUMBER-DILL SAUCE

Makes 1½ cups (600 g)

This is a fragrant, cooling sauce that works well with our Zesty Chicken Bites (page 316). We also love using it as a sauce for the Fish Roast with Cucumber-Dill Sauce (page 286).

- 1 medium cucumber, peeled in stripes and quartered lengthwise
- 3 garlic cloves, halved
- One 5.3-ounce (150 g) container plain Greek yogurt (about ⅔ cup)
- ½ cup (110 g) mayonnaise
- ¼ cup (2 g) chopped fresh dill
- Grated zest of 1 lemon
- 1 tablespoon fresh lemon juice
- 1 teaspoon Dijon mustard
- ¼ teaspoon white pepper

Process the cucumber and garlic together in a blender or food processor until finely chopped. Add the yogurt, mayonnaise, dill, lemon zest and juice, mustard, and pepper. Process until all ingredients are blended into a creamy sauce. Use immediately or store in an airtight container in the refrigerator for up to 5 days.

Serving Size 2 tablespoons; Calories 77; Protein 1 g; Carbs 2 g; Dietary Fiber 0 g; Added Sugars 0 g; Total Fat 7 g; Sat Fat 2 g; Omega-3s 500 mg; Sodium 57 mg; Potassium 54 mg

HOMESTYLE BARBECUE SAUCE
Makes 1¾ cups (455 g)

This tangy barbecue sauce can be mixed with lean ground beef to make burgers or served as a dipping sauce for Crispy Chicken Nuggets (page 310) or wings. Brush on chicken or ribs during the last 20 minutes of cooking or on steaks or pork chops for the last 5 to 10 minutes of cooking.

- One 5.3-ounce (150 g) container plain Greek yogurt (about ⅔ cup)
- ½ cup (120 ml) no-salt-added tomato sauce
- ¼ cup (40 g) finely minced onion
- 3 tablespoons Dijon mustard
- 3 tablespoons firmly packed brown sugar
- 3 tablespoons reduced-sodium Worcestershire sauce
- 2 garlic cloves, finely minced
- ½ teaspoon smoked paprika
- ⅛ teaspoon hot sauce (such as Tabasco)

Combine the yogurt, tomato sauce, onion, mustard, sugar, Worcestershire, garlic, paprika, and hot sauce in a medium bowl. Whisk until smooth. Use immediately or store in an airtight container in the refrigerator for up to 3 days.

Serving Size 2 tablespoons; Calories 29; Protein 1 g; Carbs 4 g; Dietary Fiber 0 g; Added Sugars 2 g; Total Fat 1 g; Sat Fat 0 g; Omega-3s 0 mg; Sodium 62 mg; Potassium 69 mg

HONEY MUSTARD SAUCE
Makes 1¼ cups (310 g)

This sauce brings bright flavors to pork roasts, flank steak, and grilled chicken. It also makes a delicious spread for turkey sandwiches and roasted vegetable wraps.

- ⅔ cup (160 ml) plus 2 tablespoons water
- 3 tablespoons sherry vinegar
- 2 tablespoons honey
- 3 tablespoons ground mustard
- 1 tablespoon cornstarch

1. Whisk together ⅔ cup (160 ml) of the water, the vinegar, and honey in a small saucepan over medium heat.

2. Combine the mustard and cornstarch in a small bowl; add the remaining 2 tablespoons water to make a slurry. Add the slurry to the hot honey-vinegar mixture and whisk over medium heat until it comes to a boil. Stir until thickened, 1 to 2 minutes. Serve immediately with hot foods or let cool before storing in an airtight container in the refrigerator for up to 1 month.

Serving Size 2 tablespoons; Calories 34; Protein 0 g; Carbs 4 g; Dietary Fiber 0 g; Added Sugars 3 g; Total Fat 1 g; Sat Fat 0 g; Omega-3s 0 mg; Sodium 28 mg; Potassium 5 mg

JALAPEÑO-PEACH BARBECUE SAUCE

Makes 1⅓ cups (665 g)

This sweet and spicy sauce has a hint of smokiness. It offers more heat than sweet—if you prefer less heat, use the milder green chiles. Like many sauces, this one tastes better the day after it's made. The sauce pairs beautifully with our Simply Cooked Pork Tenderloin (page 332) and our Smoky Workaday Pork Tenderloin (page 333).

- ½ cup (80 g) diced red onion
- 1 tablespoon extra virgin olive oil
- ¼ teaspoon kosher salt
- ½ teaspoon smoked paprika
- One 15.5-ounce (439 g) can sliced peaches in 100% juice, drained
- One 4-ounce (113 g) can diced green chiles or jalapeños, drained
- 1 tablespoon honey
- ½ teaspoon apple cider vinegar

1. Cook the onions, oil, and salt in a medium saucepan over medium heat until the onions start to soften and turn pale pink, 5 minutes. Add the paprika and cook, stirring constantly, for 1 minute.

2. Transfer the mixture to a blender or food processor. Add the peaches, jalapeños, honey, and vinegar, and blend until smooth.

3. Transfer the sauce back to the saucepan and simmer over low heat for 5 minutes, until gently bubbling on the surface. Serve warm or cooled. Store in an airtight container in the refrigerator for up to 1 week. To reheat, transfer to a saucepan over medium-low heat and cook until it starts to bubble gently.

Serving Size 2 tablespoons; Calories 35; Protein 0 g; Carbs 6 g; Dietary Fiber 1 g; Added Sugars 1 g; Total Fat 0 g; Sat Fat 0 g; Omega-3s 0 mg; Sodium 80 mg; Potassium 15 mg

PEANUT SAUCE

Makes 1¼ cups (340 g); ten 2-tablespoon servings

This versatile sweet and salty sauce works well with many Thai, Malaysian, or Indonesian dishes. Consider serving as a dipping sauce for our Crispy Tofu Bites (page 250) or Crispy Chicken Nuggets (page 310).

- ⅔ cup (170 g) creamy peanut butter
- ⅓ cup (80 ml) water
- 1 tablespoon toasted sesame oil
- 2 tablespoons reduced-sodium soy sauce
- 1 tablespoon fresh lime juice
- 1 tablespoon rice vinegar
- 2 teaspoons brown sugar
- 3 garlic cloves, minced
- 1 teaspoon grated fresh ginger
- ½ teaspoon ground coriander
- ¼ teaspoon cayenne

1. Heat the peanut butter, water, and oil in a small saucepan over medium heat. Whisk until the peanut butter begins to soften and emulsifies with the oil and water, about 3 minutes.

2. Add the soy sauce, lime juice, vinegar, sugar, garlic, ginger, coriander, and cayenne. Whisk until smooth, about 1 minute. If the sauce is too thick, add water, 1 tablespoon at a time, until the desired consistency is reached. Cover and let cool before serving. Store in an airtight container in the refrigerator for up to 5 days.

Serving Size 2 tablespoons; Calories 119; Protein 4 g; Carbs 5 g; Dietary Fiber 1 g; Added Sugars 2 g; Total Fat 10 g; Sat Fat 2 g; Omega-3s 10 mg; Sodium 189 mg; Potassium 10 mg

PLUM SAUCE

Makes 2 cups (480 ml)

Somewhere between a chutney and a sweet and sour sauce, this sauce pairs well with meats and any of our stir-fries such as our Simply Stir-Fried Vegetables (page 262). It also makes an excellent dipping sauce for our Crispy Chicken Nuggets (page 310) or Crispy Tofu Bites (page 250).

- One 15-ounce (425 g) can purple plums, drained, pits removed (see Tip)
- One 15-ounce (425 g) can no-sugar-added pears
- ¼ cup (60 ml) sherry vinegar
- 3 garlic cloves, minced
- Grated zest of 1 lemon
- 1 tablespoon fresh lemon juice
- 2 teaspoons reduced-sodium soy sauce or tamari
- 1 teaspoon finely minced fresh ginger
- 2 tablespoons cornstarch
- ⅓ cup (80 ml) cold water

1. Combine the plums, pears and pear juice, vinegar, garlic, lemon zest and juice, ginger, and soy sauce in a food processor or blender. Process until smooth.

2. Pour the mixture into a small saucepan. Bring to a boil; reduce the heat to a simmer.

3. Dissolve the cornstarch in the water, then stir into the plum mixture. Simmer until thickened, 10 to 12 minutes, stirring occasionally. Serve warm or at room temperature. Store in an airtight container in the refrigerator for up to 1 week.

TIP: *If you can't find canned plums, use 1 cup (160 g) pitted prunes plus 2 tablespoons water.*

Serving Size 2 tablespoons; Calories 38; Protein 0 g; Carbs 10 g; Dietary Fiber 1 g; Added Sugars 0 g; Total Fat 0 g; Sat Fat 0 g; Omega-3s 0 mg; Sodium 48 mg; Potassium 76 mg

RASPBERRY-CHIPOTLE SAUCE

Makes 2½ cups (610 g)

This tangy barbecue sauce has a lovely lingering heat from the chipotles. It's great served on burgers or as an accompaniment to grilled tri-tip. Try it on our Southwestern Beef & Bean Burgers (page 180).

- 1 tablespoon extra virgin olive oil
- 1 shallot, minced
- 3 cups (420 g) frozen red raspberries
- One 7-ounce (198 g) can chipotles in adobo, pureed
- ¼ cup (85 g) honey
- 1 teaspoon apple cider vinegar

1. Heat the oil in a saucepan over medium-low heat. Add the shallots and sauté until soft and opaque, about 5 minutes.

2. Add the raspberries, chipotle puree, honey, and vinegar, and reduce the heat to low. Simmer for 10 to 15 minutes, until the raspberries have all broken down and the sauce is gently bubbling. Serve warm or at room temperature. Store in an airtight container in the refrigerator for up to 3 weeks or in the freezer for up to 3 months. Thaw in the refrigerator and heat over low heat before serving.

Serving Size 2 tablespoons; Calories 31; Protein 1 g; Carbs 6 g; Dietary Fiber 1 g; Added Sugars 3 g; Total Fat 1 g; Sat Fat 0 g; Omega-3s 0 mg; Sodium 24 mg; Potassium 70 mg

RHUBARBECUE SAUCE

Makes 7 cups (1,845 g)

Amy created this recipe in July 2006 at her family farm in North Dakota, where rhubarb grows in great abundance. The inspiration came about as her family was gearing up to host a family reunion. They wanted to serve a meal prepared with foods from the farm, like rhubarb and honey from bees that spend their summers in North Dakota. The sauce turned out to be a big hit paired with smoked pork ribs!

2 tablespoons canola oil

1 yellow onion, diced

1 teaspoon red pepper flakes

1 cup (240 ml) water

6 garlic cloves, minced

6 cups (730 g) chopped rhubarb

1 teaspoon kosher salt

1 teaspoon freshly ground black pepper

One 12-ounce (340 g) can tomato paste

½ cup (170 g) honey (preferably clover)

½ cup (100 g) light brown sugar

¼ cup (60 ml) apple cider vinegar

2 tablespoons soy sauce

2 teaspoons prepared yellow mustard

1 teaspoon dried oregano

1 teaspoon dried thyme

¼ teaspoon hot sauce, optional

1. Heat the oil in a large saucepan over medium-high heat. Add the onions and red pepper flakes. Cook until the onions start to soften and become translucent, about 10 minutes.

2. Add the water and garlic and cook until the garlic is fragrant, about 10 minutes.

3. Add the rhubarb, reduce the heat to low, and cook until the rhubarb has softened, about 30 minutes, stirring occasionally.

4. When the rhubarb is soft and falling apart, add the tomato paste, honey, sugar, vinegar, soy sauce, mustard, oregano, thyme, and hot sauce. Cook, covered, for another 10 minutes, until the sauce is gently bubbling on the surface. Use immediately or store in the refrigerator in an airtight container for up to 1 month.

Serving Size ¼ cup (66 g); Calories 60; Protein 1 g; Carbs 13 g; Dietary Fiber 1 g; Added Sugars 9 g; Total Fat 1 g; Sat Fat 0 g; Omega-3s 0 mg; Sodium 260 mg; Potassium 235 mg

ROMESCO SAUCE

Makes 2 cups (345 g)

Romesco sauce is a classic Spanish condiment that is a wonderful accompaniment for grilled meat, fish, and vegetables. We feature it as the topping for our Spanish-Style Beef & Brown Rice Bowls (page 330).

2 Roma (plum) tomatoes, halved

1 red bell pepper, halved and seeded

¼ cup (35 g) dry-roasted, unsalted almonds

2 garlic cloves, chopped

2 tablespoons extra virgin olive oil

2 tablespoons red wine vinegar

¼ teaspoon red pepper flakes

½ teaspoon smoked paprika

¼ teaspoon kosher salt

1. Preheat oven to 450°F (230°C).

2. Place the tomatoes, cut side up, and the bell pepper, cut side down, on a rimmed baking sheet. Roast for 20 to 25 minutes, until the skin on the peppers starts to brown. Allow to cool.

3. Use a paper towel to remove as much skin from the peppers as possible. Combine the tomatoes, peppers, almonds, and garlic in a food processor. Process until smooth.

4. While running the food processor, add the oil and vinegar. Turn off the processor, scrape down the sides with a rubber spatula, and add the red pepper flakes, paprika, and salt. Process for 2 to 3 seconds until smooth. Use immediately or store in an airtight container in the refrigerator for up to 1 week.

Serving Size 2 tablespoons; Calories 33; Protein 1 g; Carbs 1 g; Dietary Fiber 1 g; Added Sugars 0 g; Total Fat 3 g; Sat Fat 0 g; Omega-3s 10 mg; Sodium 30 mg; Potassium 52 mg

SIMPLY COOKED FRESH TOMATO SAUCE

Makes 6 cups (965 g)

This sauce doesn't require the tomatoes to be peeled or seeded—we encourage using the whole tomato for added nutrition and flavor. The perfect sauce for a simple pasta topped with freshly grated Parmesan and some chopped parsley.

- 4 to 6 medium tomatoes, quartered
- ¼ cup (15 g) chopped fresh parsley
- 3 tablespoons chopped fresh thyme
- 2 tablespoons chopped fresh fennel
- 2 tablespoons chopped fresh basil
- 1 tablespoon chopped fresh oregano
- 1 teaspoon ground coriander
- 1 teaspoon sugar
- 2 tablespoons extra virgin olive oil
- 1 cup (160 g) minced onion (about 1 large onion)
- 3 garlic cloves, minced
- 1 bay leaf

1. Place the tomatoes in a blender or food processor. Pulse to form large chunks. Add the parsley, thyme, fennel, basil, oregano, coriander, and sugar. Process until the herbs and spices are incorporated.

2. Heat the oil in a heavy-bottomed saucepan or Dutch oven over medium heat. Add the onions and cook until tender but not browned, about 1 minute. Add the garlic and sauté until the garlic is fragrant and the onions are translucent, 2 to 3 minutes.

3. Stir in the tomato-herb mixture. Add the bay leaf, then increase the heat to medium-high. Stir occasionally as the sauce reaches a boil, 8 to 10 minutes.

4. Reduce the heat to low and simmer gently for 40 minutes. The sauce is done when it is thick enough to mound in a spoon. Remove the bay leaf. Use immediately or store in an airtight container in the refrigerator for up to 2 weeks.

Serving Size 2 tablespoons; Calories 44; Protein 0 g; Carbs 4 g; Dietary Fiber 0 g; Added Sugars 0 g; Total Fat 4 g; Sat Fat 0 g; Omega-3s 0 mg; Sodium 264 mg; Potassium 180 mg

SKORDALIA

Makes 2 cups (390 g)

Skordo is the Greek word for garlic. In Greece, this sauce is often used as a dip for fried fish or simply cooked vegetables. We love to use it as a creamy, fragrant topping for our Greek-Flavor Beef & Barley Bowls (page 326).

- 2 medium Yukon gold–type potatoes, diced into ½-inch (13 mm) cubes
- 1 slice whole wheat or white bread, torn into pieces
- 4 garlic cloves, minced
- ½ cup (70 g) dry-roasted unsalted almonds or toasted walnuts
- ¼ cup (60 ml) fresh lemon juice
- ¼ cup (60 ml) extra virgin olive oil
- ½ teaspoon kosher salt

1. Fill a small pot with water, add the potatoes, and bring to a simmer over medium-high heat. Cover and cook until the potatoes are soft, about 10 minutes. Remove the potatoes, reserving the cooking water.

2. Combine the cooked potatoes, ½ cup (120 ml) of the cooking water, the bread, garlic, almonds, lemon juice, oil, and salt in a blender or food processor. Blend until smooth. If the sauce is too thick, add more cooking water to achieve the desired consistency.

3. Serve at room temperature. Store in an airtight container in the refrigerator for up to 1 week.

NOTE: *You don't have to peel the potatoes for a recipe like this. About 30 percent of the fiber in a potato is contained in the peel, and the peel on most yellow skin, yellow flesh varieties like Yukon gold is very thin and tender. Eating the peel is a great way to boost your fiber intake.*

Serving Size 2 tablespoons; Calories 79; Protein 2 g; Carbs 4 g; Dietary Fiber 1 g; Added Sugars 0 g; Total Fat 6 g; Sat Fat 1 g; Omega-3s 30 mg; Sodium 71 mg; Potassium 160 mg

SWEET & SOUR SAUCE

Makes 1½ cups (400 g)

This sauce loves to be paired with our Crispy Tofu Bites (page 250), Crispy Chicken Nuggets (page 310), or Crispy Fish Sticks (page 286).

- One 8-ounce (227 g) can crushed pineapple in 100% juice
- ¼ cup (60 ml) sherry or white wine vinegar
- 1 tablespoon honey
- 1 tablespoon reduced-sodium soy sauce or tamari
- 1 tablespoon cornstarch
- 2 or 3 green onions, finely chopped

1. Drain the pineapple and reserve the juice. Add enough water to the reserved juice to make 1 cup (240 ml) and pour into a small saucepan over medium heat. Add the vinegar, honey, and soy sauce. Whisk until well blended. Bring to a simmer.

2. Dissolve the cornstarch in 2 tablespoons water in a small bowl, then whisk it into the pineapple-vinegar mixture. Bring to a boil, whisking constantly. Reduce the heat and simmer until the mixture has thickened and is smooth, about 5 minutes. Stir in the pineapple and green onions. Let cool before serving. Store in an airtight container in the refrigerator for up to 2 weeks.

TIP: *You can quickly warm up this sauce by microwaving it for 20 to 30 seconds just before serving.*

Serving Size 2 tablespoons; Calories 26; Protein 0 g; Carbs 6 g; Dietary Fiber 0 g; Added Sugars 1 g; Total Fat 0 g; Sat Fat 0 g; Omega-3s 0 mg; Sodium 104 mg; Potassium 41 mg

SWEET & TANGY RED PEPPER SAUCE

Makes 1 cup (555 g)

Fire-roasted red bell peppers in jars are convenient to have on hand to make a quick sauce for fish or roasted vegetables. The creaminess of the walnuts and the sweet, smoky flavor of the peppers and paprika also pair beautifully with our Beef & Lentil Salad Bowls (page 160).

- One 16-ounce (454 g) jar roasted red bell peppers, drained well
- ½ cup (60 g) walnuts, toasted, plus more if needed
- 2 garlic cloves
- 1 tablespoon extra virgin olive oil
- 1 tablespoon balsamic vinegar
- 1 teaspoon smoked paprika
- ¼ teaspoon cayenne
- Water, optional

Place the peppers, walnuts, garlic, oil, vinegar, paprika, and cayenne in a blender or food processor. Blend until the mixture is smooth with a bit of graininess. If the sauce is too thick, add 1 to 2 tablespoons water; if too thin, add a few more walnuts. Store in an airtight container in the refrigerator for up to 5 days.

Serving Size 2 tablespoons; Calories 94; Protein 1 g; Carbs 6 g; Dietary Fiber 3 g; Added Sugars 1 g; Total Fat 7 g; Sat Fat 1 g; Omega-3s 680 mg; Sodium 112 mg; Potassium 13 mg

TZATZIKI

Makes 2 cups (425 g)

We love to top our Greek-Flavor Beef & Barley Bowls (page 326) with this bright, tangy sauce. It's also a wonderful dip for a mezze platter with roasted vegetables, hummus, and pita.

- ½ English cucumber
- ¼ teaspoon kosher salt
- 1 cup (230 g) nonfat Greek yogurt
- 2 tablespoons red wine vinegar
- 1 garlic clove, minced
- 1 tablespoon finely chopped fresh dill

1. Grate the cucumber over a small mixing bowl and mix in the salt. Set aside for 20 minutes.

2. Drain off as much liquid as you can. In a medium bowl, combine the yogurt, vinegar, and garlic. Add the cucumber and dill. Stir to combine. Store in an airtight container in the refrigerator for up to 1 week.

Serving Size 2 tablespoons; Calories 22; Protein 1 g; Carbs 1 g; Dietary Fiber 0 g; Added Sugars 0 g; Total Fat 1 g; Sat Fat 1 g; Omega-3s 0 mg; Sodium 38 mg; Potassium 15 mg

AVOCADO SALSA

Makes 2 cups (440 g)

This mild, mellow salsa has a hint of heat from cumin. Serve alongside fish or poultry or use it to top off a spicy bowl. This salsa lends itself well to adding in a sweet element—add either ¾ cup (100 g) sliced, quartered star fruit (carambola) or fresh papaya cubes.

- 2 tablespoons avocado oil or extra virgin olive oil
- 2 tablespoons rice vinegar
- 1 tablespoon fresh lime juice
- ¼ teaspoon ground cumin
- ⅛ teaspoon kosher salt
- ⅛ teaspoon freshly ground black pepper
- 1 avocado, halved, pitted, peeled, and cubed
- 1 orange bell pepper, seeded and diced
- ¼ cup (40 g) diced red onion
- ¼ cup (4 g) chopped fresh cilantro

Whisk together the oil, vinegar, lime juice, cumin, salt, and black pepper in a medium bowl. Add the avocado, bell pepper, onion, and cilantro, and gently stir to combine. Serve immediately or cover and refrigerate for up to 2 hours before serving. Store in an airtight container in the refrigerator for up to 1 week.

NOTE: *If there was a contest to nominate a single fruit to be our Cooking à la Heart all-star fruit, we'd nominate the avocado. It contains heart-healthy unsaturated fats, potassium for promoting healthy blood pressure levels, and a wealth of dietary fiber. The unsaturated fat in avocados helps your body absorb other essential nutrients, which is why we love to pair avocados with other nutrient-rich fruits and vegetables to capture all the glorious nutrient benefits. And did we mention how much we love that naturally creamy consistency? Oh, how we adore avocados!*

Serving Size 2 tablespoons; Calories 39; Protein 0 g; Carbs 2 g; Dietary Fiber 1 g; Added Sugars 0 g; Total Fat 4 g; Sat Fat 0 g; Omega-3s 30 mg; Sodium 16 mg; Potassium 89 mg

PICO DE GALLO

Makes 4 cups (640 g)

Pico de gallo is a fresh, chunky salsa. It's easy to make, providing a convenient and delicious way to get more veggies into meals featuring tacos and burritos. Pico de gallo is perfect paired with whole grain corn chips, and it makes a vibrant, colorful topping for scrambled eggs. This sauce, like many tomato-based dishes, gets better if the flavors of the ingredients have time to blend prior to eating. Plan to let it sit in the refrigerator a few hours to a day before serving.

- 2 cups (360 g) diced red tomatoes (about 2 large tomatoes)
- 1 cup (150 g) diced yellow bell pepper (about 1 pepper)
- ½ cup (8 g) chopped fresh cilantro
- ½ cup (80 g) diced white onion
- ¼ cup (25 g) minced jalapeño chiles
- 1 tablespoon fresh lime juice
- 1 teaspoon kosher salt

Stir together the tomatoes, pepper, cilantro, onions, jalapeño, lime juice, and salt in a medium bowl. Cover and refrigerate for 1 to 2 hours before serving. Store in an airtight container in the refrigerator for up to 3 days.

Serving Size 2 tablespoons; Calories 5; Protein 0 g; Carbs 1 g; Dietary Fiber 0 g; Added Sugars 0 g; Total Fat 0 g; Sat Fat 0 g; Omega-3s 0 mg; Sodium 60 mg; Potassium 46 mg

SODIUM TIP: Using Diamond Crystal Kosher Salt will dramatically reduce the sodium in any recipe that uses kosher salt. This salt contains 50% less sodium per measure than regular kosher salt and 60% less than fine grain table salt.

PINEAPPLE SALSA WITH TOMATO & LEMON

Makes 4 cups (930 g)

This salsa is so good on our Fish Tacos (page 184). It's also wonderful tossed with Simply Cooked Brown Rice (page 230), adding subtle sweetness and a bit of heat.

- 3 cups (540 g) diced fresh tomatoes, drained (about 3 large tomatoes)
- 1 cup (115 g) diced fresh pineapple
- 10 green onions, sliced
- 1 jalapeño or serrano chile, seeded and finely chopped
- 3 tablespoons chopped fresh cilantro
- 1 teaspoon finely grated lemon zest
- 3 tablespoons fresh lemon juice
- 2 garlic cloves, finely chopped

Combine the tomatoes, pineapple, green onions, chile, cilantro, lemon zest and juice, and garlic in a large bowl. Stir gently until evenly mixed. Serve immediately or store in an airtight container in the refrigerator for up to 1 day.

Serving Size 2 tablespoons; Calories 8; Protein 0 g; Carbs 2 g; Dietary Fiber 0 g; Added Sugars 0 g; Total Fat 0 g; Sat Fat 0 g; Omega-3s 0 mg; Sodium 3 mg; Potassium 59 mg

STONE FRUIT SALSA

Makes 3 cups (830 g)

Salsas that feature fruit other than tomatoes can be so delicious. We love serving this one with grilled chicken on hot summer evenings.

- 3 peaches or nectarines, pitted and cubed
- 1 medium (200 g) cucumber, peeled and diced
- ¼ cup (4 g) chopped fresh cilantro
- ¼ cup (40 g) diced red onion
- 1 jalapeño chile, seeded and minced
- 2 tablespoons fresh lime juice

Toss the peaches, cucumber, cilantro, red onion, jalapeño, and lime juice together in a medium bowl. Serve immediately or cover and refrigerate for up to 2 hours before serving. Store in an airtight container in the refrigerator for up to 1 week.

Serving Size 2 tablespoons; Calories 11; Protein 0 g; Carbs 3 g; Dietary Fiber 1 g; Added Sugars 0 g; Total Fat 0 g; Sat Fat 0 g; Omega-3s 0 mg; Sodium 1 mg; Potassium 57 mg

STRAWBERRY SALSA

Makes 3 cups (380 g)

This sweet and hot salsa pairs well with delicate fish such as pan-seared sole fillets. Consider using half strawberries and half grapefruit, mango, or peaches to change it up from time to time.

- 2 cups (290 g) coarsely chopped fresh strawberries
- 2 green onions, chopped
- 1 small poblano chile, seeded and finely diced
- 2 tablespoons chopped fresh cilantro
- 1 tablespoon fresh lemon juice
- 1 tablespoon balsamic vinegar
- ⅛ teaspoon kosher salt

Toss the strawberries, green onions, poblano, cilantro, lemon juice, vinegar, and salt together in a medium bowl. Serve immediately or cover and refrigerate for up to 2 hours before serving. Store in an airtight container in the refrigerator for up to 1 week.

Serving Size 2 tablespoons; Calories 10; Protein 0 g; Carbs 1 g; Dietary Fiber 0 g; Added Sugars 1 g; Total Fat 0 g; Sat Fat 0 g; Omega-3s 10 mg; Sodium 10 mg; Potassium 26 mg

TOMATO-CORN SALSA

Makes 2 cups (350 g)

Corn gives this salsa a sweet foundation of flavor while fresh lime juice adds bright acidity. We feature it as a colorful topping for our Millet Curry Cakes (page 227). It's also a great accompaniment for the Cumin-Garlic Tortilla Chips (page 340).

- 1 cup (150 g) fresh white or yellow corn kernels (scraped from about 2 medium ears), cooked and cooled to room temperature
- ½ cup (90 g) diced tomato

¼ cup (40 g) diced red onion

¼ cup (4 g) chopped fresh cilantro leaves
and stems

1 tablespoon minced jalapeño or serrano chile

2 tablespoons fresh lime juice

1 tablespoon extra virgin olive oil

¼ teaspoon kosher salt

Combine the corn, tomato, onion, cilantro, jalapeño, lime juice, olive oil, and salt in a medium bowl. Transfer to an airtight container and refrigerate for 2 to 24 hours before serving to allow the flavors to blend. Store in the refrigerator for up to 3 days.

Serving Size 2 tablespoons; Calories 20; Protein 0 g; Carbs 3 g; Dietary Fiber 0 g; Added Sugars 0 g; Total Fat 1 g; Sat Fat 0 g; Omega-3s 10 mg; Sodium 32 mg; Potassium 42 mg

TROPICAL FRUIT SALSA
Makes 4 cups (885 g)

A touch of heat and sweet citrusy fruit flavors combine with the cooling flavors of cucumber and mint in this salsa. If you'd like more heat, add a second jalapeño. This recipe also works well with mango in place of the papaya and jicama in place of the cucumbers. Serve alongside any of the fish dishes starting on page 282.

1 or 2 medium papayas, peeled, seeded, and
diced

1 cup (135 g) peeled and diced cucumber
(about 1 medium)

1 cup (230 g) diced grapefruit sections
(preferably red)

½ cup (80 g) chopped red onion or shallot

1 jalapeño chile, seeded and finely chopped

2 tablespoons fresh lime juice

2 tablespoons finely chopped fresh mint

1 tablespoon champagne or sherry vinegar

1 teaspoon honey

⅛ teaspoon kosher salt

Combine the papaya, cucumbers, grapefruit, onion, jalapeño, lime juice, mint, vinegar, honey, and salt in a medium bowl. Gently stir to mix. Cover and refrigerate for at least 6 hours before serving. Store in an airtight container in the refrigerator for up to 1 week.

Serving Size 2 tablespoons; Calories 23; Protein 0 g; Carbs 6 g; Dietary Fiber 1 g; Added Sugars 0 g; Total Fat 0 g; Sat Fat 0 g; Omega-3s 20 mg; Sodium 8 mg; Potassium 76 mg

CITRUSY WALNUT GREMOLATA
Makes 1 cup (95 g)

Gremolata is a classic Italian garnish made with parsley, garlic, and lemon zest. Use it over fish or roasted vegetables, such as the Pan-Seared Crispy Catfish (page 290), Potato Turnip Gratin (page 278), or Simply Roasted Root Vegetables with Apples (page 261).

¼ cup plus 2 tablespoons (25 g) chopped fresh
flat-leaf parsley

¼ cup (30 g) finely chopped walnuts

2 tablespoons finely grated lemon zest

1 tablespoon finely grated lime zest

1 tablespoon finely grated orange zest

6 garlic cloves, minced

½ teaspoon freshly ground black pepper

Pinch of kosher salt

Whisk together the parsley, walnuts, lemon, lime, and orange zests, garlic, pepper, and salt in a small bowl until well blended. Store in an airtight container in the refrigerator for up to 1 week.

Serving Size 2 tablespoons; Calories 31; Protein 1 g; Carbs 2 g; Dietary Fiber 1 g; Added Sugars 0 g; Total Fat 2 g; Sat Fat 0 g; Omega-3s 340 mg; Sodium 16 mg; Potassium 47 mg

CUCUMBER RAITA
Makes 3½ cups (775 g)

Raitas are traditional Indian condiments that offer a cooling balance to dishes with spice or heat. This simple version can be made with Greek yogurt, but if you prefer a thinner consistency, you can add a few tablespoons milk, or use kefir in place of the yogurt. You can also add a few halved green grapes for a lovely hint of sweetness. We love to serve this with our Chicken Tikka Masala (page 309).

1½ cups (345 g) Greek yogurt

1 English cucumber, diced

⅓ cup (55 g) minced red onion

2 tablespoons fresh lemon juice

2 tablespoons extra virgin olive oil

½ teaspoon kosher salt

¼ teaspoon freshly ground black pepper

Stir together the yogurt, cucumber, onion, lemon juice, oil, salt, and pepper in a medium bowl. Use immediately or cover and refrigerate until needed. Store in an airtight container in the refrigerator for up to 3 days. Stir again before serving.

Serving Size 2 tablespoons; Calories 28; Protein 1 g; Carbs 1 g; Dietary Fiber 0 g; Added Sugars 0 g; Total Fat 2 g; Sat Fat 1 g; Omega-3s 10 mg; Sodium 40 mg; Potassium 19 mg

FRESH CRANBERRY CITRUS PEAR RELISH

Makes 3 cups (640 g)

This fresh, vibrant relish with bright citrus notes is an awesome complement to roast chicken or turkey—try it with our Herb-Roasted Turkey Breast (page 317).

2 cups (220 g) fresh or thawed frozen cranberries

1 navel orange, ends trimmed and quartered

1 ripe Bartlett pear, cored and quartered

Juice of ½ lemon

¼ cup (50 g) sugar

Combine the cranberries, orange with peel, pear, lemon juice, and sugar in a food processor. Process to create a somewhat chunky relish. Transfer to a serving bowl and serve, or refrigerate in an airtight container until ready to use. Store in the refrigerator for up to 1 week.

Serving Size 2 tablespoons; Calories 44; Protein 0 g; Carbs 11 g; Dietary Fiber 1 g; Added Sugars 8 g; Total Fat 0 g; Sat Fat 0 g; Omega-3s 0 mg; Sodium 0 mg; Potassium 17 mg

GARLIC-TOMATO CONFIT

Makes 1 cup (1,060 g)

Slow-roasting tomatoes with garlic brings out their natural sweetness. The result is a richly colored and slightly sticky paste-like sauce. This savory confit can be spread on toast, used to coat a pizza crust, or served as a topping for roasted meats.

8 medium tomatoes, cored and halved

¼ cup (60 ml) extra virgin olive oil

4 garlic cloves, minced

2 tablespoons minced fresh basil

1 tablespoon minced fresh rosemary

¼ teaspoon freshly ground black pepper

¼ teaspoon kosher salt

1. Preheat the oven to 375°F (190°C). Line a large rimmed baking sheet with parchment paper.

2. Lay the tomatoes in a single layer on the baking sheet. Mix the oil, garlic, basil, rosemary, pepper, and salt in a small bowl. Pour over the tomatoes. Roast for 1 hour, until tender.

3. Flip the tomatoes. Roast for 1 hour more, until the tomatoes are extremely soft and withered.

4. Transfer the tomatoes to large bowl. Use the back of a wooden spoon to mash them into a paste. Add any oil and garlic bits from the baking sheet and stir to combine. Use immediately or store in an airtight container in the refrigerator for up to 1 month.

Serving Size 2 tablespoons; Calories 89; Protein 1 g; Carbs 6 g; Dietary Fiber 1 g; Added Sugars 0 g; Total Fat 7 g; Sat Fat 1 g; Omega-3s 60 mg; Sodium 70 mg; Potassium 285 mg

HONEY BALSAMIC ONION JAM

Makes 1¼ cups (820 g)

This jam has a sweet-tart flavor balance. It's a delicious topping for burgers, like the Beef & Mushroom Burgers (page 178). It's also a great complement for a turkey sandwich. Use it to top warm brie paired with whole grain crackers for an appetizer or festive snack at your next party.

4 cups (640 g) diced onions

2 tablespoons extra virgin olive oil

½ teaspoon kosher salt

¼ cup (85 g) honey

¼ cup (60 ml) balsamic vinegar

½ teaspoon freshly ground black pepper

1. Combine the onions, oil, and salt in a sauté pan over medium-high heat. Sauté until the onions soften and start to brown, 10 to 15 minutes.

2. Reduce the heat to medium-low. Add the honey, vinegar, and pepper. Cook, stirring frequently, until much of the liquid evaporates and the mixture thickens, 20 to 25 minutes. Use immediately or store in an airtight container in the refrigerator for up to 1 week.

Serving Size 2 tablespoons; Calories 69; Protein 1 g; Carbs 13 g; Dietary Fiber 1 g; Added Sugars 6 g; Total Fat 3 g; Sat Fat 0 g; Omega-3s 20 mg; Sodium 84 mg; Potassium 89 mg

HOT MANGO CHUTNEY
Makes 2½ cups (620 g)

Chutneys are sauces commonly found in Indian cuisine. This chutney, which is used in our South African Lamb Pie (page 335), adds pleasing heat with a bit of sweet to dishes like a simple lentil dal or grilled chicken.

- 1 tablespoon extra virgin olive oil
- ¼ cup (40 g) diced red onion
- 2 tablespoons finely minced serrano chiles
- 1 tablespoon yellow mustard seeds
- 2 teaspoons Curry Powder (page 32), or store-bought curry powder
- 1 teaspoon red pepper flakes
- 2 cups (330 g) diced fresh mango (about 2 mangos)
- ½ cup (80 g) golden raisins
- ½ cup (120 ml) water
- 2 tablespoons fresh lime juice
- 1 tablespoon grated fresh ginger
- 1 tablespoon honey

1. Combine the oil, onion, and chiles in a medium saucepan over medium-low heat. Cook until the onions and chiles have softened, about 8 minutes. Stir in the mustard seeds, curry powder, and red pepper flakes. Cook, stirring often, until the spices are fragrant.

2. Add the mango, raisins, water, lime juice, ginger, and honey. Reduce the heat to low, cover, and cook, stirring occasionally, until the mango has softened a bit and darkened in color, 15 minutes.

3. Transfer to an airtight container and refrigerate for 2 to 24 hours before serving. Store in the refrigerator for up to 1 week.

Serving Size 2 tablespoons; Calories 30; Protein 0 g; Carbs 5 g; Dietary Fiber 1 g; Added Sugars 1 g; Total Fat 1 g; Sat Fat 0 g; Omega-3s 30 mg; Sodium 1 mg; Potassium 39 mg

ROSEMARY-SAGE GREMOLATA
Makes ¾ cup (80 g)

This topping adds vibrant flavors to pork and chicken dishes as well as whole grain sides.

- ½ cup (45 g) whole wheat bread crumbs
- 1 tablespoon extra virgin olive oil
- 2 garlic cloves, minced
- 1 tablespoon minced fresh rosemary leaves
- 1 tablespoon minced fresh sage leaves
- ⅛ teaspoon kosher salt
- Grated zest of 1 lemon

1. Combine the bread crumbs, olive oil, and garlic in a small sauté pan over medium-high heat. Sauté until the bread crumbs start to brown and the garlic is fragrant, 2 to 3 minutes. Reduce heat to low, add the rosemary and sage, and sauté to slightly wilt the herbs, 30 seconds.

2. Transfer the bread crumb mixture to a small bowl and mix in the salt and lemon zest. Store in an airtight container in the refrigerator for up to 1 week.

Serving Size 2 tablespoons; Calories 46; Protein 1 g; Carbs 5 g; Dietary Fiber 1 g; Added Sugars 0 g; Total Fat 3 g; Sat Fat 0 g; Omega-3s 30 mg; Sodium 66 mg; Potassium 35 mg

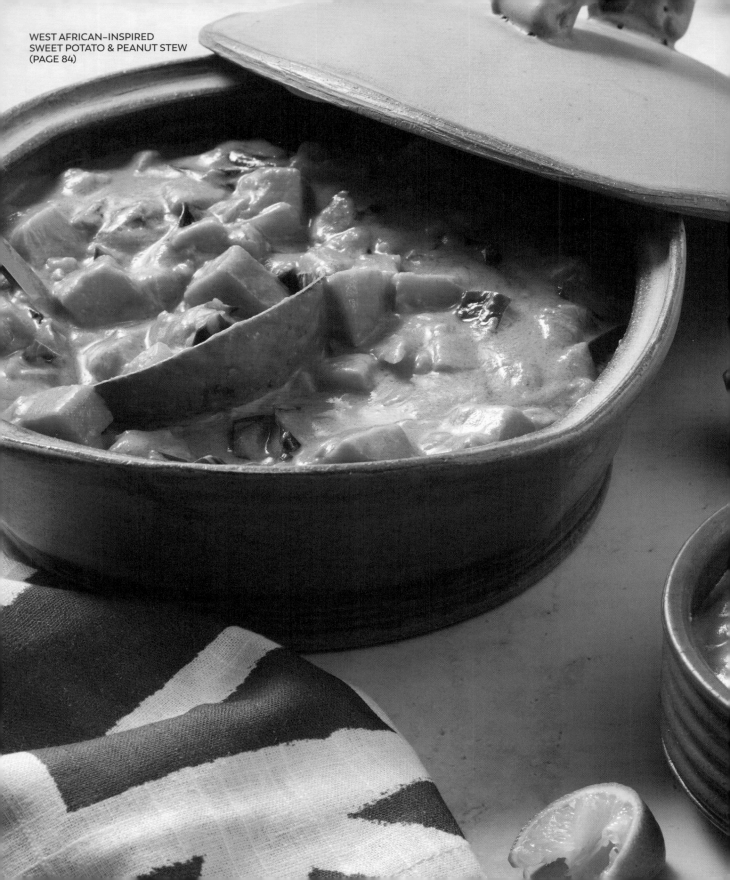

WEST AFRICAN–INSPIRED
SWEET POTATO & PEANUT STEW
(PAGE 84)

CHAPTER 5

Stocks, Soups & Stews

Stocks, Soups & Stews

Stocks & Broths

Beef Stock. 69

Chicken Stock 70

Dashi Broth 70

Fish Broth 71

Shrimp Stock 71

Vegetable Broth 72

Cold Soups

Cucumber-Grape Gazpacho 72

Cucumber-Shrimp Soup 72

Curried Peach Soup 73

Warm Soups

Borscht 73

Classic Chicken Soup 74

Creamy Asparagus Soup. 74

French Onion Soup. 75

Indian-Spiced Cauliflower &
Tomato Soup 76

Mexican Black Bean Soup. 76

Mirepoix Soupe 77

Mulligatawny Soup 78

Nordic Fish Soup. 78

Potato-Leek Soup. 79

Red Lentil & Vegetable Soup 79

Roasted Butternut Bisque 80

Roasted Poblano Soup 81

Rotisserie Chicken & Farro Soup with
Cannellini Beans 82

Thai-Inspired Shrimp Soup. 82

Tomato-Basil Soup. 83

Turkey-Vegetable Soup 84

Very Veggie Miso Soup 84

Chilis, Chowders & Stews

West African–Inspired Sweet Potato &
Peanut Stew 85

Chicken Chili Verde. 85

Cioppino 86

Midwestern Beef, Bean & Beer Chili. . . . 87

Hearty Clam Chowder. 88

Smoked Salmon & Corn Chowder. 88

Tomatillo-Pork Stew. 89

This chapter includes stocks and broths that appear as ingredients in many recipes throughout this book. Having homemade stocks and broths available in your refrigerator or freezer can make your cooking more flavorful and satisfying with less sodium, compared to the many options available in your local supermarket. What's the difference between a stock and broth? Stocks are made with bones and broths are not.

We've included a few cold soup options, many of which could also be considered smoothies if served in a glass instead of a bowl. Cold soups are wonderfully refreshing on hot summer days. Serving them in shot glasses transforms them into a fun starter or appetizer to serve at parties.

This chapter also includes soups and stews, many of which feature abundant use of vegetables as well as legumes and whole grains. Some are vegan; some are vegetarian; many contain poultry, meat, or seafood . . . and all are delicious!

We drew inspiration from many cultures around the world in putting together this chapter; we hope you discover many recipes that will find a permanent place in your culinary repertoire!

BEEF STOCK

Makes 2 quarts (2 L)

This rich, aromatic stock is the reason our French Onion Soup (page 75) gets rave reviews! It can be stored in an airtight container in the refrigerator for up to five days or frozen for up to four months. Store in large batches in the freezer to make soups. We like to store smaller portions for stews and main dishes, and we use ice cube trays so we can drop a bit of delicious beef flavor into gravies and risottos. Remove the cubes from the ice tray once they are frozen and store in an airtight container.

3 pounds (1.4 kg) meaty beef bones
   (beef shank or short ribs), rinsed

2 yellow or white onions, quartered

2 carrots, halved

2 celery stalks with leaves, cut into thirds

1 cup (70 g) white or shiitake mushrooms,
   trimmed

1 Bouquet Garni (page 30)

3 quarts (3 L) water

½ cup (120 ml) hot water

1 tablespoon balsamic vinegar

½ teaspoon kosher salt

1. Preheat the oven to 400°F (200°C). Line a large rimmed baking sheet with parchment paper.

2. Place the beef bones on the baking sheet. Roast for 30 minutes.

3. Add the onions, carrots, celery, and mushrooms. Roast for another 35 minutes, until the vegetables are caramelized and brown.

4. 10 minutes before removing the pan from the oven, add 1 quart (1 L) of the water to a stockpot or Dutch oven and set over medium-low heat.

5. Transfer the roasted bones and vegetables to the pot using a slotted spoon. Add the hot water to the baking sheet to loosen any brown bits from the parchment paper. Carefully pour the juices and bits into the stockpot. Add the bouquet garni, vinegar, salt, and the remaining 2 quarts (2 L) water; the water should cover the bones by 1 inch (2.5 cm). Turn the heat to medium-high and bring the stock just to a boil.

6. Partially cover the pot, reduce the heat to low, and allow to slowly simmer. Skim off any foam that collects on the top. Simmer for 2 to 3 hours, until the meat falls away from the bones and the bones separate from one another.

7. Remove from the heat and allow to cool slightly, about 15 minutes. Transfer the beef and bones to a plate, using the slotted spoon, to cool. Remove any meat from the bones and discard the bones. (Save the meat for another dish or enjoy as a sandwich.)

8. Line a colander with cheesecloth and place it in a large bowl. Strain the stock into the bowl and discard the vegetables and bouquet garni. Let the strained stock cool for 15 minutes, then refrigerate for 4 or more hours, until the fat congeals on the surface and broth is cold. Skim off the fat and discard.

9. Use immediately or store in an airtight container in the refrigerator for up to 3 days or in the freezer for up to 3 months.

Serving Size 1 cup (240 ml); Calories 14; Protein 2 g; Carbs 1 g; Dietary Fiber 0 g; Added Sugars 0 g; Total Fat 0 g; Sat Fat 0 g; Omega-3s 0 mg; Sodium 152 mg; Potassium 88 mg

CHICKEN STOCK

Makes 2 quarts (2 L)

Yes, you can buy chicken stock, but making your own helps you control the sodium and develop the best possible flavor. This very versatile ingredient is used in many of our recipes, including many of our chicken soup recipes. It also serves as a base for making creamy sauces for pasta dishes. Finally, it can be used in place of water for making our Simply Cooked beans and lentils.

One 3-pound (1.4 kg) chicken, quartered
2 large onions, quartered
1 medium carrot, halved
2 celery stalks with leaves, halved
1 Bouquet Garni (page 30)
½ teaspoon kosher salt
3 quarts (3 L) water
1 tablespoon white wine vinegar

1. Place the chicken, onions, carrot, and celery into a large Dutch oven or stockpot. Add the bouquet garni and sprinkle with kosher salt. Add the water and place the pot on medium-high heat until the water just reaches a boil.

2. Reduce the heat to low, add the vinegar, and partially cover. Simmer gently about 1 hour, skimming any foam that collects on the top, until a digital food thermometer reads 165°F (75°C) when inserted in the middle of a thigh (not touching bone).

3. Remove the pot from the heat and allow to cool slightly, about 15 minutes. Using a slotted spoon, transfer the chicken to a large plate. When it's cool enough to handle, debone the meat and discard the

skin. (Place the meat in an airtight container and refrigerate immediately, for future use.)

4. Line a colander with cheesecloth and place it in a large bowl. Strain the stock into the bowl and discard the vegetables and bouquet garni. Let stand for 15 minutes, then refrigerate for 4 or more hours, until the fat congeals on the surface.

5. Skim off the fat and discard. Use immediately or store in an airtight container in the refrigerator for up to 3 days or in the freezer for up to 3 months.

Serving Size 1 cup (240 ml); Calories 15; Protein 3 g; Carbs 1 g; Dietary Fiber 0 g; Added Sugars 0 g; Total Fat 0 g; Sat Fat 0 g; Omega-3s 0 mg; Sodium 134 mg; Potassium 179 mg

DASHI BROTH

Makes 6 cups (about 1.4 L)

This vegetarian broth offers an umami-rich alternative to beef broth for making soups, risottos, and so much more. Our taste buds sense umami in food due to the presence of three compounds: the amino acid glutamate and the nucleotides inosinate and guanylate. Umami increases our perception of the sodium in food, meaning you can cook with less added salt. We use this broth in our Very Veggie Miso Soup (page 84).

2 quarts (2 L) water
2 pieces (about 3 × 5 inches/7.5 × 13 cm) dashi kelp (kombu)
0.25 ounce (7 g) dried shiitake mushrooms

1. Combine the water, kelp, and mushrooms in a large stockpot over high heat. Bring to a boil, then reduce the heat to low. Simmer until the broth smells like the ocean and is a pale greenish-brown hue, 30 minutes.

2. Strain the broth, discard the kelp, and store the mushrooms for other uses. Use immediately or store in an airtight container in the refrigerator for up to 1 month or in the freezer for up to 6 months (see Headnote on page 84).

Serving Size 1 cup (240 ml); Calories 9; Protein 0 g; Carbs 2 g; Dietary Fiber 0 g; Added Sugars 0 g; Total Fat 0 g; Sat Fat 0 g; Omega-3s 0 mg; Sodium 41 mg; Potassium 65 mg

FISH BROTH

Makes 5 cups (1.2 L)

Broth made from white fish needs to be cooked for much less time than it takes to make meat or chicken stock. We chose to use white fish, which we often have on hand in the freezer and can sometimes be found at a low price. We use this broth in the Cioppino (page 86).

- 1 tablespoon extra virgin olive oil
- 2 pounds (907 g) mild-flavored white fish (such as cod, haddock or pollack), cut into 2-inch (5 cm) pieces
- 4 cups (1 L) water
- 1 cup (240 ml) white wine
- 2 leeks, cleaned (see Tip, page 79) and thinly sliced
- 1 carrot, coarsely chopped
- 1 celery stalk, coarsely chopped
- 1 teaspoon black peppercorns
- 1 teaspoon coriander seeds
- 2 whole allspice berries or whole cloves
- 1 teaspoon grated fresh ginger
- 1 tablespoon grated lemon zest
- 2 thyme sprigs
- 4 parsley sprigs
- 2 bay leaves
- ½ teaspoon kosher salt

1. Place a large heavy-bottomed saucepan or stockpot over medium heat. Add the oil to coat the bottom of the pot. Add the fish and cook, stirring constantly and flipping, until all of the pieces are warmed and slightly cooked on the outside, 2 to 3 minutes.

2. Add the water, wine, leeks, carrot, celery, peppercorns, allspice, ginger, lemon zest, thyme, parsley, bay leaves, and salt. Stir gently and increase heat to medium-high. Bring to a boil and cook for 5 to 7 minutes, stirring frequently. Reduce the heat to low and simmer for 30 minutes.

3. Remove from the heat and let cool for 20 minutes.

4. Strain the broth into a bowl and discard the solids. Use the broth immediately or refrigerate, uncovered, until cold. Store in an airtight container in the refrigerator for up to 2 days or in the freezer for up to 3 months.

Serving Size 1 cup (240 ml); Calories 20; Protein 3 g; Carbs 0 g; Dietary Fiber 0 g; Added Sugars 0 g; Total Fat 1 g; Sat Fat 0 g; Omega-3s 0 mg; Sodium 95 mg; Potassium 10 mg

SHRIMP STOCK

Makes 2½ cups (600 ml)

This quick shrimp stock works well in any recipe that calls for a seafood stock, such as fish chowder, soup, or risotto. Toasting the shells first gives the stock a burst of shrimp flavor and reduces overall cooking time. The shrimp shells can be fresh or saved in the freezer for up to a month.

- Shrimp shells and tails from 1 pound (454 g) raw shrimp
- 2 tablespoons extra virgin olive oil
- ½ cup (120 ml) white wine
- 4 cups (1 L) water
- 1 shallot or small onion, halved
- 1 teaspoon ground turmeric
- 1 teaspoon fennel seed
- 1 cup (70 g) mushrooms (of choice)
- 1 bay leaf

1. Place a large heavy-bottomed stockpot over medium-high heat. Heat the pot for 1 to 2 minutes, then add the shrimp shells and cook, stirring constantly, until they begin to stick to the bottom, 2 to 3 minutes.

2. Reduce the heat to medium and add the oil. Sauté the shells until fragrant and dark pink or toasty brown, 4 minutes.

3. Remove the pot from the heat and add the wine, stirring as you pour. Be careful of the steam! Return the pot to medium heat and simmer until the wine has evaporated, about 3 minutes.

4. Add the water, onion, turmeric, fennel seed, mushrooms, and bay leaf. Stir gently; bring to a boil, then reduce the heat to low and simmer for 20 minutes, until the stock is cloudy.

5. Remove from the heat, cover, and cool for 20 minutes.

6. Strain the stock and use immediately, or store in an airtight container in the refrigerator for up to 1 month.

Serving Size 1 cup (240 ml); Calories 81; Protein 2 g; Carbs 1 g; Dietary Fiber 0 g; Added Sugars 0 g; Total Fat 6 g; Sat Fat 1 g; Omega-3s 0 mg; Sodium 68 mg; Potassium 38 mg

VEGETABLE BROTH

Makes 2½ quarts (2.5 L)

Most recipes that call for chicken stock can be made with vegetable broth, which makes this a very versatile ingredient to always have on hand. To reduce food waste, we repurpose the vegetables that get strained from the final broth as the base for our very simple Mirepoix Soupe on page 77.

- 1 tablespoon extra virgin olive oil
- 1 white or yellow onion, cut into large chunks
- 2 carrots, cut into large chunks
- 2 celery stalks, cut into large chunks
- 1 leek, cleaned and cut into large chunks (see Tip on page 79)
- 3 quarts (3 L) water
- 1 Bouquet Garni (page 30)
- 1 teaspoon kosher salt

1. Place a large Dutch oven or stockpot over medium-high heat. Add the oil, onion, carrots, celery, and leek. Cook, stirring occasionally, until the onions start to soften and brown and the green parts of the leeks become dark green and wilted, 8 to 10 minutes.

2. Add the water, bouquet garni, and salt. Bring to a boil, then reduce the heat to low and cover. Simmer until the carrots and celery are fork-tender, 45 minutes.

3. Line a colander with cheesecloth and place it in a large bowl. Strain the broth into the bowl and discard the bouquet garni. (Save the vegetables to puree and use in our Mirepoix Soupe on page 77.) Use immediately or store in an airtight container in the refrigerator for up to 2 weeks or in the freezer for up to 2 months.

Serving Size 1 cup (240 ml); Calories 21; Protein 0 g; Carbs 3 g; Dietary Fiber 0 g; Added Sugars 0 g; Total Fat 1 g; Sat Fat 0 g; Omega-3s 0 mg; Sodium 189 mg; Potassium 115 mg

CUCUMBER-GRAPE GAZPACHO

Makes 4 servings

This nontraditional gazpacho is a refreshing addition to any summer meal. We love to serve it with grilled chicken or fish and our Fresh Chive–Yogurt Buns (page 108).

- 1 English cucumber
- 2 cups (300 g) green seedless grapes
- ½ cup (70 g) unsalted roasted almonds
- 2 green onions (green parts only)
- ¼ cup (60 ml) extra virgin olive oil
- 2 tablespoons minced fresh dill
- 2 tablespoons champagne or white balsamic vinegar
- 1 tablespoon minced fresh chives
- ½ teaspoon kosher salt

Combine the cucumber, grapes, almonds, green onions, oil, dill, vinegar, chives, and salt in a blender. Blend until smooth. Chill for 30 minutes before serving.

Per Serving: Calories 280; Protein 5 g; Carbs 19 g; Dietary Fiber 4 g; Added Sugars 0 g; Total Fat 23 g; Sat Fat 3 g; Omega-3s 110 mg; Sodium 239 mg; Potassium 261 mg

CUCUMBER-SHRIMP SOUP

Makes 8 servings

This cold soup is the perfect lunch option for a hot summer day—it doesn't require any cooking, so there's no need to heat up your kitchen. Serve with a dry white wine and fresh fruit for an easy, elegant entertaining menu.

- 1 English cucumber, diced
- 6 green onions, chopped
- 12 dill sprigs, chopped, or ½ teaspoon dried dill
- 1 pound (454 g) peeled and deveined 31/40 shrimp, cooked
- ½ teaspoon freshly ground black pepper
- Juice of 1 lemon
- 1 quart (1 L) cultured buttermilk
- Paprika
- Chopped fresh parsley

Put the cucumber in a 4-quart (3.8 L) casserole or large serving bowl. Layer the onions, dill, and shrimp on top of the cucumbers. Top with pepper and sprinkle with lemon juice, then pour over the buttermilk. Cover and refrigerate for at least 6 hours or overnight. Garnish each serving with paprika and parsley.

Per Serving: Calories 100; Protein 16 g; Carbs 9 g; Dietary Fiber 1 g; Added Sugars 0 g; Total Fat 2 g; Sat Fat 1 g; Omega-3s 60 mg; Sodium 123 mg; Potassium 296 mg

CURRIED PEACH SOUP

Makes 6 servings

This slightly sweet yet still savory soup is aromatic and cooling. Serve with your favorite chicken salad or try our Have a Plant Curried Chicken Salad (page 164) to play up the curry flavors in both dishes.

- 1 pound (454 g) ripe fresh peaches, peeled, pitted, and chopped
- 2 tablespoons butter or plant-based spread
- ½ cup (80 g) chopped onion
- 1 teaspoon Curry Powder (page 32), or store-bought curry powder
- 1 bay leaf
- 2 tablespoons whole wheat flour
- 2 cups (480 ml) Chicken Stock (page 70)
- Pinch of white pepper
- ¼ cup (60 g) plain low-fat yogurt
- Fresh mint leaves

1. Puree the peaches in a blender until smooth.

2. Combine the butter, onion, curry powder, and bay leaf in a sauté pan over medium heat. Sauté until the onions are tender, 3 to 4 minutes.

3. Remove from the heat and stir in the flour. Return to the heat, then gradually whisk in the chicken stock. Stir in the pepper and pureed peaches. Bring to a boil, reduce the heat to low, and simmer for 5 minutes to allow the flavors to combine.

4. Remove and discard the bay leaf. Refrigerate for 2 hours or until fully chilled. Serve with a dollop of yogurt and fresh mint on top.

TIPS: *You can also make this recipe using 2 cups (500 g) peaches canned in 100% juice.*

This soup can be served warm if you like. It would make a wonderful starter for a festive meal featuring roast turkey like our Herb-Roasted Turkey Breast (page 317).

Per Serving: Calories 108; Protein 4 g; Carbs 14 g; Dietary Fiber 2 g; Added Sugars 0 g; Total Fat 5 g; Sat Fat 1 g; Omega-3s 180 mg; Sodium 153 mg; Potassium 287 mg

BORSCHT

Makes 10 servings

Borscht is a vibrant and nourishing beet soup whose cultural roots connect us to Ukraine and Russia. We roast the beets first to intensify their flavor; consider wearing gloves to peel them to prevent staining your hands and nails—not to mention clothing, so wear an apron! Serve with thick slices of rye bread or Pumpernickel Bread (page 113).

- 1 pound (454 g) red beets, trimmed (about 4 medium beets)
- 3 tablespoons fresh orange juice
- 3 tablespoons extra virgin olive oil
- 1 tablespoon caraway seeds
- 2 carrots, grated
- 2 shallots, finely chopped
- 3 garlic cloves, minced
- 4 cups (1 L) water
- 4 cups (1 L) Vegetable Broth (page 72), Chicken Stock (page 70), or Beef Stock (page 69)
- 4 cups (600 g) diced yellow or white potatoes (about 3 large potatoes)
- 20 black peppercorns or ½ teaspoon freshly cracked black pepper
- 2 bay leaves
- 4 cups (280 g) shredded red or green cabbage
- 1 tablespoon balsamic vinegar
- ¼ cup (2 g) plus 2 tablespoons chopped fresh dill
- ¼ cup (15 g) chopped fresh flat-leaf parsley
- ½ teaspoon kosher salt
- Crème Fraîche (page 361)
- 2 tablespoons grated orange zest

1. Preheat the oven to 375°F (190°C).

2. To prepare the beets, wrap them tightly in a piece of foil; place on a rimmed baking sheet and roast for 45 minutes, until tender when pierced with a fork. Unwrap and allow to cool. Remove the beet skins by gently rolling and rubbing the beet between the palms of your hands; the skins will slip off easily. Grate the beets on the largest holes on your box grater into a large bowl, add 2 tablespoons of the orange juice, and stir to combine. Set aside.

3. Add 2 tablespoons of the oil and the caraway seeds to a large stockpot over medium-high heat.

Sauté the seeds, stirring continuously, until they start to pop, about 1 minute. Add the carrots, shallots, and garlic. Sauté until the carrots brighten and begin to soften, the shallots are translucent, and the garlic is fragrant, about 5 minutes.

4. Add the remaining 1 tablespoon oil and the grated beets to the pot, stirring to combine. Add the water, broth, potatoes, peppercorns, and bay leaves. Bring to a gentle simmer, cover, and reduce the heat to medium-low. Add the cabbage 5 minutes after adding the potatoes. Simmer for 15 minutes, until the cabbage has started to soften. Discard the bay leaves.

5. Stir in the vinegar, the remaining 1 tablespoon orange juice, ¼ cup (2 g) of the dill, the parsley, and salt. Simmer until the potatoes are soft and the cabbage is tender, 5 to 8 minutes. When the soup is thick, it is ready to serve.

6. Ladle the soup into bowls, add a dollop of crème fraîche, and sprinkle with the orange zest and the remaining 2 tablespoons of dill. Serve hot. Store in an airtight container in the refrigerator for up to 3 days or in the freezer for up to 2 months. Gently reheat prior to serving.

Per Serving: Calories 121; Protein 3 g; Carbs 19 g; Dietary Fiber 3 g; Added Sugars 0 g; Total Fat 5 g; Sat Fat 1 g; Omega-3s 50 mg; Sodium 390 mg; Potassium 420 mg

CLASSIC CHICKEN SOUP

Makes 10 servings

Making homemade chicken soup is rather simple. You can buy a whole chicken that's already cut up, or you can buy your favorite bone-in chicken parts. Add a few vegetables, fresh herbs, some optional whole grains, and a bit of time, and voilà—you've got a classic, comforting chicken soup.

- 1½ quarts (1.5 L) water
- 1½ quarts (1.5 L) Chicken Stock (page 70), plus more if needed
- 3 pounds (1.4 kg) bone-in, skin-on chicken parts
- 2 white or yellow onions, chopped
- 4 celery stalks, diced
- 3 carrots, diced
- 1 Bouquet Garni (page 30)

- ½ teaspoon kosher salt
- 2 cups (320 g) Simply Cooked Brown Rice, Barley, or Farro (pages 230, 223, or 226)
- ⅓ cup (20 g) chopped fresh flat-leaf parsley

1. Combine the water, chicken stock, and chicken in a large Dutch oven or stockpot over high heat. Bring to a boil, then reduce the heat to low. Cover and gently simmer until the chicken is falling off the bones, 35 to 40 minutes.

2. Remove from the heat. Remove the chicken pieces from the stock using a slotted spoon. Let cool until you can handle them. Remove and discard the chicken skin and bones. Shred or cut the chicken into bite-size pieces. Add the meat back to the stock along with the onions, celery, carrots, bouquet garni, and salt. Bring to a boil, then reduce heat to low, cover, and simmer until the vegetables are fork-tender, 35 to 40 minutes.

3. Add the rice and gently simmer to heat through, 15 to 20 minutes. If the soup is too thick, add additional chicken stock in 1-cup (240 ml) increments until the soup reaches your desired consistency. Remove from the heat and discard the bouquet garni. Serve hot, topped with a sprinkle of parsley. Store in an airtight container in the refrigerator for up to 3 days or in the freezer for up to 2 months. Gently reheat prior to serving.

Per Serving: Calories 373; Protein 32 g; Carbs 20 g; Dietary Fiber 2 g; Added Sugars 0 g; Total Fat 18 g; Sat Fat 1 g; Omega-3s 20 mg; Sodium 515 mg; Potassium 266 mg

CREAMY ASPARAGUS SOUP

Makes 6 servings

This seasonal soup is best made when asparagus are abundant and inexpensive in early spring. Serve with a crusty bread and Honey Balsamic Onion Jam (page 64) or Salmon Spring Rolls (page 188).

- 2 tablespoons butter
- 1 tablespoon extra virgin olive oil
- 1 cup (160 g) chopped shallots
- 1 celery stalk, diced
- 2 garlic cloves, minced

3 cups (375 g) chopped fresh asparagus (about 36 stalks, tough ends removed)

1 cup (420 g) peeled and diced potato (about 2 medium Yukon golds or russets)

4 cups (1 L) Vegetable Broth (page 72), plus more if needed

2 tablespoons fresh lemon juice

½ teaspoon freshly ground black pepper

¼ teaspoon kosher salt

¾ cup (180 ml) half-and-half

2 tablespoons chopped fresh dill

1. Melt the butter in a large heavy saucepan over medium-high heat. Add the oil, then add the shallots, celery, and garlic. Cook until the vegetables are soft and garlic is fragrant, about 3 minutes.

2. Add the asparagus and sauté until well coated with the butter-oil mixture, 3 minutes. Add the potatoes and broth. Bring to a boil, reduce the heat to medium-low, cover, and simmer until the asparagus are falling apart and potatoes are very tender, about 30 minutes.

3. Use an immersion blender to puree the soup in the saucepan. Or transfer to a blender or food processor, in batches if necessary, and process until smooth, then return to the saucepan. Gradually reheat over medium heat, stirring often to avoid scorching.

4. Add the lemon juice, pepper, and salt. Bring to a gentle simmer. Slowly stir in the half-and-half and cook until soup is thick and creamy, about 8 minutes. Thin with vegetable broth if the soup is too thick. Ladle into bowls, top with dill, and serve immediately. Store in an airtight container in the refrigerator for up to 3 days or in the freezer for up to 2 months. Gently reheat prior to serving.

Per Serving: Calories 165; Protein 7 g; Carbs 19 g; Dietary Fiber 2 g; Added Sugars 0 g; Total Fat 7 g; Sat. Fat 3 g; Omega-3s 0g; Sodium 85 mg; Potassium 360 mg

FRENCH ONION SOUP

Makes 8 servings

This is one of the best-loved classic French dishes served in restaurants today, a humble dish that becomes more elegant when served in ramekins with a layer of melted cheese on top.

1.5 pounds (680 g) yellow onions, halved and thinly sliced

2 tablespoons butter or plant-based spread

2 tablespoons extra virgin olive oil

3 tablespoons all-purpose flour

2 quarts (2 L) Beef Stock (page 69)

½ cup (120 ml) dry white wine (such as Chablis or Chenin Blanc)

1 teaspoon freshly ground black pepper

8 slices French bread, toasted until very crisp

2 cups (215 g) shredded Gruyère

1. Preheat the oven to 350°F (180°C).

2. Heat the butter and oil in a Dutch oven or large, heavy saucepan over low heat. Add the onions, cover, and cook until soft, 15 minutes.

3. Remove the cover, increase the heat to medium, and cook, stirring frequently, until the onions have turned a deep golden brown, 40 to 45 minutes.

4. Sprinkle the flour over the onions. Cook and stir for about 2 minutes to incorporate the flour and remove the raw flour flavor. Stir in the beef stock, wine, and pepper. Simmer, partially covered, until the soup is gently bubbling, 15 to 20 minutes.

5. Set eight 8-ounce (240 ml) flameproof ramekins or individual soup tureens on a large rimmed baking dish.

6. Use a ladle to transfer the soup to the ramekins. Top each ramekin with a slice of bread and ¼ cup (54 g) of the cheese. Bake for 15 to 20 minutes, until the cheese has melted. Set the oven to broil and when the broiler is heated, place the ramekins under the broiler for 2 minutes or until the cheese is lightly browned. Serve immediately.

TIP: *Gruyère is a traditional cheese choice, but if you like more "cheese pull," use half Gruyère for nutty flavor and*

half Monterey Jack for a delightful string of cheese that follows your spoon from the ramekin to your mouth.

Per Serving: Calories 365; Protein 19 g; Carbs 30 g; Dietary Fiber 2 g; Added Sugars 0 g; Total Fat 18 g; Sat. Fat 9 g; Omega-3s 204 mg; Sodium 600 mg; Potassium 640 mg

INDIAN-SPICED CAULIFLOWER & TOMATO SOUP

Makes 6 servings

A variety of the spices often found in Indian home kitchens—coriander, mustard seeds, turmeric, and cumin—bring bold, memorable flavors to this comforting, aromatic soup. Serve with whole wheat naan, and fresh fruit for dessert.

- 2 tablespoons peanut oil
- 1 teaspoon coriander seeds
- 1 teaspoon mustard seeds
- 1 teaspoon ground turmeric
- ½ teaspoon ground coriander
- ½ teaspoon cumin seeds
- ½ teaspoon red pepper flakes
- 1 white or yellow onion, diced
- One 28-ounce (794 g) can crushed tomatoes
- 16 ounces (454 g) fresh or frozen cauliflower florets (about 5 cups)
- 4 cups (1 L) water
- ¼ teaspoon kosher salt
- ½ teaspoon freshly ground black pepper
- ½ cup (125 g) plain yogurt, optional
- ½ cup (8 g) fresh cilantro leaves, optional

1. Combine the oil, coriander seeds, mustard seeds, turmeric, ground coriander, cumin seeds, and red pepper flakes in a medium stockpot. Turn the heat to medium and gently toast the spices until the mustard seeds begin to pop and the other spices are fragrant, 45 seconds to 1 minute.

2. Add the onions, reduce the heat to medium-low, and cook until the onions are soft, 5 to 6 minutes.

3. Add the tomatoes, cauliflower, and water. Increase the heat to high and bring to a boil. Reduce heat to low, cover, and cook until the cauliflower is soft, 25 to 30 minutes.

4. Remove from the heat and use an immersion blender to create a smooth, "creamy" soup. You can also puree the soup in a blender in batches. Return the soup to the pot and keep warm until you're ready to serve.

5. Garnish, if desired, with cilantro and yogurt, and serve. Store in an airtight container in the refrigerator for up to 3 days or in the freezer for up to 2 months. Gently reheat prior to serving.

Per Serving: Calories 113; Protein 4 g; Carbs 16 g; Dietary Fiber 6 g; Added Sugars 0 g; Total Fat 5 g; Sat Fat 1 g; Omega-3s 80 mg; Sodium 118 mg; Potassium 691 mg

MEXICAN BLACK BEAN SOUP

Makes 8 servings

This simple soup gets its rich flavor from dried Mexican chiles: the mild, aromatic ancho chile, made by drying fresh poblanos; the fruity, mildly spicy guajillo chile, made by drying fresh mirasols; and the smoky, moderately spicy chipotle chile made by drying fresh jalapeños.

Soup
- 1 pound (454 g) dried black beans, cleaned and rinsed
- Tap water
- 1 tablespoon plus 1 teaspoon kosher salt
- 1 white onion, chopped
- 2 ancho chiles, stems removed
- 2 guajillo chiles, stems removed
- 1 dried chipotle chile, stem removed
- Boiling water
- 2 quarts (2 L) water
- 2 or 3 fresh or dried avocado leaves, optional
- ½ cup (120 ml) extra virgin olive oil

Optional Toppings
- Mexican crema
- Diced avocado
- Diced white onion
- Sliced radishes
- Chopped fresh cilantro

1. Place the beans in a medium stockpot and add enough tap water so the water is at least 1 inch (2.5 cm) above the beans. Bring to a boil over high heat, then remove from the heat, add 1 teaspoon of the salt, and set aside for 1 hour to allow the beans to hydrate. (Adding the salt during the hot soak encourages the beans to take in water and hydrate more quickly.)

2. While the beans are soaking, place the ancho, guajillo, and chipotle chiles in a medium bowl and cover with boiling water. Set aside for 10 to 15 minutes to soak.

3. Drain off the soaking water from the chiles. Roughly chop the chiles.

4. Drain the soaking water from the beans and add 2 quarts (2 L) fresh water to the pot, as well as the onion, chiles, the remaining 1 tablespoon salt, and the avocado leaves, if using. Bring to a boil over high heat, then reduce the heat to low. Simmer covered for 90 minutes to 2 hours, until the beans are tender.

5. Remove the soup from the stove and remove and discard the avocado leaves. Puree the soup in batches in a blender or with an immersion blender until smooth. Return the soup to the pot if using a blender to puree, and gently reheat if necessary. Stir in the olive oil and serve warm. Garnish as desired. Store in an airtight container in the refrigerator for up to 3 days or in the freezer for up to 2 months. Gently reheat prior to serving.

NOTES: *You may notice that this soup contains far more added salt compared to other recipes in this book. Potassium-rich foods like the black beans and dried chiles require much more sodium to balance their flavor. Potassium is bitter; the added salt helps tame the bitterness, round out the mouthfeel, and enhance the flavor of the final recipe—in this case, a very delicious vegan soup.*

If you're wondering about the optional avocado leaves, think of them like bay leaves. Available from many online retailers, they add a subtle yet distinct mild licorice flavor to the soup.

Per Serving: Calories 370; Protein 14 g; Carbs 45 g; Dietary Fiber 11 g; Added Sugars 0 g; Total Fat 15 g; Sat Fat 2 g; Omega-3s 120 mg; Sodium 714 mg; Potassium 927 mg

MIREPOIX SOUPE

Makes 2 servings

This very simple soup ("soupe" in French) is one to make after you cook our Vegetable Broth, because the base for it is the pureed mirepoix (onions, carrots, celery, and leeks) used for the broth. Vadouvan, a spice blend sometimes referred to as "French curry powder," adds additional layers of flavor, while the extra virgin olive oil adds richness. Vadouvan blends vary but typically contain onion and garlic powders and ground cumin, mustard, and fenugreek seeds.

Onions, carrots, celery, and leek reserved from making Vegetable Broth (page 72)

2 tablespoons extra virgin olive oil

1 teaspoon vadouvan

¼ teaspoon kosher salt

Puree the onions, carrots, celery, and leek. Combine the olive oil and vadouvan in a small saucepan over medium heat. Heat until the spices become fragrant, 1 to 2 minutes. Stir in the pureed vegetables and salt and cook for 6 to 8 minutes, until the soup begins to gently bubble at the surface. Serve immediately.

NOTE: *It's estimated that globally nearly 40 percent of all food produced is wasted. According to ReFED, an organization that works to reduce food waste across the food system, the largest source of food waste in the United States and other developed countries is in-home waste. This recipe is an example of how to repurpose ingredients to reduce waste. We hope you'll explore other ways to reduce food waste in your home. For more information, visit refed.org.*

Per Serving: Calories 215; Protein 3 g; Carbs 21 g; Dietary Fiber 5 g; Added Sugars 0 g; Total Fat 14 g; Sat Fat 2 g; Omega-3s 150 mg; Sodium 290 mg; Potassium 143 mg

MULLIGATAWNY SOUP

Makes 6 servings

Fans of the television show Seinfeld *may smile when they see the name of this soup, but they may not be aware of its cultural heritage. Many believe this soup originated in India, but it was actually developed by cooks for the British Raj. An aromatic spice blend of mustard seeds, cloves, and curry brings a delightful depth of flavor to this dish, and the last-minute addition of coconut milk adds a rich mouthfeel.*

- 2 tablespoons extra virgin olive oil
- 1 tablespoon mustard seeds
- 4 whole cloves, or ½ teaspoon ground allspice or cardamom
- ½ cup (80 g) chopped onion
- 1 carrot, chopped
- 1 celery stalk, chopped
- 2 tablespoons all-purpose flour
- 2 teaspoons Curry Powder (page 32)
- 1 tart apple (such as Granny Smith), cored and chopped
- 1 tablespoon fresh lemon juice
- 6 cups (1.4 L) Chicken Stock (page 70), plus more if needed
- ⅓ cup (65 g) green or brown lentils, rinsed
- ⅓ cup (65 g) uncooked brown basmati rice
- 2 cups (270 g) diced cooked chicken
- ½ teaspoon kosher salt
- 1 teaspoon freshly ground black pepper
- ¾ cup (180 ml) light coconut milk
- ¾ cup (12 g) chopped fresh cilantro or mint

1. Combine the oil, mustard seeds, and cloves in a large stockpot over medium-high heat. Sauté until the mustard seeds pop but don't burn, 1 to 2 minutes.

2. Add the onion, carrots, and celery. Sauté until the onion is translucent and the color of the carrots and celery brightens, about 2 minutes. Remove and discard the cloves. Sprinkle in the flour and curry powder, stirring continuously to blend the oil and flour and coat the vegetables, about 30 seconds. Add the apple and lemon juice and cook, stirring occasionally, until the vegetables are crisp-tender, about 2 minutes.

3. Add the chicken stock 1 cup (240 ml) at a time, stirring after each addition. Increase the heat to high and bring the soup to a boil. Stir in the rice and lentils. Reduce the heat to medium-low, partially cover the pot, and simmer for 20 minutes, stirring once or twice as the lentils and rice cook and absorb the stock.

4. Add the chicken and simmer for 5 minutes, until it is well mixed in and heated through. The soup should be thick, yet fluid. Add more chicken stock, if needed, to thin.

5. Season with the salt and pepper, then slowly stir in the coconut milk. Cook about 5 minutes to bring the temperature back up.

6. Remove from the heat, ladle into bowls, and serve topped with chopped cilantro. Store in an airtight container in the refrigerator for up to 3 days or in the freezer for up to 2 months. Gently reheat prior to serving.

TIP: *For the chicken, use the meat from making our Chicken Stock (page 70).*

Per Serving: Calories 331; Protein 23 g; Carbs 32 g; Dietary Fiber 4 g; Added Sugars 2 g; Total Fat 12 g; Sat Fat 3 g; Omega-3s 140 mg; Sodium 576 mg; Potassium 486 mg

NORDIC FISH SOUP

Makes 4 servings

Simple meets delicious in 20 minutes! Select firm white fish for this elegant, tender, melt-in-your mouth fish soup topped with fresh dill. It pairs well with Scandinavian bread like rye wasabröd and our Spinach Salad with Honeycrisp Apples & Cheddar (page 148).

- 1 tablespoon extra virgin olive oil
- 2 leeks, cleaned (see Tip, page 79) and thinly chopped
- 2 carrots, thinly sliced
- 2 tablespoons whole wheat pastry flour
- 1 tablespoon Seafood Seasoning (page 37)
- 4 cups (1 L) Fish Broth (page 71)
- 1 bay leaf
- 1 pound (454 g) firm white fish fillets (such as cod, haddock, or monkfish), thinly sliced

1 cup (130 g) frozen baby peas, thawed

1 tablespoon fresh lemon juice

¼ teaspoon kosher salt

White pepper

2 tablespoons chopped fresh dill

1. Heat the oil in a large heavy-bottomed saucepan over medium-high heat. Add the carrots and leek and sauté until the carrots begin to soften and the leeks become fragrant, about 4 minutes.

2. Sprinkle the flour and seasoning over the vegetables, stirring to incorporate and coat the vegetables. Stir in the fish broth and bay leaf. Bring to a boil, reduce the heat to medium-low, and simmer for 10 minutes.

3. Add the fish and simmer for 2 to 3 minutes, then add the peas. Simmer until the peas are cooked, but not mushy and the fish easily flakes, about 5 minutes. Discard the bay leaf and add the lemon juice. Season with the salt and white pepper to taste. Ladle into bowls, garnish each with 1½ teaspoons dill, and serve hot.

Per Serving: Calories 335; Protein 33 g; Carbs 21 g; Dietary Fiber 4 g; Added Sugars 0 g; Total Fat 12 g; Sat Fat 2 g; Omega-3s 1,050 mg; Sodium 212 mg; Potassium 757 mg

POTATO-LEEK SOUP

Makes 6 servings

While leeks are in the same family as onions and garlic, they have a milder flavor that pairs well with potatoes. This soup is a wonderful starter for a meal featuring our Sheet Pan Tri-Tip Roast (page 328), but it's also great on its own for a light yet filling lunch.

2 tablespoons extra virgin olive oil

3 leeks, cleaned (see Tip) and thinly sliced

1 white onion, diced

1 celery stalk, diced

4 Yukon gold–type potatoes, cubed

3 cups (720 ml) Chicken Stock (page 70) or Vegetable Broth (page 72)

½ cup (115 g) sour cream or plain Greek yogurt

2 teaspoons kosher salt

½ teaspoon freshly ground black pepper

Chopped fresh chives

1. Combine the oil, leeks, onion, and celery in a Dutch oven or medium stockpot over medium-high heat. Sauté the vegetables until soft but not brown, 8 to 10 minutes.

2. Add the potatoes and stock and simmer, covered, until the potatoes are tender, 15 to 20 minutes. Use an immersion blender in the pot to puree the soup until smooth. Or puree in batches in a blender, then return the soup to the Dutch oven.

3. Stir in the sour cream, salt, and pepper, and cook over medium heat until the soup is bubbling gently, 12 to 15 minutes. Serve warm garnished with chives. Store in an airtight container in the refrigerator for up to 3 days or in the freezer for up to 2 months. Gently reheat prior to serving.

TIP: The best way to clean leeks and ensure you've removed all the dirt that can settle between the long leaves is to cut each leek in half from top to bottom, place it in a sink filled with cold water, and gently pull apart the long leaves, shaking the leek vigorously under water to reveal and release any dirt clinging to the leaves.

Per Serving: Calories 150; Protein 3 g; Carbs 18 g; Dietary Fiber 2 g; Added Sugar 0 g; Total Fat 8 g; Sat. Fat 2 g; Omega-3s 92 mg; Sodium 885 mg; Potassium 410 mg

RED LENTIL & VEGETABLE SOUP

Makes 6 servings

Lentils have a natural affinity with garden vegetables and aromatics such as garlic, cumin, bay leaves, and parsley. We chose red lentils because they have a hint of earthy sweetness, cook up very quickly, and become soft and creamy in texture. You can serve this as a brothy soup or puree it for a velvety, creamy soup. Serve with crusty bread and flavored olive oil for dipping, and your favorite white wine.

2 tablespoons extra virgin olive oil

2 teaspoons cumin seeds

1 teaspoon coriander seeds

1 cup (160 g) chopped white or yellow onion

1 carrot, diced

1 celery stalk, diced

4 garlic cloves, minced

4½ cups (1.1 L) Chicken Stock (page 70) or Vegetable Broth (page 72)

1½ cups (290 g) red lentils, rinsed and drained

1½ cups (210 g) diced yellow summer squash (about 1 medium)

½ cup (90 g) Simply Slow-Roasted Tomatoes (page 260) or sun-dried tomatoes (dry, not oil-packed), chopped

1 bay leaf

1 cinnamon stick

½ teaspoon kosher salt

½ teaspoon freshly ground black pepper

1 tablespoon fresh lemon juice

2 tablespoons balsamic or red wine vinegar

1 cup (180 g) diced red tomato (about 1 medium)

½ cup (30 g) chopped fresh flat-leaf parsley

1. Combine the oil, cumin, and coriander in a Dutch oven or large stockpot over medium-high heat. Sauté until the seeds pop, about 1 minute. Add the onion, carrots, celery, and garlic, and sauté until the onion is tender, the carrots and celery are softened, and the garlic is fragrant, about 3 minutes.

2. Stir in the chicken stock, lentils, squash, roasted tomatoes, bay leaf, cinnamon stick, salt, and pepper. Bring to a boil, then reduce the heat to medium-low, and partially cover. Simmer, stirring once, until lentils are tender, soft, and chewy, about 20 minutes. Remove the soup from the heat. Discard the bay leaf and cinnamon stick and stir in the lemon juice and balsamic vinegar.

3. To serve as a brothy soup, ladle into bowls and top with diced tomato and parsley.

4. To serve as a creamy soup, use an immersion blender, food processor, or blender to puree the soup. Return the pureed soup to the pot, place over medium-high heat, and cook for 5 minutes to reheat. Ladle into bowls, top with diced tomatoes and parsley, and serve. Store in an airtight container in the refrigerator for up to 3 days or in the freezer for up to 2 months. Gently reheat prior to serving.

Per Serving: Calories 264; Protein 17 g; Carbs 37 g; Dietary Fiber 17 g; Added Sugars 0 g; Total Fat 12 g; Sat Fat 2 g; Omega-3s 220 mg; Sodium 294 mg; Potassium 870 mg

ROASTED BUTTERNUT BISQUE

Makes 6 servings

Yes, this is a rich bisque—but without any cream or butter! Roasting the squash allows it to caramelize and develop its full flavor; finishing the bisque with cultured buttermilk and honey perfectly balances the flavor. To make the presentation more festive, we top the soup with diced apple, a dusting of nutmeg, and a sprinkle of toasted pepitas.

4 cups (560 g) cubed, peeled, raw butternut squash (1 medium) or frozen butternut squash cubes

4 tablespoons extra virgin olive oil

½ teaspoon ground cinnamon

Freshly ground black pepper

¼ teaspoon kosher salt

3 shallots, finely chopped

2 garlic cloves, minced

1 tart apple (such as Granny Smith, Braeburn, or Pink Lady), cored and finely diced

1 tablespoon Curry Powder (page 32)

1 teaspoon minced fresh ginger

One 15-ounce (425 g) can 100% pure pumpkin

½ cup (120 ml) apple cider

3 cups (720 ml) Vegetable Broth (page 72)

1½ cups (360 ml) cultured buttermilk or light coconut milk

1 tablespoon honey

Ground nutmeg

Lightly salted toasted pepitas (pumpkin seeds)

1. Place an oven rack in the lowest third of the oven. Preheat the oven to 400°F (200°C). Line a large rimmed baking sheet with parchment paper.

2. Pour the squash cubes into a large bowl. Add 2 tablespoons of the oil and the cinnamon, black pepper, and salt, and toss to coat. Arrange the cubes on the baking sheet in a single layer. Roast for 20 minutes, until the squash is tender and the edges are browned.

3. Combine the remaining 2 tablespoons oil, the shallots, garlic, and 1¼ cups (155 g) of the apple in a medium stockpot over medium-high heat. Sauté until the apple begins to soften, the shallots begin to turn translucent, and the garlic is fragrant, about

2 minutes. Add the roasted squash, curry powder, and ginger. Sauté to coat the apples and vegetables with the spices, about 30 seconds.

4. Add the pumpkin, apple cider, and stock, stirring after each addition. Bring to a gentle simmer, then reduce the heat to medium-low, partially cover, and simmer for 15 minutes, until flavors meld and the soup has thickened.

5. Remove the pot from the heat and use an immersion blender, food processor, or blender to puree the bisque to a smooth consistency.

6. Return the pureed bisque to the pot over medium-low heat. Slowly add the buttermilk, stirring constantly. Warm the bisque until a digital food thermometer reads 165°F (75°C) when inserted in the center of the soup.

7. Ladle into bowls, top each bowl with about 1 tablespoon of the remaining apple, a drizzle of honey, a dusting of nutmeg, and a sprinkle of pepitas. Serve hot. Store in an airtight container in the refrigerator for up to 3 days or in the freezer for up to 2 months. Gently reheat prior to serving.

Per Serving: Calories 233; Protein 4 g; Carbs 32 g; Dietary Fiber 3 g; Added Sugars 3 g; Total Fat 11 g; Sat Fat 2 g; Omega-3s 120 mg; Sodium 414 mg; Potassium 638 mg

ROASTED POBLANO SOUP

Makes 6 servings

This soup is the perfect way to add abundant vegetables—and great flavor—to any Mexican-inspired meal. If you love spicier foods, add the serrano chile, which will contribute heat as well as a subtle floral note to the soup. Mexican crema is like thin sour cream; if you can't find it, thin some sour cream with a little bit of milk so you can drizzle it on the soup as a garnish and slight cooling element. The cotija adds a bit of salt to each bite; use grated Parmesan if you can't find it.

1 white onion, halved
2 jalapeño chiles, stems removed
1 serrano chile, stem removed, optional
4 garlic cloves, unpeeled
4 cups (1 L) Chicken Stock (page 72)
4 poblano chiles from Simply Roasted Peppers (page 259)
1 bunch cilantro, ends trimmed
1 teaspoon kosher salt
6 tablespoons Mexican crema
6 tablespoons crumbled cotija

1. Place the onion, cut side down, the jalapeños, serrano (if using), and garlic in a cast-iron skillet over high heat. Sear the onion on each cut side until it turns black, and the jalapeños, serrano, and garlic flipping once, until brown spots appear on each side, 5 to 6 minutes total. Remove from the heat.

2. Pour the chicken stock into a medium pot over medium-high heat. Add the charred onions, jalapeños, serrano, poblanos, cilantro, and salt. When the garlic cloves have cooled enough, remove the skins with your fingers and drop the cloves into the pot. Gently simmer until the onions and chiles have softened and the cilantro has turned dark green, 30 minutes. Remove from the heat and let sit at room temperature for 30 to 60 minutes to cool.

3. Puree the soup in the pot using an immersion blender, or in batches in a blender, until smooth. Return it to the pot if necessary. Place over medium heat and cook until the surface is bubbling, 12 to 15 minutes.

4. Divide the soup among six bowls and drizzle each with 1 tablespoon crema and 1 tablespoon cotija. Serve hot. Store in an airtight container in the refrigerator for up to 3 days or in the freezer for up to 2 months. Gently reheat prior to serving.

Per Serving: Calories 357; Protein 27 g; Carbs 9 g; Dietary Fiber 2 g; Added Sugars 0 g; Total Fat 24 g; Sat Fat 9 g; Omega-3s 220 mg; Sodium 510 mg; Potassium 440 mg

SODIUM TIP: Using Diamond Crystal Kosher Salt will dramatically reduce the sodium in any recipe that uses kosher salt. This salt contains 50% less sodium per measure than regular kosher salt and 60% less than fine grain table salt.

ROTISSERIE CHICKEN & FARRO SOUP WITH CANNELLINI BEANS

Makes 8 servings

Using a rotisserie chicken speeds up the process of making a homemade chicken soup. If you like a lot of chicken in your soup, use the whole bird. If you want to make multiple meals out of your chicken, remove the breast and drumsticks for another meal and use the remaining meat and bones to make this soup. If you have the rind from a piece of good-quality Parmesan, add that to the soup to enrich the flavor of the broth and remove it just before serving.

> 2 quarts (2 L) water
> One 3-pound (1.4 kg) rotisserie chicken
> 3 celery stalks, diced
> 2 carrots, diced
> 1 white onion, diced
> 2 bay leaves
> 1 cup (180 g) uncooked farro
> Two 15.5-ounce (439 g) cans cannellini beans, drained and rinsed
> 2 tablespoons Italian Seasoning (page 34)
> 2 teaspoons freshly ground black pepper
> Freshly grated Parmesan

1. Combine the water, chicken, celery, carrots, onion, and bay leaves in a large stockpot over high heat. Bring to a boil, reduce the heat to medium-low, and cover. Simmer until the meat is falling off the bones, 15 to 20 minutes. Remove the chicken and set aside to cool.

2. Increase the heat to high and bring the soup to a boil. Stir in the farro, reduce the heat to medium-low, cover, and simmer for 25 to 30 minutes, until the farro is tender yet chewy.

3. When the chicken is cool enough to handle, discard the skin. Remove the meat from the bones. Shred it or cut into bite-size pieces and add it back to the soup. Add the beans, Italian seasoning, and pepper. Continue simmering until the farro is fully cooked, 25 to 30 minutes.

4. Remove the bay leaves. Ladle the soup into bowls and pass Parmesan at the table. Store in an airtight container in the refrigerator for up to 3 days or in the freezer for up to 2 months. Gently reheat prior to serving.

Per Serving: Calories 476; Protein 50 g; Carbs 29 g; Dietary Fiber 8 g; Added Sugars 0 g; Total Fat 18 g; Sat Fat 5 g; Omega-3s 120 mg; Sodium 720 mg; Potassium 450 mg

THAI-INSPIRED SHRIMP SOUP

Makes 6 servings

This elegantly garnished, highly aromatic soup is very easy to make. Your biggest challenge will likely be deciding how spicy you want it. We chose to use the Thai chile known as prik khee fah or red spur chile, which are 3 to 4 inches (7.5 to 10 cm) long and can be either red or green in color. This is the variety used to make commercial red and green chile pastes; their heat ranges from mild to hot, but they are not nearly as hot as other Thai chile varieties. Adjust the number of chiles to your personal preference and to the heat of chiles you use.

> 3 cups (720 ml) Shrimp Stock (page 71)
> One 13.5-ounce (400 ml) can light coconut milk
> ¼ cup (20 g) chopped fresh lemongrass (white part only)
> 5 fresh Thai chiles, seeded and cut lengthwise into strips
> 3 tablespoons fish sauce
> 2 tablespoons sliced peeled fresh ginger
> 1 tablespoon extra virgin olive oil
> 2 garlic cloves, minced
> 1 pound (454 g) raw peeled and deveined 31/40 shrimp, thawed if frozen
> 1 cup (70 g) thinly sliced shiitake mushroom caps
> 2 cups (390 g) Simply Cooked Brown Rice (page 230)
> ¼ cup (60 ml) fresh lime juice
> 6 tablespoons minced fresh cilantro
> Freshly ground black pepper
> Twelve 3-inch (7.5 g) slivers lemongrass (white part only)

1. Combine the stock, coconut milk, chopped lemongrass, chiles, fish sauce, and ginger in a stockpot or large saucepan. Bring the mixture to a gentle boil, reduce the heat to low, and simmer gently for 20 to 30 minutes, until flavors meld.

2. While the stock simmers, heat the oil in a large skillet over medium-high heat. Add the garlic and shrimp, and sauté until the shrimp begin to change color and firm up, 1 minute. Add the mushrooms and sauté until the garlic is fragrant, the mushrooms start to shrink and brown, and the shrimp are plump and pink, 2 more minutes. Remove from the heat.

3. Strain the soup through a fine-mesh sieve into a clean pot and discard the lemongrass, chiles, and sliced ginger. Place the pot over medium-low heat.

4. Add the shrimp-mushroom mixture and rice to the soup. Simmer gently until the soup is thoroughly heated through and is aromatic, 5 to 7 minutes. Add the lime juice just before serving. Top each bowl with a tablespoon of cilantro, a couple grinds of black pepper, and 2 lemongrass slivers laid in a crisscross on top of one another. Store in an airtight container in the refrigerator for up to 3 days or in the freezer for up to 2 months. Gently reheat prior to serving.

Per Serving: Calories 280; Protein 28 g; Carbs 27 g; Dietary Fiber 2 g; Added Sugars 2 g; Total Fat 12 g; Sat Fat 4 g; Omega-3s 180 mg; Sodium 840 mg; Potassium 526 mg

TOMATO-BASIL SOUP

Makes 6 servings

This popular comfort soup is worth making from scratch— and so very easy to do! We like using Roma tomatoes (also known as plum tomatoes) because they release less water, have very thin skins, and contain fewer and smaller seeds compared to other tomato varieties. Top this soup with Parmesan-Herb Croutons (page 172) or pair with Very Veggie Grilled Cheese Sandwiches (page 182).

- 2 tablespoons extra virgin olive oil
- 1 white onion, chopped
- 1 celery stalk, chopped
- 3 garlic cloves, minced
- 4 pounds (1.8 kg) Roma (plum) tomatoes, diced
- ⅓ cup (85 g) no-salt-added tomato paste
- 1 tablespoon brown sugar
- 3 cups (720 ml) Vegetable Broth (page 72)
- 2 tablespoons balsamic or red wine vinegar
- ½ cup (12 g) chopped fresh basil, plus 2 tablespoons for serving
- 2 tablespoons chopped fresh parsley
- 1 teaspoon dried thyme or 1 tablespoon chopped fresh thyme
- 1 tablespoon fresh lemon juice
- ¼ teaspoon kosher salt
- ¼ teaspoon freshly ground black pepper

1. Heat the oil, onions, celery, and garlic in a stockpot over medium-high heat. Sauté until the onions are translucent, the celery is softened, and the garlic is fragrant, 4 to 5 minutes.

2. Stir in the tomatoes, tomato paste, and brown sugar. Cook, stirring continuously, for 3 minutes. Add the broth and vinegar and bring to a boil. Reduce the heat to medium-low and cover. Simmer until the tomatoes are soft, 20 minutes.

3. Add ½ cup (12 g) basil, the parsley, and thyme, stir to blend, and simmer for 1 minute.

4. Remove from the heat. Use an immersion blender in the pot to puree the soup until smooth, or puree in batches in a blender and return the soup to the pot. Add the lemon juice, salt, and pepper, and heat the soup until hot and bubbly.

5. Ladle the soup into bowls and top each bowl with 1 teaspoon chopped basil. Serve hot. Store in an airtight container in the refrigerator for up to 3 days or in the freezer for up to 2 months. Gently reheat prior to serving.

Per Serving: Calories 149; Protein 4 g; Carbs 23 g; Dietary Fiber 5 g; Added Sugars 2 g; Total Fat 6 g; Sat Fat 0 g; Omega-3s 10 mg; Sodium 211 mg; Potassium 821 mg

TURKEY-VEGETABLE SOUP

Makes 8 servings

This is a perfect soup to make after roasting a large turkey breast or whole turkey. Freeze some of the soup for one of those days when you need an easy "heat & eat" dinner option.

2 quarts (2 L) Chicken Stock (page 70)

1 pound (454 g) diced red or white potatoes (about 3 medium)

2 carrots or parsnips, diced

2 celery stalks, diced

2 cups (270 g) diced cooked turkey

1 cup (165 g) frozen white or yellow corn kernels

1 teaspoon freshly ground black pepper

Chopped fresh parsley, optional

1. Bring the stock to a boil in a large stockpot over high heat. Add the potatoes, carrots, and celery. Reduce the heat to medium, partially cover, and simmer until the potatoes are fork-tender, about 15 minutes.

2. Add the turkey, corn, and black pepper. Simmer until the corn is fully cooked, about 10 minutes. Serve hot, topped with chopped parsley if desired. Store in an airtight container in the refrigerator for up to 3 days or in the freezer for up to 2 months.

Per Serving: Calories 217; Protein 15 g; Carbs 30 g; Dietary Fiber 2 g; Added Sugars 3 g; Total Fat 4 g; Sat Fat 1 g; Omega-3s 50 mg; Sodium 177 mg; Potassium 508 mg

VERY VEGGIE MISO SOUP

Makes 6 servings

Miso is a flavor-rich paste made from fermented soy-beans. Adding white (shiro) miso to dashi creates a rich, complex broth. Adding a few aromatics and lots of vege-tables turns the broth into an incredible soup to enjoy with Shrimp Fried Rice (page 296) or Tofu Fried Rice (page 232).

6 cups (1.4 L) Dashi Broth (page 70)

½ cup (140 g) white (shiro) miso

1 tablespoon reduced-sodium soy sauce

2 carrots, thinly sliced

1 cup (150 g) shelled edamame beans (green soybeans), thawed if frozen

One 2-inch (5 cm) piece ginger, quartered lengthwise

8 ounces (227 g) enoki mushrooms, divided into 6 small bunches (see Tip)

2 heads baby bok choy, chopped

One 14-ounce (397 g) package firm silken tofu, cut into ½-inch (13 mm) cubes (see Note)

2 green onions, thinly sliced diagonally

1. Combine the dashi, miso, and soy sauce in a medium stockpot over high heat. Whisk to dissolve the miso. Add the carrots, edamame, and ginger and bring to a boil. Reduce the heat to low, cover, and simmer until the carrots are soft, 8 to 10 minutes.

2. Add the mushrooms and bok choy and simmer until the bok choy stems start to soften, 2 to 3 min-utes.

3. Divide the tofu among six soup bowls. Use tongs to remove the ginger. Divide the soup among the bowls. Top with green onions and serve. Store in an airtight container in the refrigerator for up to 3 days or in the freezer for up to 2 months. Gently reheat prior to serving.

TIP: *If you can't find enoki mushrooms, feel free to use very thinly sliced white mushrooms.*

NOTE: *The easiest way to cut tofu into cubes is to lay it on a cutting board or plate. Use a sharp knife to cut the tofu in half horizontally along the "equator." Cut the block across the top into sixths in one direction and quarters in the other direction. This will create 48 small cubes.*

Per Serving: Calories 140; Protein 11 g; Carbs 18 g; Dietary Fiber 4 g; Added Sugars 0 g; Total Fat 4 g; Sat Fat 0 g; Omega-3s 600 mg; Sodium 570 mg; Potassium 580 mg

WEST AFRICAN–INSPIRED SWEET POTATO & PEANUT STEW

Makes 8 servings

This soup is an example of the saying, "What grows together goes together." It tells the story of a place, in this case West Africa, where leafy greens, sweet potatoes (or more accurately, yams), and peanuts grew in abundance and where home cooks turned those ingredients into a fantastically flavorful and very nourishing meal. Enjoy this soup with Southwest Corn Bread (page 105) for an easy, comforting meal.

- 2 tablespoons extra virgin olive oil
- 1 white or yellow onion, diced
- 2 tablespoons grated fresh ginger
- 2 teaspoons ground cumin
- ½ teaspoon cayenne
- Up to ½ cup (120 ml) water, optional
- 2 quarts (2 L) Vegetable Broth (page 72)
- 1 cup (255 g) creamy peanut butter
- One 6-ounce (170 g) can tomato paste
- 6 cups (800 g) peeled, cubed garnet sweet potatoes
- 5 ounces (142 g) dark leafy greens (such as collard greens, Swiss chard, or spinach), heavy stems removed, chopped
- 2 teaspoons kosher salt
- Juice of 2 limes
- Chopped fresh cilantro

1. Heat the oil, onion, ginger, cumin, and cayenne in a Dutch oven or large stockpot over medium-high heat. Sauté until the onions start to soften, 8 to 10 minutes. Add water as needed to prevent the ginger and onions from sticking to the bottom of the pot.

2. Stir in the broth, peanut butter, and tomato paste.

3. Add the sweet potatoes, greens, and salt. Increase the heat to high, bring to a boil, then reduce the heat to low, cover, and simmer for 30 minutes, until the sweet potatoes are fork-tender.

4. Remove from the heat, stir in the lime juice, and serve, topping with cilantro as desired. Store in an airtight container in the refrigerator for up to 3 days or in the freezer for up to 2 months. Gently reheat prior to serving.

NOTE: *While many grocery stores have signs that say "Yams" in their produce sections, these root vegetables are most likely sweet potatoes. The same is true of items labeled "candied yams" in the canned vegetable aisle. Yams grow to much larger sizes. A sweet potato may reach 1 pound (454 g) in size, but a single yam can grow to 150 pounds (68 kg)!*

Per Serving: Calories 375; Protein 12 g; Carbs 16 g; Dietary Fiber 5 g; Added Sugars 2 g; Total Fat 21 g; Sat. Fat 4 g; Omega-3s 30 mg; Sodium 860 mg; Potassium 860 mg

CHICKEN CHILI VERDE

Makes 6 servings

This is another wonderful one-pot meal that combines lean protein, nutrient-rich beans, abundant vegetables, and aromatic herbs. Serve with warm tortillas or Southwest Corn Bread (page 105).

- 1.5 pounds (680 g) boneless, skinless chicken breasts or thighs, cut into bite-size cubes
- 1 tablespoon extra virgin olive oil
- 1 tablespoon cumin seeds, crushed, or 2 teaspoons ground cumin
- 1 white onion, diced
- 2 celery stalks, diced
- 2 poblano chiles, diced
- 1 green bell pepper, seeded and cubed
- 1 jalapeño chile, minced
- 2 garlic cloves, minced
- 1 teaspoon freshly ground black pepper
- 2 bay leaves
- 4 cups (1 L) Chicken Stock (page 70)
- Two 15.5-ounce (439 g) cans cannellini beans
- 1 bunch cilantro ends, trimmed and chopped
- 2 limes, quartered

1. Heat the chicken and oil in a large Dutch oven over medium-high heat. Sauté until the chicken becomes firm and opaque, 5 to 6 minutes.

2. Add the cumin and sauté until fragrant, 1 minute. Stir in the onion, celery, and poblano. Cover and cook until the vegetables start to soften, 5 to 6 minutes.

3. Add the bell pepper, jalapeño, black pepper, and bay leaves. Stir, reduce the heat to medium, cover, and cook until softened, about 15 minutes, stirring occasionally.

4. Reduce the heat to low. Stir in the stock and beans. Cover and simmer gently for 30 minutes, stirring occasionally.

5. Remove the bay leaves, add the cilantro, stir, and simmer gently for about 5 minutes to wilt it. Serve hot with a squeeze of lime. Store in an airtight container in the refrigerator for up to 3 days or in the freezer for up to 2 months.

NOTE: A mortar and pestle is the perfect tool for crushing cumin seeds.

Per Serving: Calories 246; Protein 35 g; Carbs 18 g; Dietary Fiber 5 g; Added Sugars 0 g; Total Fat 4 g; Sat Fat 0 g; Omega-3s 40 mg; Sodium 365 mg; Potassium 560 mg

CIOPPINO

Makes 6 servings

Cioppino is a hearty seafood stew that originated in San Francisco in the late 1800s. Our version features crab, clams, shrimp, and white fish. If you choose to leave out the crab legs or the clams, add another 8 ounces (227 g) firm white fish to keep this stew hearty. Serve with a crusty French bread to sop up all the super flavorful juices.

- 2 tablespoons extra virgin olive oil
- 1 red or white onion, chopped
- 2 garlic cloves, minced
- 1 green bell pepper, seeded and sliced
- 2 carrots, chopped
- 2 cups (480 ml) Shrimp Stock (page 71) or Fish Broth (page 71)
- One 14-ounce can (400 g) crushed tomatoes
- ⅔ cup (160 ml) dry white wine
- 2 tablespoons tomato paste
- 1 tablespoon chopped fresh thyme, plus more for serving
- 1 teaspoon chopped fresh basil
- 1 teaspoon dried oregano
- ½ teaspoon red pepper flakes
- 1 bay leaf
- 1 pound (454 g) shell-on king crab, or snow crab legs or Dungeness crab, cut into 2-inch (5 cm) pieces, optional
- 1 pound (454 g) littleneck clams, scrubbed well, optional

- 8 ounces (227 g) firm white fish fillets (such as halibut, snapper, or sea bass), cut into 2- to 3-inch (5 to 7.5 cm) pieces
- 8 ounces (227 g) raw 31/40 shrimp, peeled and deveined
- 1 tablespoon fresh lemon juice
- ¼ cup (15 g) chopped fresh flat-leaf parsley
- Kosher salt and freshly ground black pepper

1. Heat the oil in a stockpot over medium-high heat. When the oil is hot and shimmering, add the onion, garlic, bell pepper, and carrots. Sauté until the onion is translucent, the garlic is fragrant, and the bell pepper and carrots brighten and begin to soften, 4 to 5 minutes.

2. Stir in the stock, tomatoes, wine, tomato paste, thyme, basil, oregano, red pepper flakes, and bay leaf. Bring to a boil. Partially cover and reduce the heat to medium-low. Simmer for 10 minutes, until the vegetables are tender and the herbs are fragrant.

3. Add the crab and clams, if using. Simmer, covered, until the crab shells turn pink and clam shells open, about 10 minutes. Add the white fish and shrimp. Simmer, covered, until the fish is opaque and flakes easily, and the shrimp are pink, about 2 to 3 minutes.

4. Remove from the heat. Discard the bay leaf and any unopened clams. Stir in the lemon juice and parsley. Season with salt and pepper. Ladle into bowls and garnish with a sprinkle of thyme; serve hot. Store in an airtight container in the refrigerator for up to 3 days or in the freezer for up to 2 months. Gently reheat prior to serving.

Per Serving: Calories 255; Protein 26 g; Carbs 12 g; Dietary Fiber 2 g; Added Sugars 0 g; Total Fat 9 g; Sat Fat 1 g; Omega-3s 510 mg; Sodium 308 mg; Potassium 598 mg

MIDWESTERN BEEF, BEAN & BEER CHILI

Makes 6 servings

Chili is an awesome one-pot meal that combines lean protein with vegetables. Pair this version with Southwest Corn Bread (page 105), corn tortillas, or tortilla chips. To make this in a slow cooker, follow steps 1 and 2, and then combine everything in the slow cooker and cook on LOW for 6 to 8 hours.

1 tablespoon extra virgin olive oil

1 white or yellow onion, chopped

1 green bell pepper, seeded and chopped

2 celery stalks, diced

2 garlic cloves, minced

2 pounds (907 g) 93% lean ground beef

Two 15-ounce (425 g) cans dark red kidney beans, drained and rinsed

12 ounces (355 ml) beer (see Tip)

1 cup (240 ml) water

One 8-ounce (227 g) can tomato sauce

One 6-ounce (170 g) can tomato paste

One 4-ounce (113 g) can diced green chiles

2 teaspoons chili powder

1 teaspoon ground cumin

1 teaspoon hot sauce

¼ teaspoon freshly cracked black pepper

Optional Garnishes

¾ cup (85 g) shredded medium or sharp cheddar

½ cup (80 g) diced white onion

½ cup (8 g) chopped fresh cilantro

⅓ cup (80 g) reduced-fat sour cream

1. Heat the oil in a large skillet or Dutch oven over medium-high heat. Add the onion, bell pepper, celery, and garlic, and sauté until the onions are soft, 10 to 12 minutes.

2. Add the ground beef and cook, stirring occasionally to break up the beef, for about 15 minutes, until browned. (Allowing some of the beef to get a hard sear will intensify the beef flavor in the final dish.)

3. Add the beans, beer, water, tomato sauce, tomato paste, chiles, chili powder, cumin, hot sauce, and black pepper. Reduce the heat to low and simmer until a digital food thermometer reads 165°F (75°C) when inserted in the center, 30 to 45 minutes. Serve hot, topped with cheddar, cilantro, onion, and/or sour cream, if desired. Store in an airtight container in the refrigerator for up to 3 days or in the freezer for up to 2 months. Gently reheat prior to serving.

NOTE: *Draining and rinsing canned beans removes up to one-third of the sodium added during canning.*

TIP: *What's the best beer to use in this recipe? We like to use light pilsners or lagers, but you can also use a dark beer like a porter or stout. Some chili aficionados like to add a teaspoon or two of cocoa powder to their chili for an extra layer of flavor; using a chocolate stout will have a similar flavor effect.*

Per Serving: Calories 333; Protein 39 g; Carbs 24 g; Dietary Fiber 6 g; Added Sugars 1 g; Total Fat 13 g; Sat Fat 5 g; Omega-3s 90 mg; Sodium 593 mg; Potassium 946 mg

HEARTY CLAM CHOWDER

Makes 4 servings

Nothing says comfort like a bowl of hot, steaming clam chowder! This New England–inspired meal in a bowl simmers hearty winter vegetables in a flavorful seafood stock seasoned with a Mediterranean herb blend. Just before serving, tender clams are added to complete the dish. Serve hot with crusty bread such as our Fresh Herb & Honey Batter Bread (page 102).

1 tablespoon extra virgin olive oil

1 large yellow onion, chopped

2 celery stalks with leaves, diced

3 garlic cloves, minced

1 tablespoon Italian Seasoning (page 34)

2 dashes hot sauce (such as Tabasco)

2 cups (480 ml) Shrimp Stock (page 71) or Fish Broth (page71)

2½ cups (375 g) diced red or white potatoes (about 2 large)

3 thyme sprigs

1 bay leaf

1½ cups (360 ml) evaporated fat-free milk

2 tablespoons whole wheat pastry flour

Two 6.5-ounce (184 g) cans chopped clams (not minced), undrained

1 teaspoon smoked paprika

Freshly ground black pepper

4 dill sprigs

1. Combine the oil, onion, celery, and garlic in a large, heavy-bottomed saucepan or Dutch oven over medium-high heat. Sauté until the onions are translucent and brown on the edges, the celery is softened, and the garlic is fragrant, about 3 minutes.

2. Stir in the Italian seasoning and hot sauce. Add the stock, potatoes, thyme, and bay leaf. Bring to a gentle boil, then reduce the heat to low and simmer until the potatoes are soft, 15 minutes. Remove the bay leaf and thyme.

3. Combine ½ cup (120 ml) of the milk and the flour in a small bowl. Add to the pot, stirring constantly. Increase the heat to high and cook until the chowder is slightly thickened, 1 to 2 minutes. Reduce the heat to medium-low and add the remaining 1 cup (240 ml) milk, the clams, and paprika. Stir and simmer

for 5 minutes, stirring gently from time to time. Cook until the chowder is thick, about 5 minutes.

4. Ladle into bowls, add a couple grinds of black pepper, and garnish each bowl with a dill sprig. Serve immediately. Store in an airtight container in the refrigerator for up to 3 days or in the freezer for up to 2 months. Gently reheat prior to serving.

Per Serving: Calories 347; Protein 34 g; Carbs 41 g; Dietary Fiber 5 g; Added Sugars 0 g; Total Fat 10 g; Sat Fat 2 g; Omega-3s 180 mg; Sodium 356 mg; Potassium 1,071 mg

SMOKED SALMON & CORN CHOWDER

Makes 6 servings

This recipe uses a very small amount of bacon to help develop the smoky flavors. Clam juice, most often sold in bottles in grocery stores, is a great way to add rich seafood flavor with very little added sodium. The addition of wine and crème fraîche help balance the flavor, ensuring the chowder isn't too sweet from the potatoes and corn. If you don't have crème fraîche, you can substitute Greek yogurt or sour cream.

1 tablespoon extra virgin olive oil

1.5 ounces (43 g) bacon (1 to 2 thin-cut strips), cut crosswise very thinly

1 onion, diced

1 celery stalk, diced

2 cups (480 ml) clam juice

1½ cups (360 ml) milk

1 pound (454 g) Yukon gold–type potatoes, diced

2 cups (330 g) frozen white or yellow corn kernels

1 teaspoon dried dill

1 teaspoon freshly ground black pepper

½ teaspoon kosher salt

6 ounces (170 g) hot-smoked salmon, broken into small pieces

3 Roma (plum) tomatoes, diced

⅓ cup (80 ml) dry white wine

¼ cup (55 g) Buttermilk Crème Fraiche (page 361), or store-bought crème fraîche

Chopped fresh chives

1. Combine the oil and bacon in a large Dutch oven or stockpot over medium-high heat. Cook until the bacon is crispy, 2 to 3 minutes. Add the onion and celery, reduce the heat to medium, and sauté until the onions are translucent and the celery softens, 7 to 8 minutes.

2. Add the clam juice, milk, and potatoes. Bring to a boil. Reduce the heat to low, cover, and cook until the potatoes can be easily pierced with a knife, 10 to 12 minutes.

3. Stir in the corn, dill, pepper, and salt. Cover and cook until the corn is heated through, about 10 minutes.

4. Gently stir in the salmon, tomatoes, wine, and crème fraîche. Cook until the salmon is warmed through and the tomatoes have started to break down, 5 minutes. (Don't let it boil.) Serve hot, topped with chopped chives. Store in an airtight container in the refrigerator for up to 3 days. Do not freeze. Gently reheat prior to serving.

Per Serving: Calories 241; Protein 13 g; Carbs 17 g; Dietary Fiber 4 g; Added Sugars 0 g; Total Fat 13 g; Sat Fat 5 g; Omega-3s 190 mg; Sodium 672 mg; Potassium 609 mg

TOMATILLO-PORK STEW

Makes 6 servings

Like their tomato cousins, tomatillos are also botanically a fruit. If you taste a small piece of raw tomatillo, it will initially make you think of a tart Granny Smith apple, but you will soon detect a bitter aftertaste. Cooking tomatillos eliminates their bitterness, leaving behind a bright acidity that adds incredible flavor to a dish like this. Serve it on its own or with Southwest Corn Bread (page 105) for sopping up the delicious sauce.

1 pound (454 g) boneless lean pork, cubed

4 tablespoons (60 ml) extra virgin olive oil

1 teaspoon cumin seeds

1 pound (454 g) tomatillos, husks removed, rinsed and quartered

1 white onion, diced

2 jalapeño chiles, minced

4 garlic cloves, minced

4 cups (1 L) Chicken Stock (page 70) or water

1 teaspoon kosher salt

2 cups (330 g) frozen white or yellow corn kernels

⅓ cup (40 g) stone-ground cornmeal or grits

½ cup (8 g) chopped fresh cilantro

1. Combine the pork, 2 tablespoons of the olive oil, and the cumin in a Dutch oven over medium-high heat. Cook, stirring occasionally, until the pork is brown and no pink is visible, 6 to 7 minutes. Remove the pork from the Dutch oven and set aside.

2. In the same Dutch oven, combine the remaining 2 tablespoons olive oil and the tomatillos. Cook over medium-high heat, stirring occasionally, until the tomatillos are browned on most sides and starting to soften, 8 to 10 minutes.

3. Reduce the heat to medium. Add the onion, jalapeños, and garlic, and cook, stirring often, until the onions start to soften, 5 to 6 minutes.

4. Add the stock and salt. Increase the heat to high, bring to a boil, then add back the pork and reduce the heat to low. Add the corn, increase the heat to medium, and cook until the stew is simmering again, 5 to 8 minutes.

5. Slowly sprinkle in the cornmeal while stirring. Cover and cook until the cornmeal has fully hydrated, the stew is thick, and the surface is gently bubbling, 18 to 20 minutes. Serve hot, topped with cilantro. Store in an airtight container in the refrigerator for up to 3 days or in the freezer for up to 2 months. Gently reheat prior to serving.

Per Serving: Calories 546; Protein 28 g; Carbs 68 g; Dietary Fiber 6 g; Added Sugars 0 g; Total Fat 19 g; Sat Fat 4 g; Omega-3s 140 mg; Sodium 612 mg; Potassium 871 mg

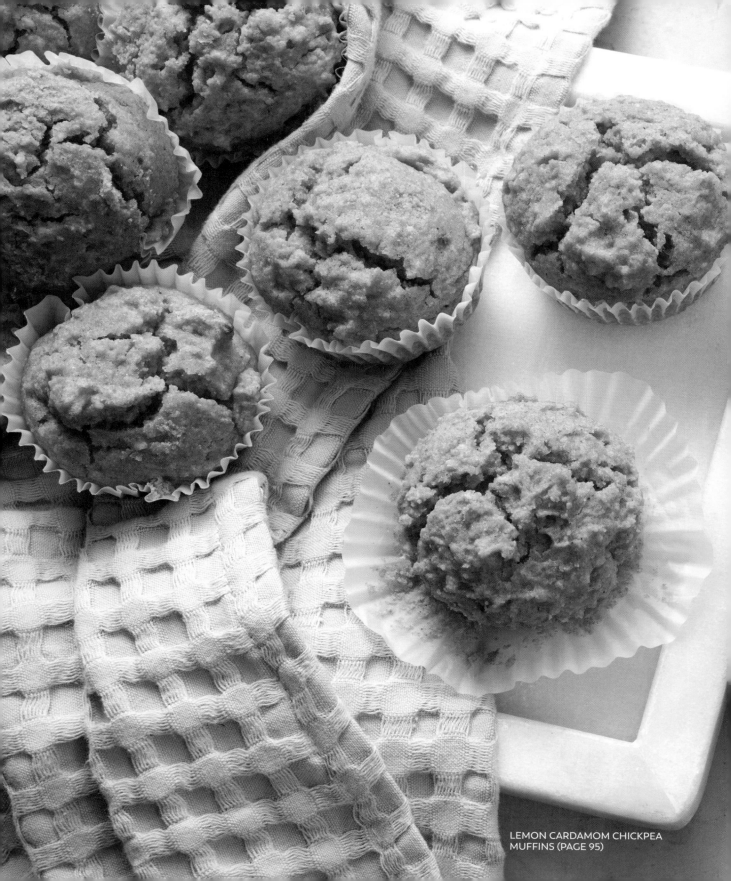

LEMON CARDAMOM CHICKPEA
MUFFINS (PAGE 95)

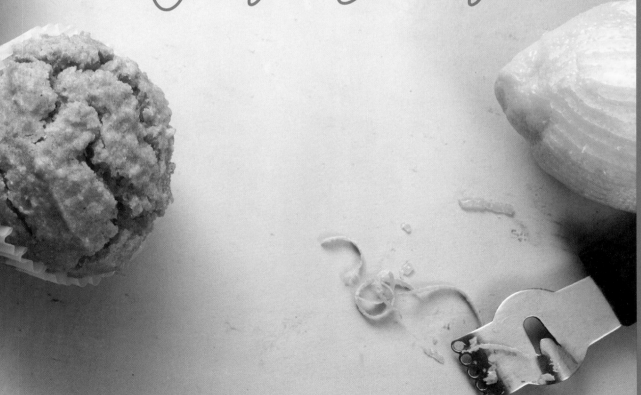

CHAPTER 6

Quick Breads & Yeast Breads

Quick Breads & Yeast Breads

Muffins & Scones

Blueberry Muffins 94

Carrot Bran Muffins 94

Lemon Cardamom Chickpea Muffins . . 95

Italian-Seasoned Corn Muffins 95

Pecan-Oat Muffins 96

Blueberry Oat Flax Scones 96

Gingery Lemon Scones 97

Light-Hearted Clotted Cream 98

Coffee Cakes & Quick Breads

Cranberry-Almond Coffee Cake 98

Rhubarb-Strawberry Coffee Cake 99

Apple-Walnut Bread 100

Banana Nut Bread 101

Cranberry-Orange Bread 101

Fresh Herb & Honey Batter Bread 102

Lemon-Blueberry Bread 102

Molasses Brown Bread 103

Nutty Apricot Cottage Cheese Bread . . 104

Pumpkin Spice Pepita Bread 104

Southwest Corn Bread 105

Zucchini-Nut Bread 106

Yeast Breads & Rolls

Beer Breadsticks with Fennel 106

Buttermilk Rolls 107

Four-Grain Sunflower Seed Bread 108

Fresh Chive Yogurt Buns 108

Harvest Crescents 109

Hearty Wheat Buns 110

Honey Whole Wheat Bread 111

Potato Dinner Rolls 112

Pumpernickel Bread 113

Whole Wheat French Baguette 114

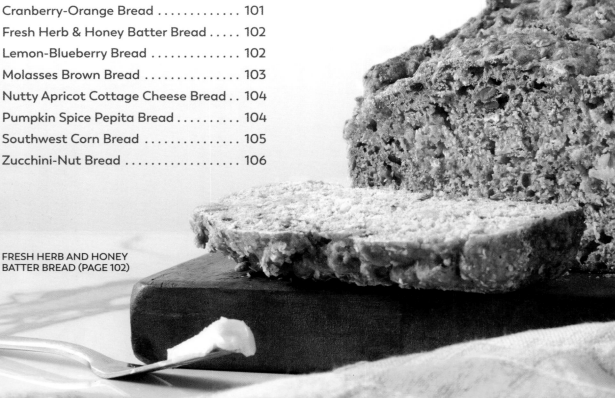

FRESH HERB AND HONEY
BATTER BREAD (PAGE 102)

Breads in all shapes, sizes, and textures are part of traditional plant-based food cultures all over the world. They can be crusty and super chewy, like a classic French baguette, or delicate and tender, like a Southern corn bread. They can be the foundation for a satisfying sandwich or used to sop up savory sauces. Or they can be a sweeter accompaniment to a favorite breakfast or brunch dish, like many of the muffins and quick breads featured in this chapter.

If you enjoy making yeast breads, we hope you'll also enjoy the mindful, meditative process of kneading dough by hand. Doing so provides a wonderful opportunity to relax and breathe deeply and slowly. Kneading helps the proteins that create gluten develop, which is what gives yeast breads their tempting textures. Baking breads at home will fill your kitchen with incredible aromas that reward your senses long before you get to taste them.

We encourage you to experiment with more whole grains in baking. Whole grains include the entire grain kernel; they haven't been refined, so their outer layer (the bran) and the nutrient-dense core (the germ) remain. Often referred to as "good" carbs, whole grains contain many heart-protecting nutrients like fiber, B vitamins, potassium, magnesium, zinc, vitamin E, and other antioxidants.

To get the most nutrition and health benefits from your baked goods, consider replacing all or part of the refined flours with whole grain options, such as whole wheat flour, whole wheat pastry flour, old-fashioned oats, cornmeal, or rye flour—all ingredients you'll find in this chapter. You'll also notice we include nut flours, which can be purchased in ground form or made by grinding roasted, unsalted nuts like almonds in a high-speed blender or food processor to a fine-grain flour consistency.

Many of our quick bread recipes use a combination of refined all-purpose flour and whole grain flours. Nearly any quick bread recipe that calls for all-purpose flour will work well if you use whole grain pastry flour, but we opted to not use it in every recipe because of the cost. If you choose to use it, rest assured that our recipes will work well and taste great! It won't work as well in yeast breads due to its lower protein content. Yeast breads typically require a higher-protein wheat flour to ensure there are enough gluten-forming proteins.

We know that many people like the flavor and texture of added sugars in quick breads and other baked goods. In many of our quick bread recipes, we've added sweeteners like granulated sugar, brown sugar, and molasses. But limiting added sugars is an important part of heart-healthy eating patterns. We encourage you to make most of your daily bread choices whole grain and unsweetened, and to bake and serve sweeter options less frequently.

Finally, this chapter isn't well suited to anyone who needs to eliminate gluten from their diet. There are many wonderful sources of gluten-free baking recipes, tips, and strategies available online and in print. For our readers with celiac disease or gluten intolerance, we hope you will appreciate the hundreds of gluten-free recipes that appear throughout this book.

BLUEBERRY MUFFINS

Makes 12 muffins

These tender, delicate muffins burst with fresh blueberry flavor. Enjoy on their own or serve with Shiitake & Spinach Quiche with Rosemary & Sage (page 125) for a brunch fit for guests.

Cooking spray

1 cup (125 g) all-purpose flour

1 cup (120 g) whole wheat flour

½ cup (100 g) plus 1 teaspoon sugar

1 tablespoon baking powder

1 teaspoon ground cinnamon

1½ cups (220 g) fresh or unthawed frozen blueberries

½ cup (120 ml) milk

¼ cup (60 g) butter or plant-based spread, melted

2 large eggs

1 teaspoon pure vanilla extract

1. Preheat the oven to 400°F (200°C). Spray a regular 12-cup muffin pan with cooking spray.

2. Combine the all-purpose flour, whole wheat flour, ½ cup (100 g) of the sugar, the baking powder, and ¾ teaspoon of the cinnamon in a medium bowl.

3. In a separate bowl, toss the blueberries with 1 tablespoon of the flour mixture. (This helps keep the blueberries suspended throughout the batter instead of settling on the bottom.)

4. In a small bowl, whisk the milk, butter, eggs, and vanilla. Add the wet mixture to the dry ingredients and stir until the batter is smooth. Fold in the berries until they are evenly distributed. (Small spots of flour may remain; that's okay. Don't overmix, or your muffins won't be tender.)

5. Using an ice cream scoop or large spoon, divide the batter evenly among the muffin cups. Mix the remaining 1 teaspoon sugar and ¼ teaspoon cinnamon in a small cup. Sprinkle the tops with the cinnamon-sugar mixture. Bake for 20 to 25 minutes, until the muffins are golden brown and a toothpick inserted in the center comes out clean.

6. Let the muffins cool in the pan for 5 minutes, then transfer to a wire rack and let cool for 10 minutes before serving. Store at room temperature, covered loosely with a kitchen towel, for up to 2 days, or in the freezer in an airtight container lined with paper towels for up to 2 months.

Serving Size 1 muffin; Calories 148; Protein 4 g; Carbs 22 g; Dietary Fiber 2 g; Added Sugars 3 g; Total Fat 5 g; Sat Fat 3 g; Omega-3s 50 mg; Sodium 50 mg; Potassium 65 mg

CARROT BRAN MUFFINS

Makes 12 muffins

Choose a bran cereal made of bran twigs (like All-Bran) to give these muffins their most robust flavor. Enjoy them as a quick "grab and go" breakfast option, or serve them with one of our entrée salads like the Chicken & Wild Rice Salad with Grapes & Candied Pecans (page 162).

Cooking spray

2 cups (115 g) finely shredded carrots (about 6 medium carrots)

1 cup (90 g) bran cereal (like Kellogg's All-Bran)

¾ cup (180 ml) milk

1 cup (120 g) whole wheat flour

1 teaspoon baking powder

½ teaspoon baking soda

½ teaspoon ground cinnamon

1 large egg, slightly beaten

2 tablespoons extra virgin olive oil

2 tablespoons brown sugar

1 tablespoon fresh lemon juice

1. Preheat the oven to 400°F (200°C). Spray a regular 12-cup muffin pan with cooking spray.

2. Combine the carrots, bran cereal, and milk in a medium bowl. Let stand for 5 minutes, until the cereal has soaked up the milk and softened a bit.

3. Combine the flour, baking powder, baking soda, and cinnamon in a large bowl.

4. Stir the egg, oil, sugar, and lemon juice into the carrot mixture. Add the liquid mixture to the dry ingredients, stirring until evenly moistened with some small lumps remaining.

5. Fill the muffin cups half-full. Bake for 20 to 25 minutes, until the muffins are dark golden brown and a toothpick inserted in the center comes out clean.

6. Let the muffins cool in the pan for 5 minutes, then transfer to a wire rack and let cool for 10 minutes before serving. Store at room temperature, covered loosely with a kitchen towel, for up to 2 days, or in the freezer in an airtight container lined with paper towels for up to 2 months.

Serving Size 1 muffin; Calories 105; Protein 3 g; Carbs 17 g; Dietary Fiber 4 g; Added Sugars 2 g; Total Fat 4 g; Sat Fat 1 g; Omega-3s 40 mg; Sodium 125 mg; Potassium 181 mg

LEMON CARDAMOM CHICKPEA MUFFINS

Makes 9 muffins

Lemon and cardamom are a classic ingredient pairing that contributes bright flavor to these moist, aromatic muffins that are great for breakfast, brunch, or snacking. We like to serve them with fruit salads like our Mixed Fruit with Yogurt-Cardamom Dressing (page 144).

Cooking spray
1 cup (150 g) canned chickpeas, drained and rinsed
½ cup (120 ml) extra virgin olive oil
½ cup (100 g) sugar
2 large eggs
Grated zest of 1 lemon
3 tablespoons fresh lemon juice
1 cup (120 g) whole wheat pastry flour
½ cup (50 g) almond flour
1 teaspoon baking powder
½ teaspoon ground cardamom
½ teaspoon kosher salt

1. Preheat the oven to 325°F (165°C). Spray a 9-cup muffin pan with cooking spray.

2. Combine the chickpeas, oil, sugar, eggs, lemon zest, and lemon juice in a food processor or blender and blend until very smooth.

3. Combine the pastry flour, almond flour, baking powder, cardamom, and salt in a medium bowl. Stir to combine. Pour in the liquid mixture and stir just enough to incorporate.

4. Spoon ⅓ cup (about 75 g) batter into each cup. Bake for 14 to 16 minutes, until a toothpick inserted into the center comes out clean.

5. Let the muffins cool in the pan for 5 minutes, then transfer to a wire rack and let cool for 10 minutes before serving. To store, see Step 6 on page 93.

TIP: You can make 12 smaller muffins with this recipe. Use ¼ cup (about 60 g) batter for each muffin and reduce the baking time to 11 to 13 minutes.

Serving Size 1 muffin; Calories 279; Protein 5 g; Carbs 27 g; Dietary Fiber 4 g; Added Sugars 11 g; Total Fat 17 g; Sat Fat 2 g; Omega-3s 120 mg; Sodium 156 mg; Potassium 66 mg

ITALIAN-SEASONED CORN MUFFINS

Makes 12 muffins

Stone-ground cornmeal gives these moist muffins a full flavor—they taste like corn, but not overpoweringly so, with a tender crumb and crunchy top.

Cooking spray
1 cup (125 g) all-purpose flour
½ cup (60 g) stone-ground cornmeal
1 tablespoon baking powder
1 tablespoon sugar
¾ teaspoon Italian Seasoning (page 34)
⅛ teaspoon garlic powder
2 large eggs
⅓ cup (80 ml) milk
1 tablespoon extra virgin olive oil
½ cup (85 g) fresh or frozen corn kernels
⅓ cup (50 g) chopped bell pepper
¼ cup (40 g) finely chopped onion

1. Preheat the oven to 400°F (200°C). Spray a regular 12-cup muffin pan with cooking spray.

2. Combine the flour, cornmeal, baking powder, sugar, Italian seasoning, and garlic powder in a medium bowl.

3. Whisk the eggs, milk, and oil in a small bowl. Gently stir the wet mixture into the dry ingredients until just combined. (Don't overmix.) Fold in the corn, pepper, and onion.

4. Using a large spoon, divide the batter evenly among the muffin cups. Bake for 20 to 25 minutes, until the muffins are light golden brown and a toothpick inserted into the center comes out clean. Let the muffins cool in the pan for 5 minutes, then transfer to a wire rack. Let cool for 5 minutes longer and serve warm. To store, see Step 6 on page 93.

Serving Size 1 muffin; Calories 96; Protein 3 g; Carbs 15 g; Dietary Fiber 1 g; Added Sugars 1 g; Total Fat 3 g; Sat Fat 1 g; Omega-3s 30 mg; Sodium 88 mg; Potassium 58 mg

PECAN-OAT MUFFINS

Makes 18 muffins

These moist, delicately flavored muffins are sweetened with honey. Topping each with a sprinkle of chopped pecans highlights their flavor within the muffin.

Cooking spray

1 cup (110 g) plus 2 tablespoons finely chopped pecans

1½ cups (140 g) old-fashioned rolled oats

½ cup (65 g) all-purpose flour

½ cup (60 g) whole wheat flour

½ teaspoon baking powder

½ teaspoon baking soda

3 tablespoons honey

3 tablespoons peanut or canola oil

1 cup (240 ml) cultured buttermilk (see Tip)

2 large eggs

1 teaspoon pure vanilla extract

1. Preheat the oven to 350°F (180°C). Spray 18 cups of two regular muffin pans with cooking spray.

2. In a dry skillet over low heat, toast 1 cup (110 g) of the pecans and the oats, stirring constantly, for about 5 to 8 minutes, until the nuts are fragrant and oats are golden brown.

3. Mix together the all-purpose flour, whole wheat flour, the baking powder, and baking soda in a large bowl. Stir in the toasted pecans and oats. Make a well in center of the dry ingredients.

4. Whisk the honey and oil together in a small bowl. In a medium bowl, whisk the honey mixture into the buttermilk, then whisk in the eggs and vanilla until well blended. Pour the wet mixture into the dry ingredients and mix only until moistened.

5. Fill the muffin cups two-thirds full. Evenly sprinkle the remaining 2 tablespoons chopped pecans over the muffins. Bake for 20 to 25 minutes, until the muffins are slightly browned and a toothpick inserted in the center comes out clean. Let the muffins cool in the pan for 10 minutes, then transfer to a wire rack and let cool for 10 minutes before serving. To store, see Step 6 on page 93.

TIP: *To use dry cultured buttermilk, add 4 tablespoons of the dry cultured buttermilk blend to the dry ingredients in Step 3. Add 1 cup water in Step 4 to the honey and oil. Proceed with Steps 4 and 5.*

Serving Size 1 muffin; Calories 147; Protein 4 g; Carbs 15 g; Dietary Fiber 2 g; Added Sugars 3 g; Total Fat 9 g; Sat Fat 1 g; Omega-3s 70 mg; Sodium 65 mg; Potassium 86 mg

BLUEBERRY OAT FLAX SCONES

Makes 12 scones

Start your day with a flaky scone made with yogurt, oats, flax, and blueberries. If you wish, swap out the blueberries for raspberries or strawberries. These are delicious served with our Light-Hearted Clotted Cream (page 98) or as an accompaniment to our Tomato-Topped Veggie-Egg Bake (page 127).

1½ cups (190 g) all-purpose flour, plus more for kneading

½ cup (45 g) old-fashioned rolled oats, plus more for sprinkling

¼ cup (50 g) sugar

2 tablespoons ground flaxseed

2 teaspoons baking powder

¼ cup (60 g) cold butter or plant-based spread, cut into pieces

1 large egg

One 5.3-ounce (150 g) container plain Greek yogurt (about ⅔ cup)

½ cup (120 ml) plain kefir or buttermilk

2 teaspoons grated lemon zest

1¼ cups (185 g) frozen blueberries or ¾ cup (120 g) dried blueberries

½ teaspoon cinnamon

1. Preheat the oven to 400°F (200°C). Line a baking sheet with parchment paper.

2. Whisk together the flour, oats, sugar, flaxseed, and baking powder in a medium bowl. Use a fork or pastry blender to cut in the butter until the mixture resembles coarse crumbs. Make a well in the center of the mixture.

3. Beat the egg in a small bowl. Transfer 1 tablespoon of egg to a second small bowl or cup and reserve for brushing the scones. Add the yogurt, kefir, and lemon zest to the egg in the first bowl. Stir to combine. Pour the wet ingredients in the first bowl into the well in the flour mixture. Using a fork, stir until just moistened. Gently fold in 1 cup (150 g) of the frozen blueberries or ½ cup (80 g) of the dried. Don't overmix; you want the dough just to come together and the berries to stay intact (which is why frozen berries work better than fresh).

4. Turn out the dough onto a lightly floured surface. Knead by folding the dough onto itself, then giving the dough a half-turn, until nearly smooth, about 10 folds. Place the dough on the baking sheet.

5. Using your hands, gently pat the dough into a 10-inch (25.5 cm) circle. Sprinkle the remaining ¼ cup (40 g) blueberries on the top, evenly spreading and slightly pushing them into the dough.

6. Score the dough ¼ inch (6 mm) deep into 12 wedges. The circle should remain intact. Brush the tops of the scones with the reserved egg. Lightly sprinkle the cinnamon and rolled oats over the top, gently pushing to secure them.

7. Bake for 20 minutes or until the scones are lightly brown. Place the baking sheet on a wire rack and let cool for 5 minutes. Transfer the scones with the parchment paper to the wire rack until completely cool, about 2 hours.

8. Cut the scones apart and serve immediately. Store in an airtight container for up to 3 days at room temperature or wrap each scone in wax paper, then store in an airtight container in the freezer for up to 2 months. Thaw at room temperature.

Serving Size 1 scone; Calories 163; Protein 5 g; Carbs 23 g; Dietary Fiber 2 g; Added Sugars 4 g; Total Fat 6 g; Sat Fat 3 g; Omega-3s 420 mg; Sodium 111 mg; Potassium 65 mg

GINGERY LEMON SCONES
Makes 16 scones

Consider serving these warm, gingery scones for brunch or in the afternoon. We make them finger food–size by shaping two 5-inch (13 cm) circles from the dough; each circle is then cut into eight wedges. They are delicious served with fruit and our Light-Hearted Clotted Cream (page 98).

- 1 large egg
- 1 tablespoon water
- ¼ cup (50 g) plus 2 tablespoons sugar
- ¼ teaspoon ground ginger
- 1½ cups (190 g) all-purpose flour, plus more for kneading
- ¼ cup (30 g) whole wheat flour
- ¼ cup (40 g) finely chopped crystallized ginger
- 2 tablespoons chia seeds
- 2 tablespoons finely grated lemon zest
- 1 teaspoon baking soda
- ¼ teaspoon kosher salt
- 1 cup (240 ml) cultured buttermilk (see Tip)
- 1 tablespoon canola oil
- 2 teaspoons fresh lemon juice

1. Preheat the oven to 350°F (180°C). Line a baking sheet with parchment paper.

2. Whisk together the egg and water in a cup to make an egg wash for the tops of the scones. Combine 2 tablespoons of the sugar with the ground ginger in a second cup to sprinkle on top of the scones.

3. Whisk together the all-purpose flour, whole wheat flour, crystallized ginger, the remaining ¼ cup (50 g) sugar, the chia seeds, lemon zest, baking soda, and salt in a large bowl. Make a well in the center.

4. Add the buttermilk, oil, and lemon juice to the dry ingredients, stirring with a fork just until blended. Don't overmix; you want the dough just to come together. (It may be slightly sticky.)

5. Turn out the dough onto a lightly floured surface. Knead a few times just until smooth and pliable. Divide into two equal parts and place both on the baking sheet.

6. Using your hands, gently pat each part into a 5-inch (13 cm) circle about ½ inch thick (13 mm). Brush the tops with the egg wash. Sprinkle with the sugar-ginger blend. Score each circle about ¼ inch (6 mm) deep into 8 wedges. The circles should remain intact.

7. Bake the scones for 15 to 17 minutes, until they are brown and firm to the touch. Place the baking sheet on a wire rack to cool for 2 minutes. Cut the scones apart and serve warm from the oven. Store in an airtight container for up to 3 days at room temperature or wrap each scone in wax paper, then store in an airtight container in the freezer for up to 2 months. Thaw at room temperature, or wrap the scone in a paper towel and heat for 8 to 10 seconds in the microwave.

TIP: *To use dry cultured buttermilk, add 4 tablespoons of the dry cultured buttermilk blend to the dry ingredients in Step 3. Add 1 cup water in Step 4 to the oil and lemon juice. Proceed with Steps 4 through 7.*

Serving Size 1 scone; Calories 97; Protein 2 g; Carbs 18 g; Dietary Fiber 1 g; Added Sugars 6 g; Total Fat 2 g; Sat Fat 0 g; Omega-3s 390 mg; Sodium 130 mg; Potassium 31 mg

LIGHT-HEARTED CLOTTED CREAM

Makes 3 cups (630 g)

This recipe can be made with dairy or plant-based whipping cream; choose what you prefer. Clotted cream contains less saturated fat than butter, which provides twice the calories and saturated fat per tablespoon. This recipe whips up so easily, and is a lovely finishing touch to serve with scones, such as Gingery Lemon Scones (page 97), or with a dessert. Or serve on its own, in a small bowl garnished with fresh berries, chocolate curls, diced candied lemon peel, or crystallized ginger.

- ½ cup (120 ml) dairy or plant-based heavy whipping cream
- 2 tablespoons confectioners' sugar
- 2 teaspoons finely grated citrus zest (see Tip)
- 2 teaspoons fresh citrus juice
- 2 cups (460 g) vanilla Greek yogurt

In a bowl, use an immersion blender, handheld mixer, or stand mixer to whip the cream until soft peaks form. Add the sugar, citrus zest, and citrus juice. Whip until the peaks are stiff, about 3 minutes. Fold in the yogurt using a wooden spoon or rubber spatula. Combine until well blended. Use immediately or store in the refrigerator in an airtight container for up to 3 days. The cream may lose some of its volume, but it will still be delicious!

TIP: *You can use any citrus fruit in this recipe for the zest and juice, but lemon will pair best with most of the scones and desserts in this book.*

NOTE: *Plant-based whipping creams can be found in the refrigerated case in your grocery store. They're made with coconut and sunflower oils, fava bean protein, and guar gum, and you can hardly tell a taste or functional difference from dairy whipping cream. There are no significant differences between the dairy version and plant-based version when it comes to calories, total fat, and saturated fat; one tablespoon of each contains 50 calories and 3.5 grams of saturated fat.*

Serving Size 2 tablespoons; Calories 40; Protein 2 g; Carbs 3 g; Dietary Fiber 0 g; Added Sugars 2 g; Total Fat 2 g; Sat Fat 2 g; Omega-3s 10 mg; Sodium 12 mg; Potassium 37 mg

CRANBERRY-ALMOND COFFEE CAKE

Makes one 8-inch (20 cm) square cake

Fresh, bright-red cranberries start to appear in many stores in early November but disappear by the end of December. Be sure to buy a couple of extra bags to tuck away in the freezer so you can make sweet or savory cranberry dishes whenever you choose. This tender, delicious tea bread–like cake brings out the cranberries' sweeter side.

Cake
Cooking spray
1½ cups (190 g) all-purpose flour
½ cup (60 g) whole wheat flour
1 tablespoon baking powder
1 tablespoon grated orange zest
½ cup (100 g) sugar
¼ cup (60 g) butter or plant-based spread, melted
1 large egg

½ cup (120 ml) milk

1 teaspoon almond extract

1½ cups (150 g) fresh or frozen cranberries, coarsely chopped

Topping

¼ cup (30 g) all-purpose flour

¼ cup (50 g) sugar

2 tablespoons sliced almonds

2 tablespoons butter or plant-based spread, melted

1. Preheat the oven to 375°F (190°C). Spray an 8-inch (20 cm) square baking pan with cooking spray.

2. To make the cake, combine the all-purpose flour, whole wheat flour, baking powder, and orange zest in a large bowl. In a small bowl, whisk together the sugar, butter, and egg. Add the milk and almond extract, and stir to combine. Stir the wet mixture into the dry ingredients and mix well. Fold in 1 cup (100 g) of the cranberries.

3. Spread the batter in the pan. Smooth and level the top with the back of wooden spoon or rubber spatula. Sprinkle the remaining ½ cup (50 g) cranberries evenly over the top, pushing them in slightly.

4. To make the topping, combine the flour, sugar, and almonds in a small bowl. Add the butter and blend using a fork until crumbly. Crumble the topping over the batter.

5. Bake for 35 to 40 minutes, until a toothpick inserted in the center comes out clean. Remove from the oven and let cool on a wire rack. Serve warm. To store, cover the baking pan and store at room temperature for up to 2 days or in the refrigerator for up to 1 week. To freeze, tightly wrap the cake in wax paper or foil, wrap with plastic wrap, and place in an airtight container for up to 3 months.

Serving Size 1 slice; Calories 153; Protein 3 g; Carbs 324 g; Dietary Fiber 2 g; Added Sugars 10 g; Total Fat 5 g; Sat Fat 4 g; Omega-3s 30 mg; Sodium 140 mg; Potassium 126 mg

RHUBARB-STRAWBERRY COFFEE CAKE

Makes one 9 × 13-inch (23 × 33 cm) cake

In her youth, Linda's duties on the farm included pulling the rhubarb, tending the strawberry bed, and making all kinds of mouthwatering goodies with them, which made her family happy! She discovered that rhubarb and strawberries play well together, and in this recipe, each enhances the other. Now it's your turn to receive raves when you make this coffee cake at home or bring it to your next gathering.

Filling

4 cups (490 g) cubed rhubarb, in ½-inch (1.25 cm) pieces

2 cups (290 g) sliced strawberries

2 tablespoons fresh lemon juice

¼ cup (50 g) granulated sugar

⅓ cup (40 g) cornstarch

Cake

Cooking spray

1½ cups (180 g) whole wheat flour

1½ cups (190 g) all-purpose flour

¾ cup (150 g) granulated sugar

1½ teaspoons baking powder

1½ teaspoons baking soda

½ teaspoon ground nutmeg

1 cup (240 ml) buttermilk

½ cup (115 g) butter or plant-based spread, melted

½ cup (120 ml) extra virgin olive oil

2 large eggs

1 teaspoon pure vanilla extract

Topping

¾ cup (90 g) coarsely chopped walnuts

¼ cup (50 g) brown sugar

¼ cup (50 g) granulated sugar

1. To make the filling, combine the rhubarb, strawberries, and lemon juice in a medium saucepan. Cook over low to medium heat, stirring frequently, until the strawberries start to soften and the rhubarb starts to break down, 5 minutes.

2. Combine the sugar with the cornstarch in a small bowl. Stir into the fruit in the saucepan. Cook over medium heat until thickened, 4 to 6 minutes. Let cool, about 20 minutes.

3. Preheat the oven to 350°F (180°C). Spray a 9 × 13-inch (23 × 33 cm) cake pan with cooking spray.

4. To make the cake, combine the all-purpose flour, whole wheat flour, sugar, baking powder, baking soda, and nutmeg in large bowl. In a medium bowl, whisk together the buttermilk, butter, oil, eggs, and vanilla. Stir the wet mixture into the dry ingredients until well blended.

5. Spread half of the cake batter into the pan. Spread the filling over the batter. Drop the remaining batter by spoonfuls over the filling. Smooth the batter evenly over the filling using a wooden spoon or rubber spatula.

6. To make the topping, combine the walnuts, brown sugar, and granulated sugar in a small bowl. Sprinkle evenly over the batter.

7. Bake for 50 to 55 minutes, until a toothpick inserted in the center comes out clean. Cool in the pan on a wire rack. Cut in a 4 × 6 pattern (2-inch/5 cm squares). Serve warm or cool. To store, cover the baking pan and place in the refrigerator for up to 3 days. To freeze, tightly wrap the cake in wax paper or foil, then wrap with plastic wrap and place in an airtight container for up to 3 months.

NOTE: *Plentiful in the spring, rhubarb can be frozen in 2-cup (245 g) or 4-cup (490 g) portions to make this and other rhubarb-laden recipes throughout the year. Not only does it taste better than commercially frozen rhubarb, it is more tender and less costly.*

Serving Size 1 slice; Calories 224; Protein 4 g; Carbs 28 g; Dietary Fiber 2 g; Added Sugars 12 g; Total Fat 12 g; Sat Fat 3 g; Omega-3s 410 mg; Sodium 154 mg; Potassium 148 mg

APPLE-WALNUT BREAD

Makes one 9 × 5-inch (23 × 13 cm) loaf

This apple-packed, walnut-studded bread boasts a to-die-for crunchy streusel top with a rich yet moist crumb. Enjoy with an afternoon cup of tea when your brain needs a break and your soul needs some soothing.

Bread

1 cup (245 g) unsweetened applesauce

½ cup (100 g) granulated sugar

⅓ cup (80 ml) canola oil

2 large eggs

3 tablespoons milk

1 tablespoon grated lemon zest

1 cup (125 g) all-purpose flour

1 cup (120 g) whole wheat flour

2 teaspoons baking powder

1 teaspoon ground cinnamon

½ teaspoon baking soda

½ teaspoon ground nutmeg

1 red apple (such as McIntosh or Jonathan), cored and diced

⅔ cup (75 g) walnuts, toasted and coarsely chopped

Topping

⅓ cup (40 g) walnuts, finely chopped

¼ cup (50 g) brown sugar

½ teaspoon ground cinnamon

1. Preheat the oven to 350°F (180°C). Line a 9 × 5-inch (23 × 13 cm) loaf pan with parchment paper. (This is most easily accomplished by using two pieces of parchment, one to run the length and up the sides and a second to run the width and up the sides.)

2. To make the bread, combine the applesauce, sugar, oil, eggs, milk, and lemon zest in a large bowl, and mix thoroughly. Sift together the all-purpose flour, whole wheat flour, baking powder, cinnamon, baking soda, and nutmeg into a second bowl. Fold the dry ingredients into the applesauce mixture until just combined. Fold in the apple and walnuts. Pour the batter into the pan and spread with a rubber spatula into the corners.

3. To make the topping, combine the walnuts, brown sugar, and cinnamon in a small bowl. Sprinkle the mixture evenly over the batter. Bake for 40 minutes.

4. Cover the pan loosely with foil. Bake for 15 to 35 minutes, until a toothpick inserted in the center comes out clean.

5. Cool in the pan for 10 minutes. Using the parchment paper, lift the loaf out of the pan onto a wire rack. Let cool for 30 minutes before slicing and serving. To store, tightly wrap the bread in wax paper or foil, then wrap with plastic wrap and place in an airtight container in the freezer for up to 3 months.

Serving Size 1 slice; Calories 206; Protein 4 g; Carbs 26 g; Dietary Fiber 2 g; Added Sugars 10 g; Total Fat 10 g; Sat Fat 1 g; Omega-3s 1,110 mg; Sodium 49 mg; Potassium 100 mg

BANANA NUT BREAD

Makes two 9 × 5-inch (23 × 13 cm) loaves

Amy has loved banana bread since childhood, but she doesn't always love the impact it has on her blood sugar. (She's had type 1 diabetes since age 7.) Her search for the "perfect" banana bread led her to develop this "nut nut" version, where almond flour and whole wheat pastry flour replace half of the all-purpose flour. The walnuts offer great flavor, interesting texture, and healthy unsaturated fats like omega-3s. Walnuts are the only nut that provides a significant amount of omega-3 fatty acids.

Cooking spray
¾ cup (150 g) sugar
½ cup (115 g) salted butter, melted
⅔ cup (150 g) plain Greek yogurt
2 large eggs
6 ripe bananas, mashed
2 cups (235 g) chopped walnuts
2 cups (250 g) all-purpose flour
1 cup (95 g) almond flour
1 cup (120 g) whole wheat pastry flour
1 tablespoon baking powder
1 teaspoon baking soda
1 teaspoon kosher salt

1. Preheat the oven to 350°F (180°C). Spray two 9 × 5-inch (23 × 13 cm) loaf pans with cooking spray.

2. Combine the sugar and butter in a large bowl. Whisk together until light and creamy, about 2 minutes. Whisk in the yogurt and eggs, then stir in the bananas and walnuts.

3. Add the all-purpose flour, almond flour, whole wheat pastry flour, baking powder, baking soda, and salt. Stir until the dry ingredients are completely incorporated into the wet mixture, but don't overmix.

4. Divide the batter evenly between the two pans. Bake for 55 to 60 minutes, until a toothpick inserted in the center comes out clean. Let each loaf cool in its pan for 10 minutes before turning out onto a wire rack. Let cool for 30 minutes before slicing and serving. Store sliced bread in a covered container at room temperature for up to 3 days or in the refrigerator for up to 1 week.

Serving Size 1 slice; Calories 233; Protein 6 g; Carbs 27 g; Dietary Fiber 3 g; Added Sugars 6 g; Total Fat 13 g; Sat Fat 3 g; Omega-3s 930 mg; Sodium 172 mg; Potassium 196 mg

CRANBERRY-ORANGE BREAD

Makes one 9 × 5-inch (23 × 13 cm) loaf

This recipe creates a tender crumb and moist loaf with a good contrast between the tartness of the cranberries and the sweet notes from the citrus. Fresh or frozen—but not thawed—cranberries work well here. This bread plus our Citrus-Mint Salad with Ginger-Lime Vinaigrette (page 143) make awesome additions to any brunch menu.

1 cup (125 g) all-purpose flour
1 cup (120 g) whole wheat pastry flour or whole wheat flour
½ cup (100 g) brown sugar
1½ teaspoons baking powder
½ teaspoon baking soda
½ teaspoon ground cinnamon
¼ teaspoon ground cloves
¼ cup (60 g) butter or plant-based spread, melted and cooled
2 large eggs
Grated zest of 1 orange (2 to 3 tablespoons)
Juice of 1 orange (¼ to ⅓ cup/60 to 80 ml)
1½ cups (150 g) firm fresh or frozen cranberries, coarsely chopped
½ cup (60 g) coarsely chopped toasted walnuts or pecans

1. Preheat the oven to 350°F (180°C). Line a 9-inch (23 cm) loaf pan with parchment paper. (This is most easily accomplished by using two pieces of parchment, one to run the length and up the sides and a second to run the width and up the sides.)

2. Sift together the all-purpose flour, whole wheat pastry flour, sugar, baking powder, baking soda, cinnamon, and cloves in a large bowl. Whisk together the butter, eggs, orange zest, and orange juice in a medium bowl. Stir the wet mixture into the dry ingredients until the flour is moistened. Add the cranberries and walnuts to the batter and mix well.

3. Pour the batter into the loaf pan. Bake for 60 minutes, until a toothpick inserted in the center comes out clean. Cool the bread in the pan on a wire rack for 5 minutes, then lift the bread out of the pan and place on the wire rack for 10 minutes to cool before serving. Serve immediately. When completely cooled, seal in an airtight container and store in the refrigerator for up to 1 week. To freeze, tightly wrap the bread in wax paper or foil, then wrap with plastic wrap and place in an airtight container in the freezer for up to 3 months.

Serving Size 1 slice; Calories 174; Protein 3 g; Carbs 27 g; Dietary Fiber 2 g; Added Sugars 12 g; Total Fat 6 g; Sat Fat 2 g; Omega-3s 370 mg; Sodium 73 mg; Potassium 78 mg

FRESH HERB & HONEY BATTER BREAD

Makes one 9 × 5-inch (23 × 13 cm) loaf

This delicious quick bread—that many assume is a yeast bread—is a crusty multigrain loaf that's fast and easy to prepare. Slide this into the oven alongside the casserole you're making and enjoy hot bread with your meal. Our Cauliflower-Walnut Casserole (page 276) is a great option for a meat-free midweek meal.

Cooking spray
1 tablespoon wheat germ
1½ cups (180 g) whole wheat flour
1 cup (125 g) all-purpose flour
½ cup (45 g) quick-cooking rolled oats
⅓ cup (110 g) plus 1 tablespoon honey
1 tablespoon finely grated orange zest
2 teaspoons baking powder
2 teaspoons chopped fresh rosemary
1 teaspoon chopped fresh thyme
½ teaspoon baking soda
1½ cups (360 ml) buttermilk

1 large egg, slightly beaten
2 tablespoons sunflower seeds, plus more for topping, optional

1. Preheat the oven to 350°F (180°C). Spray a 9 × 5-inch (23 × 13 cm) loaf pan with cooking spray. Dust the bottom and sides with the wheat germ.

2. Combine the whole wheat flour, all-purpose flour, oats, ⅓ cup (110 g) of the honey, the orange zest, baking powder, rosemary, thyme, and baking soda in a large bowl until well blended. Add the buttermilk and egg and stir just until everything is moistened. Fold in the sunflower seeds.

3. Pour the batter into the pan. Bake for about 35 minutes. If the top appears to be browning too quickly, cover the pan with foil. Check again after another 10 minutes. Bake for a total of 50 to 60 minutes, until crust is beautifully browned and feels firm to the touch.

4. Cool in the pan for 15 minutes. Remove from the pan and place on a wire rack. Brush the top of the loaf with the remaining 1 tablespoon honey and sprinkle with additional sunflower seeds, if desired. Serve immediately. To store, tightly wrap the bread in wax paper or foil, then wrap with plastic wrap and place in an airtight container in the freezer for up to 3 months.

Serving Size 1 slice; Calories 123; Protein 4 g; Carbs 24 g; Dietary Fiber 2 g; Added Sugars 7 g; Total Fat 2 g; Sat Fat 1 g; Omega-3s 40 mg; Sodium 68 mg; Potassium 102 mg

LEMON-BLUEBERRY BREAD

Makes one 9 × 5-inch (23 × 13 cm) loaf

This delicate, aromatic loaf excites the senses. It's all about lemon—the sweet and tangy lemon flavor, and the ever-so-light lemony glaze. Lemon lovers will agree: You'll want to make this again and again . . .

Bread
Cooking spray
¾ cup (95 g) all-purpose flour
¾ cup (90 g) whole wheat pastry flour or whole wheat flour
2 teaspoon baking powder

½ teaspoon baking soda

¾ cup (150 g) granulated sugar

¼ cup (60 g) butter or plant-based spread, softened

Grated zest of 1 lemon

½ cup (120 ml) milk

1 large egg; slightly beaten

2 tablespoons fresh lemon juice

1½ cups (220 g) fresh or frozen blueberries

Glaze

3 tablespoons confectioners' sugar

1 teaspoon fresh lemon juice

1. Preheat the oven to 350°F (180°C). Line a 9 × 5-inch (23 × 13 cm) loaf pan with parchment paper. Coat the parchment-lined bottom of the pan with cooking spray.

2. To make the bread, combine the flours, baking powder, and baking soda in a medium bowl. Beat the sugar, butter, and lemon zest in a large bowl until light and fluffy. Stir in the milk, egg, and lemon juice. Add the dry ingredients to the wet mixture and mix thoroughly. Gently fold in the blueberries.

3. Pour the batter into the loaf pan and bake for 40 to 50 minutes, until a toothpick inserted in the center comes out clean.

4. Meanwhile, to make the glaze, blend together the confectioners' sugar and lemon juice in a small bowl.

5. Remove the loaf from oven and let rest in the pan for 5 minutes. Lift the bread out of the pan using the parchment paper and place on wire rack. Drizzle or brush the glaze over the hot loaf. Cool on the wire rack for 10 minutes before slicing.

6. Serve immediately or completely cool before storing in an airtight container. The bread can be stored at room temperature for 2 to 3 days, in the refrigerator for 7 days, and in the freezer for 2 months.

VARIATION: *Lemon–Poppy Seed Bread*

Add 2 tablespoons poppy seeds to the dry ingredients and omit the blueberries.

Serving Size 1 slice; Calories 126; Protein 2 g; Carbs 22 g; Dietary Fiber 1 g; Added Sugars 11 g; Total Fat 4 g; Sat Fat 2 g; Omega-3s 30 mg; Sodium 71 mg; Potassium 54 mg

MOLASSES BROWN BREAD

Makes one 9 × 5-inch (23 × 13 cm) loaf

You can serve this mildly sweet, comforting bread fresh out of the oven the day you make it, and then use it as sandwich bread the next day. It is so good with egg salad and butter lettuce!

Cooking spray

½ cup (65 g) all-purpose flour

½ cup (60 g) whole wheat flour

1 teaspoon baking soda

1 teaspoon ground cinnamon

1 large egg

1 cup (90 g) bran cereal (such as Kellogg's All-Bran or bran flakes)

¾ cup (180 ml) very hot water

½ cup (80 g) raisins

⅓ cup (80 ml) molasses

2 tablespoons extra virgin olive oil

1. Adjust an oven rack to the lower middle position. Preheat the oven to 350°F (180°C). Generously coat the bottom of a 9 × 5-inch (23 × 13 cm) loaf pan with cooking spray.

2. Combine the all-purpose flour, whole wheat flour, baking soda, and cinnamon in a large bowl. Beat the egg in another large bowl until foamy. Mix in the bran cereal, water, raisins, molasses, and oil. Add the dry ingredients, stirring only until just combined.

3. Spread the batter evenly in the loaf pan. Bake for 45 minutes or until a toothpick inserted in the center comes out clean. Remove the loaf from the pan to a platter, slice, and serve hot. Cool leftover bread completely before storing in an airtight container at room temperature for 2 to 3 days.

Serving Size 1 slice; Calories 97; Protein 2 g; Carbs 19 g; Dietary Fiber 2 g; Added Sugars 5 g; Total Fat 2 g; Sat Fat 0 g; Omega-3s 30 mg; Sodium 101 mg; Potassium 212 mg

NUTTY APRICOT COTTAGE CHEESE BREAD

Makes one 9 × 5-inch (23 × 13 cm) loaf

Cottage cheese adds protein to this sweet, tender bread that can be served on its own with morning coffee or paired with a glass of milk (for extra protein) and fresh fruit (for, well, more fruit!).

Bread

1½ cups (315 g) reduced fat, small curd cottage cheese

½ cup (100 g) tightly packed light brown sugar

⅓ cup (80 ml) canola oil

2 large eggs

3 tablespoons milk

1 tablespoon grated lemon zest

1 cup (125 g) all-purpose flour

1 cup (120 g) whole wheat flour

2 teaspoons baking powder

1 teaspoon ground cinnamon

½ teaspoon baking soda

½ teaspoon ground nutmeg

1 cup (130 g) finely diced dried apricots

⅔ cup (70 g) chopped pecans, toasted

Topping

⅓ cup (35 g) pecans, finely chopped

¼ cup (50 g) brown sugar

½ teaspoon ground cinnamon

1. Preheat the oven to 350°F (180°C). Line a 9 × 5-inch (23 × 13 cm) loaf pan with parchment paper. (This is most easily accomplished by using two pieces of parchment, one to run the length and up the sides and a second to run the width and up the sides.)

2. To make the bread, combine the cottage cheese, sugar, oil, eggs, milk, and lemon zest in a large bowl and mix thoroughly. Sift together the all-purpose flour, whole wheat flour, baking powder, cinnamon, baking soda, and nutmeg into a medium bowl. Fold the dry ingredients into the cottage cheese mixture until just combined. Fold in the apricots and pecans. Pour the batter into the pan and spread with a rubber spatula into the corners.

3. To make the topping, combine the pecans, brown sugar, and cinnamon in a small bowl. Sprinkle evenly over the batter.

4. Bake for 40 minutes. Cover the pan loosely with foil. Bake for 15 to 35 minutes, until a toothpick inserted in the center comes out clean.

5. Allow the loaf to cool in the pan for 10 minutes. Using the parchment paper, lift the loaf out of the pan onto a wire rack. Let cool for 30 minutes before slicing and serving. Store in an airtight container at room temperature for 2 to 3 days.

Serving Size 1 slice; Calories 222; Protein 6 g; Carbs 28 g; Dietary Fiber 2 g; Added Sugars 9 g; Total Fat 11 g; Sat Fat 1 g; Omega-3s 520 mg; Sodium 112 mg; Potassium 189 mg

PUMPKIN SPICE PEPITA BREAD

Makes one 9 × 5-inch (23 × 13 cm) loaf

Definitely a classic autumn favorite, this bread is alluringly aromatic, spiced with cinnamon, nutmeg, ginger, and cloves. The toasted pepitas add crunch, accent the pumpkin flavor, and boost the nutrition by providing fiber as well as healthy fats. You can swap another pureed squash for the pumpkin, or use 2 teaspoons pumpkin pie spice instead of the cinnamon, nutmeg, and ginger.

Cooking spray

1¾ cups (210 g) whole wheat pastry flour, plus 1 teaspoon

1 teaspoon baking soda

2 teaspoons ground cinnamon

½ teaspoon baking powder

1 teaspoon ground ginger

½ teaspoon ground nutmeg

¼ teaspoon ground cloves

2 large eggs

1 cup (245 g) canned 100% pure pumpkin (not pumpkin pie filling)

1 cup (200 g) sugar

½ cup (120 ml) peanut or canola oil

⅓ cup (80 ml) water

4 tablespoons (30 g) pepitas (pumpkin seeds), toasted

1. Adjust an oven rack to the middle position. Preheat the oven to 350°F (180°C). Generously coat the bottom and sides of a 9 × 5-inch (23 × 13 cm) loaf pan with cooking spray. Dust the bottom of the pan with 1 teaspoon flour.

2. Combine the whole wheat pastry flour, baking soda, cinnamon, baking powder, ginger, nutmeg, and cloves in medium bowl. Whisk the eggs until lemon-colored and frothy in large bowl. Whisk in the pumpkin, sugar, oil, and water until well combined. Add the flour mixture to the pumpkin mixture, whisking until just combined. Use a spoon or rubber spatula to gently fold in 3 tablespoons of the pepitas.

3. Pour the batter into the pan. Sprinkle the remaining 1 tablespoon pepitas on top, gently pushing them down into the batter. Bake for 60 to 75 minutes, until a toothpick inserted in the center comes out clean. Let the loaf cool in the pan on a wire rack for 20 minutes. Remove from the pan and let cool completely on wire rack (for at least 2 hours) before slicing and serving or storing. To store, tightly wrap the bread in wax paper or foil, then wrap with plastic wrap and place in an airtight container. Store at room temperature for up to 2 days, in the refrigerator for up to 1 week, or in the freezer for up to 3 months.

TIP: If you can't find pepitas, you can use pecans in this bread, but we suggest mixing all of them into the batter; pecans can easily burn, which would create off-flavors in the final loaf.

Serving Size 1 slice; Calories 177; Protein 3 g; Carbs 24 g; Dietary Fiber 2 g; Added Sugars 12 g; Total Fat 8 g; Sat Fat 1 g; Omega-3s 10 mg; Sodium 84 mg; Potassium 67 mg

SOUTHWEST CORN BREAD
Makes one 8-inch (20 cm) square loaf

This corn bread gets an extra kick of flavor from the addition of Southwest Seasoning (page 37) as well as corn, onion, chiles, and pimientos. It's a wonderful addition to a meal featuring our Chicken Chili Verde (page 85).

Cooking spray
¾ cup (180 ml) milk
½ cup (115 g) plain Greek yogurt
1 large egg

1 tablespoon honey
1 cup (120 g) stone-ground whole grain yellow cornmeal
¾ cup (90 g) whole wheat flour
½ cup (65 g) all-purpose flour
2 teaspoons baking powder
1 teaspoon Southwest Seasoning (page 37)
½ teaspoon baking soda
1 cup (165 g) fresh or frozen corn kernels
½ cup (55 g) shredded Monterey Jack or cheddar
¼ cup (60 g) butter or plant-based spread, melted
¼ cup (40 g) finely diced onion
2 tablespoons canned diced green chiles, well drained
1 tablespoon chopped pimientos, well drained

1. Preheat the oven to 400°F (200°C). Spray an 8-inch (20 cm) square baking dish with cooking spray.

2. In a medium bowl, beat together the milk, yogurt, egg, and honey. Mix the cornmeal, whole wheat flour, all-purpose flour, baking powder, seasoning, and baking soda in a large bowl. Make a well in the center of the dry ingredients; pour in the wet mixture. Fold the dry ingredients into the wet ingredients until the batter is just combined and evenly moistened. Add the corn, cheese, butter, onion, chiles, and pimientos. Continue folding until the dry ingredients are just moistened. (Overmixing will make the bread tough.)

3. Pour the batter into the baking dish, then smooth out the top with a spatula. Bake for 20 to 25 minutes, until the corn bread is a light golden brown and a toothpick inserted in the center comes out clean. Let cool in the baking dish on a wire rack for 10 minutes. Serve warm. To store, tightly wrap the bread in wax paper or foil, then wrap with plastic wrap and place in an airtight container in the freezer for up to 3 months.

Serving Size 1 slice; Calories 140; Protein 4 g; Carbs 17 g; Dietary Fiber 1 g; Added Sugars 1 g; Total Fat 6 g; Sat Fat 4 g; Omega-3s 40 mg; Sodium 95 mg; Potassium 64 mg

ZUCCHINI-NUT BREAD

Makes one 9 × 5-inch (23 × 13 cm) loaf

This moist and flavorful bread tastes even better the next day. There's no need to peel the zucchini; just trim the ends. Small zucchini make a more flavorful bread, as they have a lower water content and smaller seeds, and they are more tender than larger zucchini.

Cooking spray

1 cup (125 g) all-purpose flour

1 cup (120 g) whole wheat flour

1 teaspoon baking soda

1 teaspoon ground ginger

½ teaspoon baking powder

¼ teaspoon ground nutmeg

1½ cups (185 g) shredded zucchini
(2 to 3 small zucchini)

¾ cup (150 g) sugar

2 large eggs

¼ cup (60 ml) peanut or canola oil

Grated zest of 1 lemon

1 tablespoon fresh lemon juice

½ cup (55 g) chopped toasted pecans or
walnuts

1. Move an oven rack to the low position so the top of the loaf will be in the center of the oven. Preheat the oven to 350°F (180°C). Spray the bottom of a 9 × 5-inch (23 × 13 cm) loaf pan with cooking spray.

2. Mix the all-purpose flour, whole wheat flour, baking soda, ginger, baking powder, and nutmeg in a medium bowl. In a large bowl, whisk together the zucchini, sugar, eggs, oil, lemon zest, and lemon juice. Add the dry ingredients to the zucchini mixture and gently mix until batter is just combined and evenly moistened. Fold the nuts in gently.

3. Pour the batter into the loaf pan. Smooth the top with a rubber spatula. Bake for 50 to 60 minutes, until golden brown and a toothpick inserted in the center comes out clean. Cool for 10 minutes in the pan on a wire rack. Remove the loaf from the pan and cool completely on the wire rack for 2 hours.

4. Slice and serve. To store, tightly wrap the bread in wax paper or foil, then wrap with plastic wrap and place in an airtight container. Store at room temperature for up to 2 days, in the refrigerator for up to 5 days, or in the freezer for up to 3 months.

Serving Size 1 slice; Calories 270; Protein 3 g; Carbs 21 g; Dietary Fiber 2 g; Added Sugars 9 g; Total Fat 20 g; Sat Fat 3 g; Omega-3s 60 mg; Sodium 84 mg; Potassium 82 mg

BEER BREADSTICKS WITH FENNEL

Makes 36 breadsticks

Beer makes these breadsticks fluffy, soft, and flavorful. This is because alcohol interferes with gluten formation, creating a more tender texture and crumb in yeast breads. Any type of beer except nonalcoholic versions, from lagers and pilsners to IPAs, will work well in this recipe. The fennel offers a taste of sweet anise flavor, which makes these breadsticks exceptionally memorable.

¾ cup (180 ml) warm water (105° to 115°F/40°
to 45°C)

Two 0.25-ounce (7 g) packages active dry
yeast

2 teaspoons sugar

3 cups (375 g) all-purpose flour, plus more for
kneading

2 cups (240 g) whole wheat flour

¾ cup (180 ml) beer, at room temperature

¾ cup (180 ml) extra virgin olive oil, plus more
for oiling the bowl

1 tablespoon fennel seeds, toasted and roughly
crushed

1 teaspoon kosher salt

1 large egg, slightly beaten with 1 tablespoon
water, for egg wash

⅓ cup (40 g) sesame seeds

1. Pour the warm water into a large bowl; sprinkle over the yeast and sugar. Let stand for 5 minutes for the sugar to dissolve and the yeast to proof and form bubbles.

2. Whisk together the all-purpose and whole wheat flours in a medium bowl. Whisk the beer, oil, fennel seeds, and salt into the yeast mixture. Beat in 2½ cups (310 g) of the flour mixture, then stir in just enough of the remaining flour mixture to make a soft dough. Turn out the dough onto a floured surface and knead until smooth and elastic, 5 to 6 minutes.

3. Lightly oil a large bowl and place the dough in the bowl, turning once to coat it. Cover the bowl with a damp kitchen towel. Let the dough rise in a warm place until doubled in size, about 30 minutes.

4. Preheat the oven to 350°F (180°C), and line two 12 × 17-inch (30.5 × 43 cm) baking sheets with parchment paper.

5. Punch down the dough, divide it into two parts, and cut each part into 18 equal pieces. Roll each piece of dough into a 6-inch-long (15 cm) rope. Place the ropes 1 inch (2.5 cm) apart on the baking sheets.

6. Use a pastry brush to brush the egg wash gently over the breadsticks. Sprinkle the tops with sesame seeds. Let the breadsticks rise until slightly puffed, about 10 minutes.

7. Bake for 30 to 35 minutes, until golden brown. If both baking sheets don't fit on the same rack of your oven, switch the positions of the baking sheets after about 15 minutes to ensure the breadsticks bake evenly.

8. Place the baking sheets on a wire rack to cool for 5 minutes. Transfer the breadsticks directly onto the wire rack to cool completely. Store in an airtight container at room temperature for up to 3 days or in the freezer for up to 1 month.

Serving Size 1 breadstick; Calories 116; Protein 2 g; Carbs 13 g; Dietary Fiber 1 g; Added Sugars 0 g; Total Fat 6 g; Sat Fat 1 g; Omega-3s 50 mg; Sodium 57 mg; Potassium 46 mg

BUTTERMILK ROLLS

Makes 24 rolls

Warm, yeasty, and deliciously hearty, these rolls ramp up the simplest of meals to something special. Serve with any of our warm soups in the Stocks, Soups & Stews chapter starting on page 68.

- 3 cups (360 g) whole wheat flour
- 3 tablespoons sugar
- 2 teaspoons instant or fast-acting yeast
- ½ teaspoon baking soda
- ½ teaspoon kosher salt
- 1¼ cups (300 ml) cultured buttermilk

- ½ cup (120 ml) water
- 2 tablespoons peanut or canola oil, plus more for oiling the bowl
- 1 to 1½ cups (125 to 190 g) all-purpose flour, plus more for kneading

1. Combine 1½ cups (180 g) of the whole wheat flour, the sugar, yeast, baking soda, and salt in a large bowl. Heat the buttermilk, water, and oil in a saucepan until very warm (120° to 130°F/50° to 55°C). Add the milk mixture to the dry ingredients and beat with a handheld mixer for 3 minutes at medium speed, until the dough comes together. Stir in the remaining whole wheat flour plus enough all-purpose flour to make a soft dough. Stir to incorporate.

2. Turn out the dough onto a floured surface and knead for 5 minutes, or until the dough is smooth and elastic. Lightly oil a large bowl and place the dough in the bowl, turning once to coat it. Cover the bowl with a damp kitchen towel. Let the dough rise in a warm place until doubled in size, 30 to 45 minutes.

3. Preheat the oven to 400°F (200°C). Line two baking sheets with parchment paper.

4. Punch down the dough, then divide it into 24 pieces. Shape each piece into a ball. Place 12 balls on each baking sheet, about 2 inches (5 cm) apart. Cover the dough loosely with damp kitchen towels and let rise in a warm place until almost doubled in size, 20 to 30 minutes.

5. Bake for 15 to 20 minutes, until golden brown and a digital food thermometer reads 190°F (90°C) when inserted in the center of a roll. If both baking sheets don't fit on the same rack of your oven, switch their positions after 8 to 10 minutes to ensure the rolls bake evenly.

6. Cool the rolls on the baking sheets on a wire rack for 5 minutes. Transfer the rolls directly onto the wire rack to cool completely. Store in an airtight container at room temperature for up to 3 days or in the freezer for up to 1 month.

Serving Size 1 roll; Calories 96; Protein 3 g; Carbs 18 g; Dietary Fiber 2 g; Added Sugars 2 g; Total Fat 2 g; Sat Fat 0 g; Omega-3s 10 mg; Sodium 92 mg; Potassium 86 mg

FOUR-GRAIN SUNFLOWER SEED BREAD

Makes one 9 × 5-inch (23 × 13 cm) loaf

This chewy, fiber-rich bread pairs well with the Make-Ahead Layered Salad with Eggs (page 165). It's also a wonderful breakfast bread to toast and spread with your favorite nut butter.

1 cup (120 g) whole wheat flour

½ cup (50 g) rye flour

½ cup (45 g) old-fashioned or quick-cooking rolled oats

¼ cup (30 g) fine yellow cornmeal

3 tablespoons molasses

1 tablespoon peanut or canola oil, plus more for oiling the bowl

1 teaspoon kosher salt

1 cup (240 ml) boiling water

¾ cup (95 g) sunflower seeds

¼ cup (60 ml) warm water (105° to 115°F/40° to 45°C)

One 0.25-ounce (7 g) package active dry yeast

1 to 1¼ cups (125 to 155 g) all-purpose flour

Cooking spray

1. Mix the whole wheat flour, rye flour, oats, cornmeal, molasses, oil, salt, and boiling water in a large bowl. Stir in the sunflower seeds. In a small bowl, stir together the warm water and yeast. Let sit for 5 minutes for the yeast to proof and form bubbles.

2. Stir the yeast mixture into the grain mixture. Gradually stir in the all-purpose flour, adding just enough to make a stiff dough.

3. Turn out the dough onto a floured surface and knead by hand until smooth and elastic, 4 to 5 minutes.

4. Lightly oil a large bowl and place the dough into the bowl, turning once to coat it. Cover the bowl with a damp kitchen towel and let rise in a warm place until it doubles in size, 60 to 90 minutes.

5. Punch down the dough. Then, transfer the dough to a well-floured surface and press or roll it into a 16 × 9-inch (40.5 × 23 cm) rectangle with the short side facing you. Roll the dough toward you (tucking it under as you go) into a taut, firm, cylinder-shaped loaf.

6. Turn the loaf seam side up and pinch it closed with your thumb and forefinger.

7. Spray a 9 × 5-inch (23 × 13 cm) loaf pan with cooking spray. Place the loaf seam side down in the prepared pan, pressing the loaf gently into the corners. Cover with a damp kitchen towel, and let rise again until doubled in size, 40 to 50 minutes.

8. Thirty minutes before baking, adjust an oven rack to the middle position. Preheat the oven to 375°F (190°C). Bake the loaf for 35 to 40 minutes, until deeply browned and a digital food thermometer reads 200°F (95°C) when inserted in the center of the loaf.

9. Cool the bread in the pan on a wire rack for 5 minutes. Remove the bread from the pan and cool directly on the wire rack to room temperature, about 2 hours, before slicing and serving. Wrap in wax paper and store in an airtight container at room temperature for up to 3 days or in the freezer for up to 1 month.

Serving Size 1 slice; Calories 185; Protein 6 g; Carbs 29 g; Dietary Fiber 4 g; Added Sugars 4 g; Total Fat 6 g; Sat Fat 1 g; Omega-3s 20 mg; Sodium 164 mg; Potassium 239 mg

FRESH CHIVE–YOGURT BUNS

Makes 18 buns

You'll receive compliments on these flavorful buns; the slight tang of the yogurt accented with the fresh chives make them delightfully different. Serve alongside the Creamy Asparagus Soup (page 74) or offer at your next brunch. They pair beautifully with scrambled eggs and chèvre.

1 cup (230 g) plain Greek yogurt

1¼ cups (155 g) all-purpose flour

1 cup (120 g) whole wheat flour

One 0.25-ounce (7 g) package active dry yeast

¼ cup (60 ml) warm water (105° to 115°F/40° to 45°C)

¼ cup (12 g) finely chopped fresh chives

1 large egg

2 tablespoons butter or plant-based spread, at room temperature

2 tablespoons sugar

1 teaspoon kosher salt

Cooking spray

1. Heat the yogurt in a small bowl in the microwave at 50% power for 30 seconds, until just lukewarm. Whisk the all-purpose and whole wheat flours together in medium bowl. Dissolve the yeast in the warm water in a large bowl. Let sit for 5 minutes to proof and form bubbles.

2. Add the yogurt, chives, egg, butter, sugar, salt, and 1½ cups (180 g) of the flour mixture to the yeast. Beat until smooth. Add the remaining ¾ cup (95 g) of the flour mixture and continue to beat until a smooth batter has formed. Cover with a clean kitchen towel and let rise in a warm place until doubled in size, about 45 minutes.

3. Spray 18 cups of two regular muffin pans with cooking spray. Stir down the batter, then fill the muffin cups half-full. Pat the top of the batter with floured fingers to level it. (The batter will be sticky-smooth.) Cover loosely with a kitchen towel. Let rise again until the batter reaches the tops of the cups, 20 to 30 minutes.

4. While the batter is rising, adjust an oven rack to the middle position. Preheat the oven to 400°F (200°C). Bake the buns for 15 to 20 minutes, until golden brown and a digital food thermometer reads 200°F (95°C) when inserted in the center of a bun. If both baking sheets don't fit on the same rack of your oven, bake one baking sheet at a time in the lower center rack or adjust oven racks to bake two sheets at one time, switching the positions of the baking sheets after 8 minutes to ensure the buns bake evenly.

5. Cool the buns in the pans on a wire rack for 5 minutes, then transfer the buns directly onto the wire rack to cool completely. Store in an airtight container at room temperature for up to 3 days or in the freezer for up to 1 month.

Serving Size 1 bun; Calories 95; Protein 3 g; Carbs 14 g; Dietary Fiber 1 g; Added Sugars 1 g; Total Fat 3 g; Sat Fat 2 g; Omega-3s 20 mg; Sodium 127 mg; Potassium 40 mg

HARVEST CRESCENTS
Makes 64 crescents

When the first frost of fall arrives and you're inspired to bake something comforting, you'll want to make these sweet potato and raisin crescents. This makes a large batch, perfect for fall and winter holidays when you have a large crowd gathered at your home. For convenience, you can use drained canned sweet potatoes in place of fresh. Orange sweet potatoes will produce the most beautiful color, but white sweet potatoes will also work in this recipe.

One 0.25-ounce (7 g) package active dry yeast

1½ cups (360 ml) warm water (105° to 115°F/40° to 45°C)

1 cup (225 g) butter or plant-based spread, softened

1 cup (245 g) lukewarm mashed plain sweet potatoes (about 2 medium)

½ cup (80 g) raisins or dried currants

⅓ cup (65 g) sugar

2 large eggs, slightly beaten

1½ teaspoons kosher salt

4 cups (500 g) all-purpose flour, plus more for kneading

3 to 3½ cups (360 to 420 g) whole wheat flour

Cooking spray

1. Dissolve the yeast in warm water in a large bowl; let sit for 5 minutes to proof and form bubbles.

2. Stir in ⅔ cup (150 g) of the butter, the sweet potatoes, raisins, sugar, eggs, and salt; mix thoroughly. Whisk the all-purpose and whole wheat flours together in a medium bowl. Add 3 cups (380 g) of the flour mixture to the yeast mixture; beat thoroughly. Stir in enough of the remaining flour to make the dough easy to handle.

3. Turn out the dough onto a lightly floured surface. Knead until smooth and elastic, about 5 minutes, adding enough flour to keep the dough from sticking to the surface.

4. Spray a large bowl with cooking spray, then place the dough in the bowl and lightly spray the top. Cover with a damp kitchen towel. Let rise in a warm place until doubled in size, about 1 hour. (The dough is ready if an indentation remains in the top when

poked.) Proceed to Step 5, or cover tightly and let rest in the refrigerator for 8 hours or up to 3 days. Remove from the refrigerator and bring up to room temperature before continuing.

5. Punch down the dough. Divide it into four equal parts. Roll each part into a 12-inch (30.5 cm) circle. Melt the remaining ⅓ cup (75 g) butter and brush the dough circles lightly. (You'll also use this butter to brush the tops of the crescents.)

6. Line four baking sheets with parchment paper. Cut each circle into 16 wedges using a pizza cutter or sharp knife. Gently stretch each wedge by 1 to 2 inches (2.5 to 5 cm) and then roll up each wedge, beginning at the rounded or wide end and ending at the pointed tip. Tuck the points underneath each roll. Place 16 rolls on each baking sheet; curve the ends of the rolls to form crescent shapes. Brush the tops of the crescents lightly with melted butter. Cover loosely with a kitchen towel and let rise for 1 hour.

7. While the crescents are rising, preheat the oven to 400°F (200°C).

8. Bake for 15 to 20 minutes, until deep golden brown and a digital food thermometer reads 200°F (95°C) when inserted in the center of a crescent. After 8 minutes of baking, lower the oven temperature to 350°F (180°C) to prevent the crescents from burning. Bake one baking sheet at a time in the lower center rack or adjust oven racks to bake two sheets at a time, switching the positions of the baking sheets after 8 minutes to ensure the crescents bake evenly. Repeat until all crescents are baked.

9. Cool the crescents on the baking sheets on wire racks for 5 minutes, then transfer the crescents directly to the wire racks to cool completely. Store in an airtight container or resealable zippered bag at room temperature for up to 3 days or wrapped with foil or plastic wrap and placed in a heavy-duty freezer bag in the freezer for up to 1 month.

Serving Size 1 crescent; Calories 89; Protein 2 g; Carbs 13 g; Dietary Fiber 1 g; Added Sugars 1 g; Total Fat 3 g; Sat Fat 2 g; Omega-3s 30 mg; Sodium 78 mg; Potassium 51 mg

HEARTY WHEAT BUNS
Makes 36 buns

These soft, delicious buns pair perfectly with our Classic Chicken Soup (page 74).

> 1¼ cups (300 ml) lukewarm water
>
> ⅓ cup (80 ml) honey
>
> ¼ cup (60 g) butter or plant-based spread, melted
>
> 3 tablespoons brown sugar
>
> 1 teaspoon kosher salt
>
> ¾ cup (180 ml) milk, heated to about 110°F (45°C)
>
> ½ cup (60 g) wheat germ
>
> Two 0.25-ounce (7 g) packages active dry yeast
>
> ⅓ cup (80 ml) warm water (105° to 115°F/40° to 45°C)
>
> 3 cups (360 g) whole wheat flour
>
> 1 teaspoon baking powder
>
> 3 cups (375 g) all-purpose flour
>
> Peanut or extra virgin olive oil, for oiling the bowl

1. Whisk together the lukewarm water, honey, butter, sugar, and salt in a large bowl. In a small bowl, pour the milk over the wheat germ and cool to lukewarm.

2. Add the milk mixture to the honey-butter mixture and stir to combine. In another small bowl, dissolve the yeast in the warm water to proof and form bubbles and let stand for 5 minutes.

3. Add the yeast mixture to the liquid mixture in the large bowl and mix well with a wooden spoon.

4. Whisk together the whole wheat flour and baking powder in a medium bowl. Add the flour, 1 cup (120 g) at a time, to the liquid ingredients, alternating the whole wheat flour with the all-purpose flour, until the dough is stiff enough to handle. Turn out the dough onto a floured surface and knead until smooth and elastic, about 10 minutes, adding more flour as needed.

5. Lightly oil a large bowl and place the dough in the bowl, turning once to coat it. Cover the bowl with a damp kitchen towel and let rise in a warm place until doubled in size.

6. Line three baking sheets with parchment paper. Punch down the dough and turn out onto a clean, very lightly floured surface. Using a knife, cut the dough into 4 equal sections. Cut each section into 9 pieces of dough and shape into 36 buns. Place 12 buns onto each baking sheet, about 2 inches (5 cm) apart. Cover loosely with damp kitchen towels. Let rise again until almost doubled in size, about 30 minutes.

7. While the buns are rising, preheat the oven to 350°F (180°C).

8. Bake each sheet of 12 buns for 10 to 15 minutes, until nicely browned and a digital food thermometer reads 200°F (95°C) when inserted in the center of a roll. Cool the buns on the baking sheets on wire racks for 5 minutes, then transfer the buns directly to the wire racks to cool completely. Store in an airtight container at room temperature for up to 3 days or in the freezer for up to 1 month.

Serving Size 1 bun; Calories 107; Protein 3 g; Carbs 20 g; Dietary Fiber 2 g; Added Sugars 4 g; Total Fat 2 g; Sat Fat 1 g; Omega-3s 30 mg; Sodium 68 mg; Potassium 76 mg

HONEY WHOLE WHEAT BREAD

Makes three 8 × 4-inch (20 × 10 cm) loaves

Amy started making honey whole wheat bread with her mom when she was 10 years old, first helping her mom clean wheat kernels from the wheat grown on their farm before grinding them to make flour. This soft yet firm loaf makes wonderful bread for sandwiches. Amy loves using it for open-faced fried egg sandwiches with avocado for breakfast.

4 cups (480 g) whole wheat flour

3½ teaspoons instant or fast-acting yeast

1 teaspoon kosher salt

3 cups (720 ml) milk

½ cup (170 g) honey

2 tablespoons extra virgin olive oil, plus more for oiling the bowl

1 large egg

4½ to 5 cups (565 to 625 g) all-purpose flour, plus more for kneading

Cooking spray

1. Combine 3 cups (360 g) of the whole wheat flour, the yeast, and salt in a large bowl. Whisk together the milk, honey, and oil in a microwave-safe bowl. Microwave on HIGH for about 90 seconds, until warm, then pour over the flour mixture and mix well. Add the egg and whisk well, then add the remaining whole wheat flour. Stir in the all-purpose flour, 1 cup (125 g) at a time, until the mixture forms a stiff dough. Turn out the dough onto a floured surface and knead until smooth and elastic, about 7 minutes.

2. Lightly oil a large bowl and place the dough in the bowl, turning once to coat it. Cover the bowl with a damp kitchen towel and let the dough rise in a warm place until doubled in size, 45 to 60 minutes.

3. Spray three 8 × 4-inch (20 × 10 cm) loaf pans with cooking spray. Punch down the dough, then divide into thirds. Transfer one portion of the dough at a time to a well-floured surface. Press or roll it into a 16 × 8-inch (40.5 × 23 cm) rectangle with the short side facing you. Roll the dough toward you (tucking it under as you go) into a taut, firm, cylinder-shaped loaf. Turn the the loaf seam side up and pinch it closed with your thumb and forefinger. Repeat with the remaining two pieces of dough. Place each loaf in a pan, seam side down, cover with damp kitchen towels, and let them rise until doubled in size, 30 to 45 minutes.

4. Place the loaves in a cold oven and turn on the oven to 400°F (200°C). Bake for 10 minutes, then reduce the oven temperature to 375°F (190°C) and bake for 30 minutes or until golden and a digital food thermometer reads 200°F (95°C) when inserted in the center of the loaf.

5. Cool the loaves in the pans on a wire rack for 5 minutes. Remove the loaves from the pans and let cool to room temperature directly on the wire rack for about 2 hours before slicing and serving. Wrap in plastic wrap or wax paper and store in an airtight container at room temperature for up to 3 days or in the freezer for up to 1 month.

Serving Size 1 slice; Calories 139; Protein 4 g; Carbs 27 g; Dietary Fiber 2 g; Added Sugars 4 g; Total Fat 2 g; Sat Fat 0 g; Omega-3s 20 mg; Sodium 64 mg; Potassium 106 mg

POTATO DINNER ROLLS

Makes 24 dinner rolls

Rolls like these appear frequently on Sunday dinner tables in the Red River Valley of North Dakota and in west central Minnesota where Amy and Linda grew up, respectively. The dinner rolls often were paired with roast beef or pork, steamed vegetables from the garden, simple green salads, and pickled cucumbers, beets, green beans, or asparagus. Today we serve these delicious tender rolls with our Red Lentil & Vegetable Soup (page 79) or Potato-Leek Soup (page 79), perfect for sopping up the last drop in the bowl.

- 1½ cups (225 g) russet-type potatoes, peeled and cubed (2 medium)
- 4 cups (960 ml) water
- Two 0.25-ounce (7 g) packages active dry yeast (see Tip)
- 2 large eggs, lightly beaten
- ¼ cup (60 g) butter or plant-based spread, melted
- ¼ cup (50 g) sugar
- 2 teaspoons kosher salt
- 4 to 5 cups (500 to 625 g) all-purpose flour, plus more for kneading
- 2 cups (240 g) whole wheat flour
- Cooking spray

1. Place the potatoes in a medium pot with the water. Boil the potatoes until soft and well cooked, 10 to 12 minutes. Drain well, reserving 1½ cups (360 ml) of the potato water in a large bowl. Mash the potatoes with a potato masher or fork. Measure out 1 firmly packed cup (230 g). Let cool to lukewarm. (Save any additional potatoes for thickening a soup or eating on their own.) Let the potato water cool until warm (about 110°F/45°C).

2. Dissolve the yeast in the potato water and let stand for 10 minutes to proof and form bubbles.

3. Add the eggs, butter, sugar, salt, and mashed potatoes to the yeast mixture and mix thoroughly. Add 2 cups (250 g) of the all-purpose flour and the whole wheat flour and beat until well combined. Mix in enough of the remaining all-purpose flour to make the dough easy to handle.

4. Turn out the dough onto a lightly floured surface and knead for 5 minutes or until smooth and elastic. Spray a large bowl with cooking spray, then shape the dough into a ball and place in the bowl. Spray the top of the dough with cooking spray. Cover with a damp kitchen towel and let rise at room temperature until almost doubled in size, about 45 minutes.

5. Punch down the dough and turn it out onto a clean surface, dusting with flour only if the dough is too sticky to handle. Gently cut the dough in half, then cut each half into 12 pieces, making a total of 24 pieces.

6. Line two rimmed baking sheets with parchment paper. Shape each piece of dough into a smooth, even, taut ball. If the dough sticks to your hands, dust your fingers lightly with flour. Arrange 12 rolls on each baking sheet, about 2 inches (5 cm) apart. Cover each pan loosely with a damp kitchen towel and let the dough rise until doubled in size, 30 to 40 minutes.

7. While the rolls rise, adjust an oven rack to the upper-middle position and preheat the oven to 400°F (200°C). Bake one sheet for 12 to 15 minutes, until golden brown and a digital food thermometer reads 200°F (95°C) when inserted in the center of a roll.

8. Cool the first batch of rolls on the pan on a wire rack for 5 minutes. Transfer the rolls directly to the wire rack to continue cooling or serve immediately. Bake and cool the second sheet. Store in an airtight container or resealable zippered bag at room temperature for up to 3 days or wrapped with foil or plastic wrap and placed in a heavy-duty freezer bag in the freezer for up to 1 month.

TIP: *If you only have instant yeast on hand, use 1 tablespoon instant yeast to replace the 2 packets of active dry yeast. Skip Step 2 and instead add the yeast directly to the dry ingredients in Step 3. Use the same amount of potato water.*

Serving Size 1 roll; Calories 163; Protein 5 g; Carbs 30 g; Dietary Fiber 2 g; Added Sugars 2 g; Total Fat 3 g; Sat Fat 1 g; Omega-3s 30 mg; Sodium 184 mg; Potassium 96 mg

PUMPERNICKEL BREAD

Makes 2 loaves

This bread is easy to make and very flavorful! We encourage you to enjoy one loaf directly from the oven and use the other loaf to serve with Borsht (page 73).

- 2 cups (250 g) all-purpose flour, plus more for kneading
- 1 tablespoon plus 2 teaspoons instant or fast-acting yeast
- 1 tablespoon caraway seeds, crushed
- ½ teaspoon aniseed, crushed
- ½ teaspoon fennel seeds, crushed
- 1½ cups (360 ml) very warm water (115° to 120°F/45° to 50°C)
- ½ cup (120 ml) light or mild-flavored molasses (such as Grandma's unsulphured)
- 2 tablespoons peanut or canola oil
- 1 tablespoon kosher salt
- 2 cups (255 g) dark rye flour
- ¾ to 1 cup (90 to 120 g) whole wheat flour
- Cooking spray
- Cornmeal

1. Combine the all-purpose flour, yeast, caraway seeds, aniseed, and fennel seeds in a large bowl. Whisk together the warm water, molasses, oil, and salt in a medium bowl. Add to the flour mixture. Stir with a wooden spoon for 3 minutes, until thoroughly mixed. Stir in the rye flour and as much of the whole wheat flour you can mix in with the spoon. Stir until the dough comes together and looks lumpy, yet well-mixed.

2. Turn out the dough onto a clean, floured surface and knead in the remaining whole wheat flour to form a moderately stiff, smooth, and elastic dough, 6 to 8 minutes.

3. Lightly spray a large bowl with cooking spray. Shape the dough into a ball and place it in the bowl; lightly spray the surface of dough. Cover with a damp kitchen towel and let rise in a warm place until the dough doubles in size, 90 minutes to 2 hours.

4. Spray two baking sheets with cooking spray and sprinkle lightly with cornmeal. Punch down the dough and divide it in half. Cover each dough ball with a damp kitchen towel and let rest for 10 minutes. Shape into 2 round loaves by flattening each piece of dough into a circular shape about 8 to 9 inches (20 to 23 cm) in diameter with your hands. Begin shaping the loaf by bringing the outside edges into the center and pressing in. Go around the entire circle, folding and pressing the edges into the center, repeating two to three times until you have a smooth round ball. Pinch the bottom and place the ball seam side down on the prepared pan. Repeat with the second piece of dough. Spray each ball lightly with oil or cooking spray. Cover loosely with damp kitchen towels and let rise in a warm place until nearly doubled in size, 30 to 40 minutes.

5. While the loaves are rising, preheat the oven to 350°F (180°C).

6. Bake for 35 to 40 minutes, until well browned and a digital food thermometer reads 200°F (95°C) when inserted in the center of a loaf.

7. Cool the loaves completely on a wire rack for about 2 hours before slicing and serving or storing. Wrap in wax paper and store in an airtight container at room temperature for 3 to 4 days or in the freezer for up to 1 month.

Serving Size 1 slice; Calories 86; Protein 2 g; Carbs 17 g; Dietary Fiber 1 g; Added Sugars 5 g; Total Fat 1 g; Sat Fat 0 g; Omega-3s 10 mg; Sodium 140 mg; Potassium 143 mg

SODIUM TIP: Using Diamond Crystal Kosher Salt will dramatically reduce the sodium in any recipe that uses kosher salt. This salt contains 50% less sodium per measure than regular kosher salt and 60% less than fine grain table salt.

WHOLE WHEAT FRENCH BAGUETTE

Makes 3 loaves; 36 slices

This whole wheat version of the classic French baguette is even better and crisper if baked on an ungreased, shiny, foil-lined pan with a pan of hot water on the oven rack below. Serve with Salad Niçoise (page 166).

One 0.25-ounce (7 g) package active dry yeast

1 tablespoon honey

3 cups (720 ml) lukewarm water

5 cups (625 g) all-purpose flour, plus more for kneading

1 tablespoon peanut or canola oil, plus more for oiling the bowl

1½ teaspoons kosher salt

2 cups (230 g) wheat germ

2 cups (240 g) whole wheat flour

2 tablespoons cornmeal

Cooking spray

1. In a large bowl, dissolve the yeast and honey in the lukewarm water. Let sit for 10 minutes to proof and form bubbles.

2. Mix 3 cups (375 g) of the all-purpose flour, 1 cup (125 g) at a time, into the yeast mixture. Stir the batter until all the flour is well incorporated. Cover with a damp kitchen towel and set in a warm place for 30 minutes to allow the flour to absorb the liquid.

3. Stir in the oil and salt. Add 1 cup (115 g) of the wheat germ and mix thoroughly. Mix in 1 cup (120 g) of the whole wheat flour. Repeat with the remaining 1 cup of wheat germ and the remaining 1 cup of whole wheat flour, thoroughly mixing after each addition. The dough should be stiff enough to turn out but still be sticky. Turn it out onto a floured surface and knead for 10 minutes, adding as much of the remaining 2 cups (250 g) of all-purpose flour as necessary to make the dough smooth and elastic. Shape the dough into a ball.

4. Lightly oil a large bowl and place the dough in the bowl, turning once to coat it. Cover the bowl tightly with a damp kitchen towel. Let the dough rise in a warm place until doubled in size, about 60 minutes.

5. Punch down the dough and let rise until doubled in size, 30 to 45 minutes.

6. Turn out the dough onto a floured surface. Divide it into thirds. Transfer one portion of the dough at a time to a lightly floured surface. Flatten the dough into a small circle until it is even. Fold the dough over, then lightly flour your hands. Roll the dough back and forth using the palms of both hands from the center out, making a cylinder-like shape (baguette) that is about 12 inches (30 cm) long. Repeat with the remains two portions of dough.

7. Line two baking sheets with parchment paper and sprinkle each lightly with cornmeal. Place 2 loaves on one baking sheet, about 5 inches (13 cm) apart, and place the third loaf on the second baking sheet. Slash the loaves ½-inch deep (13 mm) diagonally at 3-inch (7.5 cm) intervals with a sharp paring knife. Mist the loaves with cooking spray, cover loosely with damp kitchen towels, and let rise in a warm place until the dough is nearly doubled in size and barely springs back when poked with your knuckle, 60 to 90 minutes.

8. When the loaves have risen for about 30 minutes, adjust the oven racks to the middle and bottom positions and preheat the oven to 400°F (200°C).

9. Bring a kettle of water to a boil. Place a large baking pan on the bottom rack, then pour in boiling water. Place one pan at a time on the middle rack and bake for 15 to 20 minutes, until the crust is golden brown and a digital food thermometer reads 200°F (95°C) when inserted in the center of a loaf.

10. Transfer the loaves directly to a wire rack and let cool for 30 minutes before slicing and serving or storing. Wrap in wax paper and store in an airtight container at room temperature for up to 4 days or in the freezer for up to 1 month.

Serving Size 1 slice; Calories 116; Protein 4 g; Carbs 22 g; Dietary Fiber 2 g; Added Sugars 0 g; Total Fat 1 g; Sat Fat 0 g; Omega-3s 60 mg; Sodium 40 mg; Potassium 103 mg

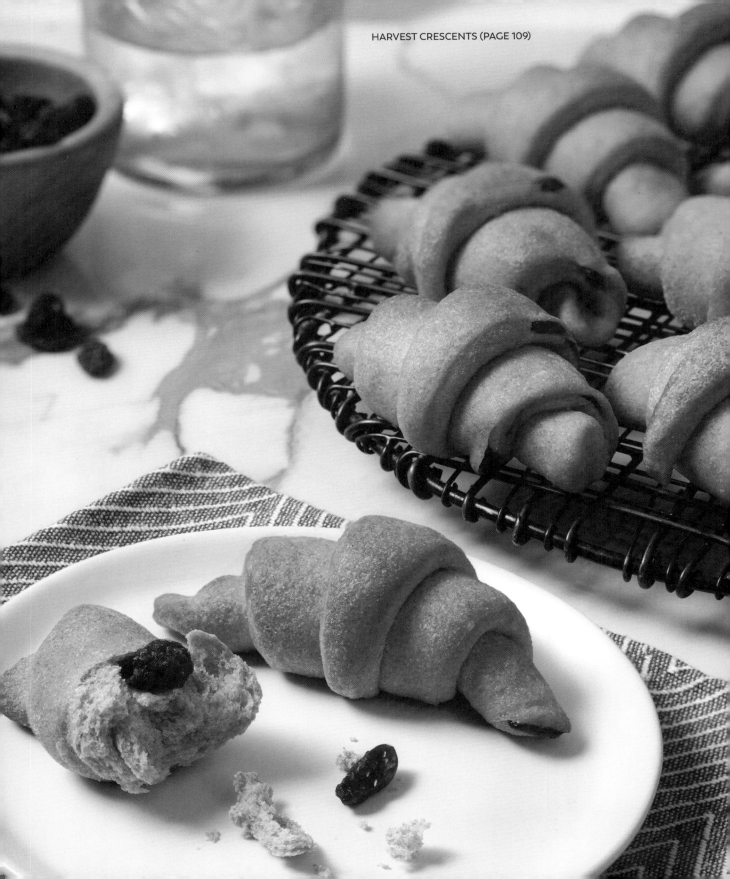

HARVEST CRESCENTS (PAGE 109)

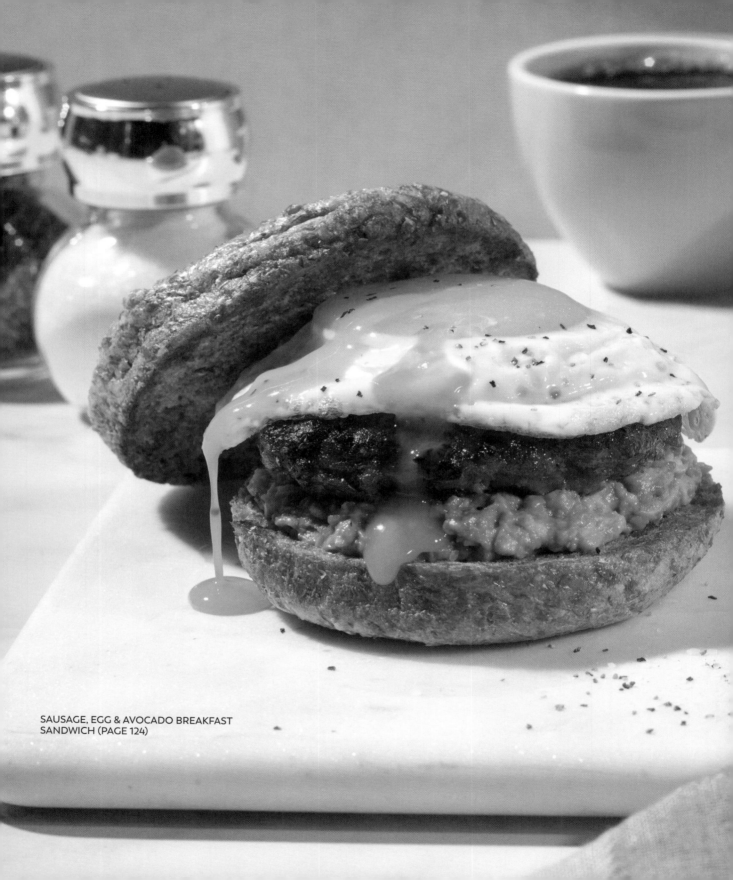

SAUSAGE, EGG & AVOCADO BREAKFAST
SANDWICH (PAGE 124)

CHAPTER 7

Breakfast & Brunch

Breakfast & Brunch

Savory

Bean & Baby Kale Frittata 119

Bulgur Breakfast Porridge
with Sausage. 120

Cheddar-Pepper Popovers 120

Garlic & Rosemary Egg Bites
with Gruyère 121

Hot Curried Egg Bites 121

Mediterranean Oats with
Cucumbers and Olives. 122

Mexican-Inspired Egg &
Veggie Skillet 122

Potato-Cheddar Breakfast
Casserole. 123

Quinoa-Veggie Egg Bites 123

Sausage, Egg & Avocado Breakfast
Sandwiches 124

Spicy Sage Breakfast Sausage 124

Shiitake & Spinach Quiche
with Rosemary & Sage 125

Spinach Scramble Pita Pockets. 127

Tomato-Topped Veggie-Egg Bake 127

Sweet

Apple-Cinnamon Compote 128

Apple-Cinnamon Pancakes 128

Apple Dutch Baby. 129

Banana Oat Blueberry
Breakfast Bars. 129

Barley with Stone Fruit 130

Carrot & Fig Oats with Pistachios 130

Chocolate Energy Bars 131

Cinnamon & Ginger Granola 131

Ginger-Pear Compote 132

Honey Whole Wheat Waffles. 132

Icelanders in America Cereal 133

Mango-Coconut Overnight Oats with
Macadamia Nuts 133

Millet Morning Cakes. 134

Mixed Berry Compote 134

Pumpkin Butter. 135

Pumpkin Spice Oats with Pecans. 135

Strawberry Pancakes. 135

Super Seeds Protein Power Bars. 136

Smoothies

Super Smoothie Secrets 137

Apricot-Chickpea Smoothie. 138

Berry-Turmeric Smoothie 138

Kefir, Spinach & Avocado Smoothie 139

Mango Tofu Soy Milk Smoothie. 139

This chapter is for breakfast and brunch lovers. We've included recipes for quick breakfast "grab and go" options like egg bites, energy bars, and smoothies, but we also incorporated many recipes for those leisurely mornings when you have time to sit and enjoy a few quiet moments. Many of these dishes reheat beautifully: On day one you can enjoy a just-prepared breakfast, and on day two you can quickly eat yummy leftovers.

We drew inspiration from many cuisines and cultures in the flavor profiles for our savory recipes, and we feature many egg recipes. Eggs are a convenient, affordable, versatile nutrient-rich food. If you're striving to eat more vegetables at breakfast, eggs are a gateway ingredient to greater vegetable consumption. The protein in eggs, dairy products like yogurt, milk, and cheese, and dark leafy greens helps extend the energy our bodies create from carbohydrates in food. Combining protein-rich foods with slow carbs from foods like whole grains and legumes can help sustain your energy level throughout the morning.

Most of our breakfast recipes make four servings, but the sweet and savory oatmeal recipes are all one-serving recipes.

If you're not a breakfast eater, we encourage you to start eating breakfast. Why? While there are many potential nutrition benefits associated with eating breakfast (e.g., a higher likelihood of meeting daily calcium, fiber, and fruit and vegetable needs), there's a growing body of research showing the significant risks of skipping breakfast, including increased risks of becoming overweight or obese, and developing type 2 diabetes and cardiovascular disease. Keep in mind that eating breakfast doesn't have to mean eating typical breakfast foods; if you fall in love with other recipes in this book, eat them for your breakfast!

BEAN & BABY KALE FRITTATA

Makes 6 servings

This recipe adapts well to many types of beans, dark leafy greens, and seasonings. Try pairing pinto beans with Swiss chard and Southwest Seasoning (page 37), or red kidney beans and spinach with Curry Powder (page 32).

- 4 shallots, thinly sliced
- 1 orange bell pepper, seeded and thinly sliced
- 3 garlic cloves, minced
- 2 tablespoons extra virgin olive oil
- 2 cups (30 g) baby kale, chopped
- 1 cup (175 g) Simply Cooked White Beans (page 241)
- 8 large eggs
- ½ cup (120 ml) milk
- 1 tablespoon Italian Seasoning (page 34)
- 2 ounces (57 g) shredded Gruyère
- Chopped fresh parsley or cilantro

1. Preheat the oven to 350°F (180°C).

2. In a 10-inch (25.5 cm) oven-safe or cast-iron skillet with a lid, sauté the shallots, bell pepper, and garlic in the oil for 3 minutes, until soft. Add the kale and sauté until wilted, about 5 minutes. Add the beans and sauté for another 2 to 3 minutes to heat them.

3. In a medium bowl, whisk together the eggs, milk, and seasoning. Pour the egg mixture into the skillet and use a spatula to spread it evenly over the vegetables. Cover and cook on medium to low heat until the sides are set but the center is still runny, about 5 minutes.

4. Remove the lid, transfer the pan to the oven, and bake for 15 to 20 minutes, until the edges brown and puff and the middle has a slight wiggle.

5. Sprinkle over the Gruyère and bake for another 3 minutes, until the cheese is just melted. Garnish with parsley, cut into 6 wedges, and serve hot. Store in a wax paper–lined airtight container in the refrigerator for up to 3 days. Do not freeze.

Per Serving: Calories 354; Protein 20 g; Carbs 35 g; Dietary Fiber 17 g; Added Sugars 0 g; Total Fat 17 g; Sat Fat 5 g; Omega-3s 530 mg; Sodium 181 mg; Potassium 916 mg

BULGUR BREAKFAST PORRIDGE WITH SAUSAGE

Makes 4 servings

In addition to eating more vegetables, we also encourage people to choose more whole grains at breakfast. Here we introduce bulgur as a savory breakfast offering with sausage, apples, raisins, and nuts. The only other item you need to complete this meal is a spoon!

- 3 cups (550 g) Simply Cooked Bulgur (page 224)
- 1 cup (240 ml) plus 1 tablespoon water
- 6 ounces (170 g) cooked chicken and apple sausage, thinly sliced or cubed
- 1 apple, cored and diced
- ¼ cup (40 g) raisins
- 2 teaspoons ground cinnamon
- ¼ cup (35 g) Savory Roasted Mixed Nuts (page 347)

1. Combine the cooked bulgur and 1 cup (240 ml) of the water in a saucepan over medium heat. Gently warm the bulgur mixture, stirring occasionally, to create a thick, warm porridge, 4 to 5 minutes.

2. Heat the sausages with 1 tablespoon water in a medium skillet over medium heat. When the water has evaporated and the sausages are nicely browned, add the apple, raisins, and 1 teaspoon of the cinnamon. Reduce the heat and cook until the apples are softened slightly and the cinnamon is fragrant, about 3 minutes.

3. To serve, divide the porridge among four bowls. Top each bowl with one-fourth of the sausage-fruit mixture, and sprinkle each bowl with ¼ teaspoon cinnamon and 1 tablespoon of the nuts.

Per Serving: Calories 338; Protein 12 g; Carbs 46 g; Dietary Fiber 7 g; Added Sugars 0 g; Total Fat 14 g; Sat Fat 3 g; Omega-3s 90 mg; Sodium 456 mg; Potassium 461 mg

CHEDDAR-PEPPER POPOVERS

Makes 6 popovers

These are an easy quick bread to make for breakfast or brunch. Fans of British fare may recognize them as similar to Yorkshire pudding. They are best served hot, right out of the oven, enjoyed on their own or served with soft scrambled eggs and fresh fruit for a lovely, leisurely breakfast or brunch. Did someone say "Mimosas!"?

- 2½ tablespoons extra virgin olive oil
- 1 cup (240 ml) milk
- 2 large eggs
- 1 cup (120 g) whole wheat pastry flour
- ½ teaspoon kosher salt
- 1 teaspoon coarsely ground black pepper
- 2 ounces (57 g) sharp white cheddar, finely grated

1. Set an oven rack in the center position. Preheat the oven to 400°F (200°C) Add ¼ teaspoon oil each to 6 cups of a regular muffin pan.

2. In a 4-cup (1L) glass measuring cup with a spout, heat the milk in the microwave for 45 seconds on HIGH until lukewarm. Whisk in the eggs and the remaining 2 tablespoons oil. (You can also make the batter in a medium bowl, but the measuring cup will make it easier to pour the batter into the muffin cups.) Whisk in the flour, salt, and pepper. It's okay if the batter is a bit lumpy.

3. Place the muffin pan in the oven to heat for 3 minutes. Carefully remove the pan from the oven. Stir the batter, then divide it evenly among the 6 muffin cups, filling each cup nearly full. Top each with about 1 tablespoon cheddar.

4. Bake for 28 to 30 minutes, until the popovers are dark brown and have risen slightly above the top of the muffin pan. Serve warm.

Serving size 1 popover; Calories 207; Protein 8 g; Carbs 17 g; Dietary Fiber 2 g; Added Sugars 0 g; Total Fat 12 g; Sat Fat 4 g; Omega-3s 100 mg; Sodium 254 mg; Potassium 142 mg

GARLIC & ROSEMARY EGG BITES WITH GRUYÈRE

Makes 6 servings

Anyone who loves the flavor of rosemary will love these egg bites, which also have a subtle nutty flavor note from Gruyère. Serve with fresh mandarin oranges, plums, or sweet, juicy apricots and Lemon Blueberry Bread (page 102) at your next brunch.

Cooking spray

1 tablespoon olive oil

2 or 3 green onions, thinly sliced

2 garlic cloves, minced

2 cups (60 g) chopped fresh spinach leaves

6 to 8 grape tomatoes, quartered

1 tablespoon minced fresh rosemary

½ teaspoon ground thyme

¼ teaspoon freshly ground black pepper

6 large eggs

½ cup (125 g) part-skim ricotta

¼ cup (25 g) grated Gruyère

1. Preheat the oven to 350°F (180°C). Coat the cups of a regular 12-cup muffin pan with cooking spray.

2. Combine the oil, green onions, and garlic in a medium skillet over medium-high heat. Sauté for 30 to 45 seconds, until the green parts of the onions become brighter in color and slightly wilted and the garlic softens. Add the spinach and sauté until wilted, 30 seconds. Stir in the tomatoes, rosemary, thyme, and pepper. Reduce the heat to medium-low and cook until any extra liquid evaporates and the herbs become aromatic, 1 minute. Distribute the vegetables evenly among the muffin cups.

3. Whisk the eggs and ricotta in a medium bowl to combine, then pour over the vegetables, filling each cup to the top.

4. Bake for 20 minutes. Top each egg bite with 1 teaspoon of the Gruyère. Bake for 5 to 10 minutes, until the egg bites are firm, rounded, and brown around their edges and the Gruyère has melted and browned. Cool in the pan on a wire rack for 10 minutes. Use a knife to loosen the egg bites, then remove each bite from its cup with a small fork. Serve warm.

TIP: *You can refrigerate or freeze the egg bites by layering them with wax paper in an airtight container. Refrigerated egg bites should be eaten within 3 days; they can be heated in a microwave for 30 seconds on MEDIUM-HIGH. Egg bites can be stored in the freezer for up to 1 month and reheated in the microwave for 60 to 90 seconds on MEDIUM-HIGH.*

Serving Size 2 egg bites; Calories 155; Protein 10 g; Carbs 4 g; Dietary Fiber 1 g; Added Sugars 0 g; Total Fat 10 g; Sat Fat 4 g; Omega-3s 160 mg; Sodium 180 mg; Potassium 150 mg

HOT CURRIED EGG BITES

Makes 6 servings

If you like heat, these egg bites are for you! Ginger and jalapeños offer a punch of flavor that will definitely help wake you up in the morning. Enjoy these egg bites with your favorite 100% juice and warm whole wheat naan.

Cooking spray

1 tablespoon olive oil

2 or 3 green onions, thinly sliced

¼ cup (35 g) finely diced red or green bell pepper

2 garlic cloves, minced

2 tablespoons minced jalapeño or serrano chile

½ teaspoon grated or minced fresh ginger

2 cups (60 g) chopped fresh spinach leaves

½ teaspoon Curry Powder (page 32)

¼ teaspoon freshly ground black pepper

6 large eggs

½ cup (125 g) part-skim ricotta

¼ cup (4 g) chopped fresh cilantro leaves

1. Preheat the oven to 350°F (180°C). Coat the cups of a regular 12-cup muffin pan with cooking spray.

2. Combine the oil, green onions, bell pepper, garlic, jalapeño, and ginger in a medium skillet over medium-high heat. Sauté until the green parts of onions become brighter in color and slightly wilted and the peppers have softened, 1 to 2 minutes. Add the spinach and sauté until wilted, 30 seconds. Stir in the curry powder and black pepper. Reduce the heat to medium-low, and cook until any extra liquid evaporates and the herbs become aromatic, 30 seconds. Distribute the vegetables evenly among the muffin cups.

3. Whisk the eggs and ricotta in a medium bowl to combine, then pour over the vegetables, filling each muffin cup to the top.

4. Bake for 25 to 30 minutes, until the egg bites are firm, rounded, and brown around their edges. Cool the egg bites in the pan on a wire rack for 10 minutes, then sprinkle with the cilantro. Use a knife to loosen the egg bites, then remove each bite from its cup with a small fork. Serve warm. See the Tip on page 121 for storage and reheating instructions.

Serving Size 2 egg bites; Calories 131; Protein 9 g; Carbs 3 g; Dietary Fiber 1 g; Added Sugars 0 g; Total Fat 8 g; Sat Fat 2 g; Omega-3s 160 mg; Sodium 91 mg; Potassium 134 mg

MEDITERRANEAN OATS WITH CUCUMBERS & OLIVES

Makes 1 serving

Like our Carrot & Fig Oats with Pistachios (page 130), this is a sophisticated take on a morning bowl of oatmeal. This recipe can also be made with whole wheat couscous by simply swapping dry couscous for the rolled oats.

½ cup (45 g) quick-cooking rolled oats
1 cup (240 ml) water, plus more if needed
½ cup (15 g) chopped fresh spinach
¼ cup (45 g) chopped fresh tomato
2 tablespoons shredded part-skim mozzarella
1 teaspoon Italian Seasoning (page 34)
Freshly ground black pepper
2 tablespoons diced cucumber
1 tablespoon chopped pitted kalamata olives
1 tablespoon extra virgin olive oil
Pinch of kosher salt

1. Combine the oats and water in a medium microwave-safe bowl. Microwave for 1 minute on HIGH power. Stir in the spinach, tomatoes, mozzarella, seasoning, and a few grinds of pepper. Microwave for up to 1 minute on HIGH, watching to make sure the oatmeal doesn't boil over. Let stand for 30 seconds before removing from the microwave.

2. The oatmeal will be thick, so stir in more water if you like a thinner consistency. Top with the cucumber and olives, and drizzle over the oil. Add a pinch of salt.

Per Serving: Calories 403; Protein 13 g; Carbs 37 g; Dietary Fiber 5 g; Added Sugars 0 g; Total Fat 23 g; Sat Fat 6 g; Omega-3s 180 mg; Sodium 222 mg; Potassium 484 mg

MEXICAN-INSPIRED EGG & VEGGIE SKILLET

Makes 4 servings

If you're striving to eat more veggies, getting multiple servings at breakfast is one smart strategy to reach your daily intake goals. This recipe provides about 2 cups of vegetables per portion, which when combined with high-quality protein from eggs is a wonderful start to any day!

1 teaspoon cumin seeds
1 tablespoon extra virgin olive oil
1 large white onion, diced
1 zucchini, diced
1 poblano chile, diced
1 jalapeño chile, diced
1 bunch cilantro, stems minced, leaves chopped for serving
½ teaspoon kosher salt
One 15-ounce (425 g) can black beans, drained and rinsed
One 14.5-ounce (411 g) can diced tomatoes with jalapeños
2 cups (330 g) frozen white corn kernels
½ teaspoon ground chipotle chile pepper
4 large eggs

1. Heat a large sauté pan or skillet over medium-high heat for 30 seconds, then add the cumin seeds. Dry-toast the cumin until it begins to perfume the air, 30 seconds. Reduce the heat to medium and add the oil, followed by the onion, zucchini, poblano, jalapeño, cilantro stems, and salt. Sauté until the vegetables have softened, the zucchini has released its moisture, and the poblano has turned a dark glossy green, 10 to 12 minutes.

2. Add the beans, tomatoes, corn, and ground chipotle. Stir well, cover, and cook until the vegetables are simmering gently, 8 to 10 minutes.

3. Use a large spoon to create four "cups" (indentations) in the vegetables. (Liquid should seep back into the cups.) Crack one egg into each cup, cover, and cook until the egg whites are opaque, 5 to 6 minutes. The yolks may still be soft; cook longer if you like your egg yolks cooked to a firmer consistency.

4. Divide the eggs and vegetables among four bowls, top with the cilantro leaves, and serve.

Per Serving: Calories 377; Protein 20 g; Carbs 56 g; Dietary Fiber 14 g; Added Sugars 0 g; Total Fat 9 g; Sat Fat 2 g; Omega-3s 260 mg; Sodium 628 mg; Potassium 947 mg

POTATO-CHEDDAR BREAKFAST CASSEROLE

Makes 6 servings

This egg bake can be assembled the night before a brunch and baked off in the morning. If you have leftovers, rest assured that it reheats beautifully in the microwave on HIGH for 2 minutes. It's great topped with Avocado Salsa (page 61) or Pico de Gallo (page 61).

> 3 tablespoons extra virgin olive oil
> 1 pound (454 g) Yukon gold–type potatoes, cubed
> 1 onion, diced
> 2 jalapeño chiles, diced
> ¼ teaspoon kosher salt
> ¼ teaspoon freshly ground black pepper
> 3 Roma (plum) tomatoes, diced
> 4 ounces (113 g) sharp or extra sharp aged white cheddar, grated
> 8 large eggs
> 1 cup (250 g) part-skim ricotta

1. Preheat the oven to 350°F (180°C). Use your fingertips or a pastry brush to cover the bottom and sides of an 8-inch (20 cm) square baking dish with 1 tablespoon of the oil.

2. Place the potatoes in a saucepan. Cover them with cold water and place over high heat. Bring to a boil, then reduce the heat to medium-low. Gently simmer until the potatoes can be pierced with a paring knife, 12 to 15 minutes.

3. Combine the remaining 2 tablespoons oil, the onion, jalapeños, salt, and pepper in a large sauté pan or skillet over medium-high heat. Sauté until the onions start to soften, about 8 minutes. Stir in the tomatoes and cook until they start to soften, another 2 to 3 minutes. Remove from the heat.

4. Drain the potatoes and spread them in the baking dish. Top with the cheddar, then cover with the vegetables. Whisk the eggs and ricotta in a medium bowl to combine, then pour over the vegetables.

5. Bake for 55 to 60 minutes, until the top is dark brown, the edges are crispy, and a digital food thermometer reads 165°F (75°C) when inserted in the center of the dish. Let cool for 15 to 20 minutes before cutting into 6 pieces and serving. Store in an airtight container in the refrigerator for up to 3 days. Do not freeze.

Per Serving: Calories 362; Protein 19 g; Carbs 19 g; Dietary Fiber 2 g; Added Sugars 0 g; Total Fat 23 g; Sat Fat 8 g; Omega-3s 230 mg; Sodium 343 mg; Potassium 157 mg

QUINOA-VEGGIE EGG BITES

Makes 4 servings (3 egg bites per serving)

These egg bites are easy to make and even easier to grab on your way out the door in the morning. Though quinoa is full of protein, the real protein star in this dish is the eggs. A ½ cup (85 g) of cooked quinoa provides 4 grams of protein, while each egg provides 7 grams. Eggs are not only a good source of protein; they also contain choline, a nutrient similar to B vitamins that has significant heart health and brain benefits.

> Cooking spray
> 12 large eggs
> ½ teaspoon kosher salt
> ½ teaspoon freshly ground black pepper
> ½ cup (75 g) finely chopped red bell pepper
> ½ cup (95 g) Simply Cooked Quinoa (page 228), cooled
> ½ cup (80 g) thawed frozen chopped spinach, excess water squeezed out
> 1 tablespoon minced garlic
> ½ cup (55 g) shredded medium cheddar

1. Preheat the oven to 350°F (180°C). Spray the cups of a regular 12-cup muffin pan with cooking spray.

2. Whisk the eggs, salt, and pepper in a 4-cup (1 L) liquid measuring cup or medium bowl. In a separate bowl, combine the bell pepper, quinoa, spinach, and garlic. Distribute the vegetables evenly among the muffin cups. Pour over the egg mixture, filling each cup about three-quarters full. Top each with a sprinkle of cheddar.

3. Bake for 25 to 30 minutes, until a digital food thermometer reads 160°F (70°C) when inserted in the center of an egg bite. Use a knife to loosen the egg bites, then remove each bite from its cup with a small fork. Serve warm or chilled. Store in an airtight container in the refrigerator for up to 5 days or in the freezer for up to 1 month.

NOTE: *Instead of spraying the individual muffin pan cups with cooking spray, you can use paper or foil muffin cup liners to make egg bites, which improves their portability as a "grab and go" breakfast option.*

Serving Size 3 egg bites; Calories 306; Protein 22 g; Carbs 5 g; Dietary Fiber 1 g; Added Sugars 0 g; Total Fat 18 g; Sat Fat 6 g; Omega-3s 360 mg; Sodium 578 mg; Potassium 65 mg

SAUSAGE, EGG & AVOCADO BREAKFAST SANDWICHES

Makes 4 servings

We like to use English muffins for these breakfast sandwiches because we love how a fried egg gently drapes over the edge of the muffin, giving a sneak peek of what's inside. Enjoy this with your morning cup of coffee or a glass of 100% fruit juice.

1 avocado, halved, pitted, peeled, and cubed

1 teaspoon minced serrano chile

1 teaspoon fresh lime juice

1 tablespoon extra virgin olive oil

4 large eggs

¼ teaspoon kosher salt

¼ teaspoon freshly ground black pepper

4 whole wheat English muffins, split and toasted

4 Spicy Sage Breakfast Sausage patties (page 124), cooked

1. Combine the avocado, chile, and lime juice in a small bowl. Mash well with a fork.

2. Heat the oil in a skillet or sauté pan over medium-high heat. Carefully add the eggs, sprinkle with the salt and pepper, cover, and cook until the whites are firm and the yolks are starting to set, 3 to 4 minutes. Cook a bit longer if you like a firm yolk.

3. Place the English muffin bottoms on a platter or individual plates. Spread each with one-quarter of the mashed avocado. Add a sausage patty and an egg, then the top of the English muffin and serve.

TIP: *These yummy sandwiches are admittedly a bit messy to eat. You can wrap each sandwich in wax paper or parchment paper: Fold a square of paper in half diagonally. Place the sandwich on the top (90-degree) corner. Wrap the sharp corners of the paper around the sandwich.*

Serving Size 1 sandwich: Calories 643; Protein 28 g; Carbs 33 g; Dietary Fiber 8 g; Added Sugars 0 g; Total Fat 45 g; Sat Fat 12 g; Omega-3s 220 mg; Sodium 567 mg; Potassium 404 mg

SPICY SAGE BREAKFAST SAUSAGE

Makes 6 patties

Lean pork can dry out quite easily, so we used a few tricks to keep the patties moist and juicy, including adding grated onion and the juice that comes with it. We feature these patties on our Sausage, Egg & Avocado Breakfast Sandwiches (page 124) and as a crumbled topping on our Sausage & Roasted Red Pepper Breakfast Pizza (page 199).

¼ cup (40 g) grated white onion, including the juice

1 tablespoon extra virgin olive oil

1 tablespoon Parmesan

1 garlic clove, finely minced

½ teaspoon Italian Seasoning (page 34)

½ teaspoon ground sage

¼ teaspoon red pepper flakes

1 tablespoon cornstarch

20 ounces (567 g) lean ground pork

¼ teaspoon kosher salt

¼ teaspoon freshly ground black pepper

1. Stir together the onion, oil, Parmesan, garlic, seasoning, sage, and red pepper flakes in a medium

bowl. Sprinkle in the cornstarch and stir to incorporate it. Add the pork and use your hands to mix everything thoroughly, but don't overwork the mixture or it will toughen the sausage texture. Divide the sausage mixture into six patties about ½ inch (13 mm) thick. Set on a baking sheet, cover with plastic wrap, and refrigerate for 30 to 60 minutes. (This allows the starch molecules in the cornstarch time to hydrate; when heated, the gelatinized cornstarch will help hold the liquid within the patties.)

2. To cook, place the patties in a cold, large, nonstick skillet. Sprinkle a bit of salt and pepper over each patty. Use half the salt and pepper so you can season the other side after flipping the patties. Turn on the heat to medium-high. Cook the patties until dark brown on the bottom, 7 to 8 minutes.

3. Flip the patties, sprinkle with the rest of the salt and pepper, and cook on the second side until a digital food thermometer reads 160°F (70°C) when inserted in the side and center of a patty, 7 to 8 minutes. Serve warm.

Serving Size 1 patty; Calories 330; Protein 16 g; Carbs 2 g; Dietary Fiber 0 g; Added Sugars 0 g; Total Fat 29 g; Sat Fat 10 g; Omega-3s 20 mg; Sodium 134 mg; Potassium 22 mg

SHIITAKE & SPINACH QUICHE WITH ROSEMARY & SAGE

Makes 6 servings

Our à la Heart approach to quiche is to replace the typically butter-rich crust with one made from our Savory Nut Crumb Topping (page 125). Serve with a fruit salad, like Watermelon, Grapefruit & Blueberry Salad (page 145).

Cooking spray

¾ cup (175 g) Savory Nut Crumb Topping (page 36)

1 tablespoon extra virgin olive oil

1 cup (70 g) sliced shiitake mushroom caps

¾ cup (120 g) finely chopped red onion

2 garlic cloves, minced

1 tablespoon balsamic vinegar

6 cups (180 g) fresh baby spinach leaves

1 cup (80 g) freshly grated Parmesan

4 large eggs

½ cup (120 ml) milk

1½ tablespoons chopped fresh sage leaves

2 teaspoons chopped fresh rosemary leaves

Freshly ground black pepper

1. Preheat the oven to 400°F (200°C). Line the bottom of a 9-inch (23 cm) pie plate with parchment paper. Coat the paper with cooking spray.

2. To make the crust, pat the nut crumb topping into the bottom and halfway up the sides of the pie plate.

3. Heat the oil in a large skillet over medium heat. Sauté the mushrooms, onions, and garlic until the onion is soft and the mushrooms are beginning to brown, 3 to 5 minutes. Stir in the vinegar, add the spinach to the skillet, and let it wilt but not fully cook, about 3 minutes. Distribute the vegetables evenly over the crust. Sprinkle over the Parmesan. Whisk the eggs in a medium bowl to combine. Add the milk, 1 tablespoon sage, and rosemary, and whisk again. Pour the egg mixture over the cheese.

4. Bake for 10 minutes. Lower the heat to 350°F (180°C) and bake for 20 to 25 minutes, until a knife inserted in the center comes out clean. Cool for 5 minutes, then sprinkle with ½ tablespoon sage and pepper. Cut into 6 wedges and serve. Store in a wax paper–lined airtight container in the refrigerator for up to 3 days. Quiche is good to eat cold or hot; to reheat, place a slice on a microwave-safe plate, cover with a paper napkin, and microwave in 20-second increments until hot.

Per Serving: Calories 294; Protein 15 g; Carbs 18 g; Dietary Fiber 3 g; Added Sugars 0 g; Total Fat 18 g; Sat Fat 5 g; Omega-3s 120 mg; Sodium 468 mg; Potassium 255 mg

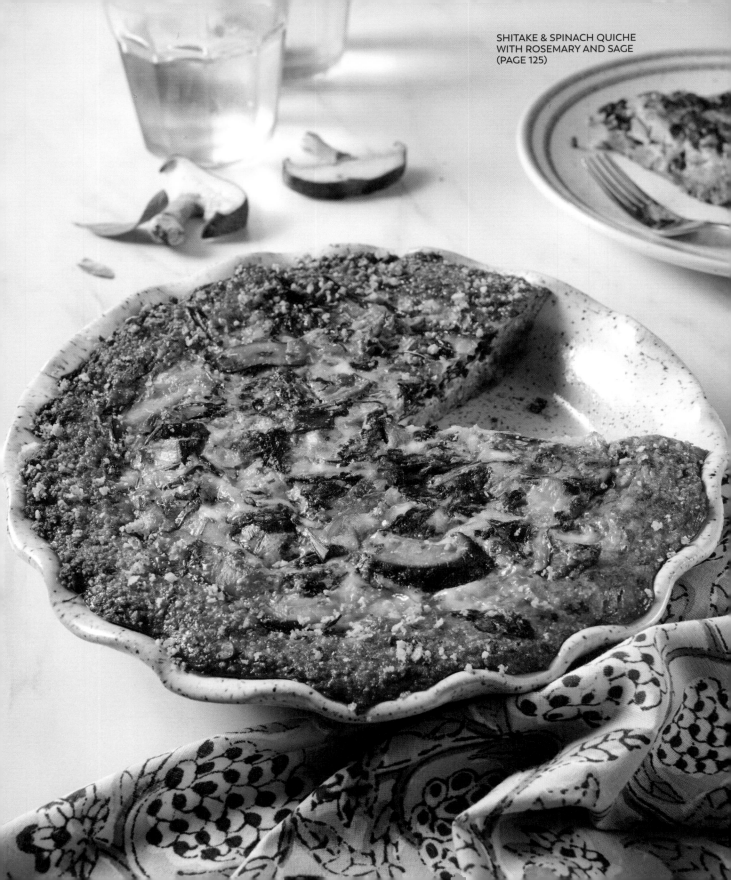

SHITAKE & SPINACH QUICHE
WITH ROSEMARY AND SAGE
(PAGE 125)

SPINACH SCRAMBLE PITA POCKETS

Makes 4 servings

This breakfast sandwich, with everything tucked into whole wheat pita pockets, incorporates frozen spinach, one of the most convenient ways to cook dark leafy greens. Serve your stuffed pita with your favorite 100% fruit juice or whole fruit for a complete breakfast that will keep you going all morning long.

- 2 tablespoons extra virgin olive oil
- 2 garlic cloves, minced
- ½ teaspoon red pepper flakes
- One 10-ounce (283 g) box frozen chopped spinach, thawed, drained, and squeezed to remove as much water as possible
- 3 Roma (plum) tomatoes, diced
- 8 large eggs, beaten
- ¼ teaspoon kosher salt
- ¼ teaspoon fresh ground black pepper
- One 5.2-ounce (150 g) package spreadable cheese (such as Boursin Garlic & Fine Herbs)
- 4 whole wheat pita pockets, halved and warmed

1. Combine the oil, garlic, and red pepper flakes in a large sauté pan over medium-high heat. Cook until the garlic is soft, 2 to 3 minutes. Add the spinach and tomatoes and cook until most of the moisture in the pan has evaporated, 4 to 5 minutes. Reduce the heat to medium. Stir in the eggs, salt, and pepper. Cook, stirring frequently until the eggs have firmed up, 4 to 5 minutes.

2. Stir in the cheese, reduce the heat to low, and cover the pan for 1 to 2 minutes to allow the cheese to fully melt.

3. Place the pita pockets on a serving platter. Fill each pita half with about ½ cup (100 g) of the mixture. Serve warm.

NOTE: *Place thawed spinach in a fine-mesh sieve or strainer and press with a fork or large spoon to remove as much water as possible.*

Serving Size 2 pockets; Calories 476; Protein 22 g; Carbs 40 g; Dietary Fiber 7 g; Added Sugars 0 g; Total Fat 26 g; Sat Fat 8 g; Omega-3s 340 mg; Sodium 613 mg; Potassium 508 mg

TOMATO-TOPPED VEGGIE-EGG BAKE

Makes 12 servings

This easy brunch recipe is a snap to make, and is also gluten-free. Serve with our Citrus, Spinach & Mushroom Salad (page 147) to complete your brunch menu.

Crust

- 2 cups (390 g) Simply Cooked Brown Rice (page 230)
- 1 cup (115 g) part-skim farmer cheese or shredded mozzarella
- 1 large egg, beaten
- Cooking spray

Filling

- 1 tablespoon extra virgin olive oil
- 1 cup (160 g) chopped white onion (1 medium)
- 8 ounces (227 g) cremini or portobello mushrooms, diced
- 1 cup (115 g) part-skim farmer cheese or shredded mozzarella
- ¼ cup (6 g) finely chopped fresh basil, plus 12 basil sprigs for serving
- 10 large eggs
- 1½ cups (360 ml) milk
- ½ teaspoon freshly ground black pepper
- ¼ teaspoon ground nutmeg
- 2 ripe tomatoes, sliced into 12 thin slices

1. To make the crust, spray a 9 × 13-inch (23 × 33 cm) baking pan with cooking spray. Stir together the rice, the first farmer cheese, and egg in a medium bowl with a fork to mix well. Press the mixture evenly in the pan and 1 to 2 inches (2.5 to 5 cm) up the sides. Cover and refrigerate for 1 hour or overnight.

2. Preheat the oven to 350°F (180°C).

3. To make the filling, heat the oil in a large sauté pan or skillet over medium heat. Sauté the onion and mushrooms until the onions are translucent and mushrooms are softened, 4 to 6 minutes. Spread the vegetables over the crust, then sprinkle evenly with the second farmer cheese and the chopped basil. Whisk the eggs, milk, pepper, and nutmeg in a medium bowl. Pour slowly over the vegetables. Gently place the tomato slices on top in a 4 × 3 or 2 × 6 pattern so each piece will have a full tomato slice.

4. Place in the oven and bake for 50 to 60 minutes, until a knife inserted into the center comes out clean. Remove and let cool for 10 minutes before serving. Cut and serve with a basil sprig alongside or on top. Store in a wax paper–lined airtight container in the refrigerator for up to 3 days. Do not freeze.

Per Serving: Calories 201; Protein 13 g; Carbs 14 g; Dietary Fiber 1 g; Added Sugars 0 g; Total Fat 10 g; Sat Fat 4 g; Omega-3s 140 mg; Sodium 270 mg; Potassium 239 mg

APPLE-CINNAMON COMPOTE
Makes 2 cups (615 g)

This apple-infused, lightly sweetened syrup works well on Apple-Cinnamon Pancakes (page 128), Honey Whole Wheat Waffles (page 132), and Apple Dutch Baby (page 129).

½ cup (120 ml) apple cider or apple juice, plus more if needed

1 tablespoon cornstarch

1 tablespoon apple cider vinegar

1 tablespoon butter or plant-based spread

1 tablespoon brown sugar

1 teaspoon ground cinnamon

½ teaspoon ground nutmeg

¼ teaspoon ground cloves

3 apples, cored and thinly sliced but not peeled

1. Combine 2 tablespoons of the apple cider with the cornstarch in a small bowl. Stir to dissolve. Mix the remaining apple cider, the vinegar, butter, brown sugar, cinnamon, nutmeg, and cloves in a medium saucepan over medium-high heat. Add the apples, stirring to mix well. Bring to a boil, reduce the heat to medium-low, cover, and simmer until the apples are soft and tender, 5 minutes.

2. Stir the cornstarch mixture into the apples. Cook, stirring constantly, until the mixture becomes thick and bubbly. If it's too thick, add 1 or 2 tablespoons of apple cider to thin it. Serve warm. Store in a glass jar with a tight-fitting lid in the refrigerator for up to 2 weeks.

Serving Size ¼ cup (77 g); Calories 60; Protein 0 g; Carbs 12 g; Dietary Fiber 2 g; Added Sugars 2 g; Total Fat 2 g; Sat Fat 1 g; Omega-3s 10 mg; Sodium 13 mg; Potassium 80 mg

APPLE-CINNAMON PANCAKES
Makes 8 servings

This recipe creates very light, fluffy pancakes that can be topped with fresh fruit like sliced bananas, or our Ginger-Pear Compote (page 132).

¾ cup (95 g) all-purpose flour

¾ cup (90 g) whole wheat flour

1 tablespoon baking powder

1 tablespoon sugar

1 teaspoon ground cinnamon

½ apple, cored and finely diced

1 cup (245 g) unsweetened applesauce

¾ cup (180 ml) milk

1 large egg, slightly beaten

2 tablespoons peanut or canola oil

1. Whisk together the all-purpose flour, whole wheat flour, baking powder, sugar, cinnamon, and apple in a large bowl. Combine the applesauce, milk, egg, and oil in a medium bowl, and stir until combined. Make a well in the center of the dry ingredients. Pour in the milk mixture and stir gently until just combined (a few lumps can remain). Do not overmix.

2. Heat a large nonstick griddle or skillet over medium heat. Use a ¼-cup (60 ml) measure to portion out the batter for each pancake. Cook until small bubbles begin to appear evenly over the surface and the edges are dry, 2 to 3 minutes. Using a thin, wide spatula, flip the pancakes and cook until the second side is golden brown, 1½ to 2 minutes longer. Serve immediately.

TIP: If you have a large griddle, you'll likely be able to cook the pancakes in two batches, but if you're using a smaller griddle or skillet and you need to cook the pancakes in three or more batches, transfer the pancakes to a wire rack set over a baking sheet in a preheated 200°F (95°C) oven to keep warm until all of them have been cooked.

Serving Size 2 pancakes; Calories 119; Protein 3 g; Carbs 17 g; Dietary Fiber 2 g; Added Sugars 2 g; Total Fat 5 g; Sat Fat 1 g; Omega-3s 30 mg; Sodium 18 mg; Potassium 115 mg

APPLE DUTCH BABY

Makes 6 servings

A cross between a pancake and a popover, this airy apple dish starts on the stovetop and finishes in the oven, all in the same pan. You'll need a 10- or 12-inch (25.5 or 30.5 cm) oven-safe skillet for this recipe. Serve topped with fresh fruit and a drizzle of real maple syrup.

- 4 tart apples, cored and thinly sliced (Braeburn, Granny Smith, or Pink Lady)
- 3 tablespoons plus 1 teaspoon fresh lemon juice
- 2 tablespoons butter or plant-based spread
- 6 large eggs
- 1 cup (240 ml) milk
- ½ cup (65 g) all-purpose flour
- ½ cup (60 g) whole wheat flour
- ½ teaspoon ground cinnamon
- 2 tablespoons honey
- Sliced strawberries
- Real maple syrup

1. Preheat the oven to 400°F (200°C).

2. Combine the apple slices with 3 tablespoons of the lemon juice in a medium bowl; toss to coat the apples. Melt the butter in a large oven-safe skillet over medium heat. Add the apples and sauté until slightly softened, 5 to 8 minutes. Turn off the heat and use a spoon or spatula to spread the apples evenly over the bottom of the skillet.

3. Whisk the eggs, milk, all-purpose flour, whole wheat flour, and cinnamon in a medium bowl until no lumps remain, 20 to 30 seconds. Let the batter rest for 5 minutes.

4. Pour the batter slowly over the apples in a circular fashion, starting on the outer rim. Place in the oven and bake for 15 to 20 minutes, until puffy, crisp, and deep golden brown. The edges will have risen above the sides of the skillet. Sprinkle with 1 teaspoon of lemon juice and drizzle with the honey. Cut into wedges and serve warm with strawberries and a drizzle of maple syrup.

Per Serving: Calories 291; Protein 10 g; Carbs 42 g; Dietary Fiber 5 g; Added Sugars 6 g; Total Fat 9 g; Sat Fat 4 g; Omega-3s 150 mg; Sodium 109 mg; Potassium 270 mg

BANANA OAT BLUEBERRY BREAKFAST BARS

Makes 32 bars

If you rarely take time to sit down for breakfast, bake up a batch of these bars so you have a convenient, filling, and nutrient-rich "grab and go" option. Paired with a coffee or latte, these bars will give you the energy you need to make it through the morning.

- 2 cups (185 g) quick-cooking rolled oats
- ½ cup (55 g) ground flaxseed
- ½ cup (60 g) whole wheat pastry flour
- 2 tablespoons chia seeds
- 1 tablespoon ground cinnamon
- 2 teaspoons baking powder
- ¼ teaspoon kosher salt
- ½ cup (120 ml) buttermilk
- ½ cup (120 ml) real maple syrup
- ⅓ cup (80 ml) warm water
- 2 tablespoons peanut or canola oil
- 2 teaspoons pure vanilla extract
- 2 bananas, mashed
- 1 cup (160 g) dried blueberries
- ½ cup (70 g) coarsely chopped almonds

1. Preheat the oven to 325°F (165°C). Line the bottom of a 9 × 13-inch (23 × 33 cm) baking pan with parchment paper; let the parchment hang over two sides.

2. Combine the oats, flaxseed, flour, chia seeds, cinnamon, baking powder, and salt in a medium bowl. Mix the buttermilk, maple syrup, water, oil, and vanilla in a large bowl. Add the mashed banana and beat well. Gradually add the dry ingredients and stir thoroughly to form a stiff dough. Sprinkle with the blueberries and almonds and fold them in until well distributed.

3. Spread the dough evenly in the baking pan. Bake for 20 to 25 minutes, until firm and golden brown. The dough in the middle of the pan will spring back when touched gently.

4. Cool the bars in the pan on a wire rack, about 30 minutes, then lift them out of the pan with the parchment paper and place on a cutting board. Cut into 32 equal bars in a 4 × 8 pattern (about 1½ ×

2-inch/4 × 5 cm squares). Store in an airtight container at room temperature for up to 4 days, or wrap each bar in wax paper, place in an airtight container, and store in the freezer for up to 2 months.

Serving Size 1 bar; Calories 103; Protein 2 g; Carbs 17 g; Dietary Fiber 2 g; Added Sugars 6 g; Total Fat 3 g; Sat Fat 0 g; Omega-3s 550 mg; Sodium 21 mg; Potassium 110 mg

BARLEY WITH STONE FRUIT

Makes 4 servings

Here we present yet another idea for incorporating whole grains into your breakfast routine. This is a great option for a workday breakfast, but if you want to include it in your next brunch menu, consider serving it with the Bean & Baby Kale Frittata (page 119).

½ cup (100 g) pearl barley or farro

2½ cups (600 ml) water

½ cup (80 g) raisins

½ cup (80 g) pitted prunes

2 or 3 fresh apricots, pitted and quartered, or ½ cup (65 g) chopped dried apricots

1 or 2 fresh peaches, pitted and chopped, or ½ cup (80 g) chopped dried peaches

1 tablespoon sherry vinegar or fresh lemon juice

1. Soak the barley in 1½ cups (360 ml) of the water in a medium saucepan overnight.

2. When you're ready to cook, add the remaining 1 cup (240 ml) water. Bring to a boil, cover, and simmer for 45 minutes, until the barley is tender.

3. Add the raisins, prunes, apricots, and peaches, and simmer until soft, 5 minutes. Just before serving, stir in the vinegar.

Per Serving: Calories 237; Protein 4 g; Carbs 58 g; Dietary Fiber 6 g; Added Sugars 0 g; Total Fat 1 g; Sat Fat 0 g; Omega-3s 10 mg; Sodium 6 mg; Potassium 583 mg

CARROT & FIG OATS WITH PISTACHIOS

Makes 1 serving

This is definitely not your grandmother's oatmeal. We hope this sophisticated approach to a sweet and savory breakfast will inspire you to try other veggies and cheeses in your morning oats.

1 cup (240 ml) milk or water, plus more if needed

½ cup (45 g) quick-cooking rolled oats

¼ cup (15 g) shredded carrots

¼ cup (35 g) chopped dried figs

1 tablespoon fresh orange juice

¼ teaspoon ground cinnamon, plus more for sprinkling, optional

2 teaspoons honey

2 tablespoons grated Manchego or crumbled soft goat cheese

1 tablespoon chopped pistachios

1. Combine the milk and oats in a medium microwave-safe bowl. Microwave for 1 minute on HIGH. Stir in the carrots, figs, orange juice, and cinnamon. Microwave again on HIGH for up to 1 minute, watching to make sure the oatmeal doesn't boil over. Let stand for 30 seconds before removing from the microwave.

2. Stir to blend well; the oatmeal will be thick. Add more milk if you like a thinner consistency. Sprinkle more cinnamon over the oatmeal if desired. Drizzle with the honey, top with the Manchego and pistachios, and enjoy.

Per Serving: Calories 529; Protein 19 g; Carbs 83 g; Dietary Fiber 8 g; Added Sugars 12 g; Total Fat 16 g; Sat Fat 6 g; Omega-3s 40 mg; Sodium 172 mg; Potassium 972 mg

CHOCOLATE ENERGY BARS

Makes 16 bars

These no-bake bars bring a healthy dose of slow carbs, unsaturated fats, omega-3s, and fiber. If you have "chocolate monsters" in your home who may be tempted to attack these as soon as you make them, be warned: They need to be chilled for 2 hours before you can dig in.

1 avocado, halved, pitted, and peeled

1 cup (145 g) pitted dates

1 cup (115 g) walnut pieces, toasted

2 tablespoons hot water

½ cup (50 g) ground almonds or superfine almond flour

⅓ cup (30 g) unsweetened cocoa powder

¼ cup (60 g) chia seeds

3 tablespoons sesame seeds

1. Line an 8-inch (20 cm) square baking pan with parchment paper, leaving a 2-inch (5 cm) overhang on all sides.

2. Place the avocado, dates, walnuts, and hot water in a food processor. Process until well blended and sticky. Add the almonds, cocoa, and chia seeds, and pulse until well combined.

3. Press the mixture in the baking pan. Top with the sesame seeds, pressing them gently into the mixture. Refrigerate until firm, about 2 hours.

4. Lift the bar out of the pan using the parchment and place on a cutting board. Cut into 16 bars (a 4 × 4 pattern, each 2 inches/5 cm square). Store by wrapping each bar in wax paper or plastic wrap, then placing in an airtight container in the refrigerator for up to 2 weeks or in the freezer for up to 2 months.

Serving Size 1 bar; Calories 145; Protein 4 g; Carbs 12 g; Dietary Fiber 4 g; Added Sugars 0 g; Total Fat 11 g; Sat Fat 1 g; Omega-3s 1,530 mg; Sodium 3 mg; Potassium 240 mg

CINNAMON & GINGER GRANOLA

Makes 20 servings

Granola makes a house smell like home. Use old-fashioned rolled oats for this recipe or your granola will be powdery. You can eat this granola with milk like cereal, use it to top a bowl of Greek yogurt and fresh fruit, or snack on it as is.

5 cups (460 g) old-fashioned rolled oats

1 cup (145 g) sliced almonds or chopped unsalted peanuts

1 cup (145 g) sesame seeds

1 cup (130 g) unsalted raw sunflower seeds or pepitas (pumpkin seeds)

1 cup (115 g) wheat germ

½ cup (170 g) honey

⅓ cup (85 g) almond or peanut butter

⅓ cup (80 ml) extra virgin olive oil

2 tablespoons ground cinnamon

1 teaspoon ground ginger

½ cup (65 g) dried cranberries

½ cup (65 g) chopped dried apricots

1. Preheat the oven to 300°F (150°C). Line two large rimmed baking sheets with parchment paper.

2. Combine the oats, almonds, sesame seeds, sunflower seeds, and wheat germ in a large bowl. Combine the honey, almond butter, and oil in a small saucepan over low heat. Stir until the ingredients are combined and the nut butter has melted, about 2 minutes. Stir in the cinnamon and ginger. Pour the wet mixture over the dry ingredients, folding and stirring until everything is completely coated. Divide the granola mixture between the two pans and spread it out evenly.

3. Bake for 15 minutes. Stir the granola and bake until the granola is golden brown, 15 minutes. Remove from the oven and allow to cool. Transfer to a large airtight container and stir in the cranberries and apricots. Store at room temperature for up to 5 days or in the freezer for up to 3 months.

Serving Size ¾ cup (75 g); Calories 336; Protein 10 g; Carbs 36 g; Dietary Fiber 7 g; Added Sugars 9 g; Total Fat 20 g; Sat Fat 2 g; Omega-3s 90 mg; Sodium 15 mg; Potassium 315 mg

GINGER-PEAR COMPOTE

Makes 2 cups (500 g)

This compote, with its intense ginger flavor and hints of lemon, is like a chutney. You can use it to top Apple-Cinnamon Pancakes (page 128) or Honey Whole Wheat Waffles (page 132), spread on Apple-Walnut Bread (page 100), or you can place a generous dollop on a piece of Apple Walnut Date Coffee Cake (page 356). It's also great paired with a wheel of triple cream Brie for a festive holiday appetizer!

> Two 15.25-ounce (432 g) cans pear halves or slices, drained and chopped
>
> 2 tablespoons diced crystallized ginger
>
> 2 tablespoons grated or finely minced fresh ginger
>
> 2 tablespoons honey
>
> ¼ teaspoon ground ginger
>
> Grated zest of 1 lemon

1. Combine the pears, crystallized ginger, fresh ginger, honey, and ground ginger in a medium saucepan over medium heat. Cook, stirring occasionally, until most of the liquid has evaporated and the pears have started to break down, 8 to 10 minutes.

2. Cool to room temperature before serving. Store in an airtight container in the refrigerator for up to 2 weeks.

TIP: *The flavor of this compote is best when it's served at room temperature.*

Per Serving: Calories 54; Protein 0 g; Carbs 14 g; Dietary Fiber 1 g; Added Sugars 6 g; Total Fat 0 g; Sat Fat 0 g; Omega-3s 0 mg; Sodium 3 mg; Potassium 64 mg

HONEY WHOLE WHEAT WAFFLES

Makes 10 waffles

If you love waffles, give this tender, light, and thoroughly delicious version a try with the Ginger-Pear Compote (see this page) or the Mixed Berry Compote (page 134). You can retain the crispy outside of the waffle by transferring cooked waffles directly from the waffle iron to a wire rack over a large baking sheet in a warm oven as you finish making the entire batch.

> Cooking spray
>
> 1½ cups (180 g) whole wheat flour
>
> ¼ cup (30 g) all-purpose flour
>
> 2 teaspoons baking powder
>
> 2 large eggs, separated
>
> 1½ cups (360 ml) milk
>
> 3 tablespoons peanut or canola oil
>
> 2 tablespoons honey

1. Preheat a 7-inch (18 cm) round waffle iron. Spray the waffle maker with cooking spray. Place a wire rack on a large baking sheet, place the baking sheet in the oven, and preheat the oven to 200°F (95°C).

2. Whisk together the whole wheat flour, all-purpose flour, and baking powder in a medium bowl. Beat the egg yolks in a small bowl until lemon colored. Add the milk, oil, and honey, and beat to combine. Gently stir into the dry ingredients. In a third bowl, beat the egg whites with a handheld mixer or whisk until stiff, then fold them into the batter with a rubber spatula.

3. Pour ⅓ cup (80 ml) batter into the waffle iron. Bake according to the manufacturer's instructions (generally until the steaming stops), about 5 minutes. Remove the waffle with a fork and place it on the wire rack in the oven. Repeat with the remaining batter, spraying the waffle maker before adding more. Serve warm.

Serving Size 1 waffle; Calories 155; Protein 5 g; Carbs 21 g; Dietary Fiber 2 g; Added Sugars 3 g; Total Fat 6 g; Sat Fat 1 g; Omega-3s 40 mg; Sodium 27 mg; Potassium 129 mg

ICELANDERS IN AMERICA CEREAL

Makes 1 serving

For Amy, the scent of cardamom immediately makes her think of her family's Icelandic baking traditions. While millet is not a traditional ingredient in Icelandic baking, our Simply Cooked Millet, when cooked with cardamom pods, honors Icelandic flavors and creates a simple breakfast perfect for any day of the year. This cereal is topped with skyr, an Icelandic cultured dairy product similar to yogurt.

½ cup (55 g) Simply Cooked Millet (page 227)

¼ cup (40 g) chopped pitted dates

¼ cup (60 ml) water

½ teaspoon grated lemon zest

Pinch of ground cardamom

One 5.3-ounce (150 g) container plain or vanilla skyr or Greek yogurt (about ⅔ cup)

Combine the millet, dates, and water in a microwave-safe bowl. Microwave on HIGH for 60 seconds. Stir in the lemon zest and cardamom, top with skyr, and enjoy.

Per Serving: Calories 331; Protein 19 g; Carbs 50 g; Dietary Fiber 4 g; Added Sugars 0 g; Total Fat 7 g; Sat Fat 4 g; Omega-3s 20 mg; Sodium 75 mg; Potassium 298 mg

MANGO-COCONUT OVERNIGHT OATS WITH MACADAMIA NUTS

Makes 1 serving

Mango, coconut, and macadamia nuts bring tropical flavors to ordinary oatmeal and transform it into something wonderful. Like all our other oatmeal recipes, it works well with dairy milk, which provides protein to balance the carbs. Plain cashew milk, which is naturally quite sweet, is especially flavorful in this recipe and could step in for dairy milk.

1 cup (240 ml) milk or water, plus more if needed

¾ cup (125 g) diced fresh or thawed frozen mango

½ cup (45 g) quick-cooking rolled oats

1 tablespoon almond butter

2 tablespoons shredded unsweetened coconut

2 tablespoons chopped roasted unsalted macadamia nuts or cashews

1. Place the milk in a wide-mouth 1-pint (475 ml) glass jar or microwave-safe bowl. Microwave on HIGH for 90 seconds. Add ½ cup (85 g) of the mango, the oats, almond butter, and 1 tablespoon of the coconut. Stir to combine, cover, and refrigerate for at least 8 hours or up to 2 days. The oats will soak up the milk, creating a thick oatmeal. Add more milk if you like a thinner consistency.

2. To enjoy cold, stir in the remaining mango and coconut and top with the macadamia nuts.

3. To eat warm, microwave on HIGH for 45 seconds. Stir, then microwave on HIGH for another 45 seconds. Let stand for 30 seconds before removing from the microwave. Top with the remaining mango and coconut and the macadamia nuts, and enjoy.

VARIATION: *Same-Day Mango-Coconut Oats*
To make this the morning you want to eat it, use a medium microwave-safe bowl. Proceed with Step 1 but microwave for 1 minute. Do not refrigerate the microwaved mixture. Instead, microwave it again on HIGH for up to 1 minute, watching to make sure the oatmeal doesn't boil over. Let stand for 30 seconds before removing from the microwave. Add more milk if you like a thinner consistency. Stir in the remaining mango and coconut, top with the macadamia nuts, and enjoy.

Per Serving: Calories 642; Protein 20 g; Carbs 69 g; Dietary Fiber 11 g; Added Sugars 0 g; Total Fat 36 g; Sat Fat 12 g; Omega-3s 110 mg; Sodium 138 mg; Potassium 990 mg

MILLET MORNING CAKES

Makes 8 cakes

This recipe provides a gluten-free alternative to traditional pancakes. We recommend serving it with Ginger-Pear Compote (page 132), but you could also top them with Pumpkin Butter (page 135) or sliced strawberries and a drizzle of real maple syrup.

- 2 cups (225 g) Simply Cooked Millet (page 227)
- 3 tablespoons extra virgin olive oil
- 2 large eggs, beaten
- 2 tablespoons millet flour
- ½ teaspoon ground cinnamon or pumpkin pie spice
- ½ teaspoon kosher salt

1. Stir together the millet, 2 tablespoons of the oil, the eggs, millet flour, cinnamon, and salt in a medium bowl.

2. Heat 1½ teaspoons of the oil in a large skillet or sauté pan over medium-high heat. When the oil is hot and shimmering, spoon in about 3 tablespoons of batter for each cake. (You should be able to fry four cakes at one time.) Cook until golden brown on the bottom, 4 to 5 minutes. Flip the cakes and cook for another 3 to 4 minutes, until golden. Transfer to a serving plate and tent with foil to keep warm.

3. Add the remaining 1½ teaspoons oil to the pan. When the oil is shimmering, use the rest of the batter to create four more cakes. Serve warm.

TIP: *You can make your own millet flour by grinding dry millet in a clean coffee grinder or blender.*

Serving Size 1 cake; Calories 106; Protein 3 g; Carbs 8 g; Dietary Fiber 1 g; Added Sugars 0 g; Total Fat 7 g; Sat Fat 1 g; Omega-3s 70 mg; Sodium 136 mg; Potassium 22 mg

MIXED BERRY COMPOTE

Makes 4 servings

This hearty whole-fruit compote has less added sugar and more antioxidants than most commercial syrups. It's an excellent topping for our Strawberry Pancakes (page 135), our Almond Lemon Cake (Variation, page 356), and is a sublime stir-in for plain Greek yogurt.

- Juice of 1 orange, plus more if needed
- 1 tablespoon cornstarch
- 4 cups (600 g) mixed fresh or frozen berries
- 1 tablespoon butter or plant-based spread
- 1 tablespoon honey
- ½ teaspoon ground cardamom

1. Combine 2 tablespoons of the orange juice with the cornstarch in a small bowl. Stir until the cornstarch is dissolved.

2. Combine the berries, the remaining orange juice, butter, honey, and cardamom in a medium saucepan over medium-high heat. Stir well and bring to a boil. Reduce the heat to medium-low and simmer, stirring occasionally until all the berries are soft, about 5 minutes.

3. Stir the cornstarch mixture into the fruit. Cook, stirring constantly, until thick and bubbly, about 2 minutes. If too thick, add a few more tablespoons orange juice. Serve warm. Store in a glass jar with a tight-fitting lid in the refrigerator for up to 2 weeks.

Per Serving: Calories 135; Protein 1 g; Carbs 27 g; Dietary Fiber 4 g; Added Sugars 4 g; Total Fat 4 g; Sat Fat 2 g; Omega-3s 180 mg; Sodium 25 mg; Potassium 126 mg

PUMPKIN BUTTER

Makes 2 cups (450 g)

This is an easy way to add pumpkin flavor—and vegetables—to pancakes, waffles, or whole grain toast. It's a great topping for Honey Whole Wheat Waffles (page 132) or Millet Morning Cakes (page 134).

- One 15-ounce (425 g) can 100% pure pumpkin (not pumpkin pie mix)
- ½ cup (120 ml) real maple syrup
- ½ teaspoon ground cinnamon
- ¼ teaspoon ground cloves
- ¼ teaspoon ground ginger
- ¼ teaspoon ground nutmeg
- ⅛ teaspoon kosher salt

Combine the pumpkin, maple syrup, cinnamon, cloves, ginger, and salt in a medium saucepan over medium heat. Cook, stirring frequently, until warmed through, 4 to 5 minutes. Serve warm. Store in an airtight container in the refrigerator for up to 2 weeks.

Serving Size 1 tablespoon; Calories 38; Protein 1 g; Carbs 9 g; Dietary Fiber 1 g; Added Sugars 6 g; Total Fat 1 g; Sat Fat 1 g; Omega-3s 0 mg; Sodium 17 mg; Potassium 23 mg

PUMPKIN SPICE OATS WITH PECANS

Makes 1 serving

What can we say? We just couldn't resist including a recipe that incorporates our other pumpkin spice recipes into one very delicious and comforting bowl of cereal!

- ½ cup (45 g) quick-cooling rolled oats
- 1 cup (240 ml) milk or water, plus more if needed
- 2 tablespoons plain yogurt
- 2 tablespoons Pumpkin Butter (see this page) or 100% pure pumpkin (not pumpkin pie mix)
- 1 teaspoon pumpkin pie spice
- 2 teaspoons real maple syrup
- 2 tablespoons chopped Pumpkin Spice Pecans (page 346) or raw pecans

1. Combine the oats and milk in a medium microwave-safe bowl. Microwave for 1 minute on HIGH. Stir, then microwave on HIGH up to 1 minute, watching to make sure the oatmeal doesn't boil over. Let stand for 30 seconds before removing from the microwave.

2. The oatmeal will be thick; add more milk if you like a thinner consistency. Stir in the yogurt, pumpkin butter, and pumpkin pie spice. Drizzle with the maple syrup, sprinkle on the chopped pecans, and enjoy.

Per Serving: Calories 423; Protein 16 g; Carbs 58 g; Dietary Fiber 5 g; Added Sugars 8 g; Total Fat 15 g; Sat Fat 5 g; Omega-3s 80 mg; Sodium 122 mg; Potassium 693 mg

STRAWBERRY PANCAKES

Makes twelve 4-inch (10 cm) pancakes

Top these thin, tender pancakes with sliced fresh strawberries, sliced bananas, blueberries, Mixed Berry Compote (page 134), or all of the above!

- 1 cup (240 ml) milk
- 1 large egg
- 1 tablespoon honey
- 1 tablespoon peanut or canola oil, plus more for the griddle
- ¾ cup (90 g) whole wheat pastry flour
- 1½ teaspoons baking powder
- ⅛ teaspoon kosher salt
- 1 cup (145 g) diced fresh strawberries

1. Whisk together the milk, egg, honey, and oil in a medium bowl. Gently whisk in the flour, baking powder, and salt until just combined.

2. Heat a large griddle or skillet over medium heat. Using a ¼-cup (60 ml) measure, portion the batter onto the griddle. Top each pancake with a generous tablespoon of strawberries. Cook until small bubbles begin to appear evenly over the surface and the edges are dry, 2 to 3 minutes. Using a thin, wide spatula, flip the pancakes and cook until the second side is golden brown, 1 to 2 minutes longer. Serve immediately.

TIPS: *You can use this recipe to make blueberry pancakes or banana pancakes. Leave the blueberries whole. To use bananas, slice one medium banana very thinly or dice them to resemble the size of blueberries.*

If you don't have a griddle that can accommodate cooking all 12 pancakes at one time, transfer the finished pancakes to a wire rack set over a baking sheet in a preheated 200°F (95°C) oven to keep warm.

Serving Size 3 pancakes; Calories 159; Protein 4 g; Carbs 25 g; Dietary Fiber 4 g; Added Sugars 4 g; Total Fat 5 g; Sat Fat 1 g; Omega-3s 50 mg; Sodium 76 mg; Potassium 58 mg

SUPER SEEDS PROTEIN POWER BARS

Makes 12 servings

These no-bake protein bars can be made in 30 minutes or less. The protein comes from the hemp, flax, chia, and pepitas, as well as the almonds. The bars offer omega-3s in the form of alpha-linolenic acid (ALA) from the hemp, chia, and flaxseed and the canola oil.

1 cup (90 g) slivered almonds, toasted

1 cup (90 g) quick-cooking rolled oats

½ cup (60 g) dried cherries

½ cup (85 g) mini dark chocolate chips

½ cup (80 g) hulled hemp seeds

½ cup (55 g) ground flaxseed

½ cup (30 g) pepitas (pumpkin seeds), toasted

¼ cup (60 g) chia seeds

¼ cup (60 ml) canola oil

¼ cup (60 ml) real maple syrup, sorghum syrup, or honey

2 tablespoons molasses

1 teaspoon pure vanilla extract

⅛ teaspoon kosher salt

1. Line a 9-inch (23 cm) square freezer-safe baking dish with parchment paper, leaving a 2-inch (5 cm) overhang on all sides.

2. Combine the almonds, oats, cherries, chocolate chips, hemp seeds, flaxseed, pepitas, and chia seeds in a medium bowl. Make a well in the center.

3. Whisk the oil, maple syrup, molasses, vanilla, and salt in a small saucepan over low heat, until the ingredients are combined well and the mixture is warm, about 2 minutes. Pour the syrup mixture into the well in the dry ingredients, stirring until the mixture is well combined and smooth. Pour into the

baking dish. Use your hands to spread the mixture evenly from edge to edge, pressing down gently, until the mixture is firmly packed and the top is level. Freeze for 15 to 20 minutes to firm the bars. Transfer the bars to a cutting board, lifting them out of the pan by the parchment. Cut in half, then cut each half into 1½-inch-wide (4 cm) bars. Store in an airtight container in the refrigerator for up to 1 week. To freeze, wrap each bar in wax paper or plastic wrap, place in an airtight container, and store in the freezer for up to 2 months.

Serving size 1 bar; Calories 248; Protein 6 g; Carbs 23 g; Dietary Fiber 4 g; Added Sugars 10 g; Total Fat 16 g; Sat Fat 3 g; Omega-3s 3,330 mg; Sodium 26 mg; Potassium 334 mg

Super Smoothie Secrets

What's the secret to a super smoothie? It's important to balance slowly digested, fiber-rich carbohydrates with ample protein to help keep your energy levels sustained. Smoothies that include mostly carbohydrates will give you a quick burst of energy, but you'll likely feel tired and sluggish within an hour or two. Our smoothie recipes are designed to give you longer-lasting energy when eaten for breakfast, but smoothies can also make great snacks or afternoon pick-me-ups.

Here's a guide to help you create great-tasting smoothies with balanced nutrition.

Table 5: Strategies to Build a Better Smoothie

PROTEIN
Aim for 20 to 30 grams of protein per smoothie.

Dairy milk, 1 cup (240 ml): 8 to 10 g

Ultra-filtered dairy milk, 1 cup (240 ml): up to 20 g

Buttermilk, 1 cup (230 ml): 8 g

Kefir, 1 cup (230 ml): 9 g

Greek yogurt, 1 cup (230 g): up to 25 g

Silken tofu, 4 ounces (113 g): 5 g

Soy milk, 1 cup (240 ml): 8 g

Other nondairy beverages: Check nutrition labels; some contain very little protein, while others may be fortified with protein from various plant sources.

Pulses (chickpeas, lentils, black beans, etc.), ½ cup (80 g): 6 to 8 g, depending on the pulse

Nut butters, 2 tablespoons: 7 g

Protein powders: Check nutrition labels. We recommend dairy milk protein, whey protein, or soy protein isolates, which have favorable amino acid profiles. One word of caution: Not all protein isolates provide all nine essential amino acids or bioavailable protein our bodies can digest, absorb, and use. While the protein will help sustain energy levels, it may not provide additional benefits.

SLOWLY DIGESTED CARBOHYDRATES
(aka Slow Carbs)

Whole grains, dry or cooked: rolled oats, cooked farro, cooked barley, cooked millet

Whole fruit, fresh or frozen: apple, pear, orange, berries

Pulses: chickpeas, lentils, black beans, cannellini beans

Vegetables: baby spinach, cucumber, red bell pepper, canned pumpkin

HEALTHY FATS

Avocados

Nuts: almonds, cashews, pecans, walnuts

Nut butters: peanut butter, almond butter, cashew butter

Seeds: chia seeds, flaxseed, hemp seeds, pepitas, poppy seeds, sesame seeds, sesame butter (tahini)

FLAVOR NOTES

Aromatics like fresh ginger and citrus zest

Fresh herbs like basil, chives, cilantro, mint; can provide additional nutrient benefits

Individual spices like cardamom, cinnamon, nutmeg, and turmeric, or the spice blends from chapter 3

APRICOT-CHICKPEA SMOOTHIE

Makes 1 smoothie

Pulses such as white beans, chickpeas, and lentils aren't commonly thought of when making smoothies, but after one taste, we think you'll reconsider. Pulses—the edible seeds of legumes—are simple carbohydrates, low in fat and high in protein, fiber, vitamins, and minerals. We like the harmony of sweet and hot provided by the coconut water and the Moroccan-Style Seasoning (page 35).

- ½ cup (80 g) frozen, drained canned, or fresh apricot halves
- ⅓ cup (50 g) canned chickpeas or cannellini beans, drained and rinsed
- ¼ English cucumber, sliced (3 ounces/85 g)
- 1 tablespoon fresh lime juice
- ½ teaspoon Moroccan-Style Seasoning (page 35)
- ½ cup (120 ml) coconut water

Combine the apricots, chickpeas, cucumber, lime juice, seasoning, and coconut water in a blender or food processor. Blend or pulse until smooth and creamy. Pour into a glass; serve and enjoy immediately.

Serving Size 1 smoothie; Calories 147; Protein 6 g; Carbs 29 g; Dietary Fiber 6 g; Added Sugars 0 g; Total Fat 2 g; Sat Fat 0 g; Omega-3s 20 mg; Sodium 149 mg; Potassium 613 mg

BERRY-TURMERIC SMOOTHIE

Makes 1 smoothie

Use whatever berry is in season, is in your fridge or freezer, or appeals to your taste. Buttermilk provides a pop of tart in this smoothie, the berries add sweetness, and the ginger and turmeric bring the flavor and some added nutrients to this meal in a glass.

- ¾ cup (115 g) frozen blueberries, raspberries, or strawberries
- ¾ cup (180 ml) cultured buttermilk
- 2 tablespoons ground flaxseed or hemp hearts
- ½ teaspoon minced fresh ginger
- ¼ teaspoon ground turmeric

Combine the berries, buttermilk, flaxseed, ginger, and turmeric in a blender or food processor. Blend or pulse until smooth and silky. Pour into a glass; serve and enjoy immediately.

NOTE: *Buttermilk, a fermented dairy product, may sound like it's high in fat, but it is just the opposite! It's what remains after cream is churned into butter, so the fat is long gone. What's left is a tangy, creamy liquid loaded with good-for-you bacteria and loads of protein.*

Serving Size 1 smoothie; Calories 215; Protein 9 g; Carbs 29 g; Dietary Fiber 7 g; Added Sugars 0 g; Total Fat 8 g; Sat Fat 2 g; Omega-3s 3,350 mg; Sodium 361 mg; Potassium 498 mg

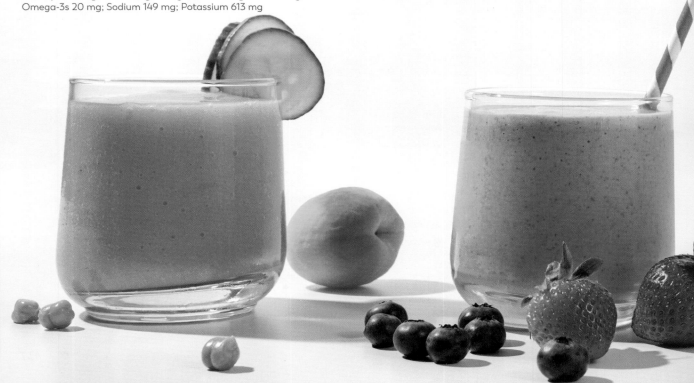

KEFIR, SPINACH & AVOCADO SMOOTHIE

Makes 1 smoothie

Kefir, a tart and tangy fermented milk beverage with a consistency similar to thin yogurt, is a wonderful base for smoothies. It contains live and active microorganisms that act as probiotics, which aid digestion and help support a healthy gut. Avocado adds healthy fats, while protein powder boosts the protein and adds body, making this smoothie Linda's favorite eye-opener.

- 2 cups (60 g) fresh baby spinach leaves
- ¾ cup (180 ml) vanilla kefir
- ½ cup (75 g) fresh or frozen berries or chopped mango, peach, or pineapple
- ½ avocado, peeled and sliced
- 1 scoop (20 g) plain or vanilla whey protein powder

Combine the spinach, kefir, berries, avocado, and protein powder in a blender or food processor. Blend or pulse until smooth and creamy. Pour into a glass; serve and enjoy immediately.

TIP: *This smoothie's thickness comes from the avocado. If you'd like a thinner consistency, add another ¼ cup (60 ml) kefir and blend again.*

Serving Size 1 smoothie; Calories 288; Protein 20 g; Carbs 23 g; Dietary Fiber 11 g; Added Sugars 0 g; Total Fat 15 g; Sat Fat 2 g; Omega-3s 180 mg; Sodium 85 mg; Potassium 645 mg

MANGO TOFU SOY MILK SMOOTHIE

Makes 1 smoothie

Silken tofu, with its high water content, is the softest tofu available and is therefore a better choice for smoothies than firm tofu. It imparts a silky texture to this smoothie. The mango provides sweetness, which is heightened by the addition of orange zest, cinnamon, and cardamom. Roasted root vegetables add additional nutrients for flavor and help to thicken the smoothie.

- 4 ounces (113 g) soft silken tofu
- ½ cup (95 g) frozen mango cubes or ½ fresh mango, peeled and chopped
- ⅓ cup (55 g) Simply Roasted Root Vegetables with Apples (page 261)
- 1 tablespoon grated orange zest
- ½ teaspoon ground cinnamon
- ¼ teaspoon ground cardamom
- ¼ to ½ cup (60 to 120 ml) soy milk

Combine the tofu, mango, vegetables, orange zest, cinnamon, and cardamom in a blender or food processor. Blend or pulse until smooth and creamy. Add soy milk to achieve the desired consistency. Pour into a glass; serve immediately.

Serving Size 1 smoothie; Calories 224; Protein 10 g; Carbs 34 g; Dietary Fiber 5 g; Added Sugars 0 g; Total Fat 7 g; Sat Fat 1 g; Omega-3s 140 mg; Sodium 96 mg; Potassium 633 mg

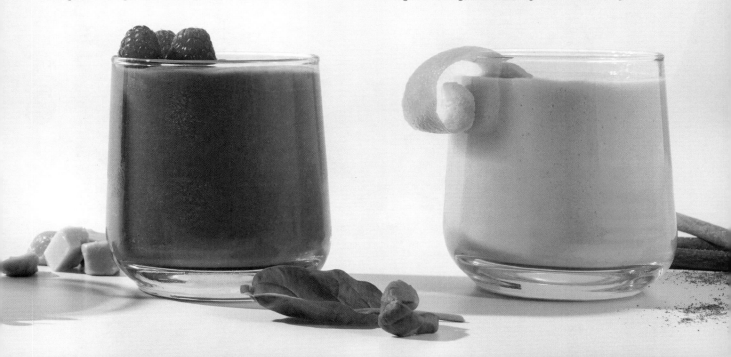

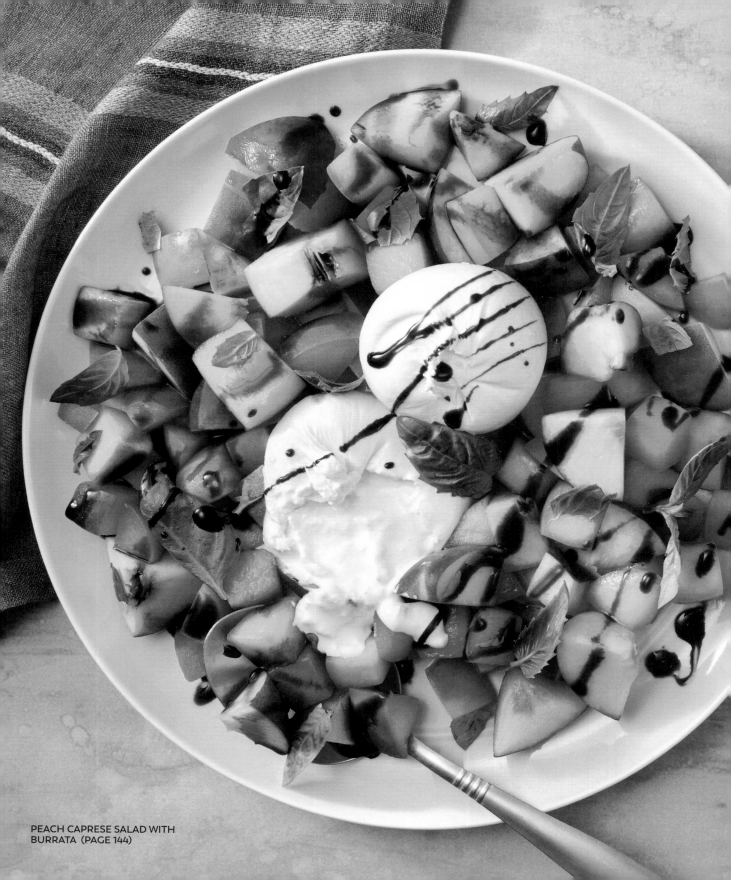

PEACH CAPRESE SALAD WITH
BURRATA (PAGE 144)

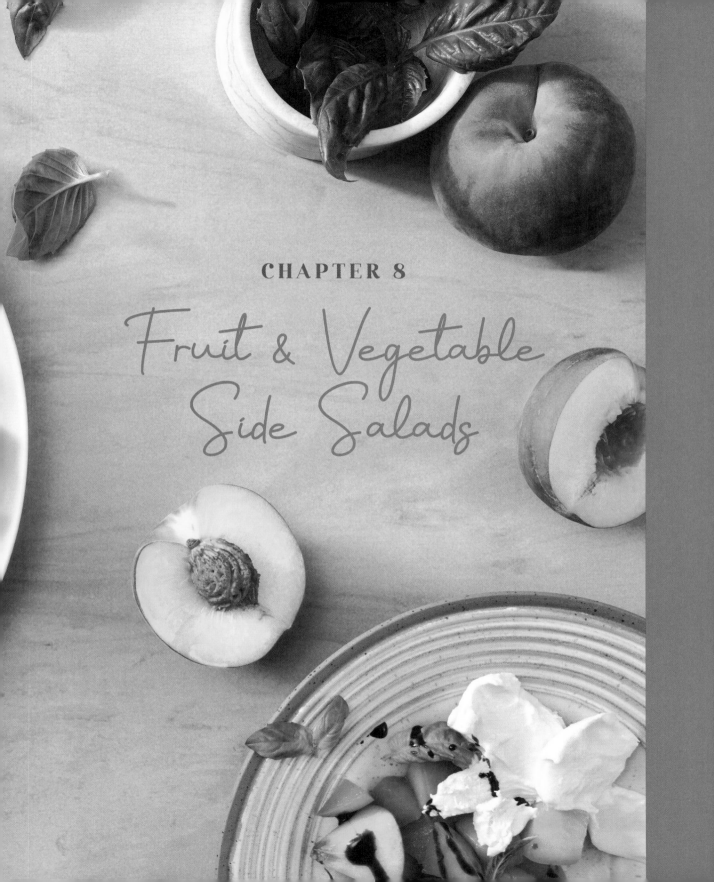

CHAPTER 8

Fruit & Vegetable
Side Salads

Fruit & Vegetable Side Salads

Fruit Salads

Citrus-Mint Salad with
Ginger-Lime Vinaigrette 143

Mixed Fruit with Yogurt-
Cardamom Dressing 144

Peach Caprese Salad with Burrata 144

Pear & Grapefruit Toss with
Citrus-Mint Dressing 144

Strawberry, Pineapple & Mint Salad . . . 145

Watermelon, Grapefruit &
Blueberry Salad 145

Fruit & Vegetable Salads

Arugula, Apple & Fennel Salad with
Gorgonzola 146

Carrot & Pineapple Couscous Salad. . . . 146

Cauliflower & Spinach Salad
with Sesame-Orange Dressing 147

Citrus, Spinach & Mushroom Salad 147

Citrusy Golden Beet Salad 148

Spinach Salad with Honeycrisp
Apples & Cheddar. 148

Vegetable Salads

Broccoli & Corn Salad. 149

Broccoli Slaw 149

Cauliflower & Kalamata Olive Salad . . . 150

Cherry Tomato Caprese Salad. 150

Creamy Cilantro Coleslaw 151

Creamy Cucumber-Dill Salad. 151

Cucumber & Tomato Salad. 152

Dilly Cucumber Salad. 152

Marinated Vegetable Salad 152

Mixed Greens & Mushroom Salad. 153

Napa Cabbage Slaw 153

Potato Salad with Red Wine
Vinaigrette 154

Radish & Cabbage Slaw 154

Wasabi-Ginger Coleslaw. 155

Wedge Salad 155

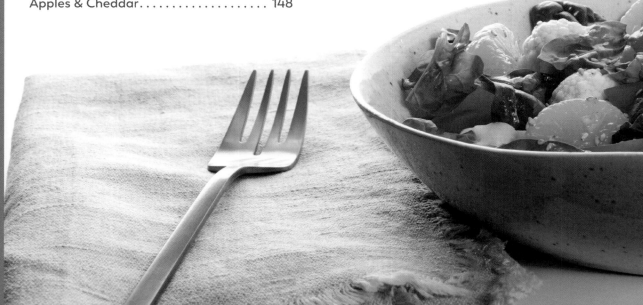

Salads can take on so many forms and flavor profiles. While most of the salads featured here use fresh fruits and vegetables, using frozen, canned, and dried products can be great, especially if you are short on time. Research shows that people who eat the most fruits and vegetables—regardless of form (fresh, fresh-cut, frozen, canned, 100% juice, or dried)—have the lowest risk of cardiovascular disease. So stock up your pantry, freezer, and refrigerator and embrace the flavor, nutrition, and health benefits as well as the convenience!

Blanching, sautéing, roasting, and grilling vegetables can enhance the flavor and create more appealing textures. Use our recipes as inspiration for finding the flavors, textures, temperatures, and ingredient combinations that you love—and that you'll want to return to time and time again.

These side salads are just as delicious for breakfast, brunch, or snacking as they are with lunch and dinner. We hope you find abundant inspiration for adding more fruits and vegetables in all their glorious forms to your meals in flavorful, enjoyable ways.

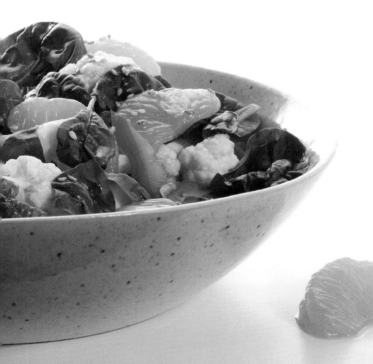

CITRUS-MINT SALAD WITH GINGER-LIME VINAIGRETTE
Makes 6 servings

This is a wonderful salad to make when citrus fruit is at its peak. It can be served as a side dish or dessert. Short on time? Buy fresh-cut citrus sections, typically found in the refrigerated area of the produce section of many grocery stores. The dressing also works well on salads made with baby greens and topped with fresh citrus or berries.

Ginger-Lime Vinaigrette

Juice of 1 lemon

2 tablespoons extra virgin olive oil

2 tablespoons sugar

1 teaspoon finely grated fresh ginger

Grated zest of 1 lime

⅛ teaspoon kosher salt

Salad

3 Cara Cara oranges, peeled and cut into supremes (see Notes)

2 navel oranges, peeled and cut into supremes

1 pink or Ruby Red grapefruit, peeled and cut into supremes

¼ cup (6 g) chopped fresh mint leaves

Whisk the lemon juice, oil, sugar, ginger, lime zest, and salt in a medium bowl. Add the oranges, grapefruit, and mint and gently toss to coat. Serve immediately.

NOTES: *A Microplane is the perfect tool for finely grating ginger.*

To make citrus supremes, cut a thin slice from the top and bottom of the fruit so it sits flat. Cut the peel from the fruit, making sure you cut off all the pith (the white part) as well as the membrane on the outside of the segments. Carefully cut out the fruit flesh of each segment (the supreme), leaving behind the membranes that separate the segments.

Per Serving: Calories 140; Protein 1 g; Carbs 25 g; Dietary Fiber 3 g; Added Sugars 4 g; Total Fat 5 g; Sat Fat 1 g; Omega-3s 40 mg; Sodium 41 mg; Potassium 158 mg

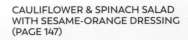

CAULIFLOWER & SPINACH SALAD WITH SESAME-ORANGE DRESSING (PAGE 147)

MIXED FRUIT WITH YOGURT-CARDAMOM DRESSING

Makes 6 servings

Loaded with color, this fruit combo provides heart-promoting fiber, phytonutrients, and antioxidants, such as vitamin C. Serve as a side salad with the Bean & Baby Kale Frittata (page 119) or the Tomato-Topped Veggie Egg Bake (page 127) for breakfast, brunch, or as a pleasant ending to a meal.

- 2 bananas, sliced
- 1 navel orange, peeled and sectioned
- 1 pear, cored and cubed
- 1 cup (150 g) red or purple seedless grapes, halved
- ½ cup (160 g) pitted prunes, diced
- 2 tablespoons fresh lemon juice
- 1 cup (245 g) Yogurt-Cardamom Dressing (page 52)
- ½ cup (60 g) coarsely chopped walnuts, toasted

Combine the bananas, orange, pear, grapes, prunes, and lemon juice in a medium bowl. Add the dressing and gently stir to coat. Just before serving, sprinkle the walnuts on top.

Per Serving: Calories 235; Protein 6 g; Carbs 40 g; Dietary Fiber 5 g; Added Sugars 3 g; Total Fat 8 g; Sat Fat 1 g; Omega-3s 930 mg; Sodium 23 mg; Potassium 523 mg

PEACH CAPRESE SALAD WITH BURRATA

Makes 4 servings

One of Amy's favorite restaurants, Mulvaney's B&L in Sacramento, California, serves this salad every summer. Anticipation builds as faithful fans await the arrival of perfectly ripe peaches from local farms. Pounce on your opportunity to make this salad as soon as you can find perfect peaches at your local market, farmstand, or farmers' market.

- 4 peaches, pitted and cubed
- 4 ounces (113 g) burrata
- ¼ cup (60 ml) balsamic vinegar
- 8 to 12 basil leaves, thinly sliced

Divide the peaches among four salad plates. Place one-quarter of the burrata on each plate. Drizzle with the vinegar and garnish with basil.

Per Serving: Calories 153; Protein 6 g; Carbs 18 g; Dietary Fiber 2 g; Added Sugars 0 g; Total Fat 6 g; Sat Fat 4 g; Omega-3s 10 mg; Sodium 49 mg; Potassium 307 mg

PEAR & GRAPEFRUIT TOSS WITH CITRUS-MINT DRESSING

Makes 8 servings

Pears deliver sweetness to add a lovely flavor balance to sometimes-tart grapefruit. Apricots and grapes offer textural contrast in this mixed fruit salad that is tossed with a yogurt-based dressing. Enjoy as a snack or sweet finish to any meal.

Salad
- 4 Bartlett pears, peeled, cut into wedges, and cored, or one 15-ounce (425 g) can Bartlett pear slices, drained
- 2 pink or Ruby Red grapefruit, peeled and sectioned, or 2 cups (460 g) jarred grapefruit sections, drained
- One 15-ounce (425 g) can apricot halves, drained
- 1 cup (150 g) red or green seedless grapes, halved

Citrus-Mint Dressing
- One 5.3-ounce (150 g) container plain Greek yogurt (about ⅔ cup)

2 tablespoons honey

2 tablespoons thinly sliced fresh mint leaves

1 tablespoon grated grapefruit, orange, lemon, or lime zest

1 tablespoon fresh grapefruit, orange, lemon, or lime juice

Combine the pears, grapefruit, apricots, and grapes in a medium bowl. Whisk the yogurt, honey, mint, zest, and juice in a small bowl. Cover both bowls and chill for at least 15 minutes, at most 2 hours. Serve the dressing on the side for drizzling on top of the fruit. If any salad or dressing remain, refrigerate covered and enjoy the next day.

Per Serving: Calories 111; Protein 3 g; Carbs 27 g; Dietary Fiber 2 g; Added Sugars 5 g; Total Fat 1 g; Sat Fat 0 g; Omega-3s 10 mg; Sodium 9 mg; Potassium 253 mg

STRAWBERRY, PINEAPPLE & MINT SALAD

Make 4 servings

This is a colorful salad with vibrant aromas. Pair with Lemon–Poppy Seed Bread (Variation, page 103) for break-fast or brunch, or serve with grilled chicken for a light lunch. If you don't want to buy and cut a whole pineap-ple, look for fresh-cut pineapple in the produce section of your local market or buy pineapple chunks canned in 100% juice. The best oil for this recipe is fruity with little or no bitterness or pungency, such as one pressed from Arbequina olives.

2 tablespoons fresh lemon juice

1 tablespoon extra virgin olive oil

1 tablespoon honey

3 cups (430 g) fresh strawberries, quartered

1 cup (115 g) cubed fresh pineapple

½ cup (15 g) fresh mint leaves, thinly sliced

Whisk the lemon juice, oil, and honey in a large bowl. Add the strawberries, pineapple, and mint, and toss to combine. Serve immediately.

NOTE: *Olive oil sensory experts refer to three sensory attributes in extra virgin olive oil: fruitiness, bitterness, and pungency or pepperiness. These positive sensory attributes vary according to the type of olive used to make the oil, along with other factors like growing conditions and fruit*

ripeness at harvest. Fruitiness refers to a fresh olive aroma; bitterness is a taste sensation perceived on the tongue; and pungency is perceived in the back of the throat. Oils that are more pungent may cause you to cough after swallowing, which is considered a good thing, since it indicates the presence of powerful health-promoting compounds.

Per Serving: Calories 100; Protein 1 g; Carbs 17 g; Dietary Fiber 3 g; Added Sugars 4 g; Total Fat 4 g; Sat Fat 1 g; Omega-3s 110 mg; Sodium 3 mg; Potassium 224 mg

WATERMELON, GRAPEFRUIT & BLUEBERRY SALAD

Makes 4 servings

This salad can easily be turned into an entrée salad by adding chickpeas and tossing it with Creamy Feta & Mint Dressing (page 49).

4 cups (610 g) cubed seedless watermelon

1 grapefruit, peeled and sectioned with membranes removed

1 avocado, halved, pitted, peeled, and cubed

1 cup (150 g) fresh blueberries

One 5- to 6-ounce (142 to 170 g) bag baby spinach (about 4 cups)

4 teaspoons balsamic vinegar

¼ cup (6 g) chopped fresh mint

Combine the watermelon, grapefruit, avocado, and blueberries in a large bowl. Divide the spinach among four plates; top with the fruit mixture. Drizzle 1 teaspoon of vinegar on each, then top each with mint.

Per Serving: Calories 192; Protein 4 g; Carbs 32 g; Dietary Fiber 9 g; Added Sugars 0 g; Total Fat 8 g; Sat Fat 1 g; Omega-3s 90 mg; Sodium 37 mg; Potassium 456 mg

ARUGULA, APPLE & FENNEL SALAD WITH GORGONZOLA

Makes 4 servings

Fennel is a celery-like vegetable that has been highly regarded in the Mediterranean diet since ancient times. It was valued for its wellness properties then, and today anyone who loves the distinctive flavor seeks out this aromatic all-star. We use fennel in this salad for its crisp, crunchy texture and licorice-like flavor.

Salad

1 red apple (such as Honeycrisp, McIntosh, Fuji, or Gala), cored and thinly sliced

1 tablespoon fresh lemon juice

1 fennel bulb, trimmed and thinly sliced, fronds chopped and reserved

½ red onion, thinly sliced

½ cup (80 g) dried blueberries or cranberries

2 cups (40 g) baby arugula

¼ cup (30 g) crumbled Gorgonzola

¼ cup (30 g) coarsely chopped toasted walnuts

Honey Lemon Dijon Dressing

3 tablespoons extra virgin olive oil

1 tablespoon apple cider vinegar

Grated zest of 1 lemon

2 tablespoons fresh lemon juice

2 teaspoons honey

1 teaspoon Dijon mustard

1 garlic clove, minced

⅛ teaspoon kosher salt

Freshly ground black pepper

1. Combine the apple and lemon juice in a medium bowl, coating the apples to keep them crisp and white. Add the fennel bulb, onion, and berries. Toss to combine.

2. Whisk together the oil, vinegar, lemon zest, lemon juice, honey, mustard, garlic, and salt in a small bowl.

3. Place the arugula in a large bowl. Add half of the dressing and toss to coat. Add the other half of the dressing to the apple-fennel mixture and toss well.

4. Divide the arugula among four salad plates. Top with the apple-fennel mixture, then sprinkle each salad with a tablespoon each of Gorgonzola and walnuts. Add pepper to taste and finish with 1 teaspoon chopped fennel fronds each. Serve.

Per Serving: Calories 275; Protein 4 g; Carbs 29 g; Dietary Fiber 5 g; Added Sugars 3 g; Total Fat 18 g; Sat Fat 3 g; Omega-3s 785 mg; Sodium 235 mg; Potassium 430 mg

CARROT & PINEAPPLE COUSCOUS SALAD

Makes 4 servings

Couscous is a North African whole grain pasta made from semolina flour, a by-product of durum wheat. It cooks up in under 15 minutes into tiny fluffy balls packed with flavor. We've put an American twist on this salad by adding pineapple tidbits and precut carrots to keep it fast and easy.

One 10-ounce (283 g) bag shredded carrots

1 teaspoon Moroccan-Style Seasoning (page 35)

One 8-ounce (227 g) can pineapple tidbits, drained

½ cup (80 g) golden raisins

Juice of 1 lemon

1 cup (155 g) Simply Steamed Couscous (page 205)

½ cup (70 g) sliced almonds, toasted

½ cup (15 g) chopped fresh mint

2 ounces (57 g) crumbled feta, optional

1. Sprinkle the carrots with the seasoning in a medium bowl. Add the pineapple, raisins, and lemon juice, and stir to combine. Chill for 1 hour.

2. Divide the couscous among four plates and top with the carrot mixture. Sprinkle with almonds and mint, and feta, if desired.

Per Serving: Calories 303; Protein 8 g; Carbs 49 g; Dietary Fiber 8 g; Added Sugars 0 g; Total Fat 11 g; Sat Fat 1 g; Omega-3s 40 mg; Sodium 309 mg; Potassium 625 mg

CAULIFLOWER & SPINACH SALAD WITH SESAME-ORANGE DRESSING

Makes 4 servings

This easy-to-prepare salad offers a variety of colors, crunchy textures, and a tangy sweetness. For something so easy to whip up, it's got big flavors.

Salad

One 11-ounce (312 g) can mandarin oranges, drained, liquid reserved

One 5- to 6-ounce (142 to 170 g) bag baby spinach (about 4 cups)

2 cups (215 g) cauliflower florets

¼ cup (35 g) chopped red bell pepper

2 tablespoons sesame seeds

Sesame-Orange Dressing

2 tablespoons reserved mandarin orange liquid

2 tablespoons toasted sesame oil

1 tablespoon white wine vinegar

1 garlic clove, minced

¼ teaspoon white pepper

Combine the oranges, spinach, cauliflower, and bell pepper in a medium bowl. Whisk together the reserved orange liquid, oil, vinegar, garlic, and white pepper. Drizzle over the vegetables, toss to combine, sprinkle with sesame seeds, and serve.

Per Serving: Calories 149; Protein 3 g; Carbs 15 g; Dietary Fiber 3 g; Added Sugars 0 g; Total Fat 9 g; Sat Fat 1 g; Omega-3s 40 mg; Sodium 52 mg; Potassium 301 mg

CITRUS, SPINACH & MUSHROOM SALAD

Makes 4 servings

Spinach and citrus fruit are not only a tasty combination, but a healthful one, too. The citrus helps our bodies absorb iron from the spinach. The spinach, mushrooms, and oranges contain fiber, magnesium, potassium, and antioxidants, like vitamin C—all champions of good heart health.

Salad

8 ounces (227 g) cremini or white mushrooms, sliced

One 5- to 6-ounce (142 to 170 g) bag baby spinach (about 4 cups)

2 navel oranges, peeled and sectioned

½ cup (80 g) thinly sliced red onion

Garlic-Lime Vinaigrette

Grated zest of 1 lime

2 tablespoons fresh lime juice

2 tablespoons extra virgin olive oil

1 teaspoon sugar

1 garlic clove, minced

Combine the mushrooms, spinach, oranges, and onion in a medium bowl. Whisk together the lime zest, lime juice, oil, sugar, and garlic in a small bowl. Pour the dressing over the salad and toss to combine. Chill for 15 minutes before serving.

Per Serving: Calories 134; Protein 3 g; Carbs 16 g; Dietary Fiber 3 g; Added Sugars 1 g; Total Fat 7 g; Sat Fat 1 g; Omega-3s 60 mg; Sodium 35 mg; Potassium 392 mg

CITRUSY GOLDEN BEET SALAD

Makes 4 servings

Golden beets are native to the Mediterranean and North Africa. They have a milder flavor than red beets and are less likely to discolor other vegetables. We pair them with lots of fresh citrus and spices native to their origin.

Salad

5 baby golden beets, trimmed, peeled, and thinly sliced

1 pink or red grapefruit, peeled, and sectioned with membranes removed

1 Cara Cara orange, peeled and sliced

1 Moro (blood) orange, peeled and sliced

1 fennel bulb, trimmed and thinly sliced, fronds reserved and minced

1 avocado, halved, pitted, peeled, and thinly sliced

2 tablespoons chopped fresh dill

Freshly ground black pepper

Cinnamon-Honey Dressing

⅓ cup (110 g) honey

½ teaspoon ground cinnamon

¼ teaspoon ground allspice

Pinch of kosher salt

⅓ cup (80 ml) white wine vinegar

¼ cup (60 ml) extra virgin olive oil

1. Arrange the beets, grapefruit, orange, fennel, and avocado in an attractive pattern on four rimmed plates.

2. Mix the fresh dill and 2 tablespoons of the fennel fronds together in a small bowl.

3. Measure the honey in a 2-cup (480 ml) glass measuring cup and microwave on HIGH for 20 to 30 seconds, until the honey is warm and thinned but not hot. Whisk in the cinnamon, allspice, salt, and vinegar. Whisk in the oil, 1 tablespoon at a time, until fully incorporated.

4. Drizzle the dressing over the salads and sprinkle each with the mixed fennel fronds and dill. Add pepper to taste and serve.

Per Serving: Calories 390; Protein 3 g; Carbs 49 g; Dietary Fiber 8 g; Added Sugars 23 g; Total Fat 23 g; Sat Fat 3 g; Omega-3s 187 mg; Sodium 135 mg; Potassium 746 mg

SPINACH SALAD WITH HONEYCRISP APPLES & CHEDDAR

Makes 4 servings

Honeycrisp apples are fantastically crisp and boast a delicate sweet-tart balance with a light berry flavor. Like the Fuji apple, their juicy sweetness comes from cells that are twice as large as those of other apples, making them a perfect eating apple. Spinach takes on new notes in this salad when mixed with sweet, crunchy apples and salty cheddar.

Salad

1 Honeycrisp apple, cored and sliced

¼ cup (35 g) dried currants, cranberries, or blueberries

¼ cup (40 g) thinly sliced red onion

One 5- to 6-ounce (142 to 170 g) bag baby spinach (about 4 cups), chopped

4 ounces (113 g) sharp cheddar, cubed (about 1 cup)

Ginger–Apple Cider Dressing

2 tablespoons extra virgin olive oil

2 tablespoons apple cider vinegar

½ teaspoon finely grated fresh ginger

⅛ teaspoon white pepper

1. Whisk together the oil, vinegar, ginger, and pepper in a medium bowl. Add the apple, currants, and onion and toss to coat. Cover and let stand for 10 to 15 minutes.

2. Place the spinach in a large bowl. Add the dressed fruits and onion and the cheddar, and toss to combine. Chill until you're ready to serve.

Per Serving: Calories 242; Protein 8 g; Carbs 16 g; Dietary Fiber 3 g; Added Sugars 0 g; Total Fat 17 g; Sat Fat 6 g; Omega-3s 100 mg; Sodium 216 mg; Potassium 156 mg

BROCCOLI & CORN SALAD

Makes 4 servings

Made from a simple trio of broccoli, corn, and red onion, this cold salad comes alive when marinated in a dressing made from lemon, oregano, and cumin. This same vegetable trio makes a tasty sheet-pan supper with chicken tenders; drizzling the lemon-herb dressing over the roasted vegetables and chicken just before serving.

Salad

2 cups (140 g) bite-size fresh broccoli florets

3 ears fresh corn or one 12-ounce (340 g) bag frozen corn kernels

½ cup (80 g) diced red onion

Lemon-Herb Dressing

3 tablespoons extra virgin olive oil

2 tablespoons apple cider vinegar

1 tablespoon fresh lemon juice

1 tablespoon chopped fresh oregano or basil

1 teaspoon ground cumin

1. Steam the broccoli until crisp-tender but still bright green, about 4 minutes. Drain and cool. Transfer to a large bowl.

2. If using fresh corn, scrape the kernels from the corn cobs; you'll need 2 cups (about 340 g) kernels. Or steam the frozen kernels according to package directions; drain and cool. Add the corn and onion to the broccoli, and mix.

3. Whisk together the oil, vinegar, lemon juice, oregano, and cumin in a small bowl. Pour over the vegetables and toss well. Cover and marinate in the refrigerator for at least 1 hour before serving. Store in the refrigerator for up to 1 week.

Per Serving: Calories 208; Protein 5 g; Carbs 25 g; Dietary Fiber 4 g; Added Sugars 0 g; Total Fat 12 g; Sat Fat 2 g; Omega-3s 140 mg; Sodium 27 mg; Potassium 441 mg

BROCCOLI SLAW

Makes 6 servings

Precut vegetables are a convenient fresh vegetable choice and serve as a shortcut to make this a quick and easy slaw. Store-bought broccoli slaw often comes with carrots and red cabbage as part of the mix. What a nice bonus! Pair with any of our tacos, such as the Portobello Street Tacos (page 184) for crunch, a little sweetness, and a lot of fresh vegetable flavor.

Slaw

One 12-ounce (340 g) bag broccoli slaw (about 6 to 8 cups)

1 apple, cored and diced into 1-inch (2.5 cm) pieces

½ cup thinly sliced red onion

¼ cup (30 g) dried cranberries

Juice of 1 lemon

Maple-Yogurt Dressing

One 5.3-ounce (150 g) container plain Greek yogurt (about ⅔ cup)

½ cup (110 g) mayonnaise

2 tablespoons apple cider vinegar

1 tablespoon real maple syrup

Combine the broccoli slaw, apple, onion, and cranberries in a large bowl. Add the lemon juice and toss to combine. Stir together the yogurt, mayonnaise, vinegar, and maple syrup in a small bowl. Add to the slaw, mix well, and refrigerate covered until ready to serve. If any slaw or dressing remains, refrigerate covered and enjoy the next day.

Per Serving: Calories 258; Protein 4 g; Carbs 20 g; Dietary Fiber 2 g; Added Sugars 7 g; Total Fat 19 g; Sat Fat 3 g; Omega-3s 1,360 mg; Sodium 291 mg; Potassium 251 mg

CAULIFLOWER & KALAMATA OLIVE SALAD

Makes 6 servings

This Greek-inspired salad contains kalamata olives, fresh lemon juice, and garlic. If you like, add a little feta to further enhance these flavors. We like to use raw fresh cauliflower for its crunch, but if you prefer a softer bite, blanch or steam the cauliflower for 2 to 3 minutes.

Salad

4 cups (430 g) thinly sliced cauliflower florets (1 medium head)

⅔ cup (100 g) chopped green bell pepper

½ cup (70 g) pitted kalamata olives, sliced

½ cup (80 g) chopped red onion

¼ cup (4 g) chopped fresh cilantro

2 tablespoons chopped pimientos, drained

Garlicky Lemon Dressing

¼ cup plus 2 tablespoons (90 ml) extra virgin olive oil

Grated zest of 1 lemon

3 tablespoons fresh lemon juice

3 tablespoons sherry vinegar

2 garlic cloves, minced

1 teaspoon sugar

¼ teaspoon white pepper

1. Combine the cauliflower, bell pepper, olives, onion, cilantro, and pimiento in a large bowl. In a jar with a tight-fitting lid, mix the oil, lemon zest, lemon juice, vinegar, garlic, sugar, and pepper. Shake well. Pour the dressing over the vegetables and mix well. Cover and refrigerate for 2 hours or overnight to allow the flavors to marry.

2. Toss again and let it sit at room temperature for 20 minutes before serving. Store with the dressing in an airtight container in the refrigerator for up to 3 days.

Per Serving: Calories 198; Protein 2 g; Carbs 10 g; Dietary Fiber 2 g; Added Sugars 1 g; Total Fat 17 g; Sat Fat 2 g; Omega-3s 110 mg; Sodium 231 mg; Potassium 292 mg

CHERRY TOMATO CAPRESE SALAD

Makes 4 servings

Many home gardeners will say a tomato fresh off the vine offers the best flavor. But thanks to talented plant breeders and hothouse technology, great-tasting tomatoes (especially grape and cherry varieties) can be found year-round in many supermarkets, which makes this salad an option any time of year.

One 16.5-ounce (468 g) container cherry or grape tomatoes, halved (about 2 ½ cups)

One 8-ounce (227 g) container bite-size fresh mozzarella balls (bocconcini)

½ cup (12 g) fresh basil leaves, thinly sliced

1 tablespoon extra virgin olive oil

1 tablespoon balsamic vinegar

¼ teaspoon flaky sea salt or kosher salt

Combine the tomatoes, mozzarella, basil, oil, vinegar, and salt in a bowl. Serve immediately.

TIPS: *The easiest way to cut basil into thin slices is to stack the leaves, roll up the stack, and cut thin slices across the roll.*

The flavor of this salad is better when served at room temperature. To make it in advance, combine all the ingredients except the basil, cover, and refrigerate. Remove from the refrigerator 20 to 30 minutes before serving. Add the basil right before serving.

Per Serving: Calories 217; Protein 11 g; Carbs 5 g; Dietary Fiber 1 g; Added Sugars 0 g; Total Fat 18 g; Sat Fat 9 g; Omega-3s 40 mg; Sodium 157 mg; Potassium 291 mg

CREAMY CILANTRO COLESLAW

Makes 8 servings

If you love fish or shrimp tacos, this is the perfect pairing. This creamy, crunchy salad also makes a great side dish for grilled chicken or Smoked Tri-Tip Roast (page 328). If you prefer less heat, reduce or eliminate the serrano pepper. Like it spicier? Add more!

Creamy Cilantro Dressing

1 bunch cilantro, ends trimmed, leaves and stems minced

½ cup (110 g) mayonnaise

Juice of 1 lime

2 teaspoons sugar

½ teaspoon kosher salt

½ teaspoon freshly ground black pepper

Coleslaw

One 10-ounce (283 g) package coleslaw mix

1 red, orange, or yellow bell pepper, seeded and diced

1 English cucumber, quartered lengthwise and diced

½ cup white onion, minced

2 serrano chiles, minced

Whisk the cilantro, mayonnaise, lime juice, sugar, salt, and pepper in a large bowl. Add the coleslaw mix, bell pepper, cucumber, onion, serrano, and cilantro. Toss to combine. Cover and refrigerate for 30 to 60 minutes before serving. Store in an airtight container in the refrigerator for up to 4 days.

Per Serving: Calories 127; Protein 2 g; Carbs 7 g; Dietary Fiber 2 g; Added Sugars 1 g; Total Fat 10 g; Sat Fat 2 g; Omega-3s 760 mg; Sodium 227 mg; Potassium 179 mg

CREAMY CUCUMBER-DILL SALAD

Makes 6 servings

Amy grew up on a farm in northeastern North Dakota. Every summer, her mom made a salad like this that she'd spoon over sliced tomatoes or serve with pan-fried walleye trout that Amy's dad would catch, and boiled baby red potatoes from their garden.

3 cucumbers, thinly sliced

½ teaspoon salt

¾ cup (180 ml) apple cider vinegar or white vinegar

½ cup (120 ml) cold water

1 small red onion or white onion, halved and thinly sliced into rings

4 teaspoons chopped fresh dill

1 teaspoon sugar

⅓ cup (75 g) mayonnaise

⅓ cup (75 g) sour cream

⅓ cup (75 g) plain Greek yogurt

Freshly ground black pepper

1. Place the cucumbers in a large bowl, sprinkle with the salt, and stir to coat. Let sit at room temperature for about 20 minutes, stirring occasionally, so the cucumbers release moisture.

2. When the cucumbers begin to look limp and are reduced in volume, drain off the liquid and rinse the cucumbers under cold running water. Shake to release as much water as possible and place the cucumbers back into the bowl.

3. Add the vinegar, water, onion, 2 teaspoons of the dill, and the sugar. Stir to coat. Refrigerate for 1 to 3 hours to allow the flavors to blend.

4. Drain the cucumbers and onion, reserving 1 tablespoon of the marinade. Whisk together the mayonnaise, sour cream, yogurt, and reserved marinade in a small bowl, then stir it into the cucumbers. Fold in the remaining 2 teaspoons dill and pepper to taste. Serve immediately or chill before serving. Store in an airtight container in the refrigerator for up to 2 days.

Per Serving: Calories 142; Protein 3 g; Carbs 6 g; Dietary Fiber 2 g; Added Sugars 1 g; Total Fat 12 g; Sat Fat 3 g; Omega-3s 700 mg; Sodium 283 mg; Potassium 267 mg

CUCUMBER & TOMATO SALAD

Makes 6 servings

Garden-fresh cucumbers and cherry tomatoes come together very simply, yet elegantly, with fresh-snipped herbs. We chose basil but rosemary, oregano, or thyme work well, too. Experiment with whatever your herb garden offers.

Salad

2 cucumbers, halved lengthwise and thinly sliced

1 pint (2 cups/300 g) cherry or grape tomatoes, halved

Lemon-Basil Dressing

2 tablespoons extra virgin olive oil

2 tablespoons fresh lemon juice

1 tablespoon chopped fresh basil leaves

Arrange the cucumbers and tomatoes on a serving dish. Whisk together the oil, lemon juice, and basil in a small bowl. Pour over the cucumbers and tomatoes and stir to combine. Serve immediately or refrigerate. Store covered in the refrigerator for up to 2 days.

Per Serving: Calories 62; Protein 1 g; Carbs 4 g; Dietary Fiber 2 g; Added Sugars 0 g; Total Fat 5 g; Sat Fat 1 g; Omega-3s 40 mg; Sodium 3 mg; Potassium 266 mg

DILLY CUCUMBER SALAD

Makes 6 servings

Growing up, Linda and her siblings picked "pickles" on their west central Minnesota farm. The joy was taking them to town for grading and weighing. The cukes in the produce aisle today would have been graded #3 or 4 and fetched very little money, as larger sizes were not highly valued. So into the kitchen a few would go to make this favored salad.

3 cucumbers, thinly sliced

½ teaspoon kosher salt

¾ cup (180 ml) apple cider vinegar or white vinegar

½ cup (120 ml) cold water

1 red onion or sweet onion (such as Vidalia or Walla Walla), halved and thinly sliced

2 teaspoons chopped fresh dill

1 teaspoon sugar

Freshly cracked black pepper

1. Place the cucumbers in a large bowl, sprinkle with the salt, and stir to coat. Let sit at room temperature for about 20 minute, stirring occasionally, so the cucumbers release moisture.

2. When the cucumbers begin to look limp and are reduced in volume, drain off the liquid and rinse the cucumbers under cold running water. Shake to release as much water as possible and place the cucumbers back into the bowl.

3. Add the vinegar, water, onion, dill, and sugar and stir to coat. Refrigerate for 1 to 3 hours, allowing the flavors to blend. Just before serving, drain the cucumbers and add black pepper to taste. The cucumbers do not stay crisp long; store covered in the refrigerator and serve the next meal or day.

Per Serving: Calories 25; Protein 2 g; Carbs 5 g; Dietary Fiber 2 g; Added Sugars 1 g; Total Fat 0 g; Sat Fat 0 g; Omega-3s 0 mg; Sodium 162 mg; Potassium 239 mg

MARINATED VEGETABLE SALAD

Makes 10 servings

This very versatile salad can be personalized with any vegetable you have on hand—perhaps your garden is flourishing with zucchini, cucumbers, tomatoes, green beans, or asparagus. Consider also using broccoli, cauliflower, cherry tomatoes, white mushrooms, snow peas, red cabbage, and/or artichoke hearts. This salad pairs well with any of our sandwiches on pages 181 and 182.

4 carrots, thinly sliced

4 celery stalks, sliced in ½-inch pieces

2 cucumbers, partially peeled (striped) and thinly sliced

1 large green or yellow bell pepper, seeded and thinly sliced

1 large red bell pepper, seeded and thinly sliced

½ red onion, thinly sliced and separated into rings

1¼ cups (300 ml) Tarragon & Thyme Vinaigrette (page 51)

1. Combine the carrots, celery, cucumbers, bell peppers, and onion in a large bowl. Add the vinaigrette and toss to coat, then cover and chill for 1 to 2 hours.

2. Use a slotted spoon to serve, or drain the marinade before serving. Keep the marinade only if you are returning the vegetables to the refrigerator. Store covered in the refrigerator for up to 1 week.

TIP: *Turn this vegetable side salad into an entrée by adding diced cooked chicken breast and cooked pasta such as rotini or penne.*

Per Serving: Calories 87; Protein 2 g; Carbs 11 g; Dietary Fiber 3 g; Added Sugars 2 g; Total Fat 4 g; Sat Fat 1 g; Omega-3s 40 mg; Sodium 86 mg; Potassium 182 mg

MIXED GREENS & MUSHROOM SALAD

Makes 4 servings

This simple go-to salad works well as a side to any meal. Keep a jar of our Herbed Red Wine Vinaigrette on hand in the fridge and this salad will come together in no time.

- 3 cups (105 g) chopped romaine lettuce
- 3 cups (75 g) chopped red leaf lettuce
- 6 green onions, thinly sliced
- 6 large white mushrooms, thinly sliced
- 1 small bunch flat-leaf parsley (leaves and stems), finely chopped
- ¼ cup (60 ml) Herbed Red Wine Vinaigrette (page 50)
- Freshly cracked black pepper

Place the lettuces, green onions, mushrooms, and parsley in a large bowl. Pour the vinaigrette over the salad and toss to combine. Add freshly cracked pepper and serve.

TIPS: *Toasted walnuts are a wonderful way to add heart-healthy fats and tempting crunch to this salad.*

Make it an entrée by adding hard-boiled eggs or roast chicken.

Per Serving: Calories 91; Protein 2 g; Carbs 6 g; Dietary Fiber 2 g; Added Sugars 1 g; Total Fat 7 g; Sat Fat 1 g; Omega-3s 90 mg; Sodium 32 mg; Potassium 389 mg

NAPA CABBAGE SLAW

Makes 6 servings

Food historians believe napa cabbage originated in China. It has an elongated shape and slightly more tender leaf than green cabbage. This light, vinegar-based coleslaw pairs perfectly with our Fresh Salmon Burgers (page 179).

- ¼ cup (60 ml) rice vinegar
- 2 tablespoons honey
- 2 tablespoons toasted sesame oil
- 2 tablespoons water
- 2 teaspoons minced fresh ginger
- ½ teaspoon red pepper flakes, or 1 small jalapeño or serrano chile, chopped
- 1 small head napa cabbage, quartered, cored and shredded
- 2 carrots, shredded
- 4 green onions, chopped

Whisk the vinegar, honey, oil, water, ginger, and red pepper flakes in a large bowl. Add the cabbage, carrots, and green onions and toss to combine. Serve immediately or refrigerate until ready to serve. Store in an airtight container in the refrigerator for up to 5 days.

TIP: *Try adding 1 tablespoon creamy peanut butter to the dressing and ¼ cup (35 g) chopped roasted peanuts to the salad for a boost of healthy fat and flavor!*

Per Serving: Calories 95; Protein 3 g; Carbs 12 g; Dietary Fiber 2 g; Added Sugars 6 g; Total Fat 5 g; Sat Fat 1 g; Omega-3s 90 mg; Sodium 107 mg; Potassium 390 mg

POTATO SALAD WITH RED WINE VINAIGRETTE

Makes 6 servings

This potato salad includes garden-fresh green beans and green onions with a vinaigrette dressing in place of the typical creamy mayonnaise-based dressing. We like to use baby red or gold potatoes. Dressing the potatoes with vinaigrette when they're warm helps them absorb more flavor. For optimal flavor, serve this salad at room temperature.

- 2 pounds (907 g) small red-skin (about 6 to 7) or Yukon gold (about 3 to 5) potatoes
- 6 ounces (170 g) green beans, trimmed, cut into 1-inch (2.5 cm) pieces, and blanched and drained (1 cup/150 g)
- ½ cup (80 g) thinly sliced green onions (about 6)
- ¼ cup (15 g) minced fresh parsley
- ½ cup (120 ml) extra virgin olive oil
- ¼ cup (60 ml) red wine vinegar
- 1 tablespoon Dijon mustard
- 1 teaspoon sugar
- ½ teaspoon celery seed
- ¼ teaspoon kosher salt
- Freshly ground black pepper

1. Boil the potatoes just until tender, 15 to 20 minutes.

2. Drain, then quarter the potatoes while still hot. Arrange them in an 11 × 7-inch (28 × 18 cm) glass baking dish. Add the green beans, green onions, and parsley

3. Whisk together the oil, vinegar, mustard, sugar, celery seed, salt, and pepper in a small bowl. Pour over the vegetables while the potatoes are still warm. Toss gently. Marinate for 30 minutes or longer at room temperature before serving. Store in an airtight container in the refrigerator for up to 5 days.

TIP: *To make ahead, allow the salad to marinate in the refrigerator. Remove 30 minutes before serving.*

Per Serving: Calories 270; Protein 3 g; Carbs 25 g; Dietary Fiber 4 g; Added Sugars 1 g; Total Fat 18 g; Sat Fat 3 g; Omega-3s 156 mg; Sodium 225 mg; Potassium 680 mg

RADISH & CABBAGE SLAW

Makes 6 servings

Serve this slaw as a side salad or use it to top a seared ahi tuna sandwich.

Sesame-Lime Dressing
- ¼ cup (60 ml) toasted sesame oil
- 3 tablespoons rice vinegar
- 2 tablespoons sesame seeds, toasted
- 1 teaspoon finely grated lime zest
- 1 tablespoon fresh lime juice
- ¼ teaspoon red pepper flakes
- ¼ teaspoon white pepper
- ⅛ teaspoon kosher salt

Slaw
- 4 cups (290 g) shredded cabbage or coleslaw mix with carrots
- 1 cup (115 g) radishes, trimmed and very thinly sliced
- 6 green onions, chopped
- ½ cup (70 g) pitted black olives, sliced

Whisk together the oil, vinegar, sesame seeds, lime zest and juice, red pepper flakes, pepper, and salt in large bowl. Add the cabbage, radishes, green onions, and olives and stir to combine. Serve immediately or cover and refrigerate until ready to serve. Store in an airtight container in the refrigerator for up to 5 days.

Per Serving: Calories 135; Protein 2 g; Carbs 7 g; Dietary Fiber 3 g; Added Sugars 0 g; Total Fat 12 g; Sat Fat 2 g; Omega-3s 16 mg; Sodium 165 mg; Potassium 180 mg

POTATO SALAD WITH RED WINE VINAIGRETTE (PAGE 154)

WASABI-GINGER COLESLAW

Makes about 4 cups (615 g)

This coleslaw loves to be paired with seafood. We feature it as the perfect topping for our ahi burgers (page 177), but it's also great with shrimp tacos and as an accompaniment to bowls featuring whole grains, legumes, and grilled fish or shrimp.

½ cup (110 g) mayonnaise

2 tablespoons fresh lemon juice

1 tablespoon grated fresh ginger

1 tablespoon white (shiro) miso

1 tablespoon prepared wasabi

14 ounces (6 cups/397 g) tri-color coleslaw mix or thinly sliced cabbage

¼ cup (40 g) minced red or white onion

Whisk together the mayonnaise, lemon juice, ginger, miso, and wasabi in a medium bowl. Stir in the coleslaw mix and onion. Cover and chill until ready to serve. Store in an airtight container in the refrigerator for up to 3 days.

TIP: *We use white miso here due to its mild flavor and lower sodium content compared to other types of miso.*

Serving Size 1 cup (154 g); Calories 245; Protein 2 g; Carbs 12 g; Dietary Fiber 3 g; Added Sugars 0 g; Total Fat 21 g; Sat Fat 3 g; Omega-3s 1,517 mg; Sodium 440 mg; Potassium 265 mg

WEDGE SALAD

Makes 4 servings

If you love blue cheese dressing, you're a likely fan of the classic wedge salad. Our version features a blue cheese vinaigrette, which contains less saturated fat and sodium but not less flavor than a standard blue cheese dressing, and Smoky Pecan Bits in place of bacon. Serve this salad with a grilled or pan-seared lean steak like a filet mignon, Simply Roasted Potatoes (page 260), and a glass of Cabernet Sauvignon for a special, celebratory meal.

1 head iceberg lettuce, quartered into wedges

¾ cup (170 g) Blue Cheese Vinaigrette (page 48)

4 green onions, thinly sliced

2 tomatoes, diced

½ cup (55 g) Smoky Pecan Bits (page 173)

Place 1 iceberg wedge on each of four plates. Drizzle 3 tablespoons of the vinaigrette over each wedge. Divide the green onions and tomatoes evenly among the salads, top with the pecan bits, and serve.

Per Serving: Calories 374; Protein 5 g; Carbs 13 g; Dietary Fiber 4 g; Added Sugars 2 g; Total Fat 35 g; Sat Fat 5 g; Omega-3s 390 mg; Sodium 206 mg; Potassium 469 mg

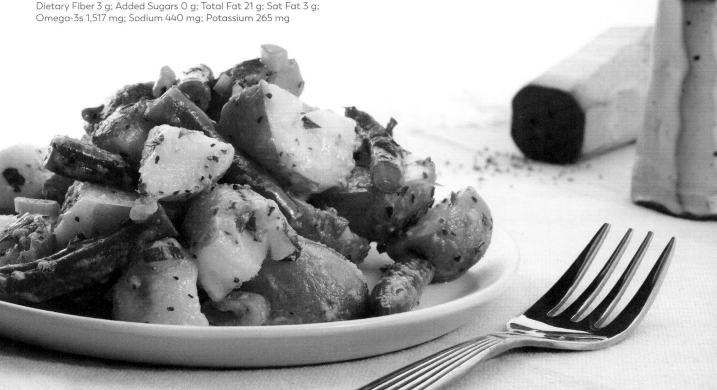

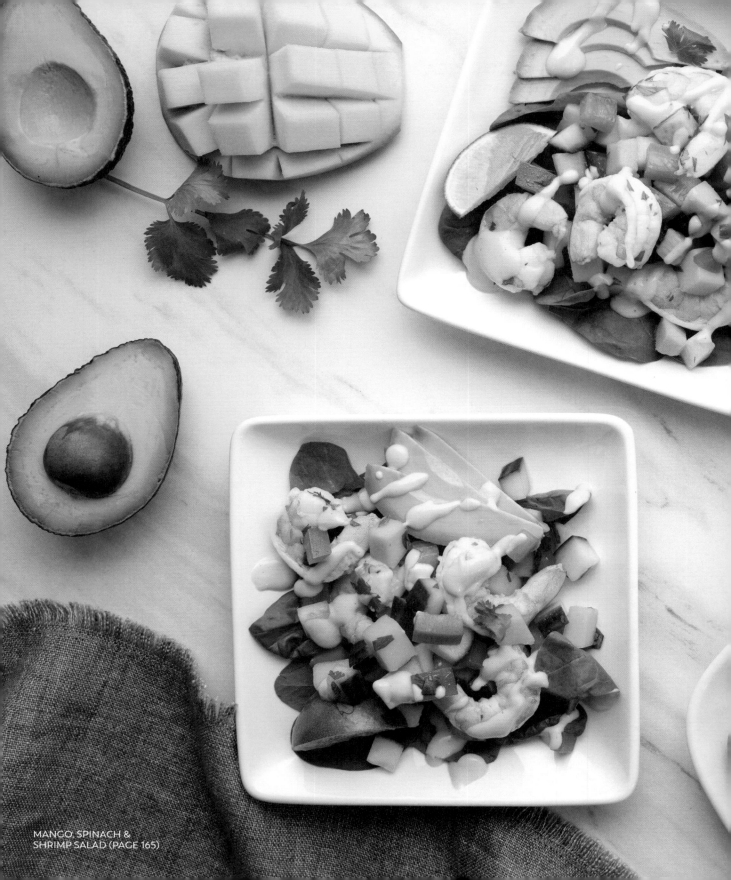

MANGO, SPINACH &
SHRIMP SALAD (PAGE 165)

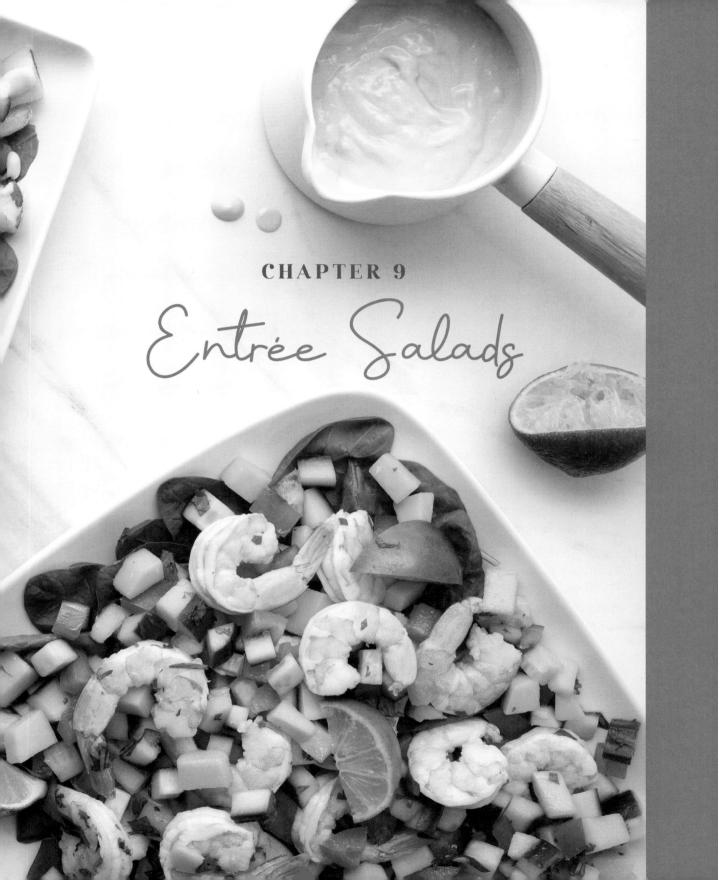

CHAPTER 9

Entrée Salads

Entrée Salads

Salads with Meat or Fish

Autumn Wild Rice & Chicken Bowls 159

Beef & Lentil Salad Bowls. 160

Bulgur-Tomato Salad with
Tuna & Mint 160

Chicken Caesar Salad 161

Chicken Lentil Spinach Bowls 161

Chicken Waldorf Tomato Blossoms
with Feta & Dill 162

Chicken & Wild Rice Salad with
Grapes & Candied Pecans 162

Cilantro-Lime Chicken & Corn Salad . . . 163

Crab, Asparagus & Avocado Salad 163

Have A Plant Curried Chicken Salad . . . 164

Make-Ahead Layered Salad
with Eggs 165

Mango, Spinach & Shrimp Salad. 165

Pan-Seared White Fish, Arugula
& Roasted Tomato Salad 166

Salade Niçoise. 166

Southeast Asian–Style Shrimp & Napa
Cabbage Salad with Rice Noodles 167

Wild Crab Salad. 168

Salads with Plant Protein

Cooking à la Heart Salad 168

Crispy Tofu with Lentils &
Mixed Greens. 169

Four-Bean Salad. 169

Lentil & Brown Rice Salad with
Fresh Thyme. 170

Lentil Caprese Salad 170

Lentil & Mixed Greens Salad with
Goat Cheese 170

Wild Rice & Chickpea Salad 171

Zoodle Tofu Bowls. 171

Salad Accompaniments

Crunchy Italian-Flavored Chickpeas . . . 172

Parmesan-Herb Croutons 172

Smoky Pecan Bits. 173

Spicy Candied Pecans 173

salads can take on so many forms and flavor profiles. For this chapter, we created a wide variety of entrée salads, some with animal protein and others with plant protein. Many are inspired by Mediterranean cuisine, like the classic French Salade Niçoise (page 166), but we've also included salads with Asian and Latin flavor profiles, like Southeast Asian–Style Shrimp & Napa Cabbage Salad with Rice Noodles (page 167) and Cilantro-Lime Chicken & Corn Salad (page 163).

Many recipes in this chapter are bowl concepts. We say "concepts" because bowls are endlessly customizable. Use our recipes as jumping-off points; you can alter the ingredients and proportions to create the perfect bowls for yourself and your family, choosing the vegetables, whole grains, animal and/or plant protein sources, and dressings that fit the mood or use the ingredients in your pantry and refrigerator. Want a zestier green? Choose arugula instead of baby spinach. Thinking about adding some sweetness to a bowl? Throw in some grapes! Hungry for more protein? Add chicken and chickpeas to your bowl. Have fun creating bowls that feed your body and your soul.

You will quickly notice that every recipe in this chapter includes vegetables. We often feature dark leafy greens as star players, but sometimes we only use vegetables in a supporting role to add color, flavor, or texture. Many salads also feature fruit, whole grains, and legumes. The dressings and vinaigrettes most often include extra virgin olive oil, but some incorporate Greek yogurt, mayonnaise, or peanut butter for a creamy, flavorful base.

Finally, while we call this chapter Entrée Salads, you can of course enjoy these in smaller portions as sides.

AUTUMN WILD RICE & CHICKEN BOWLS

Makes 4 servings

This salad features so many appealing textures, from chewy wild rice and dried cranberries to crunchy raw vegetables and nuts. The red wine vinegar–based dressing adds bright flavor notes to the chicken and chickpeas.

2 cups (330 g) Simply Cooked Wild Rice (page 234)

Grated zest of 1 lemon

One 5-ounce (142 g) bag mixed greens (about 4 cups)

1 cup (100 g) chopped celery (about 2 stalks)

1 cup (70 g) sliced cremini or white mushrooms

1 cup (160 g) chopped red onion (about 1 large onion)

2 cups (270 g) diced cooked chicken breast

One 15-ounce (425 g) can chickpeas, drained and rinsed

½ cup (120 ml) Herbed Red Wine Vinaigrette (page 50)

½ cup (65 g) dried cranberries

¼ cup (30 g) Spicy Candied Pecans (page 173)

Divide the wild rice among four bowls. Sprinkle over the lemon zest. Top with the mixed greens, then add rows or layers of celery, mushrooms, and onion. Add the chicken and chickpeas to each bowl. Drizzle 2 tablespoons vinaigrette over each bowl, then top each with 2 tablespoons cranberries and 1 tablespoon pecans. Serve.

TIP: You can also serve this salad family-style by combining all the ingredients in a large bowl, tossing well, and asking diners to serve themselves.

Serving Size 1 bowl; Calories 550; Protein 32 g; Carbs 54 g; Dietary Fiber 9 g; Added Sugars 2 g; Total Fat 24 g; Sat. Fat 3 g; Omega-3s 360 mg; Sodium 245 mg; Potassium 670 mg

BEEF & LENTIL SALAD BOWLS

Makes 4 servings

Beef and lentils pair up to provide protein in this easy-to-assemble entrée salad that features a bright, red wine vinegar–based dressing that perfectly complements the flavors of the other ingredients. If you bring home extra steak from a restaurant, this recipe is a great way to turn it into something exciting and new.

½ cup (120 ml) extra virgin olive oil

⅓ cup (80 ml) fresh lime juice

2 tablespoons red wine vinegar

½ teaspoon hot sauce

½ cup (8 g) chopped fresh cilantro

¼ cup (40 g) chopped green onions

1½ cups (285 g) Simply Cooked Lentils (page 247)

½ cup (50 g) diced celery

½ cup (65 g) diced cucumber

¼ cup (35 g) diced bell pepper

One 2-ounce (57 g) jar diced pimientos, drained

6 cups (210 g) mixed salad greens or fresh baby spinach leaves

8 ounces (227 g) cooked lean beef (such as flank or sirloin steak), thinly sliced

4 ounces (113 g) toasted walnuts, chopped

2 ounces (57 g) creamy blue cheese, broken into small pieces with a fork

1. Whisk together the oil, lime juice, vinegar, hot sauce, cilantro, and green onions in a small bowl. Combine the lentils, celery, cucumber, pepper, and pimiento in a large bowl. Add half the dressing and toss well to coat. Cover and refrigerate for at least an hour to allow the flavors to meld.

2. When you're ready to serve, combine the greens with the rest of the dressing and toss well to coat. Divide the greens among four bowls. Top each bowl with one-fourth each of the lentil mixture, steak, walnuts, and blue cheese.

Serving Size 1 bowl; Calories 687; Protein 29 g; Carbs 20 g; Dietary Fiber 10 g; Added Sugars 0 g; Total Fat 56 g; Sat Fat 10 g; Omega-3s 2,820 mg; Sodium 235 mg; Potassium 650 mg

BULGUR-TOMATO SALAD WITH TUNA & MINT

Makes 4 servings

Nutty bulgur, a vibrant vinegar-based dressing, leafy greens, and canned tuna come together to create a very flavorful, healthful meal in a bowl. Enjoy on its own or pair with fresh pita bread for sopping up extra dressing.

3 cups (550 g) Simply Cooked Bulgur (page 224)

⅔ cup (150 g) plain Greek yogurt

½ cup (40 g) thinly sliced green onions

½ cup (12 g) chopped fresh mint leaves

¼ cup (15 g) finely chopped fresh parsley

1 tablespoon grated lemon zest

2 tablespoons fresh lemon juice

1 tablespoon white wine vinegar or red wine vinegar

1 teaspoon Dijon mustard

1 tomato, diced

¾ cup (100 g) diced cucumber or zucchini

6 cups (210 g) mixed salad greens

Two 5-ounce (142 g) cans tuna, drained

1 lemon, quartered

1. Combine the bulgur, yogurt, onions, 6 tablespoons (9 g) of the mint, the parsley, lemon zest and juice, vinegar, and mustard in a large bowl. Add the tomato and cucumber. Toss, cover, and chill for at least 1 hour.

2. Just before serving, toss again. To serve, divide the greens among four bowls. Top with equal amounts of bulgur salad and of tuna. Sprinkle each bowl with the remaining mint and garnish with a lemon wedge.

Per Serving: Calories 214; Protein 15 g; Carbs 30 g; Dietary Fiber 5 g; Added Sugars 0 g; Total Fat 5 g; Sat Fat 1 g; Omega-3s 130 mg; Sodium 187 mg; Potassium 426 mg

CHICKEN CAESAR SALAD

Makes 4 servings

The chicken served with many Caesar salads is often dry, requiring a lot of dressing to make it moist and juicy. This recipe creates tender, flavorful chicken that is great on its own but also a welcome addition to the salad. This chicken is also good in a pita pocket with some lettuce and a spoonful of our À la Heart Caesar Dressing (page 47).

Chicken

2 tablespoons extra virgin olive oil

1 pound (454 g) chicken tenders or boneless, skinless chicken breasts, cut into bite-size pieces

1 garlic clove, minced

2 tablespoons fresh lemon juice

2 teaspoons minced fresh oregano or thyme

½ teaspoon freshly ground black pepper

Salad

12 cups (420 g) chopped romaine lettuce

1 cup (240 g) À la Heart Caesar Dressing (page 47)

1 cup (90 g) Parmesan-Herb Croutons (page 172)

2 ounces (57 g) freshly shaved or shredded Parmesan

1. Heat 1 tablespoon of the oil in a large sauté pan over medium-high heat. When the oil starts to shimmer, add the chicken and sauté until no longer pink, 7 to 8 minutes.

2. Add the remaining 1 tablespoon of oil and the garlic, reduce the heat to medium-low, and cook, stirring frequently, until the garlic is aromatic, 1 to 2 minutes. Add the lemon juice, oregano, and pepper, and cook just long enough to wilt the oregano, 30 to 45 seconds. Remove from the heat and set aside to cool.

3. Combine the lettuce and dressing in a large bowl. Divide the lettuce among four plates or shallow bowls. Divide the chicken, croutons, and Parmesan among the four salads and serve.

Per Serving: Calories 500; Protein 38 g; Carbs 24 g; Dietary Fiber 5 g; Added Sugars 0 g; Total Fat 28 g; Sat Fat 7 g; Omega-3s 307 mg; Sodium 715 mg; Potassium 800 mg

CHICKEN LENTIL SPINACH BOWLS

Makes 4 servings

Rotisserie chicken makes creating these bowls quick and easy. Yes, rotisserie chicken contains much more sodium than chicken you'd cook at home, but sometimes convenient options reduce stress, which is also important for heart health.

½ cup (120 ml) extra virgin olive oil

⅓ cup (80 ml) fresh lime juice

2 tablespoons red wine vinegar

½ teaspoon hot sauce

½ cup (8 g) chopped fresh cilantro

1 green onion, thinly sliced

1½ cups (285 g) Simply Cooked Lentils (page 247)

1 celery stalk, diced

½ cup (65 g) diced cucumber

¼ cup (35 g) diced bell pepper

10 ounces (285 g) grape tomatoes, halved

6 cups (180 g) fresh baby spinach leaves

12 ounces (340 g) skinned, deboned, rotisserie chicken, chopped

2 ounces (57 g) Swiss cheese or Parmesan, diced

1. Whisk together the oil, lime juice, vinegar, hot sauce, cilantro, and green onions in a small bowl. Combine the lentils, celery, cucumber, and pepper in a large bowl, add half the dressing, and toss well to coat. Cover and refrigerate for at least an hour to allow the flavors to meld.

2. To serve, combine the tomatoes and spinach with the rest of the dressing and toss well to coat. Divide the spinach-tomato mixture among four bowls. Top each bowl with equal amounts of the lentil mixture, the chicken, and the cheese.

Per Serving: Calories 552; Protein 32 g; Carbs 21 g; Dietary Fiber 9 g; Added Sugars 0 g; Total Fat 37 g; Sat Fat 8 g; Omega-3s 280 mg; Sodium 577 mg; Potassium 762 mg

CHICKEN WALDORF TOMATO BLOSSOMS WITH FETA & DILL

Makes 4 servings

Replacing some of the mayonnaise in this chicken salad with Greek yogurt adds protein, calcium, and potassium; the dill and lemon zest add flavor, tang, and tartness; and the feta adds a bit of saltiness—all tasty, healthful changes to the traditional Waldorf salad. Serving the salad in tomato "blossoms" creates a gorgeous presentation perfect for a party!

- 1½ cups (190 g) diced meat from Roast Chicken with Lemon & Thyme (page 313) or rotisserie chicken
- 1 apple, cored and chopped
- ⅔ cup (150 g) plain Greek yogurt
- ½ cup (50 g) chopped celery
- ⅓ cup (75 g) mayonnaise
- 1 tablespoon chopped fresh dill
- 1 teaspoon grated lemon zest
- Freshly ground black pepper
- 4 Boston, Bibb, or butter lettuce leaves
- 4 tomatoes (see Tip)
- ¼ cup (40 g) crumbled feta
- ¼ cup (30 g) toasted walnuts, coarsely chopped
- 4 dill sprigs

1. Combine the chicken, apple, yogurt, celery, mayonnaise, dill, lemon zest, and pepper to taste in a medium bowl. Cover and chill for 1 hour or more to allow the flavors to meld.

2. Place a lettuce leaf on each of four plates. Cut each tomato into six sections from the bottom almost to the stem and place each on a lettuce leaf. (The tomato will look more like a water lily than an upright pocket.)

3. Scoop one-fourth of the salad (about ¾ cup/100 g) into each opened tomato, turning it into a blossom. Sprinkle each with 1 tablespoon each feta and walnuts and top with a dill sprig.

TIP: *Look for the largest, most beautiful ripe tomatoes you can find at your local market to create your "blossoms."*

Per Serving: Calories 337; Protein 20 g; Carbs 10 g; Dietary Fiber 2 g; Added Sugars 0 g; Total Fat 25 g; Sat Fat 5 g; Omega-3s 1,770 mg; Sodium 402 mg; Potassium 298 mg

CHICKEN & WILD RICE SALAD WITH GRAPES & CANDIED PECANS

Makes 4 servings

It's common to combine chicken and wild rice to make a hot casserole, but here we pair them to make a delicious cold summer salad. We include grapes for a bit of juicy sweetness and spicy candied pecans for an unexpected pop of heat and crunch, creating an adventurous new dish from the familiar.

- ⅔ cup (145 g) mayonnaise
- ⅔ cup (150 g) plain Greek yogurt
- Grated zest of 1 lemon
- 2 tablespoons fresh lemon juice
- 3 cups (380 g) chicken, cut into bite-size pieces, from Roast Chicken with Lemon & Thyme (page 313)
- 2 cups (330 g) Simply Cooked Wild Rice (page 234)
- ½ cup (40 g) finely sliced green onions
- ½ cup (75 g) finely chopped bell pepper
- ½ teaspoon white pepper
- 1½ cups (225 g) seedless green grapes, halved
- ¾ cup (85 g) chopped pecans, from Spicy Candied Pecans (page 173)
- 4 cups (140 g) mixed salad greens

1. Mix the mayonnaise, yogurt, lemon zest, and lemon juice in a small bowl. Combine the chicken, rice, onions, bell pepper, and white pepper in a medium bowl. Fold in the mayonnaise mixture. Cover and refrigerate for 2 to 3 hours.

2. Just before serving, fold in the grapes and pecans. To serve family-style, place the mixed greens at the bottom of a large bowl and top with the chicken salad. For individual salads, divide the mixed greens and chicken salad evenly among four plates.

Per Serving: Calories 650; Protein 31 g; Carbs 18 g; Dietary Fiber 4 g; Added Sugars 1 g; Total Fat 52 g; Sat Fat 8 g; Omega-3s 2,376 mg; Sodium 415 mg; Potassium 630 mg

CILANTRO-LIME CHICKEN & CORN SALAD

Makes 4 servings

This salad is a summer sensation when sweet corn is at its peak! We recommend shredding the chicken, rather than cutting it into cubes, to create more surface area for the tangy lime dressing to soak into. Serve as an entrée salad with tortillas or tortilla chips, or offer it along with another summer salad like our Cucumber & Tomato Salad (page 152) and our Simply Cooked Black Beans (page 241).

- 1 pound (454 g) chicken tenders
- ¼ cup (60 ml) plus 1 tablespoon extra virgin olive oil
- 4 ears corn, shucked
- ¼ cup (60 ml) fresh lime juice (about 2 limes)
- ½ teaspoon kosher salt
- ½ teaspoon freshly ground black pepper
- ½ cup (8 g) minced fresh cilantro leaves and stems

1. Heat 1 tablespoon of the oil in a large sauté pan over medium heat. Add the chicken and cook for 5 minutes on each side, until a digital food thermometer reads 165°F (75°C) when inserted in the thickest part of a tender. Transfer the chicken to a bowl and use two forks to shred it into bite-size pieces.

2. While the chicken cooks, bring a large pot of water to a boil over high heat. Add the corn and cook for 10 minutes. Set the corn aside to cool slightly before cutting off the kernels.

3. Whisk the remaining ¼ cup (60 ml) oil, the lime juice, salt, and pepper in a large bowl. Add the shredded chicken, corn, and cilantro and stir well. Serve immediately.

TIP: *You can use a chef's knife to cut the corn off the cob, but there are also inexpensive tools called corn cutters or corn peelers that make the process a bit easier. No matter how you cut the corn off the cob, we recommend using a knife to gently scrape the cob after cutting off the kernels to remove as much corn "milk" as possible. This contributes a slight creaminess to the dressing.*

Per Serving: Calories 385; Protein 29 g; Carbs 22 g; Dietary Fiber 3 g; Added Sugars 0 g; Total Fat 21 g; Sat Fat 3 g; Omega-3s 170 mg; Sodium 350 mg; Potassium 620 mg

CRAB, ASPARAGUS & AVOCADO SALAD

Makes 4 servings

There are so many great food and flavor pairings in this recipe, we hardly know where to begin! Crab, avocado, asparagus, and lemon come together in this light yet flavor-packed salad. Offer extra Avocado Lemon Dill Aïoli on the side for those who want a little more on their salad.

- 24 fresh asparagus spears, trimmed, or two 8-ounce (227 g) bags frozen asparagus spears
- Ice water
- 2 cups (480 ml) Avocado Lemon Dill Aïoli (page 43)
- ½ cup (40 g) finely chopped green onions
- 2 tablespoons sriracha
- 2 teaspoons Dijon mustard
- 8 ounces (227 g) lump crab meat or thawed frozen cooked crab meat, separated into chunks
- One 12-ounce (340 g) jar roasted red pepper strips, drained
- 6 cups (210 g) mixed salad greens
- 1 avocado, halved, pitted, peeled, and sliced
- 1 lemon, quartered
- ½ cup (70 g) slivered almonds, toasted
- 48 Southwest Pita Chips (page 340)

1. Steam the asparagus until bright green and tender-crisp, about 2 minutes. Drain and plunge into ice water to cool. Drain, pat dry, and cut into bite-size pieces.

2. Whisk together 1 cup (240 ml) of the aïoli, the green onions, sriracha, and mustard in a medium bowl. Add the asparagus, crab, and roasted peppers and toss until well combined.

3. Line four serving dishes with the mixed greens. Top with fanned avocado slices. Add a scoop of the crab salad on top of or alongside the avocado. Add a lemon wedge and sprinkle with 1 tablespoon of toasted slivered almonds. Serve with pita chips and the remaining aïoli on the side.

Per Serving: Calories 358; Protein 18 g; Carbs 33 g; Dietary Fiber 14 g; Added Sugars 1 g; Total Fat 19 g; Sat Fat 2 g; Omega-3s 130 mg; Sodium 832 mg; Potassium 837 mg

HAVE A PLANT CURRIED CHICKEN SALAD

Makes 8 servings

This recipe includes chicken, but a greater proportion of the ingredients comes from fruits and vegetables in various forms (fresh, frozen, canned, dried, and 100% juice). It's an example of how you can increase your intake of plant-based foods without giving up the flavors, textures, and nutrition properties of animal-based foods. The salad can be served on lettuce leaves, or as a sandwich filling— it's especially good in whole wheat pita pockets.

1 tablespoon extra virgin olive oil

1 pound (454 g) chicken tenders

¾ cup (165 g) mayonnaise

3 to 4 tablespoons Curry Powder (page 32)

One 20-ounce (567 g) can pineapple chunks in 100% juice, drained, juice reserved

2 cups (300 g) red or green seedless grapes, halved

3 celery stalks, diced

1 red, yellow, or orange bell pepper, seeded and diced

1 cup (135 g) roasted unsalted cashews, chopped

4 green onions, sliced

½ cup (80 g) golden raisins

Butter lettuce leaves

1. Heat the oil in a large sauté pan over medium-high heat. Add the chicken and cook for 5 minutes on each side, until a digital food thermometer reads 165°F (75°C) when inserted in the thickest part of the chicken. Transfer the chicken to a cutting board and cut into bite-size pieces.

2. Whisk together the mayonnaise, curry powder to taste, and ¼ cup (60 ml) of the reserved pineapple juice in a large bowl. Add the chicken, pineapple, grapes, celery, pepper, cashews, onions, and raisins. Stir gently to combine, then chill for at least 30 minutes before serving.

3. To serve, place the lettuce leaves on eight salad plates and top each with 1 cup (225 g) of the chicken salad. Store in an airtight container in the refrigerator for up to 3 days.

TIP: *We've suggested a range of curry powder amounts so you can make this according to your preference. If you really love curry, use the full 4 tablespoons; if you want a little less curry flavor, use less.*

Per Serving: Calories 530; Protein 15 g; Carbs 43 g; Dietary Fiber 4 g; Added Sugars 0 g; Total Fat 35 g; Sat Fat 6 g; Omega-3s 1,590 mg; Sodium 606 mg; Potassium 620 mg

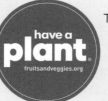

The Have A Plant movement was launched in 2019 by the Produce for Better Health Foundation (PBH), the United States' "only national 501(c)3 non-profit organization whose mission is to achieve increased daily consumption of fruits and vegetables" to promote public health. This salad exemplifies many of its principles, including the benefits of enjoying fruits and vegetables of all forms. PBH also understands the power of eating inclusive dietary patterns that don't exclude any food groups; rather, they emphasize plant-based ingredients that create delicious foods and beverages every day. You can learn more about Have A Plant at fruitsandveggies.org.

MAKE-AHEAD LAYERED SALAD WITH EGGS

Makes 12 servings

In Linda's family, this was an often-made salad put together on a summer morning right after breakfast before they all headed out to till the fields, hoe the garden, or mend fences. Made with a variety of vegetables, it's the perfect one-dish meal to have waiting in the fridge when you've had a busy day. Add fresh Buttermilk Rolls (page 107) or Hearty Wheat Buns (page 110) and a glass of milk or ice water to round out the meal.

One 9- to 10-ounce (255 to 283 g) bag mixed greens

1 red onion, diced

3 celery stalks, diced

1 bell pepper, seeded and diced

6 hard-boiled large eggs, peeled and chopped

2 cups (270 g) frozen green peas, thawed under running water and drained

Two 5.3-ounce (150 g each) containers plain Greek yogurt (about 1⅓ cups)

¾ cup (165 g) mayonnaise

2 tablespoons chopped fresh dill

½ teaspoon freshly cracked black pepper

8 ounces (227 g) shredded part-skim mozzarella

1. In a 9 × 13-inch (23 × 33 cm) pan, layer the greens, onion, celery, bell pepper, eggs, and peas. Combine the yogurt, mayonnaise, dill, and black pepper in a small bowl. Spread the mixture over the layered vegetables (as if frosting a cake). Top with mozzarella.

2. Refrigerate overnight. Cut into squares and serve.

3. Store in an airtight container in the refrigerator for up to 2 days.

Per Serving: Calories 228; Protein 11 g; Carbs 8 g; Dietary Fiber 2 g; Added Sugars 0 g; Total Fat 17 g; Sat Fat 5 g; Omega-3s 810 mg; Sodium 301 mg; Potassium 208 mg

MANGO, SPINACH & SHRIMP SALAD

Makes 4 servings

This salad is so well-liked because of its easy preparation, visual appeal, freshness, and beautiful combination of greens, fruit, and shrimp. Linda and her daughter, Alicia, serve it as their annual main dish on Mother's Day. Because it's mid-May and the rhubarb is flourishing at the edge of the garden, either Rhubarb-Strawberry Coffee Cake (page 99) or Strawberry-Rhubarb Bars (page 359) are served later along with their coffee and conversation.

One 16-ounce (454 g) bag frozen cooked, peeled shrimp, thawed and drained

1 mango, pitted, peeled, and diced

1 English cucumber, diced

1 red bell pepper, seeded and diced

½ cup (8 g) chopped fresh cilantro

One 5- to 6-ounce (142 to 170 g) bag baby spinach (about 4 to 6 cups)

2 cups (480 ml) Avocado Lime Cilantro Aïoli (page 44)

1 avocado, halved, pitted, peeled, and sliced

1 lime, halved

1. Combine the shrimp, mango, cucumber, pepper, and cilantro in a large bowl.

2. To assemble the salads, divide the spinach among four plates, top with the shrimp mixture, and drizzle each plate with ¼ cup (60 ml) of the aïoli. Add the avocado slices to each plate; squeeze half the lime over the top.

3. Quarter the remaining half lime and add a wedge to each plate. Serve the remaining aïoli on the side.

Per Serving: Calories 415; Protein 34 g; Carbs 21 g; Dietary Fiber 7 g; Added Sugars 0 g; Total Fat 23 g; Sat Fat 4 g; Omega-3s 930 mg; Sodium 265 mg; Potassium 935 mg

PAN-SEARED WHITE FISH, ARUGULA & ROASTED TOMATO SALAD

Makes 4 servings

This warm salad is loaded with fresh ingredients and vibrant flavors. Plate it as you go. Start with the arugula, add the roasted tomatoes, and finally the marinated and pan-seared fish fillets. Serve with fresh-from-the-oven Whole Wheat French Baguettes (page 114) or another warm whole grain bread you love.

- ½ cup (120 ml) white wine
- ¼ cup (60 ml) fresh lemon juice
- 6 tablespoons (90 ml) extra virgin olive oil, plus more for oiling the pan
- 1 tablespoon minced fresh tarragon or 1 teaspoon dried tarragon
- 1 garlic clove, minced
- 1 pound (454 g) white fish fillets (such as cod, flounder, haddock, halibut, sea bass, or tilapia)
- 2 tomatoes, sliced ½ inch (13 mm) thick
- One 9 to 10-ounce (255 to 283 g) bag arugula
- 3 tablespoons (45 g) butter or plant-based spread
- ½ cup (65 g) all-purpose flour
- 1 tablespoon chopped fresh basil or 1 teaspoon dried basil
- 1 tablespoon fresh marjoram or 1 teaspoon dried marjoram
- 1 tablespoon chopped fresh thyme leaves or 1 teaspoon dried thyme
- 1 teaspoon white pepper
- 1 cup (240 ml) Tarragon & Thyme Vinaigrette (page 51)

1. Adjust an oven rack to the middle position. Preheat the oven to 400°F (200°C).

2. Whisk the wine, lemon juice, 1 tablespoon of the oil, tarragon, and garlic in a 7 × 11-inch (18 × 28 cm) glass baking dish. Add the fish fillets in a single layer; flip them to coat both sides. Refrigerate for 30 minutes.

3. Place the tomato slices in a single layer on an oiled, rimmed baking pan. Brush the tomatoes with 1 tablespoon of the oil and roast for 10 minutes, until they start to release much of their juice. Flip the slices over, brush with tablespoon oil and roast for 10 minutes, until they start to caramelize slightly. Divide the arugula among four plates and add the tomatoes.

4. While the tomatoes are roasting, cook the fish. Heat the last 3 tablespoons of oil and the butter in a large skillet over medium heat. Whisk together the flour, basil, marjoram, thyme, and pepper in a small bowl; pour onto a large plate. Remove the fish fillets from the marinade and dredge until entirely coated with the flour mixture. Place in the skillet and cook for 4 to 6 minutes per side, until the fish is firm and opaque, and flakes easily with a fork (time will depend on the thickness of the fillets). A digital food thermometer should read 145°F (65°C) when inserted in the thickest part of the largest fillet. Break the fish into large chunks and divide among the four plates, over the tomatoes.

5. Spoon 2 to 3 tablespoons vinaigrette over the fish and salad; serve any remaining vinaigrette on the side.

Per Serving: Calories 478; Protein 25 g; Carbs 20 g; Dietary Fiber 3 g; Added Sugars 0 g; Total Fat 31 g; Sat Fat 9 g; Omega-3s 530 mg; Sodium 154 mg; Potassium 938 mg

SALADE NIÇOISE

Makes 4 servings

Salade Niçoise originated in the French city of Nice. It's traditionally made with green beans, potatoes, hard-boiled eggs, olives, anchovies, and tuna, and dressed with olive oil. Here, we've added more vegetables, and used canned sardines and our vibrant Herbed Red Wine Vinaigrette.

- 8 ounces (227 g) green beans, trimmed
- Ice water
- 4 baby red-skin potatoes
- 1½ cups (360 ml) Herbed Red Wine Vinaigrette (page 50)
- 1½ heads romaine lettuce, torn into bite-size pieces
- 1 small red onion or large shallot, diced
- 2 small globe red (or 2 medium Roma) tomatoes, quartered

Two 3-ounce (85 g) cans sardines or one 5-ounce (142 g) can tuna, drained

4 large hard-boiled eggs, peeled and quartered

8 radishes, trimmed and sliced

½ cup (70 g) pitted Niçoise olives, sliced

Freshly ground black pepper

1. Cover the potatoes with cold water in a small saucepan. Bring to a simmer over medium-high heat and cook until fork-tender, about 5 minutes. Drain and let cool. Thinly slice the potatoes and place in a medium bowl. Add 2 tablespoons of the vinaigrette, toss gently to combine, and refrigerate for at least 30 minutes.

2. Blanch or steam the green beans until bright green and crisp-tender, 3 to 4 minutes. Drain and immediately plunge into ice water to chill. When cold, drain and pat dry.

3. To serve, divide the lettuce among four plates. Arrange the onion, green beans, potatoes, tomatoes, sardines, eggs, and radishes in a pattern of your choosing over the lettuce. Drizzle or lightly spoon 2 to 3 tablespoons of the vinaigrette over each salad, then sprinkle with olives and pepper. Pour the remaining vinaigrette into a cruet or small bowl and serve on the side.

Per Serving: Calories 369; Protein 23 g; Carbs 43 g; Dietary Fiber 10 g; Added Sugars 1 g; Total Fat 13 g; Sat Fat 3 g; Omega-3s 900 mg; Sodium 516 mg; Potassium 1,731 mg

SOUTHEAST ASIAN–STYLE SHRIMP & NAPA CABBAGE SALAD WITH RICE NOODLES

Makes 4 servings

This salad makes a great quick and easy weeknight dinner. We took a few shortcuts, like using precut napa cabbage, frozen fully cooked shrimp, and fast-cooking rice noodles. This recipe also adapts well to using other fresh vegetables. We use fresh snow peas, but you could also add thinly sliced carrots, cucumbers, or bean sprouts.

Salad

8 ounces (227 g) vermicelli rice noodles

One 10-ounce (283 g) bag thinly shredded napa or green cabbage (about 4 cups)

One 16-ounce (454 g) bag frozen cooked, peeled shrimp, thawed

4.5 ounces (128 g) fresh snow peas, strings removed, halved diagonally (about 1½ cups)

¼ cup (4 g) chopped fresh cilantro

1 lime, quartered

Peanut-Lime Dressing

¼ cup (65 g) creamy peanut butter

3 tablespoons fresh lime juice

2 tablespoons fish sauce

1 tablespoon toasted sesame oil

1 tablespoon reduced-sodium soy sauce or tamari

1 teaspoon finely grated fresh ginger

2 garlic cloves, minced

1 teaspoon sugar

1. Bring a large pot of water to a boil. Add the noodles, cover, and turn off the heat. After 3 to 4 minutes, loosen the noodles with a fork. Drain in a colander and rinse under cold running water. Continue draining as you prepare the dressing.

2. Combine the peanut butter, lime juice, fish sauce, sesame oil, soy sauce, ginger, garlic, and sugar in a large bowl. Stir until smooth.

3. Add the cabbage, shrimp, snow peas, and noodles to the dressing and toss well. Divide among four plates, sprinkle each with 1 tablespoon of the cilantro, and add a lime wedge to each plate.

Per Serving: Calories 510; Protein 38 g; Carbs 60 g; Dietary Fiber 5 g; Added Sugars 2 g; Total Fat 12 g; Sat Fat 2 g; Omega-3s 85 mg; Sodium 925 mg; Potassium 720 mg

WILD CRAB SALAD

Makes 4 servings

Wild-caught claw crab meat can be purchased ready-to-eat, fully cooked, and pasteurized. You can find it in 8-ounce (227 g) containers in the refrigerated section of your grocery store. Shelf-stable canned crab is also wild-caught crab, and it's often less expensive. Either works well in this salad.

Salad

Two 8-ounce (227 g) cans premium claw
  crab meat

One 8-ounce (227 g) can sliced water
  chestnuts, drained and coarsely chopped

1 red bell pepper, seeded and diced

2 celery stalks, diced

½ cup (70 g) pitted kalamata olives, halved

4 green onions, sliced

1 tablespoon fresh lemon juice

One 5 to 6-ounce (142 to 170 g) bag mixed
  greens (baby greens, spring mix, 50/50
  blend)

Creamy Dijon Dressing

1 cup (230 g) plain Greek yogurt

¾ cup (165 g) mayonnaise

¼ cup (15 g) minced fresh parsley

1 teaspoon Dijon mustard

1 garlic clove, minced

1. Combine the crab, water chestnuts, pepper, celery, olives, and green onions in a medium bowl. Sprinkle with lemon juice. Refrigerate while you prepare the dressing.

2. Combine the yogurt, mayonnaise, parsley, mustard, and garlic in a blender and blend until smooth.

3. Add the dressing to the salad and toss gently to combine. Refrigerate until you're ready to serve.

4. Divide the greens among four plates. Top each with one-quarter of the crab salad and serve.

Per Serving: Calories 454; Protein 18 g; Carbs 15 g; Dietary Fiber 4 g; Added Sugars 0 g; Total Fat 37 g; Sat Fat 6 g; Omega-3s 2,300 mg; Sodium 860 mg; Potassium 388 mg

COOKING À LA HEART SALAD

Makes 12 cups (210 g)

This salad is a true mélange of foods we hope you'll eat more often to promote good health—fruits, vegetables, whole grains, pulses, nuts, seeds, and dairy! And yes, this recipe makes a lot; it's a great option for potlucks or for when you need something handy in the fridge for busy weeks when cooking isn't an option.

Creamy À la Heart Dressing

Two 5.3-ounce (150 g each) containers plain
  Greek yogurt (about 1⅓ cups)

½ cup (110 g) mayonnaise

Grated zest of 1 lemon

1 tablespoon fresh lemon juice

1 tablespoon red wine vinegar

2 teaspoons Curry Powder (page 32)

1 teaspoon dried tarragon

½ teaspoon chili powder

½ teaspoon ground ginger

½ teaspoon paprika

½ teaspoon ground turmeric

Salad

2 cups (175 g) chopped fresh broccoli, florets
  and stems

2 cups (390 g) Simply Cooked Brown Rice
  (page 230)

One 15.5-ounce (439 g) can chickpeas or kidney
  beans, drained and rinsed

2 celery stalks, chopped

6 green onions, sliced

1 bell pepper, seeded and diced

¾ cup (120 g) golden raisins

½ cup (50 g) bite-size pieces fresh green beans

1½ cups (120 g) shredded Parmesan or
  Romano cheese

½ cup (45 g) slivered almonds

½ cup (65 g) unsalted sunflower seeds

1. Whisk together the yogurt, mayonnaise, lemon zest, lemon juice, vinegar, curry powder, tarragon, chili powder, ginger, paprika, and turmeric in a large bowl. Add the broccoli, rice, celery, onions, bell pepper, chickpeas, raisins, and green beans. Toss well to coat. Cover and chill for 2 to 3 hours in the refrigerator.

2. Just before serving, add the Parmesan, almonds, and sunflower seeds. Toss again and serve. Store in an airtight container in the refrigerator for up to 4 days.

Serving Size 1 cup (18 g); Calories 300; Protein 11 g; Carbs 28 g; Dietary Fiber 5 g; Added Sugars 0 g; Total Fat 17 g; Sat Fat 4 g; Omega-3s 555 mg; Sodium 460 mg; Potassium 400 mg

CRISPY TOFU WITH LENTILS & MIXED GREENS

Makes 4 servings

Our Crispy Tofu Bites are a wonderful textural complement to perfectly cooked lentils and crisp mixed greens. A simple cilantro-lime vinaigrette brightens the flavors.

¼ cup (60 ml) extra virgin olive oil

3 tablespoons fresh lime juice

1 tablespoon sherry vinegar or red wine vinegar

¼ teaspoon hot sauce

¼ cup (4 g) chopped fresh cilantro

2 tablespoons chopped green onion

1½ cups (285 g) Simply Cooked Lentils (page 247)

½ cup (50 g) diced celery

½ cup (65 g) diced cucumber

¼ cup (35 g) diced bell pepper

One 2-ounce (57 g) jar diced pimientos, drained

4 cups (140 g) mixed salad greens

4 cups (990 g) Crispy Tofu Bites (page 250)

1. Whisk together the oil, lime juice, vinegar, hot sauce, cilantro, and green onion in a large bowl. Add the lentils, celery, cucumber, pepper, and pimiento to the bowl and toss well to coat. Cover and refrigerate for at least an hour to allow the flavors to blend.

2. To serve, place 1 cup (35 g) salad greens in each of four shallow bowls or plates. Top each with one-quarter of the lentil salad mixture and 1 cup (250 g) tofu bites, and serve.

Per Serving: Calories 682; Protein 29 g; Carbs 63 g; Dietary Fiber 14 g; Added Sugars 1 g; Total Fat 36 g; Sat Fat 5 g; Omega-3s 220 mg; Sodium 825 mg; Potassium 463 mg

FOUR-BEAN SALAD

Makes 8 servings

This salad is usually available in Linda's kitchen today because the four kinds of beans used in the recipe are her family's favorites and are reminiscent of past impromptu family picnics. A hastily packed "picnic basket" (actually a wide-rim woven willow laundry basket) would often hold this salad packed in mason jars, along with peanut butter sandwiches and a whole watermelon.

Rosemary-Cider Vinaigrette

½ cup (120 ml) extra virgin olive oil

⅓ cup (80 ml) apple cider vinegar

2 tablespoons chopped fresh rosemary, thyme, or oregano

1 tablespoon sugar

½ teaspoon freshly ground black pepper

Salad

One 15.5-ounce (439 g) can butter beans, drained and rinsed

One 15.5-ounce (439 g) can cannellini or white navy beans, drained and rinsed

One 15.5-ounce (439 g) can chickpeas, drained and rinsed

One 15.5-ounce (439 g) can dark red kidney beans, drained and rinsed

2 celery stalks, diced

¾ cup (45 g) chopped parsley

½ cup (80 g) diced onion

1. Whisk together the oil, vinegar, rosemary, sugar, and pepper in a large bowl. Add the butter beans, cannellini beans, chickpeas, kidney beans, celery, parsley, and onion. Toss gently. Cover and refrigerate for 3 hours or overnight, if possible.

2. Toss gently again before serving. Serve cold or at room temperature. Store in an airtight container in the refrigerator for up to 1 week.

Per Serving: Calories 353; Protein 12 g; Carbs 41 g; Dietary Fiber 13 g; Added Sugars 4 g; Total Fat 16 g; Sat Fat 2 g; Omega-3s 120 mg; Sodium 432 mg; Potassium 500 mg

LENTIL & BROWN RICE SALAD WITH THYME

Makes 6 servings

This Mediterranean-inspired salad is great served with our Four-Grain Sunflower Seed Bread (page 108). Leftovers create a wonderful filling for a wrap the next day; try the Horseradish-Dijon Aïoli (page 44) as a sauce to smear on the inside of your wrap before you add the filling.

Lemon Vinaigrette

½ cup (120 ml) extra virgin olive oil

Grated zest and juice of 1 lemon

2 tablespoons water

1 tablespoon red wine vinegar

1 garlic clove, minced

1 teaspoon sugar

½ teaspoon freshly ground black pepper

Salad

2 cups (380 g) Simply Cooked Lentils (page 247)

1 cup (195 g) Simply Cooked Brown Rice (page 230)

2 tablespoons chopped fresh thyme

1 bay leaf

1 tomato, diced

1 celery stalk, diced

½ cup (30 g) chopped fresh flat-leaf parsley

¼ cup (35 g) diced bell pepper

¼ cup (40 g) diced red onion

½ teaspoon freshly ground black pepper

6 cups (210 g) mixed greens

½ cup (25 g) chopped fresh chives

1. Whisk together the oil, lemon zest, lemon juice, water, vinegar, garlic, sugar, and black pepper in a large bowl. Stir in the lentils, brown rice, thyme, and bay leaf, cover, and refrigerate for 1 to 2 hours.

2. When you're ready to serve, remove the bay leaf, then add the tomato, celery, parsley, bell pepper, onion, and black pepper. Mix well. Serve over mixed greens, and top with chopped chives. Store in an airtight container in the refrigerator for up to 4 days.

Per Serving: Calories 288; Protein 6 g; Carbs 23 g; Dietary Fiber 8 g; Added Sugars 1 g; Total Fat 20 g; Sat Fat 3 g; Omega-3s 170 mg; Sodium 88 mg; Potassium 402 mg

LENTIL CAPRESE SALAD

Makes 4 servings

The addition of lentils to the classic caprese turns a starter salad into a complete meal. Serve with our crusty Fresh Herb & Honey Batter Bread (page 102) to make a memorable meal.

Balsamic Vinaigrette

¼ cup (60 ml) extra virgin olive oil

3 tablespoons balsamic vinegar

1 tablespoon fresh lemon juice

1 large garlic clove, minced

1 teaspoon Italian Seasoning (page 34)

½ teaspoon freshly ground black pepper

Salad

2 cups (380 g) Simply Cooked Lentils (page 247)

One 8-ounce (227 g) container bite-size fresh mozzarella balls (bocconcini), drained

1½ cups (225 g) grape tomatoes, halved

¾ cup (20 g) fresh basil leaves, thinly sliced

Whisk together the oil, vinegar, lemon juice, garlic, seasoning, and pepper in a medium bowl. Add the lentils, mozzarella, tomatoes, and basil, toss to combine, and serve.

Per Serving: Calories 405; Protein 16 g; Carbs 22 g; Dietary Fiber 10 g; Added Sugars 0 g; Total Fat 29 g; Sat Fat 10 g; Omega-3s 120 mg; Sodium 36 mg; Potassium 426 mg

LENTIL & MIXED GREENS SALAD WITH GOAT CHEESE

Makes 4 servings

This is the perfect salad for a warm summer day. A simple cilantro-lime vinaigrette heightens the flavors of the fresh vegetables, while the goat cheese adds a creamy contrast to the lentils and greens. Our Zucchini-Nut Bread (page 106) is a sweet finish.

Cilantro-Lime Vinaigrette

¼ cup (60 ml) extra virgin olive oil

3 tablespoons fresh lime juice

1 tablespoon sherry vinegar or red wine vinegar

¼ teaspoon hot sauce

¼ cup (4 g) chopped fresh cilantro

2 tablespoons chopped green onion

Salad

2 cups (380 g) Simply Cooked Lentils (page 247)

½ cup (50 g) diced celery

½ cup (65 g) diced cucumber

¼ cup (35 g) diced bell pepper

One 2-ounce (57 g) jar diced pimientos, drained

4 cups (140 g) mixed salad greens

2 ounces (57 g) soft goat cheese, crumbled

1. Whisk together the oil, lime juice, vinegar, hot sauce, cilantro, and green onion in a large bowl. Add the lentils, celery, cucumber, bell pepper, and pimientos to the bowl and toss well to coat. Cover and refrigerate for at least an hour to allow the flavors to blend.

2. Serve over mixed greens, topped with the goat cheese.

Per Serving: Calories 284; Protein 9 g; Carbs 20 g; Dietary Fiber 10 g; Added Sugars 0 g; Total Fat 19 g; Sat Fat 5 g; Omega-3s 130 mg; Sodium 120 mg; Potassium 424 mg

WILD RICE & CHICKPEA SALAD

Makes 4 servings

The unusual pairing of chewy wild rice with creamy chickpeas creates a beautiful contrast of textures, while the aromatic herbs in the dressing perfectly complement the ingredients and add tanginess. This salad can stand on its own for a meal or be topped with sliced grilled chicken breast.

2 cups (330 g) Simply Cooked Wild Rice (page 234)

One 15.5-ounce (439 g) can chickpeas, drained and rinsed

1 cup (100 g) chopped celery (about 2 stalks)

1 cup (160 g) diced red onion (1 medium onion)

1 cup (70 g) sliced cremini or white mushrooms

Grated zest of 1 lemon

1 cup (240 ml) Herbed Red Wine Vinaigrette (page 50)

One 5- to 6-ounce (142 to 170 g) bag mixed greens or baby arugula

1 tablespoon minced fresh rosemary or tarragon, optional

1. Combine the wild rice, chickpeas, celery, onion, mushrooms, lemon zest, and vinaigrette in a large bowl. Cover and refrigerate for 1 to 2 hours to allow the flavors to blend.

2. Serve over greens and top with rosemary, if desired.

Per Serving: Calories 235; Protein 11 g; Carbs 43 g; Dietary Fiber 10 g; Added Sugars 0 g; Total Fat 3 g; Sat Fat 0 g; Omega-3s 120 mg; Sodium 439 mg; Potassium 411 mg

ZOODLE TOFU BOWLS

Makes 4 servings

Zucchini spirals (aka zoodles) star alongside tofu in this bowl, served as a cold Vietnamese-inspired salad. This salad can be transformed into a stir-fry by stir-frying the vegetables in a wok or hot skillet for 1 minute or so, then adding the marinade, followed by the tofu. Hot or cold, this dish evokes umami, the fifth element of taste.

Marinated Tofu

8 ounces (227 g) extra firm tofu, cut into 1-inch (2.5 cm) cubes

3 tablespoons reduced-sodium soy sauce or tamari

2 teaspoons toasted sesame oil

2 garlic cloves, minced

1 teaspoon honey

¼ teaspoon red pepper flakes

1 tablespoon fresh lime juice

Bowls

2 teaspoons toasted sesame oil

12 ounces (340 g) spiral-cut zucchini (aka zoodles)

2 cups (145 g) shredded lettuce or baby greens

¾ cup (90 g) thinly sliced carrots

1 cup (105 g) mung bean sprouts

4 green onions, chopped

¼ cup (4 g) chopped fresh cilantro

1. Place the tofu in a single layer in a shallow 8-inch (20 cm) round baking dish. Whisk together the soy sauce, sesame oil, garlic, honey, and red pepper flakes in a small bowl. Pour 1 tablespoon of the marinade over the tofu and toss so all sides are coated. Add the lime juice to the remaining marinade. Marinate the tofu for 10 minutes.

2. To make the bowls, heat 1 teaspoon of the sesame oil in a large skillet or wok over medium heat, then add the zucchini. Cook over medium heat, stirring frequently, until hot and softened, about 5 minutes. Transfer the zucchini to a plate to cool.

3. Increase the heat to medium-high and add the remaining 1 teaspoon sesame oil to the same skillet; add the tofu. Sauté until golden brown, about 3 minutes. Transfer to a separate plate to cool.

4. Divide the zucchini among four shallow bowls or rimmed plates. Arrange ½ cup (35 g) shredded lettuce around the zucchini in each bowl. Place the carrots on one half of the zucchini and the bean sprouts on the other. Drizzle 2 teaspoons of the reserved marinade mixture over each bowl. Add the tofu in the center and sprinkle with green onions and cilantro and serve

Serving Size 1 bowl; Calories 174; Protein 11 g; Carbs 17 g; Dietary Fiber 5 g; Added Sugars 1 g; Total Fat 8 g; Sat Fat 1 g; Omega-3s 90 mg; Sodium 460 mg; Potassium 445 mg

CRUNCHY ITALIAN-FLAVORED CHICKPEAS

Makes 4 servings

In addition to being a crunchy topping for salads, these little morsels are also a satisfying snack or delicious nibble to put out with nuts, olives, veggies with dip, and other items for happy hour.

One 15.5-ounce (439 g) can chickpeas, drained, rinsed

2 tablespoons extra virgin olive oil

1 tablespoon Italian Seasoning (page 34)

1 tablespoon freshly grated Parmesan

¼ teaspoon garlic powder

¼ teaspoon cayenne

¼ teaspoon kosher salt

1. Preheat the oven to 250°F (120°C). Cover a large rimmed baking sheet with a single layer of paper towels.

2. Place the chickpeas on the paper towels and gently swirl the baking sheet to get the chickpeas to roll around, to remove as much moisture as possible. Remove the paper towels. Bake for 45 minutes, until crunchy on the outside but still chewy on the inside.

3. While the chickpeas are baking, combine the oil, seasoning, Parmesan, garlic powder, cayenne, and salt in a medium bowl.

4. Add the chickpeas and stir well to coat. Line the baking sheet with parchment paper and spread out the chickpeas.

5. Increase the oven temperature to 425°F (220°C).

6. Bake the chickpeas for 10 to 12 minutes, until golden brown. Transfer to a plate or shallow container to cool. Enjoy immediately or store in an airtight container at room temperature for 2 to 3 days.

Per Serving: Calories 223; Protein 8 g; Carbs 26 g; Dietary Fiber 7 g; Added Sugars 0 g; Total Fat 10 g; Sat Fat 1 g; Omega-3s 100 mg; Sodium 376 mg; Potassium 143 mg

PARMESAN-HERB CROUTONS

Makes 4 cups (350 g)

Making your own croutons is a great way to use up those last few slices of whole wheat bread, and it guarantees your croutons will have more fiber, more heart-healthy fats, and less salt than most store-bought croutons. This savory salad topping is equally good as a garnish for soup or base for poultry stuffing.

10 slices (280 g) whole wheat bread

¼ cup (60 ml) extra virgin olive oil

2 tablespoons freshly grated Parmesan

1 tablespoon Italian Seasoning (page 34)

1. Preheat the oven to 300°F (150°C). Line a rimmed baking sheet with parchment paper.

2. Brush both sides of the bread slices with oil. Combine the Parmesan and herbs in a small bowl, then sprinkle the slices with the mixture. Cut the slices into ½-inch (13 mm) cubes. Spread on the baking sheet in a single layer. Bake for 15 minutes or until the croutons are crispy and dry, stirring after about 8 minutes.

3. Place the baking sheet on a wire rack to cool completely. Store in an airtight container at room temperature for up to 1 week or in the freezer for up to 3 months.

Serving Size ½ cup (44 g); Calories 155; Protein 5 g; Carbs 16 g; Dietary Fiber 2 g; Added Sugars 0 g; Total Fat 8 g; Sat Fat 1 g; Omega-3s 100 mg; Sodium 182 mg; Potassium 101 mg

SMOKY PECAN BITS
Makes 1 cup (110 g)

If you love bacon bits on salads, these will give you the smoky flavor and crunchy texture you crave without all the sodium and saturated fat. You can serve them whole, or chopped to resemble the size and shape of bacon bits. Our favorite use for them is on our Wedge Salad (page 155).

- 1 cup (110 g) pecan halves
- 1 tablespoon extra virgin olive oil
- 1 teaspoon ground chipotle chile powder
- ¼ teaspoon kosher salt

1. Preheat the oven to 350°F (180°C). Cover a small baking pan with parchment paper.

2. Combine the oil, paprika, and salt in a small bowl. Add the pecans and toss well to coat. Spread on the baking pan in a single layer. Bake for 8 to 10 minutes, until the pecans have started to darken slightly in color.

3. Cool to room temperature. Chop if desired, and serve. Store in an airtight container at room temperature for up to 1 week.

Serving Size ¼ cup (28 g); Calories 223; Protein 3 g; Carbs 4 g; Dietary Fiber 3 g; Added Sugars 0 g; Total Fat 23 g; Sat Fat 2 g; Omega-3s 300 mg; Sodium 120 mg; Potassium 113 mg

SPICY CANDIED PECANS
Makes 2 cups (225 g)

If you love foods that offer a little sweet with a little heat, these pecans are perfect for you. Easy to make and easier to eat, they are a wonderful topping for salads and bowls like our Autumn Wild Rice & Chicken Bowls (page 159) and our Chicken & Wild Rice Salad with Grapes & Candied Pecans (page 162).

- 2 cups (220 g) pecan halves
- 2 tablespoons real maple syrup
- ½ teaspoon cayenne
- ½ teaspoon red pepper flakes
- ½ teaspoon kosher salt
- ¼ teaspoon ground ginger

1. Preheat the oven to 350°F (180°C). Cover a large baking sheet with parchment paper.

2. Combine the pecans, syrup, cayenne, red pepper flakes, ginger, and salt in a medium bowl. Toss well to coat. Spread the pecans on the baking sheet in a single layer. Bake for 10 minutes.

3. Stir, then bake for 7 to 8 minutes, until the pecans have developed a dark brown color and hard, crunchy exterior.

4. Cool to room temperature and serve. Store in an airtight container at room temperature for up to 1 week.

Serving Size: ¼ cup (28 g); Calories 204; Protein 3 g; Carbs 7 g; Dietary Fiber 3 g; Added Sugars 3 g; Total Fat 20 g; Sat Fat 2 g; Omega-3s 270 mg; Sodium 121 mg; Potassium 128 mg

> **SODIUM TIP:** Using Diamond Crystal Kosher Salt will dramatically reduce the sodium in any recipe that uses kosher salt. This salt contains 50% less sodium per measure than regular kosher salt and 60% less than fine grain table salt.

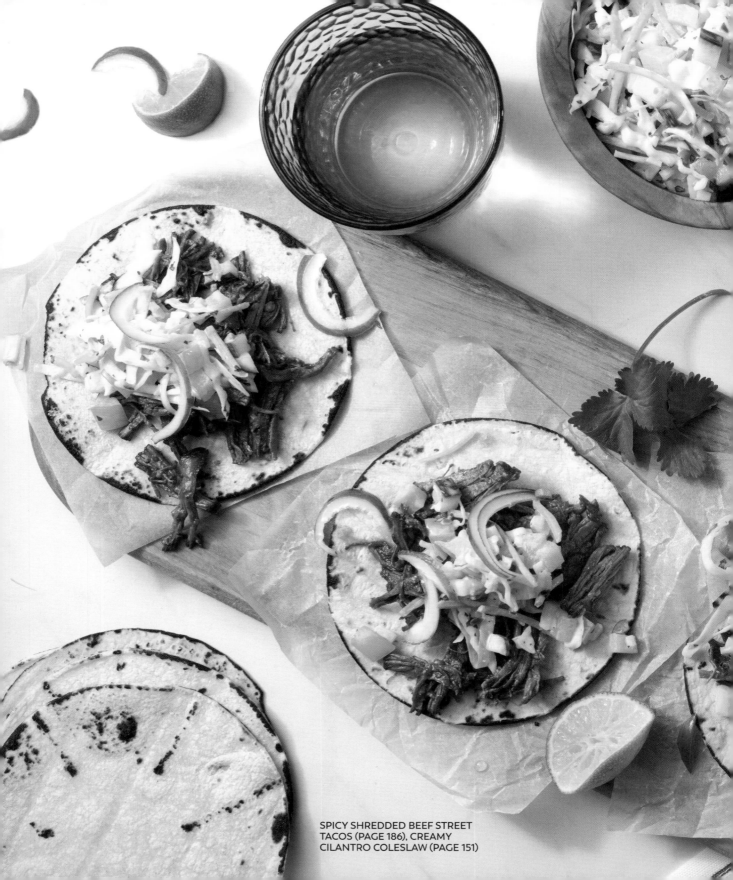

SPICY SHREDDED BEEF STREET
TACOS (PAGE 186), CREAMY
CILANTRO COLESLAW (PAGE 151)

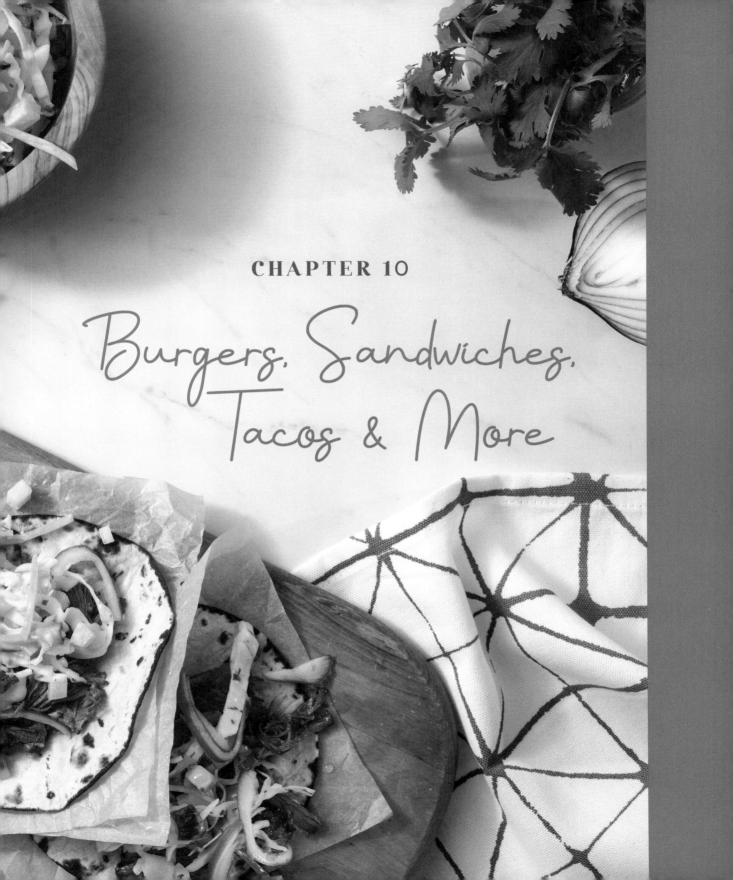

CHAPTER 10

Burgers, Sandwiches,
Tacos & More

Burgers, Sandwiches, Tacos & More

Burgers

Ahi Burgers with Wasabi-Ginger Slaw . . 177

Beef & Mushroom Burgers 178

Chickpea Burgers 178

Fresh Salmon Burgers 179

Pork Banh Mi Burgers 180

Southwestern Beef & Bean Burgers. . . . 180

Sandwiches

Super Savory Sloppy Joes 181

Tofu Sloppy Joes 182

Very Veggie Grilled Cheese
Sandwiches 182

Tacos

Beef & Mushroom Taco Filling 183

Fish Tacos 184

Portobello Street Tacos. 184

Shrimp Tacos 185

Spicy Shredded Beef Street Tacos 186

And More

Chicken & Bean Burritos 186

Pork Lettuce Wraps 187

Salmon Spring Rolls 188

Seared Lamb Pita Pockets
with Cucumber Mint Yogurt Sauce. 189

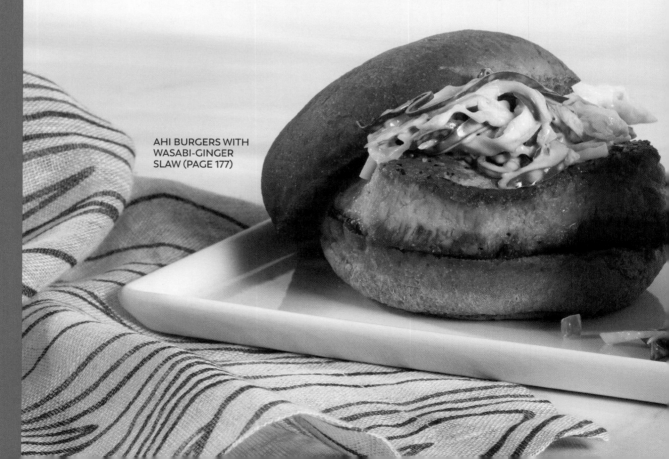

AHI BURGERS WITH
WASABI-GINGER
SLAW (PAGE 177)

Many people believe that if they want to eat heart healthy, they'll need to give up their favorite foods, like burgers. In this chapter, we show you how to use sources of healthy protein, including blends of animal and plant protein, to create delicious, crave-worthy foods—these options are healthful and also delicious. We also offer strategies like right-sizing the animal protein to no more than 4 ounces (113 g) per serving, using produce in abundance in the fillings and toppings, and choosing whole grain buns and tortillas when possible.

In addition, we offer suggestions for pairing these handheld heroes with sauces and sides that create memorable meals. We hope you'll use these recipes as inspiration for creating plant-forward favorites you return to time and time again.

AHI BURGERS WITH WASABI-GINGER SLAW

Makes 4 burgers

Barely seared ahi tuna steaks pair perfectly with crunchy yet creamy Wasabi-Ginger Coleslaw. The pungent wasabi cuts through the richness of the ahi, creating a memorable feel-good burger fit for any feast.

4 whole wheat burger buns

2 tablespoons extra virgin olive oil

1 teaspoon freshly ground black pepper

Four 4-ounce (113 g) ahi tuna steaks

4 cups (615 g) Wasabi-Ginger Coleslaw (page 155)

1. Brush the cut sides of the buns with 1 tablespoon of the oil, then place cut side down in a large skillet or sauté pan over medium heat to gently toast. Keep warm.

2. Sprinkle the pepper on both sides of the tuna steaks. Place a large skillet or cast-iron pan over high heat. Add the remaining 1 tablespoon oil and swirl to distribute it evenly. Add the tuna steaks and sear for 1 minute. Flip and sear for 1 minute on the other side. (The goal is to cook the tuna on each side just until the outer ¼ inch [6 mm] of the tuna turns from pink to beige. If you don't like rare tuna, feel free to cook the tuna for longer.)

3. To assemble the burgers, place a tuna steak on each bun bottom, add a generous scoop of slaw, and cover with the bun top.

Serving Size 1 burger; Calories 620; Protein 36 g; Carbs 46 g; Dietary Fiber 4 g; Added Sugars 0 g; Total Fat 32 g; Sat Fat 5 g; Omega-3s 1,690 mg; Sodium 848 mg; Potassium 609 mg

BEEF & MUSHROOM BURGERS

Makes 4 burgers

Research conducted by The Culinary Institute of America and the University of California, Davis, shows that most people prefer beef and mushroom blends to all-beef, because the mushrooms enhance the aroma, flavor, and texture of the final dish. Mushrooms offer an additional benefit: They contain umami compounds that help offset flavor loss when less salt is used in cooking. The key for the best flavor and texture is to cook the mushrooms prior to adding them to the ground beef; doing so reduces the moisture content of the mushrooms and makes their texture meatier.

2 tablespoons extra virgin olive oil or peanut oil

8 ounces (227 g) white mushrooms, finely diced

1 teaspoon ground thyme

½ teaspoon freshly ground black pepper

1 pound (454 g) 93% lean ground beef

1. Heat the oil in a skillet over medium-high heat for 1 minute. Add the mushrooms, thyme, and pepper, and sauté until the mushrooms start to soften and release their liquid, about 5 minutes. Transfer to a medium bowl and cool in the refrigerator for least 10 minutes.

2. Mix the beef and mushrooms together. Use your hands to mix well, then form into four patties about ¾ inch (2 cm) thick.

3. Cook over medium-high heat, 5 to 6 minutes per side, flipping once, until a digital food thermometer reads 160°F (70°C) when inserted through the side into the center of the thickest burger.

TIP: Top the burgers with your favorite toppings. We love to serve them with lettuce, tomato, and avocado or our Honey Balsamic Onion Jam (page 64). If you like cheese on your burgers, Swiss is an obvious choice, but Brie is also a lovely option, especially if using the onion jam.

Serving Size 1 burger (burger only, no bun); Calories 214; Protein 26 g; Carbs 2 g; Dietary Fiber 0 g; Added Sugars 0 g; Total Fat 11 g; Sat Fat 3 g; Omega-3s 90 mg; Sodium 79 mg; Potassium 646 mg

CHICKPEA BURGERS

Makes 3 burgers

We are very fond of using chickpeas (aka garbanzo beans), not only because of their outstanding nutrient profile (high in fiber and iron, a good source of protein, low in fat) but also because they're so versatile and affordable. Here we use them to make burgers by combining them with aromatic vegetables like onions and garlic, spices such as coriander and cumin, and Greek yogurt or tahini to help bind these tasty ingredients. Pair the finished burger with the usual works—top it with baby spinach, sliced tomatoes and red onions, and crumbled feta. We like to slather our whole grain buns with Honey Balsamic Onion Jam.

One 15.5-ounce (439 g) can chickpeas, drained and rinsed (see Note)

3 tablespoons minced red onion

1 garlic clove, minced

1 large egg

¼ cup (60 g) plain Greek yogurt or sesame tahini

2 tablespoons chopped fresh cilantro

1 teaspoon Dijon mustard

½ teaspoon ground coriander

½ teaspoon ground cumin

¼ teaspoon red pepper flakes

⅓ cup (75 g) Garlic & Herb Bread Crumbs (page 33)

1 tablespoon extra virgin olive oil

3 whole grain hamburger buns

Suggested Toppings

Baby greens

Sliced tomatoes

Sliced red onions

Crumbled feta

Honey Balsamic Onion Jam (page 64)

1. Line a platter or large plate with wax paper or parchment paper.

2. Smash the chickpeas in a medium bowl using the back of a fork to create a coarse consistency, or pulse them in a food processor or blender until coarsely ground. Stir in the onion and garlic with a fork. Whisk together the egg, yogurt, cilantro, mustard, coriander, cumin, and red pepper flakes in a large bowl. Stir in the chickpea mixture with a fork. Stir in the bread crumbs until well blended and the mixture holds its shape.

3. Shape the mixture into three 1-inch-thick (2.5 cm) patties. Continue to work the patties by hand, squeezing and shaping, until they firmly hold together. Place the patties on the platter.

4. Heat the oil in a large skillet over medium-high heat. When the oil is shimmering, gently add the patties and cook until firm and golden brown on the bottom, about 4 minutes. Flip and cook on the second side for another 4 minutes, until brown and crispy on the outside with a firm, chewy center. The burgers are done when a digital food thermometer reads 145°F (65°C) when inserted through the side and into the center.

5. Serve warm on the buns with your choice of toppings.

NOTE: *We suggest saving the aquafaba, the liquid drained from the chickpeas, which can be whipped to the consistency of meringue like egg whites. With a small amount of added sugar or honey and flavorings of your choice (such as vanilla bean), it can be used in place of whipped cream and served with any of the fruit crisps, cakes, puddings, or galettes found in the Desserts chapter.*

Serving Size 1 burger; Calories 450; Protein 20 g; Carbs 63 g; Dietary Fiber 14 g; Added Sugars 0 g; Total Fat 16 g; Sat Fat 3 g; Omega-3s 130 mg; Sodium 760 mg; Potassium 242 mg

FRESH SALMON BURGERS

Makes 4 burgers

These tender, juicy, bursting-with-flavor burgers are so easy to make! Serve them topped with Pineapple Salsa with Tomato & Lemon and spread a little Horseradish-Dijon Aïoli on the whole grain burger buns.

- 1 pound (454 g) boneless, skinless salmon fillets, cut into ¼-inch (6 mm) cubes
- 3 tablespoons plain Greek yogurt
- 2 tablespoons chopped fresh herbs (chervil, cilantro, parsley, and/or dill)
- 2 tablespoons fresh lemon juice or pineapple juice

- 1 tablespoon chopped fresh thyme
- 2 teaspoons Dijon mustard
- 1 garlic clove, minced
- ¼ teaspoon kosher salt
- ¼ teaspoon freshly ground black pepper
- 1 tablespoon extra virgin olive oil
- 4 whole grain buns
- 2 cups (70 g) baby greens
- 1 cup (230 g) Pineapple Salsa with Tomato & Lemon (page 62), optional
- ½ cup (140 g) Horseradish-Dijon Aïoli (page 44), optional

1. Line a platter or large plate with wax paper or parchment paper.

2. Gently mix the salmon, yogurt, herbs, lemon juice, thyme, mustard, garlic, salt, and pepper in a large bowl. Divide and shape the mixture into four 1-inch-thick (2.5 cm) patties. Continue to work the patties by hand, squeezing and shaping, until they firmly hold. Place the patties on the platter. Refrigerate for 10 to 15 minutes, until you're ready to cook.

3. To grill the burgers, brush the grill grate with the oil. Preheat the grill to medium-high (about 400°F/200°C). Add the burgers and grill for 4 to 5 minutes. Carefully flip the burgers and grill for another 4 to 5 minutes, until patties are firm, lightly brown, and have visible grill marks. Toast the buns in the grate, cut side down, if desired.

4. To broil the burgers, lightly oil a wire rack placed over a rimmed baking pan, and place the pan 5 to 6 inches (13 to 15 cm) under the broiler. Heat the broiler on HIGH. Broil for 4 minutes on each side, flipping once. (The burgers will have marks from the wire rack.)

5. To cook in a skillet, heat the oil in a large skillet over medium-high heat. When the oil is shimmering, gently add the burgers. Cook until crisp and golden brown on the bottom, about 4 minutes. Flip and cook on the second side for 4 minutes, until the burgers are brown and crispy on the outside with a firm, chewy center.

6. The burgers are done when a digital food

thermometer reads 145°F (65°C) when inserted through the side and into the center.

7. Place the burgers on the bun bottoms. Top with greens, and salsa if using. Spread aïoli, if using, on the top bun. Close the burgers and serve immediately.

Serving Size 1 burger; Calories 413; Protein 30 g; Carbs 31 g; Dietary Fiber 5 g; Added Sugars 0 g; Total Fat 18 g; Sat Fat 4 g; Omega-3s 2,900 mg; Sodium 512 mg; Potassium 643 mg

PORK BANH MI BURGERS

Makes 4 burgers

This recipe combines the classic flavors of a Vietnamese banh mi sandwich with the comfort and ease of a burger. The patties can be made in advance and refrigerated for up to 24 hours before grilling. If you don't have a grill, use a grill pan or sauté pan to cook them on your stovetop over medium-high heat.

Burgers

1 pound (454 g) lean ground pork

2 tablespoons lemongrass paste (such as Gourmet Garden; see Tip)

1 tablespoon grated fresh ginger

1 tablespoon reduced-sodium soy sauce

1 teaspoon minced garlic

Pickled Carrots

1 cup (55 g) shredded carrots

½ cup (120 ml) fresh lime juice (about 3 limes)

½ teaspoon kosher salt

To Serve

4 hamburger buns (brioche, if possible)

1 bunch cilantro, ends trimmed

¼ English cucumber, thinly sliced

1 jalapeño chile, thinly sliced, optional

¼ cup (60 ml) Roasted Garlic Aïoli (page 45) or mayonnaise, optional

1. Combine the pork, lemongrass paste, ginger, soy sauce, and garlic in a medium bowl. Form the mixture into four patties approximately 4 inches (10 cm) in diameter. Place on a baking sheet, cover, and refrigerate for at least 30 minutes to allow the flavors to develop.

2. While the burgers are chilling, preheat the grill to 350°F (180°C).

3. While the grill is heating, prepare the pickled carrots. Combine the carrots, lime juice, and salt in a small glass bowl. Cover and place in the refrigerator to quick-pickle for 15 to 20 minutes.

4. When the grill is hot, place the patties on the grill. Cook for 5 to 8 minutes per side, until a digital food thermometer reads 160°F (70°C) when inserted in through the side and into the center. (The total cooking time will depend on the type of grill; use a thermometer to determine doneness.) Transfer the burgers to a clean plate.

5. Drain off the excess liquid from the carrots. Build the burgers by placing a patty on a bun bottom. Top each patty with ¼ cup (15 g) pickled carrots, 5 or 6 cilantro sprigs, 3 or 4 cucumber slices, a few jalapeño slices for extra heat, and aïoli, if desired. Top with the bun top and serve immediately.

TIP: *Many stores carry lemongrass paste in the refrigerated area of the produce section near or with the fresh herbs. If you can't find lemongrass paste, you can make your own: Combine the white part of 1 fresh lemongrass stalk, trimmed and chopped, with a few teaspoons of extra virgin olive, peanut, or corn oil in a food processor or high-powered blender; blend until relatively smooth. This should result in just enough lemongrass paste for this recipe.*

Serving Size 1 burger; Calories 500; Protein 28 g; Carbs 43 g; Dietary Fiber 3 g; Added Sugars 0 g; Total Fat 23 g; Sat Fat 7 g; Omega-3s 465 mg; Sodium 690 mg; Potassium 555 mg

SOUTHWESTERN BEEF & BEAN BURGERS

Makes 6 servings

Adding pureed beans to lean ground beef creates very tender, moist burgers. This is also a wonderful budget-friendly option—a single pound of ground beef typically costs three to four times the cost of one pound of cooked beans. The burgers can be cooked on the stovetop in a sauté pan, skillet, or grill pan. If you grill them, we recommend grilling at a slightly lower temperature than you would use to grill an all-beef burger to ensure the beans don't burn.

1 pound (454 g) 93% lean ground beef

One 15-ounce (425 g) can pinto beans, drained, rinsed, and mashed

1 tablespoon Southwest Seasoning page 37)

Six 1-ounce (28 g) pepper Jack slices

6 whole wheat hamburger buns

3 poblano chiles from Simply Roasted Peppers (page 259)

1. Combine the ground beef, beans, and seasoning in a medium bowl. Use your hands to mix well, then form into six patties approximately ½ inch thick (13 mm).

2. Place a large skillet or sauté pan over medium-high heat for 2 to 3 minutes. Preheat the pan for 2 to 3 minutes before adding the patties. Cook for 5 minutes per side, until a digital food thermometer reads 160°F (70°C).

3. During the last two minutes of cooking, place a slice of cheese on each burger, allowing the cheese to melt as the burgers finish cooking. (Cover the pan to help the cheese melt more quickly.)

4. Place the burgers on the bun bottoms. Top each burger with half of a poblano pepper, then the bun top. Serve immediately.

Serving Size 1 burger; Calories 472; Protein 32 g; Carbs 46 g; Dietary Fiber 5 g; Added Sugars 0 g; Total Fat 18 g; Sat Fat 8 g; Omega-3s 120 mg; Sodium 721 mg; Potassium 575 mg

SUPER SAVORY SLOPPY JOES

Makes 8 servings

This veggie-filled beef dish is a wonderful way to make everyone in the family happy with a comforting, savory, and familiar meal. Have leftovers? The mixture also works well as a pasta sauce. You can also turn leftovers into chili by adding kidney beans, corn kernels, and ground cumin.

1 pound (454 g) 93% lean ground beef

1 cup (70 g) diced cremini or white mushrooms

½ teaspoon kosher salt

1 teaspoon freshly ground black pepper

1 cup (240 ml) red wine (Merlot, Syrah, or Zinfandel) or low-sodium beef broth

1 large white onion, finely diced

1 celery stalk, finely diced

1 carrot, finely diced

1 jalapeño chile, finely diced, or one 4-ounce (113 g) can diced jalapeños, drained

2 to 3 garlic cloves, minced

One 12-ounce (340 g) can tomato paste

1½ cups (360 ml) water

1 tablespoon honey

1 tablespoon Worcestershire sauce

1 teaspoon chili powder

½ cup (40 g) freshly grated Parmesan

8 hamburger buns

1. Place a large skillet or Dutch oven over medium-high heat. Add the ground beef and cook, stirring occasionally to break up the beef, until the beef is fully browned with no pink remaining, 10 minutes.

2. Reduce the heat to medium, add the mushrooms, salt, and pepper, and cook, stirring occasionally, until the mushrooms have softened, 5 minutes.

3. Add the red wine and stir to remove any brown bits on the bottom of the pan.

4. Reduce the heat to low. Stir in the onion, carrots, celery, jalapeno, and garlic. Cover and cook, stirring occasionally, until all the vegetables have softened, 25 to 30 minutes.

5. Stir in the tomato paste, water, honey, Worcestershire sauce, and chili powder. Cover and cook until the mixture is bubbling gently on the surface, 15 minutes.

6. Stir in the Parmesan, cover, and cook for 1 minute to let the cheese to melt into the sauce.

7. Spoon ⅔ cup (170 g) of the mixture onto each hamburger bun bottom, cover with the top, and serve immediately. Store covered in the refrigerator for up to 2 days.

TIP: *If you're short on time and you have a food processor, pulse the onion, celery, carrot, jalapeño, and garlic until finely chopped. This will save not only prep time but also cooking time, as the vegetables will soften much more quickly.*

Per Serving: Calories 322; Protein 21 g; Carbs 38 g; Dietary Fiber 3 g; Added Sugars 2 g; Total Fat 7 g; Sat Fat 3 g; Omega-3s 110 mg; Sodium 535 mg; Potassium 392 mg

TOFU SLOPPY JOES

Makes 6 servings

This vegetarian version of the classic kids' favorite offers wonderful aroma with lots of umami. Serve with Savory Sweet Potato Fries (page 272) and your favorite dipping sauce. Finish the meal with a Blueberry Crisp (page 353).

- 2 tablespoons reduced-sodium soy sauce
- 1 tablespoon Tofu Seasoning (page 38)
- 14 ounces (397 g) firm or extra firm tofu, drained and diced or crumbled
- 1 tablespoon extra virgin olive oil
- 8 green onions, chopped
- 1 cup (70 g) chopped cremini or white mushrooms
- ½ cup (75 g) chopped green bell pepper
- 2 cloves garlic, minced
- 2 cups (635 g) Simply Cooked Fresh Tomato Sauce (page 59)
- 1 tablespoon chili powder
- 1 teaspoon ground cumin
- ½ teaspoon freshly ground black pepper
- 6 slices sourdough bread or 6 whole grain hamburger buns

1. Combine the soy sauce and seasoning in a medium bowl. Add the tofu, then prick it with a small fork for better marinade absorption. Gently stir. Set aside for 15 minutes to let the marinade penetrate the tofu.

2. Heat the oil to a large skillet over medium-high heat. Sauté the green onions for 1 minute. Add the mushrooms, bell pepper, and garlic, and sauté until the green onions and bell pepper are softened and the garlic and mushrooms are fragrant, about 3 minutes.

3. Add the tofu and marinade. Sauté until the tofu begins to brown, 2 to 3 minutes. Stir in the tomato sauce, chili powder, and cumin. Reduce the heat to medium-low and cook at a gentle simmer for 3 to 4 minutes, until thickened and heated through. Serve hot on sourdough bread as an open-face sandwich or on hamburger buns. Store in an airtight container in the refrigerator for up to 4 days. To reheat, measure a portion into a microwave-safe bowl, cover with a paper towel, and microwave in 30-second increments on HIGH until hot.

Per Serving: Calories 181; Protein 11 g; Carbs 21 g; Dietary Fiber 3 g; Added Sugars 0 g; Total Fat 7 g; Sat Fat 1 g; Omega-3s 160 mg; Sodium 360 mg; Potassium 380 mg

VERY VEGGIE GRILLED CHEESE SANDWICHES

Makes 4 servings

These sandwiches, with their beautiful color and tempting cheese pull, are yummy on their own, or served with our Tomato Jam (page 343) or Tomato-Basil Soup (page 83). Customize them as you like, using other vegetables you have on hand like yellow summer squash, orange or yellow bell peppers, poblano peppers, mushrooms, Swiss chard, or broccoli. The vegetable-cheese mixture for these sandwiches also makes great filling for an omelet.

- 1 zucchini, diced
- ½ red bell pepper, diced
- ½ cup (30 g) shredded carrot
- ½ cup (80 g) diced red onion
- 3 tablespoons extra virgin olive oil
- 1 cup (30 g) chopped fresh baby spinach leaves
- 1 green onion, thinly sliced
- 1 garlic clove, minced
- ¼ teaspoon red pepper flakes
- ½ cup (125 g) part-skim ricotta
- 4 ounces (113 g) shredded part-skim mozzarella
- 2 tablespoons mayonnaise
- 1 tablespoon freshly grated Parmesan
- 8 slices whole grain bread

1. Combine the zucchini, bell pepper, carrot, red onion, and 1 tablespoon of the oil in a large nonstick sauté pan over medium-high heat. Cook until the vegetables start to soften, 8 to 10 minutes.

2. Add the spinach, green onion, garlic, and red pepper flakes and sauté until the spinach has wilted and turned dark green, 1 to 2 minutes. If there's visible moisture in the pan, reduce the heat and cook for a minute or two longer until the liquid has evaporated.

3. Transfer the vegetables to a bowl. Add the ricotta and mozzarella and stir to combine.

4. Combine the mayonnaise, 1 tablespoon of the remaining oil, and the Parmesan in a small bowl. Lay out the bread slices. Spread 1½ teaspoons of the mayo mixture on each slice.

5. Heat the remaining 1 tablespoon of oil in a large sauté pan, skillet, or griddle over medium-high heat. Place 2 slices of the bread, mayo mixture up, in the pan. Top each with one-quarter of the vegetable-cheese mixture. Top with a second slice of bread, mayo mixture down, and cook until the bread on the bottom is golden brown and crispy, 2 to 3 minutes. Flip the sandwiches and cook until the other side is golden brown, 2 to 3 more minutes. Transfer to plates to keep warm. Repeat to cook the other two sandwiches. Cut each sandwich in half and serve hot.

TIP: *Save time and water by wiping out the sauté pan you used to sauté the vegetables with a paper towel and reusing that pan to cook your sandwiches.*

Serving Size 1 sandwich; Calories 378; Protein 13 g; Carbs 40 g; Dietary Fiber 6 g; Added Sugars 0 g; Total Fat 21 g; Sat Fat 4 g; Omega-3s 510 mg; Sodium 433 mg; Potassium 437 mg

BEEF & MUSHROOM TACO FILLING

Makes 4 cups (1,150 g)

Get ready for Taco Tuesday with a batch of this beef and mushroom taco filling. Serve in corn or flour tortillas with your favorite taco toppings. We love shredded lettuce, diced white onion, Pico de Gallo (page 61), and Avocado Salsa (page 61) on our tacos.

> 2 tablespoons extra virgin olive oil or peanut oil
>
> 8 ounces (227 g) cremini mushrooms, finely diced
>
> 1 white onion, finely diced
>
> 1 pound (454 g) 93% lean ground beef
>
> One 14.5-ounce (411 g) can no-salt-added diced tomatoes
>
> ¼ cup (30 g) Taco Seasoning (page 38) or one 1-ounce (28 g) packet reduced-sodium taco seasoning

Heat the oil in a skillet over medium-high heat for 1 minute. Add the mushrooms and sauté until they release their moisture and start to soften, 5 minutes. Add the onion and cook until soft, 5 minutes. Add the beef and cook, stirring occasionally to break it up, until browned with no visible pink remaining, 5 minutes. Stir in the tomatoes and their liquid and the seasoning. Reduce the heat to low, cover, and simmer for 10 minutes, until a digital food thermometer reads 165°F (75°C) when inserted into the mixture. Serve immediately. Store covered in the refrigerator for up to 2 days or freeze and then thaw in the refrigerator. Reheat on the stovetop over medium heat until the mixture reaches 165°F (75°C).

Serving Size ½ cup (575 g); Calories 154; Protein 13 g; Carbs 7 g; Dietary Fiber 2 g; Added Sugars 0 g; Total Fat 8 g; Sat Fat 2 g; Omega-3s 60 mg; Sodium 97 mg; Potassium 475 mg

FISH TACOS

Makes 12 tacos

Fish tacos are fun to make, flavorful, and never boring. This recipe provides a starting point to use whatever fish you have on hand, choose seasonings that best fit the tastes of your guests, and cook the fish using your oven or grill. Get your guests involved in assembling their own custom creations. Our Creamy Cilantro Coleslaw (page 151), Avocado Salsa (page 61), and Tropical Fruit Salsa (page 63) offer great variety in taste and texture and make great accompaniments.

1 pound (454 g) fresh or thawed frozen skinless white fish fillets (cod, sole, halibut, or flounder), ½ inch thick (13 mm)

2 tablespoons fresh lime or lemon juice

1 tablespoon extra virgin olive oil or avocado oil

1 garlic clove, minced

1 teaspoon chili powder

½ teaspoon ground cumin

½ teaspoon white pepper

Cooking spray

Twelve 6-inch (15 cm) whole wheat flour tortillas

1. Arrange the fish in a single layer in an 8-inch (20 cm) square baking dish. Whisk together the lime juice, oil, garlic, chili powder, cumin, and pepper. Pour over the fish and turn to coat. Gently rub the marinade into the fish with your fingers. Cover and refrigerate the fish for 30 to 35 minutes, turning once.

2. Drain and discard the marinade.

3. **To oven-roast the fish,** preheat the oven to 400°F (200°C). Line a baking sheet with parchment paper. Place the fish on the baking sheet and roast for 10 to 15 minutes.

4. **To grill the fish on a charcoal grill,** spray the grill rack with cooking spray and heat the coals to medium. Place the fish on the rack and grill for 6 to 8 minutes.

5. **To grill the fish on a gas grill,** spray the grill rack with cooking spray and heat the grill to high. Reduce the heat to medium. Place the fish on the rack, close the cover. and grill for 6 to 8 minutes.

6. The fish is done when it flakes easily with a fork and a digital food thermometer reads 145°F (65°C) when inserted in the thickest part of a fillet. Transfer the fish to a cutting board.

7. Stack the tortillas and wrap in foil. While the fish is cooking, warm them in the oven or on the grill.

8. Cut or flake the fish into bite-size pieces. Serve in the warm tortillas.

VARIATION: Fish Tacos with Ginger & Lemongrass
Replace the chili powder and cumin with 1 tablespoon grated fresh ginger and 2 teaspoons lemongrass paste (see Tip, page 180).

VARIATION: Fish Tacos with Garlic & Basil
Increase the garlic to 2 cloves, and replace the chili powder and cumin with 3 tablespoons finely chopped fresh basil.

Serving Size 2 tacos; Calories 307; Protein 20 g; Carbs 37 g; Dietary Fiber 0 g; Added Sugars 0 g; Total Fat 9 g; Sat Fat 3 g; Omega-3s 170 mg; Sodium 475 mg; Potassium 605 mg

PORTOBELLO STREET TACOS

Makes 12 tacos

Portobellos are the meatiest of the mushrooms, providing an earthy, satisfyingly flavorful filling for these soft tacos. Creamy Cilantro Coleslaw adds bright flavor and Chipotle Aïoli contributes smokiness.

2 tablespoons extra virgin olive oil

4 large portobello mushroom caps, cleaned, sliced into ½-inch (6 mm) strips

1 red bell pepper, seeded and sliced

2 tablespoons balsamic vinegar

2 garlic cloves, minced

½ cup (8 g) cilantro leaves, finely minced

12 small flour "street taco" tortillas, warmed

1 cup (200 g) Creamy Cilantro Coleslaw (page 151)

½ cup (140 g) Chipotle Aïoli (page 44)

1. Heat the oil in a large sauté pan or skillet over high heat. When the oil is sizzling but not smoking, add the mushrooms and pepper, lower the heat to medium-high, and sauté until tender, 4 to 6 minutes. The vegetables should sizzle loudly. Shake the pan occasionally, and allow some of the vegetables to become charred.

2. Add the vinegar and garlic. Stir for 2 minutes, then remove from the heat. Stir in the cilantro.

3. To assemble the tacos, fill a warm tortilla with a few portobello strips and some peppers. Top with slaw and aïoli and serve immediately.

VARIATION: *Taco Bowls*

Omit the tortillas. Into each of four shallow bowls, spoon ¾ cup to 1 cup (165 g to 220 g) Creamy Cilantro Coleslaw (page 151). Evenly divide the vegetable mixture among the bowls. Drizzle each with Chipotle Aïoli (page 44) and sprinkle with cilantro. Serve immediately.

Serving Size 3 tacos; Calories 384; Protein 8 g; Carbs 37 g; Dietary Fiber 5 g; Added Sugars 1 g; Total Fat 23 g; Sat Fat 5 g; Omega-3s 930 mg; Sodium 401 mg; Potassium 552 mg

SHRIMP TACOS

Makes 8 tacos

The flavor mash-up in these tacos originates from the Cajun Seasoning, which adds a distinctive note to the shrimp prior to cooking. The orange-balsamic vinaigrette provides a bright, delicious, citrus tang, and the Persian Fresh Herb Mix contributes crunch with incredible bursts of freshness.

- 1 pound (454 g) fresh or thawed frozen 31/40 shrimp, peeled and deveined
- 2 tablespoons Cajun Seasoning (page 30)
- 1 teaspoon grated orange zest
- ⅓ cup (80 ml) fresh orange juice
- 2 tablespoons balsamic vinegar
- 2 tablespoons toasted sesame oil
- 1 tablespoon chopped fresh oregano or 1 teaspoon dried oregano
- Eight 6-inch (15 cm) soft corn tortillas or whole wheat flour tortillas
- 2 cups (65 g) Persian Fresh Herb Mix (page 35)
- 1 avocado, halved, pitted, peeled, and cut into 8 slices
- 2½ tablespoons toasted sesame seeds

1. Rinse the shrimp, drain, and pat dry with paper towels. Place in a large bowl and sprinkle with the seasoning. Toss to coat and let sit for 5 minutes.

2. Whisk together the orange zest, orange juice, vinegar, 1 tablespoon of the oil, and the oregano.

3. Preheat the oven to 200°F (95°C). Stack the tortillas, wrap in foil, and place in the oven to warm.

4. Heat the remaining 1 tablespoon of oil in a large skillet over medium-high heat. Add the shrimp and sauté for 3 minutes, until the thickest part of the shrimp (opposite end of the tail) has turned from translucent to opaque. The shrimp will be firm, white, and orange-colored on the outside. (A single shrimp is difficult to test for doneness with a digital food thermometer, but if you skewer 3 or 4 through the thickest part, they are fully cooked when the thermometer reads 145°F/65°C.) Immediately remove the shrimp from the heat.

5. Place 2 tortillas on each of four plates and divide the shrimp evenly among the tortillas. Top each with ¼ cup (8 g) of the herb mix and a slice of avocado. Rewhisk the dressing, then drizzle each taco with 1 tablespoon. Sprinkle each with 1 teaspoon sesame seeds and serve immediately.

Serving Size 2 tacos; Calories 320; Protein 26 g; Carbs 20 g; Dietary Fiber 4 g; Added Sugars 0 g; Total Fat 16 g; Sat Fat 2 g; Omega-3s 150 mg; Sodium 145 mg; Potassium 580 mg

SPICY SHREDDED BEEF STREET TACOS

Makes about 6 cups (1,500 g) beef

Oven-braising lean beef is a wonderful way to create a tender, flavorful filling for street tacos. You can use Mexican lager, American pilsner, or an IPA for the beer in the braising liquid.

Beef Filling

8 dried chipotle chiles, stems removed

3 tablespoons extra virgin olive oil

2 tablespoons white vinegar

1 tablespoon kosher salt

One 2.5- to 3-pound (1.1 to 1.4 kg) lean beef roast (see Tip)

1 large white onion, diced

One 12-ounce (355 ml) bottle or can beer

1 cup (240 ml) water

Tacos

24 small (4-inch/10 cm) soft corn or flour tortillas, warmed

Simply Quick-Pickled Red Onions (page 259)

Creamy Cilantro Coleslaw (page 151)

1. Place the chiles in a small saucepan, cover with water, and place over high heat. Bring to a boil, then turn off the heat, cover, and let them steep and soften for 30 minutes to 1 hour.

2. Preheat the oven to 350°F (180°C).

3. Drain the chiles and combine them with 2 tablespoons of the oil, the vinegar, and salt in a food processor or blender. Blend until smooth.

4. Heat the remaining 1 tablespoon of oil in a large Dutch oven over medium-high heat. Add the beef and sear on all sides, to create a dark brown crust, 2 minutes per side. Remove from the heat and add the chile puree, onion, beer, and water.

5. Cover the pot and braise the roast in the oven for 2½ to 3 hours, until very tender. (A smaller roast will take about 2½ hours while a larger roast will take 3 hours to become tender.)

6. Remove the beef and shred it using two forks. If there are a lot of large, long shreds, chop them with a chef's knife. Return the beef to the pot, if necessary,

and stir to evenly incorporate it into the braising liquid. If needed, place the pot over low heat to reheat the beef.

7. To assemble the tacos, place a spoonful of beef in each tortilla and top with a few pickled red onions and some coleslaw. Serve immediately. Store the beef, covered, in the refrigerator for up to 3 days and reheat on the stovetop over medium heat until the mixture reaches 165°F (75°C).

TIP: *The following types of beef roasts are lean cuts of beef: chuck tender, eye of round, top round, bottom round, and sirloin.*

Serving Size ½ cup (125 g) beef; Calories 313; Protein 30 g; Carbs 17 g; Dietary Fiber 2 g; Added Sugars 0 g; Total Fat 12 g; Sat Fat 3 g; Omega-3s 50 mg; Sodium 552 mg; Potassium 248 mg

CHICKEN & BEAN BURRITOS

Makes 6 burritos

This recipe is part of our "cook once, eat twice" strategy. It uses chicken from the Roast Chicken with Lemon & Thyme to make a hand-held second meal of burritos. The chicken is moistened by simmering it in a sauce of reduced seasoned Chicken Stock. We then add flavorful Refried Beans and sprinkle with Asiago. We suggest serving these with Avocado Salsa and Pico de Gallo.

Six 8-inch (20 cm) whole wheat tortillas

1 cup (240 ml) Chicken Stock (page 70), plus more if needed

3 garlic cloves, minced

1 teaspoon ground turmeric

½ teaspoon ground cumin

2 cups (270 g) shredded meat from Roast Chicken with Lemon & Thyme (page 313), thawed if frozen

1 cup (260 g) Refried Beans (page 243)

6 tablespoons (45 g) shredded Asiago

4 cups (140 g) shredded lettuce

3 cups (540 g) chopped tomatoes

½ cup (70 g) sliced black olives

2 cups (440 g) Avocado Salsa (page 61)

2 cups (320 g) Pico de Gallo (page 61)

1. Preheat the oven to 200°F (95°C). Stack the tortillas, wrap in foil, and heat in the oven until the filling is ready.

2. Combine the chicken stock, garlic, turmeric, and cumin in a medium saucepan over medium-high heat. Bring to a boil, reduce the heat to medium-low, and simmer until the liquid is reduced to ½ cup (120 ml), 3 to 5 minutes.

3. Add the chicken and heat to blend the flavors together, about 3 minutes. Stir in the refried beans and cook until the mixture has thickened, about 4 minutes, and a digital food thermometer reads 165°F (75°C) when inserted in the center of the filling. Add a little more chicken stock if the filling is too thick.

4. Lay out the tortillas on a work surface. Spoon ¼ to ⅓ cup (50 to 65 g) of the filling just below the center of each tortilla, toward the edge closest to you. Avoid the urge to overfill; allow room for the other ingredients. Sprinkle with 1 tablespoon cheese and top with ½ to ⅔ cup lettuce, ½ cup tomatoes, and 1 to 1½ tablespoons black olives. Fold the edge closest to you up to enclose the filling, fold the sides in, roll up, and tuck in the edges. Place the burrito seam side down on a serving plate, or wrap the burrito in parchment paper or wax paper for later. Serve with avocado salsa and pico de gallo on the side.

Serving Size 1 burrito; Calories 418; Protein 22 g; Carbs 45 g; Dietary Fiber 12 g; Added Sugars 0 g; Total Fat 18 g; Sat Fat 4 g; Omega-3s 150 mg; Sodium 590 mg; Potassium 751 mg

PORK LETTUCE WRAPS
Makes 4 servings

Need a new take on Taco Tuesday? This aromatic pork and vegetable mixture is a wonderful dinner option when you want something light yet satisfyingly flavorful. You can top Simply Cooked Brown Rice (page 230) or Simply Cooked Millet (page 227) with this mixture when you want something slightly more filling. Or you can have the best of both worlds by spooning some rice or millet into the lettuce leaves before adding the pork mixture.

1 tablespoon peanut oil

4 green onions, thinly sliced

3 garlic cloves, minced

1 tablespoon finely grated or minced fresh ginger (see Tip)

1 pound (454 g) lean ground pork

2 carrots, grated

2 tablespoons reduced-sodium soy sauce

1 tablespoon toasted sesame oil

½ teaspoon kosher salt

2 tablespoons fresh lime juice

¼ cup (35 g) roasted peanuts, finely chopped

½ cup (15 g) fresh mint leaves, thinly sliced, or fresh cilantro leaves

1 head butter or iceberg lettuce or 2 romaine hearts, leaves separated

1. Heat the peanut oil in a large sauté pan or skillet over high heat for 1 minute, swirling the pan to evenly distribute the oil. Add half of the green onions, the garlic, and ginger, and stir-fry until the green onions start to soften and there is an aroma of ginger and garlic, 1 to 2 minutes. Add the pork and cook, stirring frequently to break it up, until completely browned, 5 to 6 minutes.

2. Add the carrots, soy sauce, sesame oil, and salt, reduce the heat to medium-low, and cook until the carrots are softened, 2 minutes.

3. Transfer the mixture to a bowl, cover, and refrigerate for 20 to 30 minutes, until cool but not cold.

4. When you're ready to serve, stir in the lime juice, the remaining green onions, the peanuts, and mint. Spoon into lettuce leaves and serve.

TIP: A Microplane is the perfect tool for finely grating ginger.

Per Serving: Calories 400; Protein 26 g; Carbs 9 g; Dietary Fiber 3 g; Added Sugars 0 g; Total Fat 30 g; Sat Fat 9 g; Omega-3s 190 mg; Sodium 715 mg; Potassium 675 mg

SODIUM TIP: Using Diamond Crystal Kosher Salt will dramatically reduce the sodium in any recipe that uses kosher salt. This salt contains 50% less sodium per measure than regular kosher salt and 60% less than fine grain table salt.

SALMON SPRING ROLLS

Makes 8 spring rolls

We love make-ahead meals when you cook once and eat twice. No cooking is required to make these wraps if you do a little planning. We suggest making these with spring roll wrappers (rice paper sheets), but you could also use four whole wheat tortillas and make four wraps instead of eight spring rolls.

1 cup (270 g) Peanut Sauce (page 56)

2 tablespoons rice vinegar

Eight 8-inch (20 cm) round spring roll wrappers

1 cup (55 g) shredded carrots (about 2 medium carrots)

8 green onions, cut lengthwise into thin slices

1 English cucumber, halved crosswise and cut into thin strips

8 ounces (227 g) Simply Broiled Salmon (page 298), flaked or broken into small pieces

1 pear or apple, cored and diced, or 1 mango, peeled, pitted, and diced

⅓ cup (5 g) chopped fresh cilantro leaves

2 tablespoons fresh lime juice

⅛ teaspoon kosher salt

Freshly cracked black pepper

1. Whisk ½ cup (135 g) of the peanut sauce with the rice vinegar in a small bowl.

2. Pour 1 inch (2.5 cm) warm water into a 9-inch (23 cm) pie plate. Dip a spring roll wrapper in the warm water and soak for 10 seconds; the wrapper should still feel firm. (Don't let the wrapper soak too long, as it will continue to soften and may tear when rolling; the moisture in the fillings will help keep the wrapper soft.) Remove from the water and place on a damp paper towel or on a serving plate.

3. Layer about 2 tablespoons of the carrots and 2 or 3 strips each of green onion and cucumber below the center of the wrapper, about 1 inch (2.5 cm) above the edge closest to you. Add a few pieces of salmon, 2 tablespoons of the fruit, and a sprinkle of cilantro and lime juice. Drizzle 1 tablespoon of the peanut sauce over the filling. Add a pinch of salt and a grind of black pepper. Fold the bottom edge of the wrapper up to encase all the filling. Fold in the sides, roll and

continue to tuck in the sides as you roll. Place the roll seam side down on the plate and cut in half diagonally.

4. Assemble the rest of the rolls. Serve with the remaining peanut sauce on the side. These taste best the day they are made but can be stored in an airtight container in the refrigerator for up to 2 days.

Serving Size 2 spring rolls; Calories 311; Protein 10 g; Carbs 37 g; Dietary Fiber 5 g; Added Sugars 1 g; Total Fat 15 g; Sat Fat 3 g; Omega-3s 730 mg; Sodium 310 mg; Potassium 468 mg

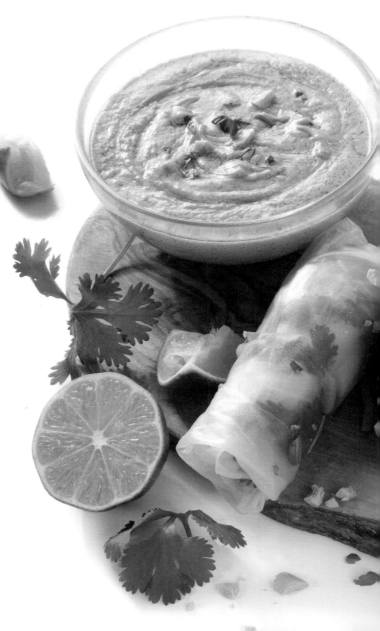

SEARED LAMB PITA POCKETS WITH CUCUMBER MINT YOGURT SAUCE

Makes 4 servings

This is a very versatile recipe. You can serve the lamb, yogurt sauce, and lettuce in pita pockets, or you can top a red leaf lettuce salad with the lamb and use the yogurt sauce for dressing. You can also build a bowl with Simply Cooked Sorghum (page 229) and Simply Cooked Lentils (page 247). Have fun finding the presentation that best suits your mood and eating style!

Lamb

2 tablespoons extra virgin olive oil

1 tablespoon fresh lemon juice

1 teaspoon dried oregano

½ teaspoon kosher salt

½ teaspoon freshly ground black pepper

1 pound (454 g) lamb sirloin steak, trimmed of all visible fat and cut into 1-inch (2.5 cm) cubes

SALMON SPRING ROLLS

Cucumber Mint Yogurt Sauce

One 5.3-ounce (150 g) container plain Greek yogurt (about ⅔ cup)

¾ cup (100 g) grated English cucumber

2 tablespoons thinly sliced fresh mint leaves

1 tablespoon fresh lemon juice

¼ teaspoon kosher salt

To Assemble

4 whole wheat pita pockets, halved

8 red leaf lettuce leaves

1. Whisk together the oil, lemon juice, oregano, salt, and pepper in a large glass bowl. Add the lamb and toss with a spoon to evenly coat. Set aside to marinate for at least 15 minutes.

2. While the lamb is marinating, make the sauce: Combine the yogurt, cucumber, mint, lemon juice, and salt in a small bowl.

3. Heat a large sauté pan or skillet over high heat. Add the lamb and marinade. Cook the lamb undisturbed for 2 minutes, stir once, then continue to cook undisturbed for 2 minutes, until the color changes from dark red to brown.

4. Place a lettuce leaf in each pita half, then top each with one-eighth of the lamb and a spoonful of the sauce. Serve immediately, with the remaining sauce on the side.

Serving Size 2 pita pockets; Calories 465; Protein 44 g; Carbs 30 g; Dietary Fiber 5 g; Added Sugars 1 g; Total Fat 19 g; Sat Fat 6 g; Omega-3s 230 mg; Sodium 670 mg; Potassium 495 mg

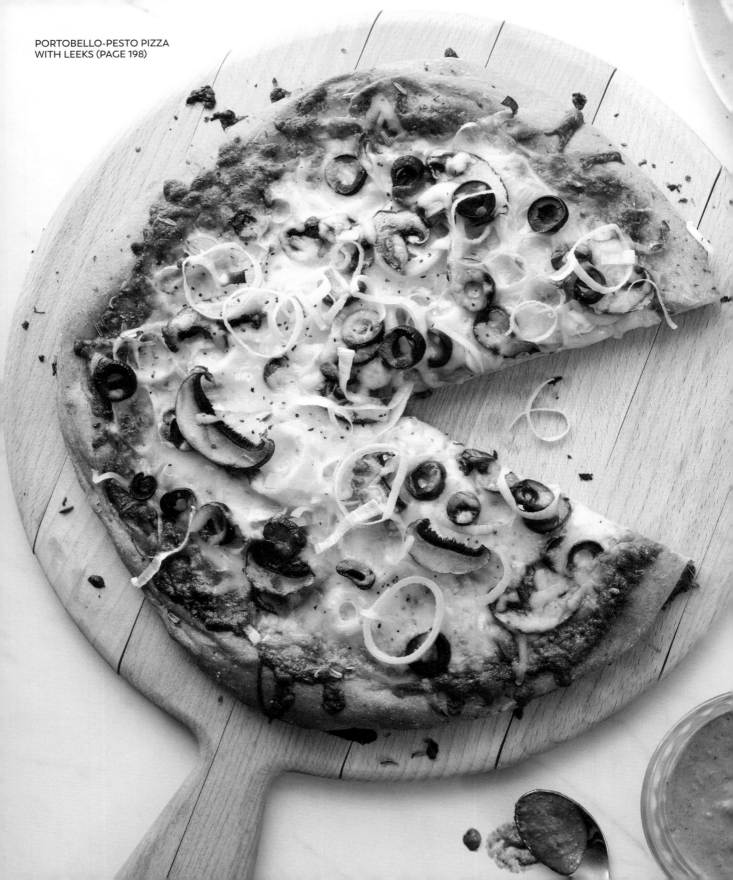

PORTOBELLO-PESTO PIZZA
WITH LEEKS (PAGE 198)

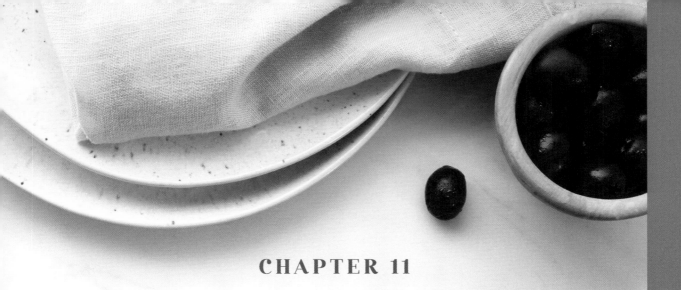

CHAPTER 11

Pizzas, Piadine & Flatbreads

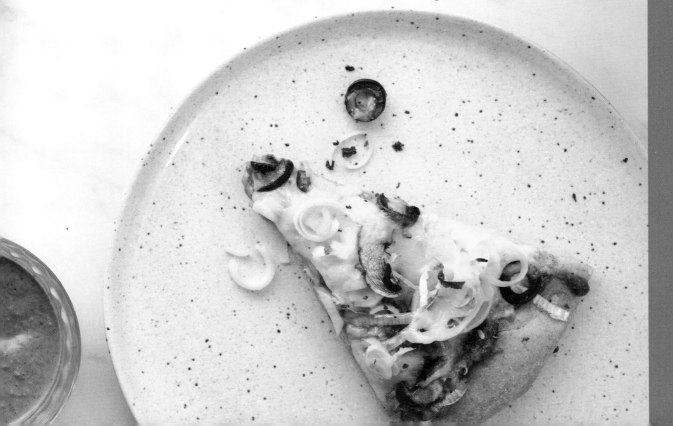

Pizzas, Piadine & Flatbreads

Pizza Dough

À la Heart Classic Pizza Dough........ 194

Honey Whole Wheat
Potato Pizza Dough.................. 194

Whole Wheat–Herb Pizza Dough...... 195

SMOKED SALMON
FLATBREAD WITH DILL
(PAGE 200)

Pizzas, Piadine & Flatbreads

Chicken-Pesto Pizza.................. 196

Gorgonzola & Beef Piadine
with Arugula Salad.................. 196

Margherita Pizza 197

Portabello-Pesto Pizza with Leeks..... 198

Prosciutto & Pear Piadine
with Balsamic Drizzle 198

Sausage & Roasted Red Pepper
Breakfast Pizza..................... 199

Smoked Salmon Flatbread with Dill.... 200

Very Veggie Pizza 200

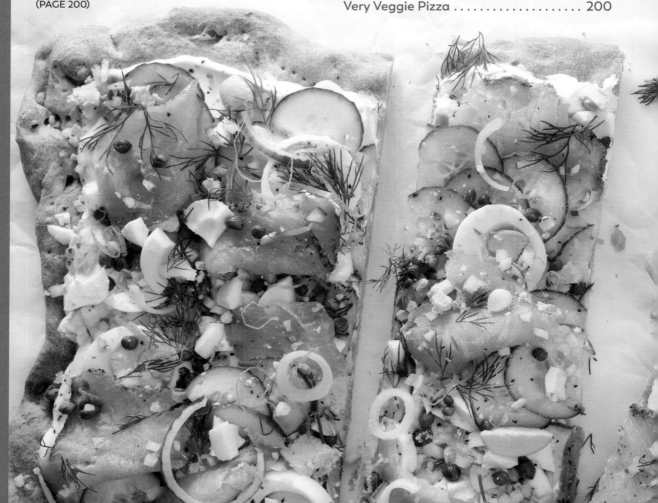

Pizza is a favorite food for many of us. It's a simple food with endless options for customization. In this chapter, we offer you three different crusts that incorporate whole grain flour. Each version includes extra virgin olive oil, which creates a more pliable dough—there's no need to struggle with a dough that won't easily stretch or roll out to your desired size and shape. We've also reduced the amount of salt in our dough compared to more traditional dough recipes, since we wanted to save room for the salt that comes from other pizza ingredients like cheese.

The recipes are based on the weight of the dough. Here's a chart on how the dough ball sizes translate.

We provide options for turning the dough into various shapes beyond the typical round pizza, including smaller piadine, an Italian term for flatbread. Each piadina is essentially a personal pizza with a thin crust. Piadine are intended to be folded up and eaten like a taco, sandwich, or New York slice.

We also offer a flatbread recipe where the dough is shaped into a large rectangle; don't worry about the shape being perfect. Imperfection suggests an artisan—you!—made it.

You'll notice our recipes emphasize vegetable toppings. We don't omit meat toppings, but we limit the amount of meat and maximize the veggies. We even include a recipe that puts fruit—pears—on piadine with prosciutto.

Table 6: Pizza Dough Ball Sizes

THIS RECIPE	MAKES	WHICH CAN BE TURNED INTO
À la Heart Classic Pizza Dough	Two 10-ounce (283 g) dough balls	• Two 12-inch (30.5 cm) thin pizza crusts • Two 8 × 14-inch (20 × 35.5 cm) rectangular flatbreads • Six 7-inch (18 cm) flatbreads, piadine, or pita breads
Honey Whole Wheat Potato Pizza Dough	Three 10-ounce (283 g) dough balls	• Three 12-inch (30 cm) thin pizza crusts • Three 8 × 14-inch (20 × 35.5 cm) rectangular flatbreads • Nine 7-inch (18 cm) flatbreads or piadine
Whole Wheat– Herb Pizza Dough	One 14-ounce (397 g) dough ball	• One 10 × 15-inch (25 × 38 cm) thin pizza crust • Four 7-inch (18 cm) flatbreads or piadine

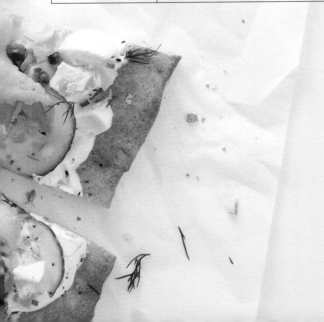

In most cases, we use cheeses made with part-skim milk (to reduce saturated fat) or fresh cheeses, which contain more water by weight, to limit the sodium per serving. But limiting saturated fat and sodium in no way limits flavor! So what are you waiting for? Go forth and make some pizza!

À LA HEART CLASSIC PIZZA DOUGH

Makes two 10-ounce (283 g) dough balls

This pizza dough follows a very standard recipe with one exception; half the all-purpose flour is replaced with whole wheat flour. This dough can be used to make any of the pizzas or flatbreads in this chapter.

- 1 cup (240 ml) warm water (110° to 115°F/43°C to 46°C)
- One 0.25-ounce (7 g) packet active dry yeast
- 2 tablespoons plus 1 teaspoon extra virgin olive oil
- ½ teaspoon Diamond Crystal Kosher Salt
- 1 cup (120 g) whole wheat flour
- 1 cup (125 g) all-purpose flour, plus more for dusting

1. Combine the water and yeast in a small bowl. Gently stir and set aside to proof the yeast and form bubbles for 2 to 3 minutes.

2. In a large bowl or the bowl of a stand mixer fitted with the paddle attachment, combine 2 tablespoons of the oil and the salt. Mix in the whole wheat flour. Add the yeast-water mixture and mix well.

3. If you're working by hand, stir in ¾ cup (95 g) of the all-purpose flour until the dough is sticky but starts to pull away from the sides of the bowl. Turn out the dough onto a clean surface and knead in the remaining ¼ cup (30 g) of the all-purpose flour. Knead for at least 2 minutes, until all the flour is incorporated and a smooth, supple dough has formed.

4. If using a stand mixer, switch to the dough hook attachment. Stir in 1 cup (125 g) of the all-purpose flour, then use the dough hook to knead the dough for at least 2 minutes, until all the flour is incorporated and a smooth, supple dough has formed.

5. Shape the dough into a smooth ball. Use the remaining 1 teaspoon of oil to lightly oil a medium bowl. Transfer the dough to the bowl and roll it around a few times to coat it. Cover with a kitchen towel and set in a warm spot for the dough to rise until double in size, about 60 minutes.

6. Punch down the dough and divide it into two

10-ounce (283 g) balls. Use immediately or store in airtight containers in the refrigerator for up to 3 days. Remove from the refrigerator at least an hour before using so the dough can warm up and become pliable enough to stretch without tearing. The dough can be frozen for up to a month; thaw at room temperature for 3 hours prior to use.

Serving Size ¼ of a dough ball; Calories 155; Protein 4 g; Carbs 23 g; Dietary Fiber 2 g; Added Sugars 0 g; Total Fat 6 g; Sat Fat 1 g; Omega-3s 50 mg; Sodium 70 mg; Potassium 70 mg

HONEY WHOLE WHEAT POTATO PIZZA DOUGH

Makes three 10-ounce (283 g) dough balls

This dough was created for two of our pizza recipes, the Sausage & Roasted Red Pepper Breakfast Pizza (page 199) and the Very Veggie Pizza (page 200). The starch in russet potatoes (or other starchy potatoes) helps bind water, creating a pliable dough that's very easy to roll out.

- 1 cup (240 ml) warm water (110° to 115°F/43° to 46°C; see Tip)
- One 0.25-ounce (7 g) package active dry yeast
- 1 cup (230 g) plain mashed russet-type potatoes
- 2 tablespoons plus 1 teaspoon extra virgin olive oil
- 1 tablespoon honey
- 1 teaspoon Diamond Crystal Kosher Salt
- 2 cups (240 g) whole wheat flour
- ½ cup (65 g) all-purpose flour

1. Combine the water and yeast in a small bowl. Gently stir and set aside to proof the yeast and form bubbles for 2 to 3 minutes.

2. In a large bowl or the bowl of a stand mixer fitted with the paddle attachment, combine the potatoes, 2 tablespoons of the oil, the honey, and salt. Mix in 1 cup (120 g) of the whole wheat flour. Add the yeast-water mixture and mix well.

3. If kneading by hand, add the remaining 1 cup (120 g) of whole wheat flour and mix until the dough is sticky but starts to pull away from the sides of the bowl. Turn out the dough onto a clean surface and knead in the all-purpose flour. Knead for at least 2 minutes, until all the flour is incorporated and a smooth, supple dough has formed.

4. If you're using a stand mixer, switch to the dough hook attachment. Add the remaining 1 cup (120 g) of whole wheat flour and the all-purpose flour, and mix and knead the dough for at least 2 minutes, until all the flour is incorporated and a smooth, supple dough has formed.

5. Shape the dough into smooth ball. Use the remaining 1 teaspoon of olive oil to lightly oil a medium bowl. Transfer the dough to the bowl and roll it around a few times to coat. Cover with a kitchen towel and set in a warm spot for the dough to rise and double in size, 60 to 90 minutes.

6. Punch down the dough and divide into three 10-ounce (283 g) balls. Use immediately or store in airtight containers in the refrigerator for up to 3 days. Remove from the refrigerator at least an hour before using so it can warm up and become pliable enough to stretch without tearing. The dough can be frozen for up to a month; thaw at room temperature for 3 hours prior to use.

TIP: *If you're cooking potatoes specifically for this recipe, reserve and use the potato water to proof the yeast.*

Serving Size ¼ of a dough ball; Calories 135; Protein 4 g; Carbs 22 g; Dietary Fiber 3 g; Added Sugars 1 g; Total Fat 4 g; Sat Fat 0.5 g; Omega-3s 40 mg; Sodium 90 mg; Potassium 120 mg

WHOLE WHEAT-HERB PIZZA DOUGH

Makes four 3.5-ounce (100 g) dough balls

This recipe uses whole wheat pastry flour, which is made with soft (low-protein) wheat, to produce a lighter, softer-textured dough. We use a partial packet of active dry yeast (a full packet contains 2¼ teaspoons); don't be tempted to use it all or your dough will rise too much. This recipe is perfect for making the flatbreads (piadine) for the Gorgonzola & Beef Piadine with Arugula Salad (page 196).

⅔ cup (160 ml) warm water
(110° to 115°F/43° to 46°C)

1¼ teaspoons active dry yeast

2 tablespoons plus 1 teaspoon extra virgin olive oil

2 teaspoons Italian Seasoning (page 34)
½ teaspoon Diamond Crystal Kosher Salt
½ teaspoon sugar
1¾ cups (210 g) whole wheat pastry flour

1. Combine the water and yeast in a small bowl. Gently stir and set aside to proof the yeast and form bubbles for 2 to 3 minutes.

2. In a large bowl or the bowl of stand mixer fitted with the paddle attachment, combine 2 tablespoons of the oil, the seasoning, salt, and sugar. Mix in 1 cup (120 g) of the flour. Add the yeast-water mixture and mix well. If you're using a stand mixer, switch to the dough hook attachment before adding more flour.

3. If kneading by hand, add ½ cup (60 g) of the flour and mix until the dough is sticky but starts to pull away from the sides of the bowl. Turn out the dough onto a clean flat surface and knead in the remaining ¼ cup (30 g) flour. Knead the dough for at least 2 minutes, until all the flour is incorporated and a smooth, supple dough has formed.

4. If using a stand mixer, switch to the dough hook attachment. Add the remaining ¾ cup (90 g) of flour and knead the dough for at least 2 minutes, until all the flour is incorporated and a smooth, supple dough has formed.

5. Shape the dough into a smooth ball. Use the remaining 1 teaspoon of oil to lightly oil a medium bowl. Transfer the dough to the bowl and roll it around a few times to coat. Cover with a kitchen towel and set in a warm spot for the dough to rise and double in size, about 45 minutes.

6. Punch down the dough and divide into four 3.5-ounce (100 g) balls. Use immediately or store in airtight containers in the refrigerator for up to 3 days. Remove from the refrigerator at least 1 hour before using so the dough can warm up and become pliable enough to stretch without tearing. The dough can also be frozen for up to 2 months; thaw at room temperature for 3 hours prior to use.

Serving Size 1 dough ball; Calories 290; Protein 7 g; Carbs 41 g; Dietary Fiber 6 g; Added Sugars 1 g; Total Fat 11 g; Sat Fat 1 g; Omega-3s 75 mg; Sodium 140 mg; Potassium 195 mg

CHICKEN-PESTO PIZZA

Makes one 12-inch (30.5 cm) pizza

You could make this pizza with chicken from our Chicken Caesar Salad (page 161), our Simply Roasted Peppers (page 259), and our Basil Pesto (page 45), but we created this recipe specifically for busy people who need a few shortcuts. Feel free to use a prebaked commercial pizza crust, if you like.

Extra virgin olive oil

One 10-ounce (283 g) ball Honey Whole Wheat Potato Pizza Dough (page 194)

⅓ cup (80 g) store-bought basil pesto

1 cup (260 g) jarred roasted red bell pepper strips, drained

½ cup (80 g) thinly sliced red onion

1 cup (115 g) shredded part-skim mozzarella

Two 3-ounce (85 g) chicken Italian sausages, cooked and thinly sliced

Freshly ground black pepper

Red pepper flakes, optional

1. Adjust an oven rack to the middle position. Preheat the oven to 425°F (220°C). Set out a 15-inch (38 cm) square piece of parchment paper and a large, flat baking sheet or pizza pan.

2. Oil your hands, then transfer the dough ball to the center of the parchment. Rotate the paper as you use your hands to work the dough into a 10-inch (25.5 cm) circle. Oil a rolling pin, then roll out the dough to a 12-inch (30.5 cm) circle. Use kitchen shears to trim the parchment paper about ½ inch (13 mm) from the edge of the dough. Transfer the dough, on the parchment, to the baking sheet.

3. Spread the pesto to the edges of the crust. Add the roasted peppers and onions, then sprinkle on the cheese. Top with the sausage and freshly ground pepper.

4. Bake for 18 to 20 minutes, until the crust has turned dark brown and the cheese is melted and golden brown. Cut into 8 pieces and serve immediately, topped with red pepper flakes if desired.

Serving Size 2 slices; Calories 360; Protein 16 g; Carbs 27 g; Dietary Fiber 3 g; Added Sugars 1 g; Total Fat 21 g; Sat Fat 6 g; Omega-3s 160 mg; Sodium 620 mg; Potassium 240 mg

GORGONZOLA & BEEF PIADINE WITH ARUGULA SALAD

Makes 4 piadine

Piadine are Italian flatbreads meant to be folded over to create a sandwich. This version incorporates tangy Gorgonzola and a small amount of deli roast beef topped with a beautiful arugula salad that's simply dressed with lemon juice and extra virgin olive oil. You can eat your piadina with a knife or fork or fold it up and eat it like a big taco.

2 tablespoons extra virgin olive oil, plus more for oiling

Four 3.5-ounce (100 g) balls Whole Wheat–Herb Pizza Dough (page 195)

4 ounces (113 g) crumbled Gorgonzola

2 tablespoons milk

8 ounces (227 g) thinly sliced low-sodium deli roast beef

Freshly ground black pepper

6 cups (120 g) baby arugula

2 tablespoons fresh lemon juice

1 ounce (28 g) shaved Parmesan

1. Adjust one oven rack to the middle position and another to the lowest position. Preheat the oven to 425°F (220°C). Set out two 15 × 20-inch (38 × 51 cm) pieces of parchment paper and two large baking sheets.

2. Oil your hands, then place a dough ball on one half of one piece of parchment. Use your hands to work the dough into a 4-inch (10 cm) circle. Oil a rolling pin, then roll the dough into a 7-inch (18 cm) circle. Set a second dough ball on the other side of the parchment and repeat to create a second 7-inch (18 cm) circle. Roll out 2 more circles on the second sheet of parchment. Transfer the piadine, still on the parchment, to the baking sheets.

3. Place one baking sheet on each oven rack and bake for 5 minutes. Switch the baking sheets and bake for position 5 minutes, until the piadine are golden brown on the edges. Remove from the oven and allow to cool slightly.

4. While the piadine are cooling, combine the Gorgonzola and milk in a small microwave-safe bowl and microwave on HIGH for 30 to 40 seconds. Stir to create a creamy sauce with some Gorgonzola crumbles still visible. Divide the sauce evenly among the four piadine; spread with a spoon, distributing it within ½ inch (13 mm) from the edge.

5. Top each piadina with 2 ounces (57 g) roast beef, gently folding and piling the beef on top of the sauce. Add a few grinds of pepper.

6. Combine the arugula, lemon juice, and olive oil in a medium bowl. Use your fingers to toss the arugula, coating it. Add the Parmesan, then use tongs to gently toss again. Divide the salad among the four piadine and serve.

TIP: You can bake off the piadine and store them in an airtight container at room temperature for up to 3 days prior to topping them.

Serving Size 1 piadina; Calories 580; Protein 32 g; Carbs 46 g; Dietary Fiber 6 g; Added Sugars 1 g; Total Fat 31 g; Sat Fat 10 g; Omega-3s 190 mg; Sodium 830 mg; Potassium 520 mg

MARGHERITA PIZZA

Makes one 12-inch (30.5 cm) pizza

This scrumptious pizza with toppings fresh from the garden will remind you of a caprese salad. But enjoy it piping hot, right from the oven! If you want to save some time, use a prebaked 12-inch (30.5 cm) 100% whole grain thin pizza crust.

- 1 tablespoon plus 1 teaspoon extra virgin olive oil
- One 10-ounce (283 g) ball À la Heart Classic Pizza Dough (page 194)
- 1 tablespoon Italian Seasoning (page 34), plus more for sprinkling
- 3 garlic cloves, minced
- ⅔ cup (16 g) chopped fresh basil leaves
- 2 Roma (plum) tomatoes, thinly sliced
- 6 ounces (170 g) thinly sliced fresh mozzarella
- Freshly ground black pepper
- ½ cup (25 g) chopped fresh basil leaves

1. Adjust an oven rack to the middle position. Preheat the oven to 450°F (230°C). Set out a 15-inch (38 cm) square piece of parchment paper and a large, flat baking sheet or pizza pan.

2. Oil your hands and a rolling pin with 1 tablespoon of the oil. Place the dough in the center of the parchment. Rotate the paper as you use your hands to work the dough into a 10-inch (25.5 cm) circle, then use the rolling pin to roll out the dough to a 12-inch (30.5 cm) circle. Use kitchen shears to trim the parchment about ½ inch (13 mm) from the edges of the dough. Transfer the dough, still on the parchment, to the baking sheet. Use a fork to prick the crust 6 to 8 times.

3. Bake for 6 minutes. Remove from the oven, brush with the remaining 1 teaspoon oil, and sprinkle with the seasoning and garlic. Scatter over half the chopped basil and add the tomato slices in a single layer. Top with the mozzarella, nestling some slices between the tomato slices and placing some slices slightly overlapping the tomatoes. Add the remaining chopped basil, and sprinkle with fresh pepper and additional seasoning.

4. Bake for 14 to 16 minutes, until the cheese is melted in the center and brown in some spots, the crust is golden brown, and the pizza is fragrant and hot. Let stand for 5 minutes before garnishing with fresh basil sprigs, cutting into 8 slices, and serving.

NOTE: Choosing a ready-made whole grain thin crust can enhance the nutrition quality of your pizza. A thin crust keeps the carb count manageable, and often contains less sodium per serving than a slice of bread. There are several off-the-shelf or refrigerated pizza dough brands to choose from that are made from sprouted whole grains and have added flax or chia for added omega-3 fats, yet are reduced in sodium.

Serving Size 2 slices; Calories 320; Protein 13 g; Carbs 26 g; Dietary Fiber 3 g; Added Sugars 0 g; Total Fat 19 g; Sat Fat 7 g; Omega-3s 105 mg; Sodium 240 mg; Potassium 265 mg

PORTOBELLO-PESTO PIZZA WITH LEEKS

Makes one 12-inch (30.5 cm) pizza

If you're a mushroom lover or you cook for one, plan to make this pizza! The mushrooms take on the role of meat while the leeks add a mild onion flavor, and the olives provide a bit of salty brininess.

Extra virgin olive oil

One 10-ounce (283 g) ball À la Heart Classic Pizza Dough (page 194)

½ cup (130 g) Spinach Pesto (page 46)

2 cups (225 g) shredded part-skim mozzarella

3 tablespoons chopped fresh oregano leaves, plus more for sprinkling on top (or 1 tablespoon dried)

1 tablespoon fennel seeds

2 leeks, cleaned (see Tip, page 79) and thinly sliced

8 ounces (227 g) portobello mushrooms, sliced

½ cup (70 g) sliced pitted black olives

Freshly ground black pepper

1. Adjust an oven rack to the middle position. Preheat the oven to 450°F (230°C). Set out a 15-inch (38 cm) square piece of parchment paper and a large, flat baking sheet or pizza pan.

2. Oil your hands, then transfer the dough to the center of the parchment. Rotate the paper as you use your hands to work the dough into a 10-inch (25.5 cm) circle. Oil a rolling pin and roll out the dough to a 12-inch (30.5 cm) circle. Use kitchen shears to trim the parchment about ½ inch (13 mm) from the edges of the dough. Transfer the dough, still on the parchment, to the baking sheet. Use a fork to prick the crust 6 to 8 times.

3. Bake the crust for 6 minutes. Remove from the oven and spread the pesto over the entire crust with the back of a spoon. Sprinkle the oregano and fennel seeds evenly over the pesto, followed by 1 cup (115 g) of the mozzarella, the leeks, mushrooms, and olives. Top with the remaining 1 cup (115 g) of mozzarella. Sprinkle with additional oregano and a few grinds of black pepper.

4. Bake for 14 to 16 minutes, until the cheese is melted, the crust is golden brown, and the mushrooms are reduced and wrinkled. Let stand for 5 minutes before cutting into 8 slices. Serve warm.

Serving Size 2 slices; Calories 490; Protein 22 g; Carbs 36 g; Dietary Fiber 5 g; Added Sugars 0 g; Total Fat 30 g; Sat Fat 9 g; Omega-3s 270 mg; Sodium 725 mg; Potassium 515 mg

PROSCIUTTO & PEAR PIADINE WITH BALSAMIC DRIZZLE

Makes 3 piadine

We were so tempted to write this recipe using fresh figs instead of canned pears, but we opted for a year-round recipe instead. If you can get fresh figs in season, do try this recipe with them. Prosciutto and figs are a classic flavor combination. If you use fresh figs or fresh pears, apple juice makes a great stand-in for the pear canning liquid. You can omit the juice altogether, but the Gorgonzola will be more likely to "escape" unless your piadina is folded over and tightly compressed!

1 tablespoon extra virgin olive oil, plus more for oiling your hands

One 10-ounce (283 g) ball À la Heart Classic Pizza Dough (page 194), divided into three 3.3-ounce (94 g) balls

4 ounces (113 g) crumbled Gorgonzola

One 15.25-ounce (432 g) can sliced pears in 100% juice, drained and chopped, 2 tablespoons juice from the canned pears reserved

3 tablespoons chopped hazelnuts, optional

3 ounces (85 g) sliced prosciutto

6 cups (180 g) fresh baby spinach leaves

1 tablespoon balsamic glaze

1. Arrange one oven rack to to the middle position and another to the lowest position. Preheat the oven to 425°F (220°C). Set out two 15 × 20-inch (38 × 51 cm) pieces of parchment paper and two large baking sheets.

2. Oil your hands, then place a dough ball on one half of one piece of parchment. Use your hands to work the dough into a 4-inch (10 cm) circle. Oil a rolling pin and roll the dough into a 7-inch (18 cm) circle. Set a second dough ball on the other side of the parchment and repeat to create a second 7-inch

(18 cm) circle. Roll out 1 more circle on the second piece of parchment with the third ball of dough. Transfer the piadine, still on the parchment, to the baking sheets.

3. Place one baking sheet on each oven rack and bake for 5 minutes. Switch the baking sheets and bake for 5 minutes, until the piadine are golden brown on the edges. Remove from the oven and let cool slightly.

4. Combine the Gorgonzola and pear juice in a small microwave-safe bowl and microwave on HIGH for 30 to 40 seconds. Stir to create a creamy sauce with some Gorgonzola crumbles still visible. Divide the sauce evenly among the three piadine, spreading it with a spoon to within ½ inch (13 mm) from the edge. Top each piadina with about ½ cup (110 g) pears, 1 tablespoon hazelnuts, if desired, and 1 ounce (28 g) prosciutto, gently draped to create folds rather than lying flat.

5. Combine the spinach and 1 tablespoon oil in a medium bowl. Use your fingers to toss the spinach, coating it with oil, then divide the spinach among the three piadine. Drizzle with the balsamic glaze and serve.

TIP: *If you can't find syrupy balsamic glaze in your local market, you can cook down balsamic vinegar over medium heat until it is reduced by half.*

Serving Size 1 piadina; Calories 545; Protein 23 g; Carbs 53 g; Dietary Fiber 7 g; Added Sugars 0 g; Total Fat 27 g; Sat Fat 10 g; Omega-3s 190 mg; Sodium 980 mg; Potassium 495 mg

SAUSAGE & ROASTED RED PEPPER BREAKFAST PIZZA

Makes one 10-inch (25 cm) pizza

Anyone who loves leftover pizza for breakfast will also likely love this pizza, created especially for enjoying at breakfast or brunch. An egg takes the place of pizza sauce and our Spicy Sage Breakfast Sausage is the featured meat. Serve with fresh fruit or 100% fruit juice.

Extra virgin olive oil

One 10-ounce (283 g) ball Honey Whole Wheat Potato Pizza Dough (page 194)

1 large egg

¼ teaspoon Diamond Crystal Kosher Salt

1 Spicy Sage Breakfast Sausage patty (page 124), cooked and crumbled

¼ cup (65 g) red bell peppers from Simply Roasted Peppers (page 259), cut into thin strips

⅓ cup (80 g) part-skim ricotta

¼ teaspoon Italian Seasoning (page 34)

Freshly ground black pepper

Freshly grated Parmesan, optional

Red pepper flakes, optional

1. Adjust an oven rack to the middle position. Preheat the oven to 450°F (230°C). Set out a 15-inch (38 cm) square piece of parchment paper and a large, flat baking sheet or pizza pan.

2. Oil your hands, then place the dough in the center of the parchment. Rotate the paper as you use your hands to work the dough into a 10-inch (25.5 cm) circle. Use kitchen shears to trim the parchment paper about ½ inch (13 mm) from the edge of the dough. Transfer the dough, still on the parchment, to the baking sheet.

3. Use a fork to beat the egg and salt in a small bowl. Pour the egg onto the pizza dough and use the back of a spoon to spread it so it covers nearly all the crust. Evenly distribute the sausage and roasted peppers on the crust, then use a small spoon to dollop on the ricotta. Sprinkle with the seasoning and grind some pepper on top.

4. Bake for 17 to 18 minutes, until the crust is dark brown and the ricotta has started to turn brown in spots.

5. Use a pizza cutter to cut into 4 pieces. Serve warm, sprinkled with Parmesan and red pepper flakes, if desired.

Serving Size 2 slices; Calories 245; Protein 12 g; Carbs 24 g; Dietary Fiber 3 g; Added Sugars 1 g; Total Fat 11 g; Sat Fat 3 g; Omega-3s 105 mg; Sodium 250 mg; Potassium 255 mg

SMOKED SALMON FLATBREAD WITH DILL

Makes 4 servings as an entrée or 8 as an appetizer

This recipe can be served as an appetizer or an entrée at breakfast, brunch, lunch, or dinner—it's a very versatile recipe fit for any smoked salmon lover. It's also a great make-ahead recipe; bake the flatbread and prep the ingredients in advance, then assemble the flatbread in a few minutes when you're ready to serve.

Extra virgin olive oil

One 10-ounce (283 g) ball À la Heart Classic Pizza Dough (page 194)

⅓ cup (75 g) Crème Fraîche (page 361) or sour cream

2 hard-boiled large eggs, peeled and chopped

¼ English cucumber, thinly sliced

2 tablespoons minced red onion

1 tablespoon capers, drained

¼ teaspoon Diamond Crystal Kosher Salt

¼ teaspoon freshly ground pepper

4 ounces (113 g) cold-smoked salmon

1 tablespoon chopped fresh dill or 2 tablespoons chopped fresh chives

1 teaspoon grated lemon zest

1. Adjust an oven rack to the middle position. Preheat the oven to 450°F (230°C). Set out a 15-inch (38 cm) square piece of parchment paper and a large, flat baking sheet.

2. Oil your hands, then place the dough ball in the center of the parchment. Use your hands and/or an oiled rolling pin to work the dough into a rectangle approximately 8 × 14 inches (20 × 35.5 cm). Use kitchen shears to trim the parchment paper about ½ inch (13 mm) from the edges of the dough. Transfer the flatbread, still on the parchment, to the baking sheet. Use a fork to prick the crust 12 to 15 times.

3. Bake for 14 to 15 minutes, until the edges start to turn dark brown. Place the baking sheet on a wire rack and cool for 10 to 15 minutes before adding the toppings.

4. Spread the crème fraîche on the crust, then evenly distribute the eggs, cucumber, onion, and capers on top. Sprinkle on the salt and pepper. Add the smoked salmon, gently draping and folding it to create some height. Sprinkle the dill and lemon zest on top, cut into 8 or 16 pieces, and serve.

Serving Size ¼ of a flatbread (for an entrée); Calories 265; Protein 14 g; Carbs 26 g; Dietary Fiber 3 g; Total Fat 12 g; Sat Fat 3 g; Omega-3s 250 mg; Sodium 800 mg; Potassium 225

VERY VEGGIE PIZZA

Makes one 12-inch (30.5 cm) pizza

This pizza is all about the veggies. Use the ingredients below or choose your favorite vegetables to create your own very veggie masterpiece. Serve with a tossed salad and your favorite beer or wine.

1 tablespoon extra virgin olive oil, plus more for oiling

One 10-ounce (283 g) ball Honey Whole Wheat Potato Pizza Dough (page 194)

1 teaspoon very finely minced garlic

¼ teaspoon Diamond Crystal Kosher Salt

2 tablespoons freshly grated Parmesan

1 cup (30 g) chopped fresh baby spinach leaves

½ red bell pepper, diced

¼ cup (40 g) thinly sliced red onion

8 to 10 grape or pear tomatoes, halved

8 ounces (227 g) sliced fresh mozzarella

Freshly ground black pepper

¼ cup (6 g) thinly sliced fresh basil leaves

1 tablespoon chopped fresh oregano, or 1 teaspoon dried oregano, crushed

1. Adjust an oven rack to the middle position. Preheat the oven to 425°F (220°C). Set out a 15-inch (38 cm) square piece of parchment paper and a large, flat baking sheet or pizza pan.

2. Oil your hands, then place the dough ball in the center of the parchment. Rotate the paper as you use your hands to work the dough into a 10-inch (25.5 cm) circle. Oil a rolling pin and roll out the dough to a 12-inch (30.5 cm) circle. Use kitchen shears to trim the parchment paper about ½ inch (13 mm) from the edges of the dough. Transfer the dough, still on the parchment, to the baking sheet.

3. Combine 1 tablespoon oil, the garlic, and salt in a small bowl. Spoon the mixture onto the dough and spread to the edges. Sprinkle with the Parmesan.

4. Bake for 6 minutes, then remove from the oven. Discard the parchment and place the crust directly on the baking sheet. Increase the oven temperature to 450°F (230°C).

5. Sprinkle the crust with the spinach and bell pepper, then evenly distribute the onion and tomatoes. Top with the mozzarella slices and 3 to 4 grinds of black pepper.

6. Bake for 15 to 18 minutes more, until the crust is brown on the edges and the cheese has some golden-brown spots. Let sit for 4 to 5 minutes before topping with the basil and oregano and cutting into 8 slices.

Serving Size 2 slices; Calories 225;
Protein 16 g; Carbs 26 g; Dietary Fiber
4 g; Added Sugars 1 g; Total Fat 20 g;
Sat Fat 9 g; Omega-3s 100 mg;
Sodium 435 mg;
Potassium 300 mg

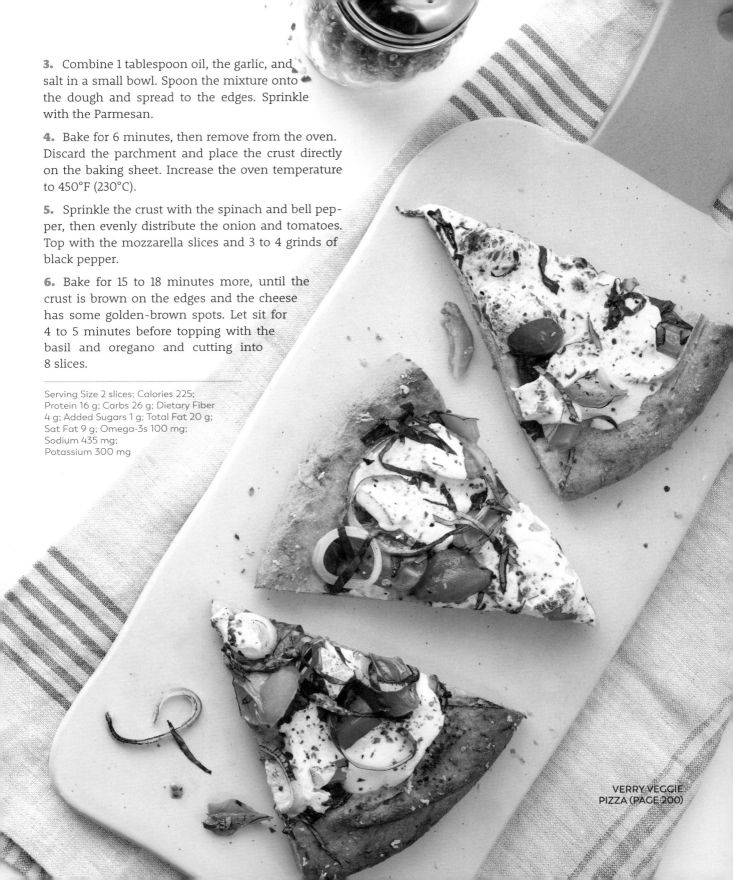

VERRY VEGGIE
PIZZA (PAGE 200)

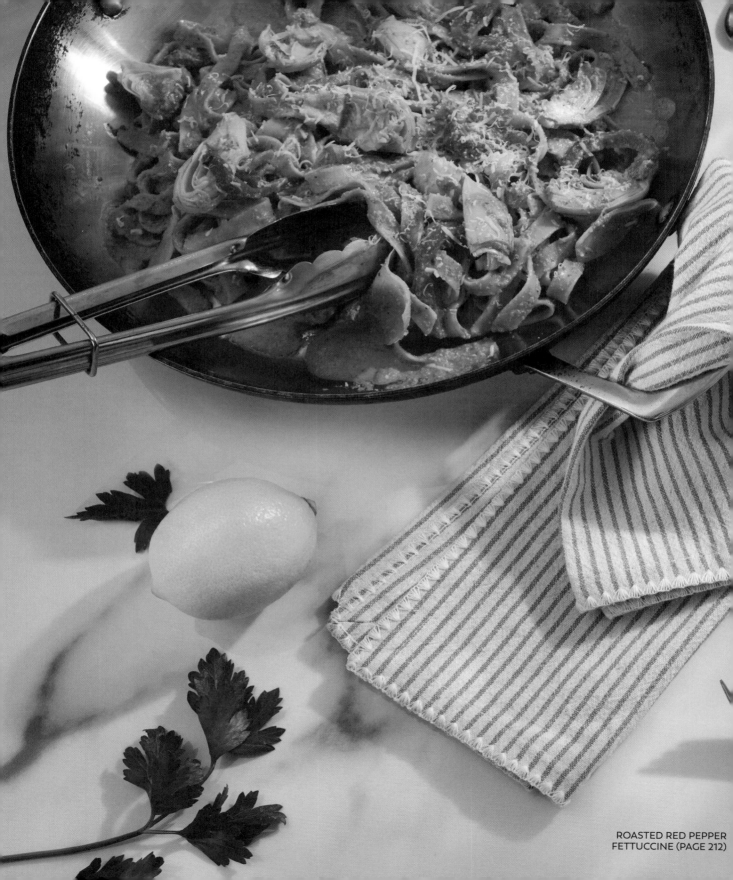

ROASTED RED PEPPER
FETTUCCINE (PAGE 212)

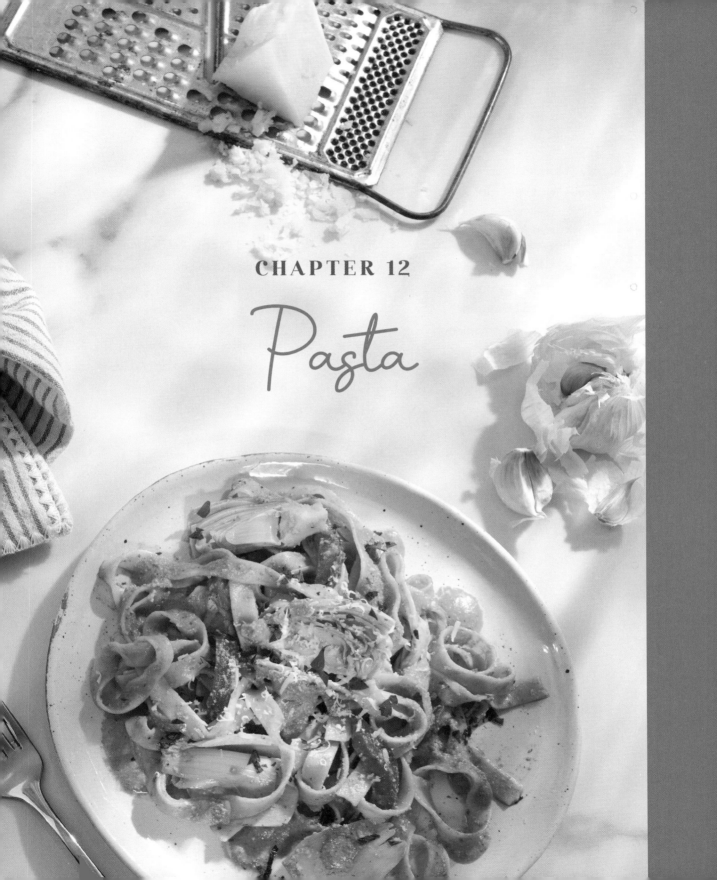

CHAPTER 12

Pasta

Pasta

Simply Steamed Couscous 205

Couscous with Vegetables &
Pine Nuts 206

À la Heart Mexican-Inspired
Mac & Cheese 206

Angel Hair with Tomatoes & Basil 207

Cheesy Mushroom Manicotti 207

Creamy Spinach Lasagna 208

Greek Orzo Salad with Spinach
& Tomatoes 209

Italian Pasta Salad 210

Orzo with Peas & Parmesan 210

Pasta Primavera 211

Penne with Spicy North African–Style
Carrot Sauce & Goat Cheese 211

Rice Noodles with Snow
Peas & Shrimp 212

Roasted Red Pepper Fettuccine 212

Roasted Vegetable Lasagna 213

Shrimp & Vegetable Pasta Bake 214

Singapore-Inspired
Chicken Rice Noodles 214

Spaghetti with Meat Sauce 215

Stir-Fried Vegetable & Farfalle Bowl . . . 216

Summer Vegetable Pasta Toss 217

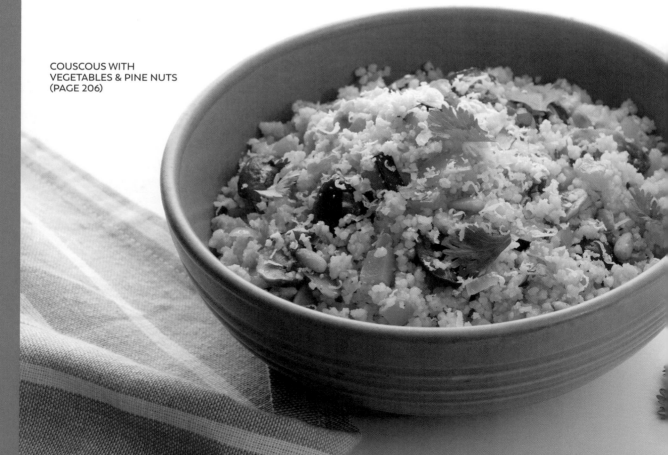

COUSCOUS WITH
VEGETABLES & PINE NUTS
(PAGE 206)

Pasta has a long history and a place in food cultures around the world, from Asia to the Mediterranean. While many may associate pasta with Italy, there are different kinds of noodles made with all types of grains in kitchens around the globe. From couscous in North Africa, wide egg noodles in Eastern Europe, the endless shapes of Italian pasta, Japanese buckwheat soba, dense and chewy Chinese lo mein noodles, and the delicate rice noodles of Southeast Asia, there are endless opportunities for exploring culinary tradition and creativity in pasta.

What exactly is pasta? The most classic versions are made with wheat flour (typically a higher protein content wheat like durum wheat) and liquid (sometimes egg and water), but many food cultures traditionally only make pasta with water. Home cooks in the Calabria region of Italy are known for making many shapes of pasta with just semolina (coarsely ground high-protein wheat flour) and water. Eggs were a very precious source of protein in Calabria, so instead of using them for their daily pasta, women saved the eggs for special occasions like family meals on Sundays or baking special treats for celebratory occasions.

While pasta has a long history, innovation continues today. Thanks to brilliant food scientists and consumer demand for gluten-free options, there are companies selling noodles of all shapes and sizes made with beans, lentils, and chickpeas. There's a pasta shape, size, and ingredient composition for every use, occasion, and dietary requirement.

One of the culinary blessings of pasta is its versatility. It can be eaten hot or cold, paired with endless sweet or savory ingredients, and, in most cases, reheated and enjoyed again the next day. For this chapter, we created recipes that use various types of pasta with an emphasis on whole grain wheat pastas. They are widely available, less expensive than newer alternatives, and perform as well as their refined counterparts in most recipes. One thing we discovered during recipe development is that whole grain pastas perform best when cooked al dente¸ and they often taste better when paired with umami-rich ingredients like mushrooms, onions, tomatoes, and lean beef as well as hard aged cheeses and sauces like soy sauce and miso. We hope you enjoy cooking and eating these pasta recipes!

SIMPLY STEAMED COUSCOUS
Makes 3 cups (470 g)

Couscous requires no cooking! It's a pasta sold as tiny grains in two varieties that differ in size. Israeli and Lebanese couscous grains are slightly smaller than a pea. Moroccan couscous is much smaller. Most couscous is made with refined flour; we recommend selecting a whole grain couscous to receive the fiber benefits.

2 cups (480 ml) water
1 cup (190 g) instant whole wheat couscous
¼ teaspoon kosher salt
1 tablespoon extra virgin olive oil

1. Bring the water to a boil in a medium saucepan. Add the couscous, stir, remove the pan from the heat, and cover. Allow to sit for 5 minutes, until the couscous has absorbed all the water. Add the salt, drizzle with the oil, and fluff with a fork.

2. To store, package ½- to 1-cup (80 to 155 g) portions in freezer bags. Press out as much air as you can, seal, label, and freeze for up to 6 months. Thaw in the refrigerator overnight or place in a bowl of warm water, massaging every few minutes to break up the grains.

Serving Size 1 cup (157 g); Calories 267; Protein 8 g; Carbs 45 g; Dietary Fiber 7 g; Added Sugars 0 g; Total Fat 6 g; Sat Fat 1 g; Omega-3s 30 mg; Sodium 74 mg; Potassium 0 mg

COUSCOUS WITH VEGETABLES & PINE NUTS

Makes 4 servings

This side dish comes together quickly, especially if you've already made Simply Steamed Couscous and use pre-cut vegetables. Serve with Lemon Chicken with Smoked Paprika (page 312) or rotisserie chicken for an easy worknight meal.

- 1 tablespoon extra virgin olive oil
- 1 orange bell pepper, seeded and diced
- 1 small onion or shallot, chopped
- 3 garlic cloves, chopped
- 1 zucchini, cubed
- 1 cup (70 g) sliced white or cremini mushrooms
- 3 cups (470 g) Simply Steamed Couscous (page 205)
- ½ cup (120 ml) Vegetable Broth (page 72) or dry white wine
- 1 tablespoon Italian Seasoning (page 34)
- ¼ cup (35 g) sliced pitted black olives
- ¼ cup (20 g) freshly grated Parmesan
- ¼ cup (35 g) toasted pine nuts
- ¼ cup (4 g) chopped fresh cilantro leaves
- Freshly ground black pepper

1. Heat the oil in a large skillet over medium-high heat until it shimmers, about 1 minute. Add the bell pepper, onion, and garlic. Cook, stirring constantly, until the vegetables glisten and start to soften, 3 minutes.

2. Stir in the zucchini and mushrooms. Reduce the heat to medium. Add the couscous, broth, and seasoning. Stir occasionally, scraping up all the bits from the bottom of the pan. Cook until the mixture is creamy and thick and the vegetables are fork-tender, 6 to 8 minutes.

3. Remove from the heat. Stir in the olives, Parmesan, and pine nuts. Transfer to a serving dish, top with cilantro, and serve hot.

Per Serving: Calories 360; Protein 11 g; Carbs 44 g; Dietary Fiber 7 g; Added Sugars 0 g; Total Fat 16 g; Sat Fat 3 g; Omega-3s 90 mg; Sodium 218 mg; Potassium 418 mg

À LA HEART MEXICAN-INSPIRED MAC & CHEESE

Makes 6 servings

If you love mac and cheese but you don't love all the saturated fat and sodium that can come with it, this is the recipe for you. We created a creamy sauce with milk, pureed sweet corn and beans, and a little cheese. We use whole grain pasta, and found many ways to incorporate vegetables, like our Simply Roasted Peppers, to contribute great flavor. The pièce de resistance is a crunchy mixture of tortilla chip crumbs, Cotija, and cilantro. Serve with our Habanero Chicken Wings (page 311) and your favorite Mexican beer.

- Cooking spray
- 1 teaspoon cumin seeds
- 2 tablespoon extra virgin olive oil
- 1 white onion, diced
- 2 jalapeño chiles, diced
- 8 ounces (227 g) whole wheat, lentil, or chickpea penne or rotini
- 2 cups (480 ml) milk
- One 15.5-ounce (439 g) can pinto beans, drained and rinsed
- 1 cup (165 g) frozen white corn kernels
- 2 poblano chiles from Simply Roasted Peppers (page 259)
- 8 ounces (227 g) Monterey Jack, shredded
- 2 Roma (plum) tomatoes, diced
- ½ cup (30 g) finely crushed tortilla chips or fresh whole wheat bread crumbs
- ¼ cup (30 g) grated Cotija or freshly grated Parmesan
- ½ cup (8 g) minced fresh cilantro leaves

1. Preheat the oven to 350°F (180°C). Spray a 9-inch (23 cm) square baking dish with cooking spray. Bring a large pot of water to a boil.

2. Heat a large sauté pan or skillet over medium-high heat for 30 seconds, then add the cumin. Dry-toast until the cumin is fragrant, about 30 seconds. Add the oil and onions, reduce the heat to medium, and cook until the onions are soft, 5 to 6 minutes. Add the jalapeños and cook until they start to soften and their green color brightens, 2 to 3 minutes. Remove from the heat.

3. Cook the pasta until al dente, according to package directions. Drain and transfer to a large bowl.

4. While the pasta is cooking, combine the milk, beans, corn, and poblanos in a blender. Blend until smooth. Transfer to a large saucepan over medium heat. Cook, stirring occasionally, until the mixture starts to bubble slightly, 5 to 6 minutes. Reduce the heat to low, add the Cotija, and stir to melt.

5. Add the sauce to the pasta. Stir in the tomatoes, then transfer to the baking dish. Combine the tortilla chips, Cotija, and cilantro in a small bowl. Stir well, then sprinkle over the top of the mac and cheese.

6. Bake for 30 minutes, until the top is bubbling and golden brown. Serve hot. Store covered in the refrigerator for up to 3 days. Leftovers are best reheated in the microwave.

Per Serving: Calories 451; Protein 23 g; Carbs 45 g; Dietary Fiber 4 g; Added Sugars 0 g; Total Fat 21 g; Sat Fat 10 g; Omega-3s 160 mg; Sodium 533 mg; Potassium 621 mg

ANGEL HAIR PASTA WITH TOMATOES & BASIL

Makes 4 servings

This simple summer meal comes together in minutes. It's ideal for the gardener who's overwhelmed by overzealous tomato and basil plants, and also perfect for those who have access to farmers' markets with peak summer produce. This pasta pairs beautifully with roast chicken or grilled shrimp.

- 8 ounces (227 g) angel hair pasta
- 2 cups (360 g) diced fresh tomatoes or halved cherry tomatoes
- 1 cup (25 g) loosely packed fresh basil leaves, cut into thin slices (see Tip, page 150)
- ¼ cup (60 ml) extra virgin olive oil
- 4 garlic cloves, finely minced
- 1 teaspoon salt

Cook the pasta until al dente, according to package directions. Drain, then toss with the tomatoes, basil, oil, garlic, and salt, and serve.

Per Serving: Calories 359; Protein 10 g; Carbs 46 g; Dietary Fiber 3 g; Added Sugars 0 g; Total Fat 15 g; Sat Fat 2 g; Omega-3s 120 mg; Sodium 239 mg; Potassium 324 mg

CHEESY MUSHROOM MANICOTTI

Makes 4 servings

The easiest way to stuff manicotti shells is to put the cheese filling in a plastic bag and snip off a corner. Gather the top of the bag. Hold an uncooked manicotti shell in one hand and with the other, squeeze the filling into the shell through the corner. You're a pro!

- 2 tablespoons extra virgin olive oil
- 8 ounces (227 g) portobello mushrooms, trimmed and coarsely chopped
- ½ cup (80 g) chopped onion
- 3 garlic cloves, minced
- 4 cups (1,270 g) Simply Cooked Fresh Tomato Sauce (page 59)
- ½ cup (30 g) chopped fresh parsley
- 3 tablespoons finely chopped fresh basil
- 2 tablespoons Italian Seasoning (page 34)
- ½ teaspoon freshly ground black pepper
- 1 cup (246 g) part-skim ricotta
- 2 cups (225 g) shredded part-skim mozzarella
- One 5- to 6-ounce (142 to 170 g) bag baby spinach (about 4 cups), torn into small pieces
- 2 large eggs
- ½ cup (40 g) freshly grated Parmesan
- One 8-ounce (227 g) package large whole wheat manicotti shells (12 to 14 shells)

1. Preheat the oven to 350°F (180°C). Line a 9 × 13-inch (23 × 33 cm) baking dish with foil and brush the bottom with 1 tablespoon of the oil.

2. Heat the remaining 1 tablespoon oil in a medium skillet over medium heat. Sauté the mushrooms, onion, and garlic until the mushrooms begin to shrink, the onions are translucent, and the garlic is fragrant, 3 minutes. Stir in 2 cups (635 g) of the tomato sauce, the parsley, 2 tablespoons of the basil, the seasoning, and pepper. Simmer until hot and well blended, 15 minutes.

3. Ladle 2 cups (480 ml) of the vegetable-tomato sauce into the baking dish and evenly distribute it over the bottom using the back of a spoon.

4. Combine the ricotta, 1 cup (113 g) of the mozzarella, the spinach, eggs, Parmesan, and the remaining 1 tablespoon basil in a large bowl. The mixture will be soft but thick. Fill a plastic bag with the filling and stuff the manicotti shells with it (see headnote). Arrange the manicotti in the baking pan; continue until all the shells are stuffed.

5. Spread any remaining cheese mixture and the remaining sauce around and over the top of the shells. Cover and bake for 30 minutes. Check for adequate liquid. The pasta will absorb most of the sauce, so if the pasta is very dry, add water in ½-cup (120 ml) increments.

6. Re-cover and bake for 30 minutes. The pasta is done when it's hot, bubbly, and steamy, and a digital food thermometer reads 165°F (75°C) when inserted in the center of the dish.

7. Top with the remaining 1 cup (113 g) mozzarella. Re-cover the pan and let rest for 10 minutes. Spoon any extra sauce from the pan over the manicotti when serving.

8. Store in an airtight container in the refrigerator for up to 4 days or in a freezer- and oven-safe airtight container in the freezer for up to 2 months. Reheat in the oven.

Serving Size 3 manicotti; Calories 675; Protein 39 g; Carbs 63 g; Dietary Fiber 9 g; Added Sugars 1 g; Total Fat 32 g; Sat Fat 13 g; Omega-3s 345 mg; Sodium 680 mg; Potassium 1,110 mg

CREAMY SPINACH LASAGNA

Makes 8 servings

This lasagna includes a rich tomato sauce made with fresh spinach and three types of cheese. It satisfies the hungriest of appetites. Serve with our Marinated Vegetable Salad (page 152) adding a tangy crunch to complement this creamy vegetarian entrée.

2 tablespoons extra virgin olive oil

1 white or yellow onion, chopped

2 garlic cloves, minced

Two 14.5-ounce (411 g) cans no-salt-added petite diced tomatoes

2 tablespoons Italian Seasoning (page 34)

1 teaspoon honey

Freshly cracked black pepper

One 9- to 10-ounce (255 to 283 g) bag baby spinach leaves (about 4 to 6 cups)

One 15-ounce (425 g) container reduced-fat ricotta

2 large eggs

9 ounces (255 g) no-boil whole wheat lasagna noodles (9 sheets)

2 cups (225 g) shredded part-skim mozzarella

1 cup (80 g) freshly grated Parmesan

1. Preheat the oven to 350°F (180°C). Line a 9 × 13-inch (23 × 33 cm) baking dish with foil.

2. Heat the oil in a medium skillet over medium heat. Sauté the onion until soft, about 4 minutes. Add the garlic and sauté until fragrant, 2 to 3 minutes. Stir in the tomatoes, seasoning, honey, and pepper. Reduce the heat and simmer, stirring occasionally, until well blended and bubbling hot, 20 minutes.

3. Add the spinach one handful at a time, stirring until wilted, 2 minutes.

4. Combine the ricotta with the eggs in a medium bowl, beating until smooth.

5. To assemble the lasagna, follow the chart on the next page. After layer 11, cover and bake the lasagna for 30 minutes.

6. Uncover, top with layers 12 and 13 of cheese, and return to the oven for 10 to 15 minutes, until the cheeses are melted and the lasagna is bubbling. Let rest

for 5 minutes before cutting into 8 pieces and serving hot. Store in an airtight container in the refrigerator for up to 5 days and reheat in the microwave, or store in an airtight freezer- and oven-safe container in the freezer for up to 2 months and reheat in the oven.

Per Serving: Calories 315; Protein 21 g; Carbs 20 g; Dietary Fiber 3 g; Added Sugars 1 g; Total Fat 17 g; Sat Fat 8 g; Omega-3s 100 mg; Sodium 486 mg; Potassium 215 mg

Creamy Spinach Lasagna Assembly Guide

LAYER	INGREDIENT
1	3 lasagna noodles
2	⅓ of the tomato sauce
3	½ of the ricotta-egg mixture
4	½ cup (55 g) mozzarella
5	3 lasagna noodles
6	⅓ of the tomato sauce
7	½ of the ricotta-egg mixture
8	½ cup (55 g) mozzarella
9	3 lasagna noodles
10	⅓ of the tomato sauce
11	½ cup (40 g) Parmesan
12	1 cup (115 g) mozzarella
13	½ cup (40 g) Parmesan

GREEK ORZO SALAD WITH SPINACH & TOMATOES

Makes 8 servings

This salad is so beautiful—the bright green of the spinach and vibrant red of the tomatoes provide appealing contrasts to the creamy color of the orzo. It's a great salad to have on hand for easy meals during a busy week. A bonus is that it travels well; it doesn't require refrigeration when going from home to work or on an outside adventure to a local park. Pair with roasted chicken, baked fish, or grilled shrimp.

1 cup (170 g) whole wheat or regular orzo

⅓ cup (80 ml) extra virgin olive oil

2 tablespoons red wine vinegar

1 tablespoon honey

1 teaspoon Dijon mustard

1 garlic clove, minced

1 teaspoon kosher salt

½ teaspoon freshly ground black pepper

½ teaspoon ground oregano

4 cups (120 g) fresh baby spinach leaves, chopped

2 cups (300 g) grape tomatoes, halved

4 ounces (113 g) finely crumbled feta

1. Prepare the orzo according to the package directions. Drain.

2. Whisk together the oil, vinegar, honey, mustard, garlic, salt, pepper, and oregano in a large bowl. Stir in the orzo to combine. Place in the refrigerator to cool.

3. Once the mixture has cooled, gently stir in the spinach, tomatoes, and feta. Cover, then refrigerate for 30 minutes to allow the flavors to blend before serving. Store in an airtight container in the refrigerator for up to 1 week.

TIP: Adding the warm orzo to the vinaigrette helps it absorb the flavors, but it's best to wait to add the spinach until the orzo cools down so the spinach doesn't wilt.

Per Serving: Calories 210; Protein 6 g; Carbs 18 g; Dietary Fiber 2 g; Added Sugars 2 g; Total Fat 13 g; Sat Fat 3 g; Omega-3s 100 mg; Sodium 305 mg; Potassium 125 mg

ITALIAN PASTA SALAD

Makes 10 servings

The next time you're asked to bring a dish to a family, church, school, book club, or community potluck, bring this. Nearly everyone loves familiar, comforting pasta salads that can be customized in endless ways. Craving some smoky flavor? Awesome! Use a smoked cheese like smoked Gouda in place of the mozzarella. Hate olives? Leave them out. You have our permission to make this salad your own.

- One 16-ounce (454 g) box whole wheat rotini or shells
- 1 cup (120 g) thinly sliced carrots (about 3 carrots)
- 2 zucchini, trimmed and thinly sliced
- Ice water
- 1 cup (80 g) diced red onion (1 large onion)
- One 6-ounce (170 g) jar marinated artichoke hearts, drained and quartered, 2 tablespoons marinade reserved
- 4 ounces (113 g) part skim mozzarella, cubed
- ½ cup (70 g) sliced pitted black olives
- ¼ cup (20 g) shredded Parmesan or pecorino
- ¼ cup (60 ml) extra virgin olive oil
- 2 tablespoons white wine vinegar or red wine vinegar
- 2 garlic cloves, minced
- 1½ teaspoons ground mustard
- 1 teaspoon dried basil
- 1 teaspoon dried oregano
- ½ cup (30 g) chopped fresh parsley or basil
- Juice of 1 lemon

1. Bring a large pot of water to a boil. Cook the pasta until al dente, about 10 minutes. Drain, reserving ¼ cup (60 ml) of the pasta water. Rinse the pasta under cold water. Drain, then transfer to a large bowl.

2. Place a steamer basket in a large saucepan with a lid. Steam the carrots for 15 minutes. Add the zucchini and steam for 5 to 10 minutes, until just crisp-tender. Chill the vegetables in ice water, then drain.

3. Add the zucchini, carrots, onion, artichokes, mozzarella, olives, and Parmesan to the pasta.

4. Whisk together the oil, reserved pasta water, reserved artichoke marinade, vinegar, garlic, mustard, basil, and oregano in a small bowl. Add to the pasta mixture and toss to combine.

5. Cover and chill for 1 hour or up to overnight. Just before serving, sprinkle with the parsley and lemon juice. Store in an airtight container in the refrigerator for up to 5 days.

Per Serving: Calories 189; Protein 6 g; Carbs 19 g; Dietary Fiber 3 g; Added Sugars 0 g; Total Fat 11 g; Sat Fat 3 g; Omega-3s 60 mg; Sodium 231 mg; Potassium 201 mg

ORZO WITH PEAS & PARMESAN

Makes 6 servings

Orzo is a wonderful ingredient to have in your pantry. It cooks quickly and can be used in so many ways. This orzo dish can be served either warm or cold, but we like it better chilled. Like most pasta dishes, the flavor gets better as the pasta absorbs the sauce and the flavors blend.

- 1 cup (170 g) whole wheat or regular orzo pasta
- 3.5 ounces (95 g) fresh sugar snap peas, strings removed, sliced diagonally into halves or thirds (1½ cups)
- ½ cup (40 g) grated Parmesan
- ¼ cup (6 g) chopped fresh mint
- 3 tablespoons pine nuts, toasted
- Grated zest of 1 lemon
- 2 tablespoons fresh lemon juice
- 2 tablespoons extra virgin olive oil
- 1 teaspoon white wine vinegar
- ½ teaspoon kosher salt
- ½ teaspoon freshly ground black pepper

1. Cook the orzo according to package directions, adding the snap peas to the cooking water about 7 minutes into cooking. Drain, rinse with cold water, and drain again.

2. Combine the Parmesan, mint, pine nuts, lemon zest and juice, oil, vinegar, salt, and pepper in a medium bowl. Add the orzo mixture, stirring to coat all ingredients. Serve immediately or cover and chill until you're ready to serve. Store in an airtight container in the refrigerator for up to 4 days.

Per Serving: Calories 184; Protein 7 g; Carbs 19 g; Dietary Fiber 2 g; Added Sugars 0 g; Total Fat 9 g; Sat Fat 2 g; Omega-3s 50 mg; Sodium 242 mg; Potassium 81 mg

PASTA PRIMAVERA

Makes 8 servings

This classic springtime pasta dish features a whole host of sautéed garden-fresh vegetables. A light basil sauce beautifully pairs the pasta with asparagus, cherry tomatoes, and spring peas. Serve the vegetables atop the pasta or tossed together, as we've done. Add a simple green salad and a hot crusty bread, such as our Whole Wheat French Baguettes (page 114).

- 8 ounces (227 g) whole wheat spaghetti, bucatini, or fettucine
- 3 tablespoons extra virgin olive oil
- 3 shallots, finely chopped
- 2 garlic cloves, minced
- 10 asparagus spears, trimmed and cut into 2-inch (5 cm) pieces
- 10 white mushrooms, thinly sliced (2½ cups/175 g)
- 1 orange bell pepper, seeded and diced
- 1 cup (150 g) cherry tomatoes, halved
- ¾ cup (180 ml) Vegetable Broth (page 72)
- 3 tablespoons finely chopped fresh basil
- ½ teaspoon kosher salt
- ¼ teaspoon white pepper
- 1 cup (130 g) frozen petite or baby peas, thawed
- ¼ cup (15 g) chopped fresh parsley
- ½ cup (40 g) freshly grated Parmesan

1. Cook the pasta until al dente, according to package directions. Drain the pasta and return to the pot. Drizzle in 1 tablespoon of the oil. Toss with a fork to coat the strands.

2. Heat the remaining 2 tablespoons oil in a wok or large skillet over medium heat. Add the shallots and garlic and stir constantly until the shallots are softened and the garlic is fragrant, about 1 minute.

3. Add the asparagus, mushrooms, and bell pepper. Stir constantly until the asparagus is bright green, the mushrooms begin to shrink, and the bell pepper softens, about 3 minutes.

4. Add the tomatoes, broth, 2 tablespoons of the basil, the salt, and white pepper. Simmer until the sauce is reduced slightly to concentrate the flavors,

about 3 minutes. Add the peas and stir until heated through, about 1 minute.

5. Add the pasta and toss to combine. Add the parsley, the remaining 1 tablespoon of basil, and the Parmesan. Toss again and serve. Store in an airtight container in the refrigerator for up to 4 days. Reheat in a saucepan over medium heat, adding broth if necessary.

Per Serving: Calories 151; Protein 6 g; Carbs 17 g; Dietary Fiber 3 g; Added Sugars 0 g; Total Fat 7 g; Sat Fat 2 g; Omega-3s 60 mg; Sodium 173 mg; Potassium 321 mg

PENNE WITH SPICY NORTH AFRICAN–STYLE CARROT SAUCE & GOAT CHEESE

Makes 4 servings

This is the perfect recipe to make if you've got extra Spicy North African–Style Carrot Dip in your refrigerator. The dip gets turned into a luscious pasta sauce with the simple addition of some pasta cooking water and a bit of mild, creamy goat cheese.

- 8 ounces (227 g) whole wheat or lentil penne pasta
- 1½ cups (375 g) Spicy North African–Style Carrot Dip (page 343)
- 5 ounces (142 g) soft goat cheese, broken into small pieces
- Chopped fresh flat-leaf parsley, optional

1. Cook the pasta until al dente, according to package directions. Drain, reserving ½ cup (120 ml) of the pasta cooking water.

2. While the pasta is cooking, gently warm the carrot dip in a large skillet over low heat. Stir in the pasta water, then add the pasta and toss to combine. Top with goat cheese, sprinkle on parsley, if desired, and serve.

Per Serving: Calories 421; Protein 14 g; Carbs 26 g; Dietary Fiber 5 g; Added Sugars 0 g; Total Fat 31 g; Sat Fat 10 g; Omega-3s 130 mg; Sodium 300 mg; Potassium 334 mg

RICE NOODLES WITH SNOW PEAS & SHRIMP

Makes 4 servings

This dish is perfect for an easy weeknight dinner—using precooked shrimp and quick-cooking rice noodles means you can get a light, bright, flavorful dinner on the table in about 15 minutes. We're confident this is a recipe you'll turn to frequently!

8 ounces (227 g) thin rice noodles

1 tablespoon reduced-sodium soy sauce

1 tablespoon white (shiro) miso

1 tablespoon toasted sesame oil

2 teaspoons rice vinegar

¼ teaspoon kosher salt

¼ teaspoon freshly ground black pepper

2 tablespoons peanut oil or extra virgin olive oil

2 green onions, chopped

2 tablespoons minced or grated fresh ginger

2 garlic cloves, minced

1 zucchini, halved lengthwise and sliced into half-moons

6 ounces (170 g) snow peas, ends trimmed, halved diagonally (about 3 cups)

1 pound (454 g) frozen cooked peeled 31/40 shrimp, thawed

¼ to ½ cup (60 to 120 ml) Shrimp Stock (page 71) or Fish Broth (page 71), optional

½ cup (8 g) chopped fresh cilantro or mint

½ cup (15 g) chopped fresh mint leaves

1. Bring a large stockpot of water to a boil. Cook the noodles according to package directions.

2. Meanwhile, stir together the soy sauce, miso, sesame oil, vinegar, salt, and pepper in a small bowl.

3. Heat the peanut oil in a large sauté pan or skillet over medium-high heat for 1 minute. Add the green onions, garlic, and ginger and stir-fry until they start to soften and the garlic and ginger are fragrant, 1 to 2 minutes. Add the zucchini and snow peas and stir-fry until the zucchini starts to soften and the peas are dark green, 3 to 4 minutes. Remove from the heat.

4. When the noodles have 2 minutes left to cook, return the vegetables to medium-high heat and add the shrimp and the soy sauce mixture. Cook until warmed through, 1 to 2 minutes.

5. Drain the noodles and toss with the shrimp-vegetable mixture. If you want a bit more sauce, add ¼ to ½ cup (60 to 120 ml) broth to the pan and heat for another minute or so. Toss again, then serve, garnishing with cilantro and mint.

NOTE: *Due to its fatty acid content, sesame oil easily goes rancid when stored at room temperature after opening. To maintain the freshness and quality of the oil, always store it in the refrigerator.*

Per Serving: Calories 435; Protein 34 g; Carbs 53 g; Dietary Fiber 3 g; Added Sugars 0 g; Total Fat 11 g; Sat Fat 2 g; Omega-3s 90 mg; Sodium 520 mg; Potassium 595 mg

ROASTED RED PEPPER FETTUCCINE

Makes 4 servings

Fettuccine, a type of pasta popular in Roman and Tuscan cuisines, is widely available in whole wheat varieties. We've taken this flat, thick pasta and added roasted red peppers, artichokes, and nutty pecorino. Simply delicious! Serve with a spring greens salad, crusty bread, and your favorite ale.

2 red bell peppers from Simply Roasted Peppers (page 259); cut into thin 2-inch-long (5 cm) strips

1 cup (90 g) sliced almonds, toasted

¼ cup (60 ml) extra virgin olive oil

2 tablespoons chopped fresh basil

2 garlic cloves, minced

1 tablespoon fresh lemon juice

1 tablespoon red wine vinegar

½ teaspoon cayenne

8 ounces (227 g) whole wheat fettuccine

One 9-ounce (255 g) jar water-packed artichoke hearts, drained and quartered

½ cup (40 g) freshly grated pecorino

¼ cup (15 g) chopped fresh parsley

1. Blend ½ cup (130 g) of the pepper strips with the almonds, oil, basil, garlic, lemon juice, vinegar, and cayenne in a food processor until smooth.

2. Cook the pasta until al dente, according to package directions. Drain, reserving ½ cup (120 ml) of the pasta water. Transfer the pasta to a large serving bowl. Add the pasta water, pepper mixture, artichokes, and the remaining red pepper strips. Toss to combine. Top with pecorino and sprinkle with parsley. Serve hot.

Per Serving: Calories 519; Protein 17 g; Carbs 49 g; Dietary Fiber 11 g; Added Sugars 0 g; Total Fat 30 g; Sat Fat 5 g; Omega-3s 140 mg; Sodium 221 mg; Potassium 512 mg

ROASTED VEGETABLE LASAGNA

Makes 8 servings

The sweet smokiness of the roasted vegetables balances the creamy ricotta-based sauce in this lasagna. Serve with a simple green salad and your favorite red wine. A Pinot Noir from Oregon's Willamette Valley or the Carneros region of the Napa Valley pairs beautifully with this dish.

- Cooking spray
- 6 tablespoons (90 ml) extra virgin olive oil
- 2 zucchini, trimmed and diced
- One eggplant, trimmed, peeled, and coarsely chopped
- 1 red bell pepper, seeded and diced
- 1 white onion, chopped
- 3 garlic cloves, minced
- 2 tablespoons thinly sliced fresh basil leaves (see Tip, page 150)
- One 15-ounce (425 g) container reduced-fat ricotta
- 2 large eggs
- 1 teaspoon ground marjoram
- 1 teaspoon ground thyme, or dried lemon thyme if available
- ⅓ cup (40 g) all-purpose flour
- 2½ cups (600 ml) milk
- One 9- to 10-ounce (255 to 283 g) bag baby spinach, coarsely chopped
- ½ cup (40 g) freshly grated Parmesan
- 9 ounces (255 g) no-boil whole wheat lasagna noodles (9 sheets)
- 8 ounces (227 g) shredded part-skim mozzarella

1. Preheat the oven to 350°F (180°C). Line a large, rimmed baking sheet with parchment paper. Line a 9 × 13-inch (23 × 33 cm) baking pan with foil; spray the foil with cooking spray.

2. Combine the zucchini, eggplant, bell pepper, onion, garlic, and basil with 3 tablespoons of the oil in a large bowl. Toss well, then spread the vegetables in a single layer on the baking sheet. Roast for 20 to 30 minutes, until the vegetables begin to soften and brown.

3. Mix the ricotta, eggs, marjoram, and thyme in a medium bowl.

4. Heat the remaining 3 tablespoons oil in a medium saucepan over medium-low heat. Whisk in the flour (it will be thick). Gradually add the milk, ½ cup (120 ml) at a time, whisking after each addition. Whisk constantly until the mixture begins to boil and thicken, about 5 minutes. Remove from the heat and add the chopped spinach a handful at a time. When incorporated, stir in the Parmesan.

5. Lay out half of the lasagna noodles in the baking pan. (If there are an odd number of noodles in the box, you can break one apart to use in each noodle layer.) Top with half of the ricotta mixture, half of the vegetable mixture, half of the mozzarella, and half of the spinach-cheese sauce. Layer on the remaining noodles, ricotta, and vegetable mixture. Spoon the remaining sauce over the vegetables. Cover and bake for 40 minutes.

6. Uncover the pan and top with the remaining mozzarella. Return to the oven and bake for another 5 minutes, until the lasagna is hot and bubbly. Let rest for 10 minutes, then cut into pieces and serve hot. Store in an airtight container in the refrigerator for up to 5 days and reheat in the microwave, or store in an airtight freezer- and oven-safe container in the freezer for up to 2 months and reheat in the oven.

Per Serving: Calories 404; Protein 22 g; Carbs 29 g; Dietary Fiber 5 g; Added Sugars 0 g; Total Fat 23 g; Sat Fat 8 g; Omega-3s 180 mg; Sodium 329 mg; Potassium 522 mg

Roasted Vegetable Lasagna Assembly Guide

LAYER	COMPONENT
1	½ of the noodles
2	½ of the ricotta mixture
3	½ of the vegetable mixture
4	½ of the spinach-cheese sauce
5	½ of the mozzarella
6	½ of the noodles
7	½ of the ricotta mixture
8	½ of the vegetable mixture
9	½ of the spinach-cheese sauce
10	½ of the mozzarella

SHRIMP & VEGETABLE PASTA BAKE

Makes 8 servings

Shrimp, peas, and mushrooms combine with a creamy sauce and whole wheat pasta to create a delicious baked pasta dish perfect for a casual family meal.

Cooking spray

16 ounces (454 g) whole wheat penne, shells, or rotini

¼ cup (60 ml) extra virgin olive oil

1 cup (70 g) sliced cremini mushrooms

½ cup (80 g) finely diced onion

1 tablespoon minced fresh oregano

1 tablespoon minced fresh thyme

1 teaspoon red pepper flakes

¼ cup (30 g) all-purpose flour

1½ cups (360 ml) reduced-fat milk

1 cup (135 g) frozen peas, thawed

½ cup (40 g) freshly grated Parmesan

½ teaspoon freshly ground black pepper

1 pound (454 g) frozen cooked, peeled, 31/40 shrimp, thawed

1 red bell pepper, seeded and diced

1. Preheat the oven to 350°F (180°C). Spray a 9 × 13-inch (23 × 33 cm) baking dish with cooking spray.

2. Cook the pasta in boiling water for 4 minutes, or half the amount of time on the package directions. Drain, reserving ½ cup (120 ml) of the pasta water. Rinse the pasta with cold water and drain again. Return to the pasta pot.

3. Heat the oil in a medium saucepan over medium heat. Add the mushrooms, onion, oregano, thyme, and red pepper flakes. Sauté until the onions are softened, translucent, and brown on the edges, 3 minutes. Add the flour, stirring constantly, until thickened, about 1 minute. Add 2 tablespoons of the reserved pasta water, if need be, to prevent browning. Carefully add the milk and stir until the mixture comes to a gentle boil and thickens, about 4 minutes. Stir in the peas, cheese, and black pepper. Cook for 1 minute, then remove from the heat.

4. Combine the shrimp, bell pepper, and cooked vegetables, and sauce with the pasta. Transfer to the baking dish. Cover and bake for 30 minutes. Uncover and bake for 15 minutes, until the pasta is hot and bubbling. Store in an airtight container in the refrigerator for up to 4 days and reheat in the microwave, or store in an airtight freezer- and oven-safe container in the freezer for up to 2 months and reheat in the oven.

Per Serving: Calories 268; Protein 15 g; Carbs 31 g; Dietary Fiber 4 g; Added Sugars 0 g; Total Fat 10 g; Sat Fat 2 g; Omega-3s 90 mg; Sodium 499 mg; Potassium 318 mg

SINGAPORE-INSPIRED CHICKEN RICE NOODLES

Makes 4 servings

Singaporean food culture includes many iconic dishes, and Chicken Rice is at the top of the list. More accurately called Hainanese Chicken Rice, the dish features gently poached sliced chicken breast atop rice fortified with chicken fat and accompanied by a spicy red chile sauce. Other accompaniments are determined by the chef's interpretation. This playful adaptation includes an intense ginger-garlic sauce, and rice noodles instead of rice.

Chile Sauce

4 ounces (113 g) red Fresno chiles, diced

1.5 ounces (43 g) orange habanero or Scotch bonnet chiles, diced

¼ cup (60 ml) water

2 tablespoons extra virgin olive oil

1 teaspoon white vinegar

½ teaspoon kosher salt

Ginger-Garlic Sauce

4 ounces (113 g) peeled fresh ginger, cut into large chunks

¼ cup (30 g) roughly chopped peeled garlic

2 tablespoons extra virgin olive oil

Chicken

1 pound (454 g) chicken tenders

3 cups (720 ml) Chicken Stock (page 70)

1 ounce (28 g) fresh ginger, thinly sliced

Noodles

8 ounces (227 g) stir-fry rice noodles

To Serve

2 ripe red tomatoes, quartered

1 English cucumber, thinly sliced

1 green onion, thinly sliced diagonally

Fresh cilantro leaves, chopped

1. To make the chile sauce, combine the Fresno chiles, habaneros, water, oil, vinegar, and salt in a small saucepan over medium-low heat. Cover and cook, stirring occasionally, until the chiles soften, 25 to 30 minutes. Set aside.

2. To make the ginger-garlic sauce, combine the ginger, garlic, and oil in a food processor. Process to create a thick paste. Transfer to a small saucepan over low heat and cook until warmed but not browned, stirring occasionally, 10 to 12 minutes. Set aside.

3. To make the chicken, combine the chicken, stock, and ginger in a large sauté pan or saucepan. Bring to a boil, then reduce the heat to low, cover, and simmer for 8 to 10 minutes, until a digital food thermometer reads 165°F (75°C) when inserted in the thickest part of a tender. Transfer the chicken to a cutting board and thinly slice.

4. Remove and discard the ginger slices, then bring the stock to a boil over high heat. Add the noodles, reduce the heat to medium, and simmer until the noodles are tender but still firm, 4 to 6 minutes.

5. Evenly divide the noodles and any remaining broth among four shallow bowls. Top with chicken and garnish with tomatoes, cucumber, green onions, and cilantro. Serve with the sauces on the side.

TIP: Stir-fry rice noodles are wider and thicker than thin rice noodles. If you can't find stir-fry rice noodles, feel free to use thin rice noodles. You won't need to cook them; they can simply be soaked in the warm chicken stock for 4 to 5 minutes. They'll have the same flavor, but they won't stand up to the sauces quite as well as thicker noodles.

Per Serving: Calories 611; Protein 25 g; Carbs 51 g; Dietary Fiber 4 g; Added Sugars 0 g; Total Fat 34 g; Sat Fat 5 g; Omega-3s 920 mg; Sodium 1,048 mg; Potassium 898 mg

SPAGHETTI WITH MEAT SAUCE

Makes 6 servings

To elevate the flavor and reduce the amount of sodium in this familiar family favorite, we encourage you to use Simply Cooked Fresh Tomato Sauce. Sprinkle your plated spaghetti with our Garlic & Herb Bread Crumbs for an added burst of flavor and crunch.

2 tablespoons extra virgin olive oil

1 cup (70 g) sliced white or cremini mushrooms

½ cup (80 g) diced onion

3 garlic cloves, chopped

½ teaspoon red pepper flakes

1 pound (454 g) 93% lean ground beef

2 cups (360 g) chopped fresh tomatoes (about 2 large tomatoes)

2 cups (635 g) Simply Cooked Fresh Tomato Sauce (page 59)

¼ cup (15 g) chopped fresh parsley

1 tablespoon Italian Seasoning (page 34)

1 bay leaf

1 teaspoon freshly ground black pepper

12 ounces (340 g) whole wheat spaghetti

1 cup (220 g) Garlic & Herb Bread Crumbs (page 33)

Freshly grated Parmesan

1. Heat the oil in a large skillet or Dutch oven over medium-high heat. Sauté the mushrooms, onion, garlic, and red pepper flakes until the mushrooms and onions have softened a bit and the garlic is fragrant, 4 to 5 minutes. Add the beef and cook, stirring occasionally to break up the beef, until lightly browned, about 6 minutes.

2. Add the tomatoes, tomato sauce, parsley, seasoning, bay leaf, and pepper. Bring to a boil, then reduce the heat to medium-low, and cover. Simmer about 30 minutes, until the sauce has thickened.

3. While the sauce is cooking, cook the pasta in boiling water according to package directions. Drain the pasta and divide among serving bowls. Serve the sauce over the pasta, dust with the bread crumbs, and sprinkle with Parmesan. Serve hot. Store pasta and sauce in separate airtight containers in the refrigerator for up to 4 days. To reheat, plate the spaghetti on a microwave-safe plate, top with sauce, cover, and microwave in 30-second increments on HIGH until hot.

Per Serving: Calories 423; Protein 26 g; Carbs 42 g; Dietary Fiber 7 g; Added Sugars 0 g; Total Fat 18 g; Sat Fat 4 g; Omega-3s 150 mg; Sodium 245 mg; Potassium 829 mg

STIR-FRIED VEGETABLE & FARFALLE BOWL

Makes 6 servings

The vegetables in this delicious bowl are coated with balsamic vinegar instead of soy sauce, eliminating a great deal of sodium without sacrificing flavor. This bowl is so versatile—you can add tofu cubes, shrimp, or leftover chicken or steak. There's no wrong way to customize your bowl, so make it to fit your preferences!

1 tablespoon extra virgin olive oil

4 green onions, sliced

3 garlic cloves, minced

1 tablespoon minced fresh ginger

¼ teaspoon red pepper flakes

One 12- to 14-ounce (340 to 397 g) bag fresh or frozen stir-fry vegetable blend (carrots, broccoli, and snow peas; about 4½ cups)

¼ cup (60 ml) balsamic vinegar

8 ounces (227 g) whole wheat farfalle, cooked, drained, and cooled

2 tablespoons toasted sesame oil

½ cup (8 g) chopped fresh cilantro leaves and stems

2 tablespoons toasted sesame seeds

Juice of 1 lime

1. Heat the olive oil in a large skillet over medium heat. Sauté the green onions, garlic, ginger, and red pepper flakes until the onions start to soften, 2 to 3 minutes. Add the vegetables, stirring continuously to thaw (if frozen) and blacken in spots, about 4 minutes.

2. Add the vinegar and pasta and cook until the pasta is hot and coated with the sauce, 3 minutes. Remove from the heat, add the sesame oil and cilantro, and toss to combine.

3. Divide among six bowls. Top with sesame seeds and a squeeze of lime juice.

Per Serving: Calories 207; Protein 4 g; Carbs 20 g; Dietary Fiber 3 g; Added Sugars 0 g; Total Fat 13 g; Sat Fat 1 g; Omega-3s 50 mg; Sodium 187 mg; Potassium 232 mg

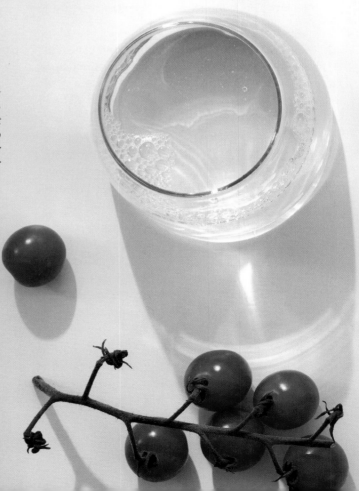

SUMMER VEGETABLE PASTA TOSS

Makes 6 servings

This vegetable-pasta dish is like our classic Pasta Prima-vera (page 211), but served cold. Both dishes are chock-full of vegetables and paired with long pasta, but this is sure to satisfy on a muggy summer evening. We think you'll be pleased with the results of pairing zoodles (zucchini spirals) and linguine, enlivened by fresh basil and parsley.

- 3 tablespoons extra virgin olive oil
- 8 ounces (227 g) sliced cremini mushrooms
- 2 garlic cloves, minced
- 10 ounces (283 g) cherry tomatoes, halved
- 8 ounces (227 g) linguine, cooked, drained, and cooled
- 2 cups (220 g) spiral-cut zucchini (aka zoodles)
- ½ cup (40 g) freshly grated Parmesan
- ¼ cup (6 g) chopped fresh basil
- ¼ cup (15 g) chopped fresh parsley
- ¼ cup (35 g) pine nuts, toasted
- ½ teaspoon kosher salt
- ½ teaspoon freshly ground black pepper

1. Heat 1 tablespoon of the oil in a large sauté pan or skillet over medium heat. Sauté the mushrooms and garlic until the mushrooms begin to brown and the garlic is fragrant, 6 minutes. Add the tomatoes and sauté until they start to release their juices, 1 to 2 minutes.

2. Transfer the vegetable mixture to a large bowl. Add the linguine and toss gently to coat. Add the zucchini, Parmesan, basil, parsley, pine nuts, salt, and pepper. Toss to combine; drizzle with the remaining 2 tablespoons oil and serve immediately.

Per Serving: Calories 215; Protein 6 g; Carbs 16 g; Dietary Fiber 2 g; Added Sugars 0 g; Total Fat 15 g; Sat Fat 3 g; Omega-3s 80 mg; Sodium 207 mg; Potassium 430 mg

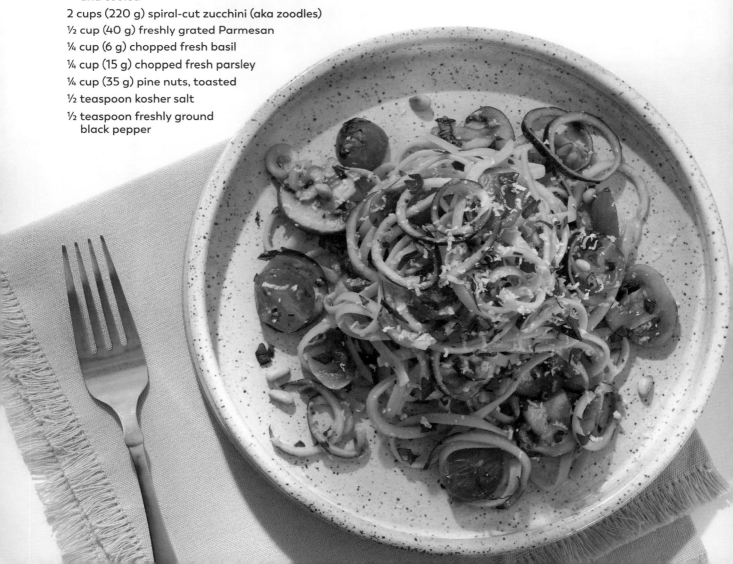

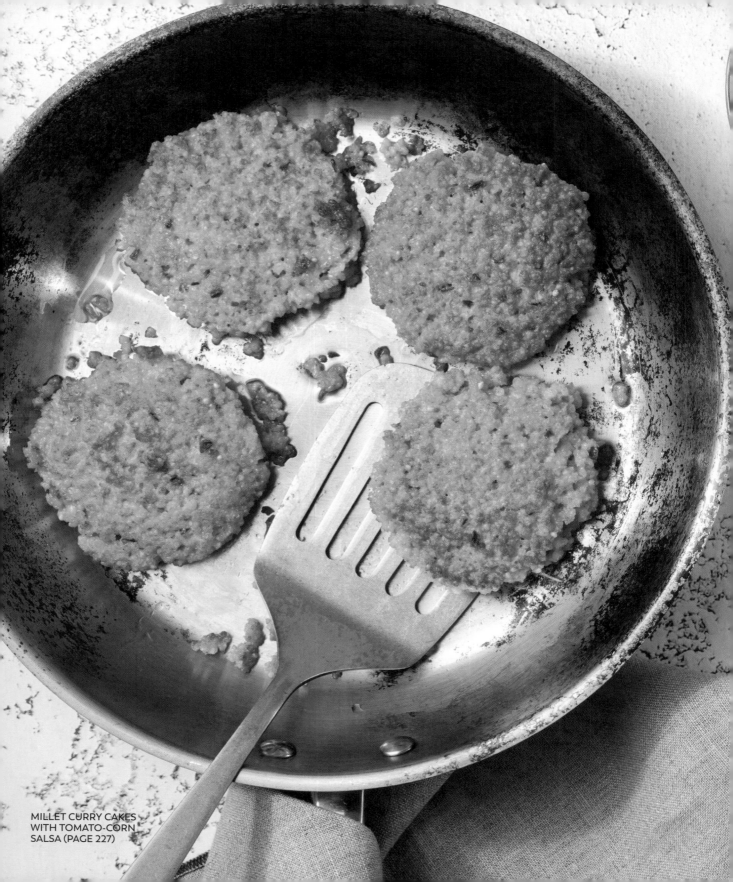

MILLET CURRY CAKES
WITH TOMATO-CORN
SALSA (PAGE 227)

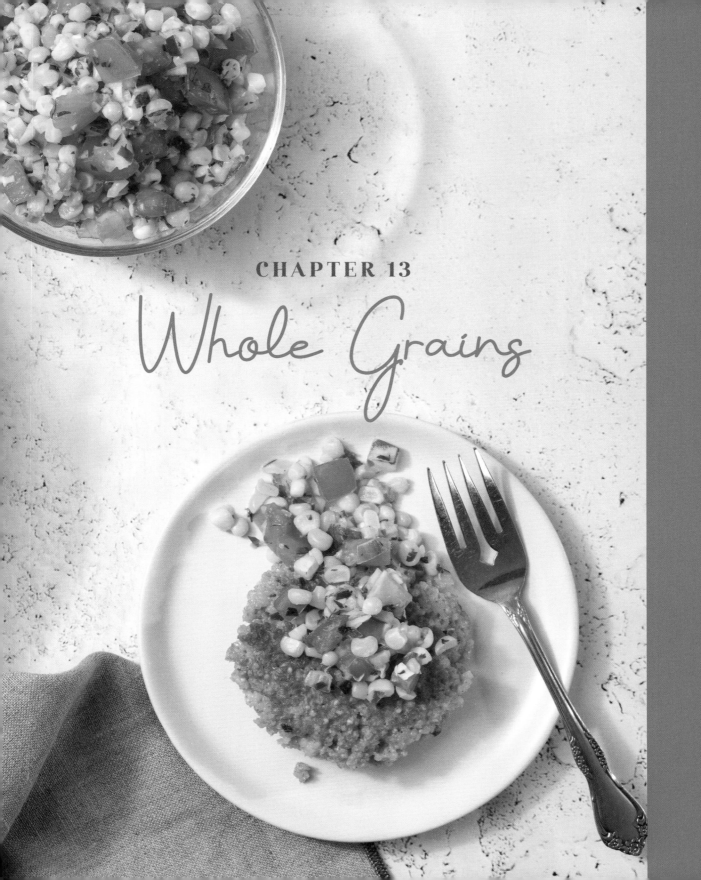

CHAPTER 13

Whole Grains

Whole Grains

Cooking Whole Grains 221

Barley
Simply Cooked Barley 223
Roasted Mushroom–Barley Pilaf 223

Bulgur
Simply Cooked Bulgur 224
Bulgur Sauté with Pomegranate &
Pistachios 224
Bulgur & Tomato Salad with Mint 224
Tabbouleh 225
Turkish-Inspired Bulgur–Sweet
Potato Patties 225

Farro
Simply Cooked Farro 226
Farro with Roasted Grapes 226

Millet
Simply Cooked Millet 227
Millet Curry Cakes with
Tomato-Corn Salsa 227

Quinoa
Simply Cooked Quinoa 228
Quinoa & Black Bean Medley 228

Sorghum
Simply Cooked Sorghum 229
Savory Sorghum Porridge 229

Rice
Simply Cooked Brown Rice 230
Brown Rice with Pine Nuts &
Roasted Butternut Squash 230
Mediterranean Rice Bake with
Eggplant & Tomatoes 231
Mock Risotto with Zucchini 231
Persian-Inspired Rice Pilaf with
Cherries & Pistachios 232
Tofu Fried Rice 232
Vegetable-Almond Rice
with Parmesan 233
Vegetable Fried Rice 233

Wild Rice
Simply Cooked Wild Rice 234
Wild Rice with Mushrooms,
Tarragon & Pine Nuts 234
Wild Rice with Sausage & Sage 235

Whole grains are yet another category of nutrient-rich, health-promoting foods that offer adventurous cooks endless inspiration. They all provide a bit more beneficial fiber than their processed counterparts, and they can also offer more interesting flavors and textures. Many people refer to the nuttier flavor and chewier texture of whole grains, which we love. We also love how well these ingredients stand up in mixed dishes; they don't get lost among other ingredients. You know they're there by their flavor, texture, and appearance.

As we developed recipes for this chapter, we loved finding great flavor pairings, determining which ingredients—fruits, vegetables, legumes, and herbs—can turn a humble grain into an extraordinary dish. Whole grains themselves are so versatile, and so we've also included them in many other chapters in various forms, including whole grain flours for baking.

There are so many types of cereals, grasses, grains, and rice that the Whole Grains Council (a nonprofit consumer advocacy group working to increase consumption of whole grains for better health) considers whole grains—from amaranth and corn to millet, sorghum, and wild rice. It may even surprise you that foods like oatmeal and popcorn are considered whole grains. We chose to mostly feature better-known options that are versatile in their use and widely available at most supermarkets, like barley, quinoa, brown rice, and wild rice. We also included a few lesser-known options, like farro and sorghum, to help expand your repertoire. Doing the research and recipe development for this book prompted Amy to try millet for the first time; it's now a staple in her kitchen! As a Minnesota native, Linda has great access to and loves cooking with wild rice. You'll see many of her wild rice recipes in this chapter as well as in the Entrée Salads chapter.

If you can't find these whole grains at your local market, you can buy them from online sources. No matter where or how you shop, we encourage you to keep them on hand, to use our Simply Cooked recipes often, and to keep precooked whole grains in your freezer to make it quicker and easier to assemble the healthful, delicious recipes featured in this chapter.

Cooking Whole Grains

While there are many newer appliances you can use to cook whole grains, we chose to focus on stovetop cooking, because nearly everyone has a stove and a pot with a lid. With that said, if you prefer the convenience of a rice cooker, Instant Pot, or other appliance, refer to the owner's manual for best practices for various whole grains.

Other Cooking Methods for Rice

Most whole grains typically come in one form, which makes stovetop cooking instructions easier to provide. But rice comes in so many forms. For example, cooking Arborio rice to make risotto is very different from cooking long-grain rice. Here is guidance for cooking various types of rice using other common kitchen equipment.

- Oven: Cooking rice in the oven when other foods are baking is an efficient use of energy. Carefully combine the rice and boiling liquid in a baking dish. Stir, cover tightly, and bake at 350°F (180°C) for 25 to 30 minutes for long-grain white rice, 30 to 40 minutes for parboiled rice, and 1 hour for whole grain brown rice. Remove from the oven, fluff with fork, and serve.

- Microwave: Combine the rice and liquid (see Table 7 on page 222) in a deep 2½- to 3-quart (2.5 to 3 L) microwave-safe baking dish and cover tightly. For medium- or long-grain rice, microwave on HIGH (100% power) for 5 minutes or until boiling; reduce to MEDIUM (50% power) and microwave for 15 minutes (20 minutes for whole grain brown rice or parboiled brown rice; 30 minutes for wild rice) or until the water is absorbed. Let stand for 5 minutes before fluffing with a fork and serving.

- Rice Cooker: Follow the manufacturer's instructions for your rice cooker. Combine all of the ingredients in the rice cooker. Turn on the rice cooker; it will stop cooking automatically by sensing a rise in temperature and change in moisture content that occurs when the rice has absorbed the liquid and is fully cooked. For the proportion of rice to liquid, follow the guidelines in Table 7 below.

Table 7: Grain Cook Times & Yields

GRAIN (1 CUP UNCOOKED)	LIQUID	STOVETOP COOK TIME	COOKED YIELD
Barley, pearl (200 g)	3 cups (720 ml)	50 minutes	3½ cups (550 g)
Buckwheat groats, aka kasha (165 g)	2 cups (480 ml)	15 minutes	3½ cups (590 g)
Bulgur, aka cracked wheat (140 g)	2 cups (480 ml)	20 minutes	3 cups (545 g)
Farro* (180 g)	4 cups (960 ml)	25–30 minutes	2½ cups (490 g)
Couscous, quick-cooking (190 g)	2 cups (480 ml)	5 minutes	3 cups (470 g)
Oats, rolled, quick-cooking (90 g)	2 cups (480 ml)	1–5 minutes	2 cups (470 g)
Millet (180 g)	2 cups (480 ml)	20–25 minutes	4 cups (450 g)
Quinoa (190 g)	2 cups (480 ml)	20–25 minutes	3 cups (555 g)
Sorghum* (200 g)	6 cups (1.4 L)	55–65 minutes	2½ cups (500 g)
Arborio, aka risotto (180 g)	1½ cups (360 ml)	20 minutes	3 cups (615 g)
Basmati (200 g)	2 cups (480 ml)	40 minutes soak and cook	3 cups (475 g)
Brown, whole-grain (190 g)	1¼ cups (300 ml)	40–45 minutes	3 to 4 cups (585 to 780 g)
Brown, parboiled (190 g)	2¼ cups (530 ml)	30 minutes	3 to 4 cups (465 to 620 g)
White, parboiled/precooked instant (95 g)	1 cup (240 ml)	5 minutes	2 cups (330 g)
White, long-grain (185 g)	2 cups (480 g)	15 minutes	3 to 4 cups (475 to 630 g)
White, medium-grain (195 g)	2 cups (480 g)	15 minutes	3 cups (560 g)
White, short-grain (200 g)	1¼ cups (300 g)	15 minutes	3 cups (560 g)
Wild,* whole grain (160 g)	3 cups (720 g)	50–60 minutes	3 to 4 cups (490 to 655 g)

*Farro, sorghum, and wild rice must be washed thoroughly before cooking.

SIMPLY COOKED BARLEY

Makes 3½ cups (550 g)

Barley is a grain that is sold in hulled or pearl varieties. Hulled barley has had the outer husk of the grain removed, leaving the rest of the grain intact. This makes it a great whole grain choice, although it does take longer to cook than pearl barley. Pearl barley undergoes further processing, including polishing, which gives it a lighter color. It's not considered a whole grain; it cooks more quickly and has a more tender texture than hulled barley. But both are great choices due to their soluble fiber content.

- 3 cups (720 ml) water
- 1 cup (185 g) hulled or pearl barley
- ⅛ teaspoon kosher salt
- 1 tablespoon extra virgin olive oil

1. Bring the water and barley to a boil in a medium saucepan. Reduce the heat to low, cover, and simmer until the barley is tender and chewy but not mushy, 35 to 50 minutes.

2. Add the salt and drizzle with oil. Fluff with a fork. Prepared barley keeps in an airtight container in the refrigerator for up to 5 days.

3. To store, package ½- to 1-cup (80 to 160 g) portions in freezer bags. Press out as much air as you can, seal, label, and freeze for up to 6 months. Thaw in the refrigerator overnight, or place in a bowl of warm water, massaging every few minutes to break up the kernels.

Serving Size 1 cup (157 g); Calories 233; Protein 7 g; Carbs 39 g; Dietary Fiber 9 g; Added Sugars 0 g; Total Fat 5 g; Sat Fat 1 g; Omega-3s 90 mg; Sodium 33 mg; Potassium 239 mg

ROASTED MUSHROOM–BARLEY PILAF

Makes 4 servings

We recommend using hulled barley for this recipe—it's dense, chewy texture pairs well with the mushrooms. This pilaf is a great side dish to pair with roast chicken or turkey.

- 1 pound (454 g) cremini mushrooms
- 2 tablespoons extra virgin olive oil
- 2 tablespoons chopped fresh thyme
- 2 garlic cloves, minced
- ¼ teaspoon freshly ground black pepper
- One 5- to 6-ounce (142 to 170 g) bag baby spinach leaves (about 4 cups)
- 2 tablespoons balsamic vinegar
- 2 cups (315 g) Simply Cooked Barley (page 223)
- ½ cup (120 ml) Vegetable Broth (page 72), plus more if needed
- ¼ cup (35 g) pine nuts, toasted

1. Adjust an oven rack to the middle position. Preheat the oven to 400°F (200°C). Line a large baking sheet with parchment paper.

2. Place the mushrooms in a large bowl. Add the oil, thyme, garlic, and pepper. Using your hands, massage the mushrooms until well coated. Transfer to the baking sheet; roast for 10 minutes, until the mushrooms start to soften and release some moisture.

3. Add half of the spinach to the baking sheet and roast for 5 minutes or until the spinach has wilted. Remove from the oven and gently stir with a wooden spoon. Add the remaining spinach and roast for 3 to 5 minutes more, until the mushrooms are browned, all the spinach is wilted, and the liquid is mostly evaporated.

4. While the mushrooms are roasting, prepare the barley. Place the barley in a large, deep skillet. Stir in the broth and turn the heat to medium-low. Cover and cook, stirring occasionally, until the barley is heated, 10 minutes. Add more broth if the barley gets too dry.

5. Add the roasted mushrooms and spinach to the skillet. Mix well and heat thoroughly to allow the flavors to blend, 4 to 5 minutes. Top with pine nuts and serve.

Per Serving: Calories 475; Protein 13 g; Carbs 62 g; Dietary Fiber 14 g; Added Sugars 0 g; Total Fat 20 g; Sat Fat 3 g; Omega-3s 170 mg; Sodium 85 mg; Potassium 875 mg

SIMPLY COOKED BULGUR

Makes 3 cups (550 g)

Bulgur is an affordable quick-cooking whole grain made from wheat. Use it as a savory base in a whole grain bowl, topped with roasted vegetables, a creamy, flavorful pesto or aïoli, and a few nuts or seeds. Bulgur also makes a great grain for breakfast bowls. Try our Bulgur Breakfast Porridge with Sausage (page 120).

2 cups (480 ml) water
1 cup (140 g) coarse bulgur
1 tablespoon extra virgin olive oil
⅛ teaspoon kosher salt

1. Combine the water and bulgur in a medium saucepan and bring to a boil. Reduce the heat to low, cover, and simmer until the bulgur is tender, about 12 minutes.

2. Drain off any excess liquid, cover, and allow to steam for 5 minutes. Add the oil and salt then and with a fork. Use immediately or spread on a rimmed baking sheet to cool.

3. To store, package in ½- to 1-cup (90 to 180 g) portions in freezer bags. Press out as much air as you can, seal, label, and freeze for up to 4 months. Thaw in the refrigerator overnight or place in a bowl of warm water, massaging every few minutes to break up the grains.

Serving Size 1 cup (183 g); Calories 202; Protein 6 g; Carbs 35 g; Dietary Fiber 6 g; Added Sugars 0 g; Total Fat 5 g; Sat Fat 1 g; Omega-3s 40 mg; Sodium 45 mg; Potassium 191 mg

BULGUR SAUTÉ WITH POMEGRANATE & PISTACHIOS

Makes 4 servings

Pomegranate seeds (arils) are bursting with a sweet-tart flavor and lots of bold color. They offer a lovely pop of flavor and an interesting texture in this dish, which can be eaten as a side or used as a filling for pita pockets with Greek yogurt, pesto, and a few mixed greens.

1 tablespoon extra virgin olive oil
1 cup (160 g) finely chopped onion
    (about 1 medium onion)

2 garlic cloves, minced
1 tablespoon chopped fresh oregano
1 pint (300 g) cherry tomatoes, halved
2 cups (365 g) Simply Cooked Bulgur
    (page 224)
1 cup (175 g) pomegranate arils
½ cup (60 g) unsalted roasted pistachios

1. Heat a large skillet over medium-high heat. Add the oil and heat for 20 seconds, then add the onions and sauté until the onions are translucent and very lightly brown on the edges, about 5 minutes.

2. Reduce the heat to medium. Stir in the garlic and cook until it starts to soften, 1 minute. Stir in the oregano and tomatoes and cook until warm, about 2 minutes. Stir in the bulgur, reduce the heat to medium-low, cover, and cook until hot, stirring occasionally, for 5 minutes. Gently stir in the pomegranate arils and pistachios and serve.

TIP: Create an inviting Mediterranean mezze platter by placing a bowl of the bulgur sauté in the center of a large wooden board, surrounded with warm pita pockets and separate smaller bowls of kalamata olives, green onions, Greek yogurt, Tabbouleh (page 225), and Classic Hummus (page 245). Add pistachios and small clusters of grapes to complete the platter.

Per Serving: Calories 273; Protein 8 g; Carbs 35 g; Dietary Fiber 7 g; Added Sugars 0 g; Total Fat 13 g; Sat Fat 2 g; Omega-3s 80 mg; Sodium 27 mg; Potassium 584 mg

BULGUR & TOMATO SALAD WITH MINT

Makes 4 servings

This contemporary take on a classic Middle Eastern salad is so simple to prepare. It's an ideal salad to make at the start of the week and use as a base for other meals throughout the week, as the flavors continue to improve as it sits in the fridge. It's great served with fresh pita bread and Classic Hummus (page 245). We also feature it in our Bulgur-Tomato Salad with Tuna & Mint (page 160).

3 cups (550 g) Simply Cooked Bulgur
    (page 224)
⅔ cup (150 g) plain Greek yogurt
½ cup (40 g) thinly sliced green onions

4 tablespoon (6 g) chopped fresh mint leaves

¼ cup (15 g) finely chopped fresh parsley

1 tablespoon grated lemon zest

2 tablespoons fresh lemon juice

1 tablespoon white or red wine vinegar

1 teaspoon Dijon mustard

1 tomato, diced

¾ cup (100 g) diced cucumber or zucchini

2 cups (70 g) mixed salad greens

1. Combine the bulgur, yogurt, onions, 3 tablespoons of the mint, the parsley, lemon zest, lemon juice, vinegar, and mustard in a large bowl. Add the tomato and cucumber. Toss, cover, and chill for at least 1 hour.

2. Just before serving, toss again. Serve on a bed of mixed greens, with the remaining tablespoon mint sprinkled over the top.

Per Serving: Calories 182; Protein 9 g; Carbs 29 g; Dietary Fiber 5 g; Added Sugars 0 g; Total Fat 4 g; Sat Fat 1 g; Omega-3s 50 mg; Sodium 86 mg; Potassium 403 mg

TABBOULEH

Makes 6 servings

This simple salad of vegetables, parsley, mint, and bulgur is a classic Eastern Mediterranean dish. Contrary to what many think, bulgur is not the star in tabbouleh—the parsley is. Be sure to use fresh lemon juice, not bottled, for the best flavor when you make this recipe.

3 cups (550 g) Simply Cooked Bulgur (page 225)

¾ cup (45 g) finely chopped fresh parsley

1 green onion, thinly sliced

¼ cup (6 g) finely chopped fresh mint

1 tablespoon finely chopped fresh oregano

¼ cup plus 2 tablespoons (90 ml) fresh lemon juice

¼ cup plus 2 tablespoons (90 ml) extra virgin olive oil

¼ teaspoon kosher salt

Freshly cracked black pepper

¾ cup (100 g) finely chopped English cucumber

2 Roma (plum) tomatoes, finely chopped, excess water drained

2 cups (70 g) chopped romaine lettuce

Plain Greek yogurt, optional

1. Combine the bulgur, parsley, onion, mint, and oregano in a large bowl. Add the lemon juice, oil, salt, and pepper, and mix well. Refrigerate for 2 to 4 hours, until fully chilled.

2. Just before serving, stir in the cucumber and tomatoes. Serve over romaine and top with a dollop of yogurt, if desired.

Per Serving: Calories 232; Protein 4 g; Carbs 19 g; Dietary Fiber 4 g; Added Sugars 0 g; Total Fat 17 g; Sat Fat 2 g; Omega-3s 140 mg; Sodium 58 mg; Potassium 293 mg

TURKISH-INSPIRED BULGUR– SWEET POTATO PATTIES

Makes 24 patties

These patties can be made as a savory breakfast, served as a side at a meal, enjoyed as a snack on the go, or broken apart and used as crunchy salad or bowl toppers. A small amount of sugar intensifies the flavors of the spices and helps them infuse into the bulgur and sweet potato.

4 cups (960 ml) water

2 cups (265 g) cubed sweet potato (about 2½ medium sweet potatoes)

One 3-inch (7.5 cm) cinnamon stick

1 bay leaf

1½ cups (275 g) Simply Cooked Bulgur (page 224)

½ cup (8 g) finely chopped fresh cilantro

1 teaspoon chili powder

1 teaspoon ground cumin

1 teaspoon smoked paprika

½ teaspoon sugar

¼ teaspoon kosher salt

¼ teaspoon freshly ground black pepper

¼ cup (60 ml) balsamic vinegar

1. Combine the water, sweet potato, cinnamon, and bay leaf in a medium saucepan over medium-high heat. Simmer until the sweet potatoes are fork-tender, about 20 minutes. Drain, discard the spices, and allow to cool to room temperature.

2. If baking with one baking sheet, adjust the oven rack to the middle; if baking with two, adjust one rack in the upper third and one in the lower third of the oven. Preheat the oven to 400°F (200°C). Line two baking sheets with parchment paper.

3. When the potatoes have cooled enough to handle, transfer them to a medium bowl. Add the bulgur, cilantro, chili powder, cumin, paprika, sugar, salt, and pepper. Use your hands to mix until sticky and thoroughly combined.

4. With wet hands, scoop out 2 tablespoons of the mixture and roll it into a ball. Place the ball in the palm of your hand, then press into a thin, flat patty using the fingers of your opposite hand. (Thicker patties will be soft and tender; thin patties will be light and crispy.) Place the patty on a baking sheet, then repeat with the remaining mixture. Bake for 30 to 60 minutes, until the patties are dry and starting to crisp on the edges. If the baking sheets are on different racks, switch their positions after 15 to 20 minutes to ensure the patties bake evenly. Drizzle balsamic vinegar on only the patties you are serving and serve warm.

5. Store in an airtight container in the refrigerator for up to 5 days. To freeze, place layers of patties in an airtight freezer container, separated with wax paper. Label and store in the freezer for up to 2 months. Thaw in the refrigerator overnight. To reheat, place on a microwave-safe plate, cover, and heat in 30-second increments on HIGH until hot. Drizzle with balsamic vinegar and serve.

Serving Size 2 patties; Calories 50; Protein 1 g; Carbs 10 g; Dietary Fiber 2 g; Added Sugars 0 g; Total Fat 1 g; Sat Fat 0 g; Omega-3s 10 mg; Sodium 71 mg; Potassium 145 mg

SODIUM TIP: Using Diamond Crystal Kosher Salt will dramatically reduce the sodium in any recipe that uses kosher salt. This salt contains 50% less sodium per measure than regular kosher salt and 60% less than fine grain table salt.

SIMPLY COOKED FARRO
Makes 2½ cups (425 g)

Farro, a whole grain that is part of the wheat family, is often associated with Italian cuisine. With its chewy texture and nutty flavor, it can be used in place of rice, incorporated into warm and cold entrées, salads, and sides like our Farro with Roasted Grapes (page 226), and even used in desserts like our Cherry-Farro Pudding Parfaits (page 359).

> 1 cup (180 g) farro, rinsed and thoroughly drained
> 1 tablespoon extra virgin olive oil
> 4 cups (960 ml) water
> ¼ teaspoon kosher salt

1. Combine the farro and oil in a large saucepan over medium-high heat. Stirring constantly, gently toast the farro for 2 minutes, until fragrant. Carefully add the water and salt. Bring to a boil, reduce the heat to medium, cover, and cook until the farro is chewy yet tender, 30 minutes. Drain off any excess water, then serve.

2. Store in an airtight container in the refrigerator for up to 7 days. To freeze, package in ½- to 1-cup (85 to 170 g) portions in freezer bags. Press out as much air as you can, seal, label, and freeze for up to 4 months. Thaw in the refrigerator overnight or place in a bowl of warm water, massaging every few minutes to break up the grains.

Serving Size 1 cup (170 g); 1 cup Calories 274; Protein 10 g; Carbs 48 g; Dietary Fiber 5 g; Added Sugars 0 g; Total Fat 6 g; Sat Fat 1 g; Omega-3s 40 mg; Sodium 115 mg; Potassium 139 mg

FARRO WITH ROASTED GRAPES
Makes 6 servings

Roasted grapes offer a sweet contrast to the chewy nuttiness of the farro. Pair with Tuscan-Inspired Pork (page 333) and a simple green salad or steamed broccolini for an easy weeknight dinner that will transport your taste buds to Italy.

> 2 cups (300 g) red or green seedless grapes, halved
> 3 tablespoons extra virgin olive oil

1 tablespoon minced fresh rosemary

1 white onion, diced

2½ cups (425 g) Simply Cooked Farro (page 226)

½ teaspoon kosher salt

Juice of ½ lemon

1. Preheat the oven to 400°F (200°C). Line a rimmed baking sheet with parchment paper.

2. Combine the grapes, 1 tablespoon of the oil, and the rosemary in bowl. Toss to combine. Spread out the grapes on the baking sheet. Roast for 20 minutes or until the skin on some of the grapes starts to blister.

3. Meanwhile, heat the remaining 2 tablespoons of oil in a sauté pan or skillet and cook the onions over medium heat. Sauté until soft and opaque, 10 minutes. Add the farro and salt, cover, and cook until the farro is warmed through, about 5 minutes.

4. Add the grapes and lemon juice, stir to combine, and serve.

Per Serving: Calories 351; Protein 9 g; Carbs 55 g; Dietary Fiber 5 g; Added Sugars 0 g; Total Fat 12 g; Sat Fat 2 g; Omega-3s 100 mg; Sodium 184 mg; Potassium 130 mg

SIMPLY COOKED MILLET

Makes 4 cups (450 g)

Millet is a family of tiny grains whose seeds are similar in size to mustard seeds. The pale yellow millet seeds have a mild, sweet flavor and—bonus!—they cook quickly. We cook them here with whole cardamom pods to honor their use in Indian cuisine. We also feature this amazing whole grain in our Icelanders in America Cereal (page 133) and Millet Curry Cakes with Tomato-Corn Salsa (page 227).

1 cup (200 g) millet

2 cups (480 ml) water

4 green cardamom pods

½ teaspoon kosher salt

1. Gently toast the millet in a medium saucepan over medium heat, stirring frequently with a wooden spoon, until you start to smell a nutty, corn-like aroma, 3 to 4 minutes. (The millet won't change in color.)

2. Carefully add the water, cardamom, and salt, and increase the heat to high. Bring to a boil, then reduce the heat to low, cover, and cook for 20 minutes, until the millet is light and fluffy and all the water has been absorbed.

3. Remove and discard the cardamom, fluff the millet with a fork, and serve. Store in the refrigerator for up to 3 days or in the freezer for up to 2 months. Thaw in the refrigerator before reheating.

NOTE: *The United Nations declared 2023 the International Year of Millets to increase awareness of millet's nutrition benefits as well as its ability to grow in ever-changing climate conditions around the world, helping to promote food security in many regions.*

Serving Size 1 cup (113 g); 1 cup Calories 60; Protein 2 g; Carbs 12 g; Dietary Fiber 1 g; Added Sugars 0 g; Total Fat 1 g; Sat Fat 0 g; Omega-3s 10 mg; Sodium 201 mg; Potassium 35 mg

MILLET CURRY CAKES WITH TOMATO-CORN SALSA

Makes 8 cakes

These cakes are very tender with a mild curry flavor. They can be served as an appetizer or side dish.

2 cups (225 g) Simply Cooked Millet (page 227)

2 large eggs, beaten

3 tablespoons extra virgin olive oil

2 tablespoons millet flour (see Tip)

1 tablespoon minced jalapeño or serrano chile

½ teaspoon Curry Powder (page 32)

½ teaspoon kosher salt

Tomato-Corn Salsa (page 227) for serving

Combine the millet, eggs, 2 tablespoons of the oil, the millet flour, jalapeño, curry powder, and salt in a medium bowl. Heat 1½ teaspoons of the remaining oil in a large skillet or sauté pan over medium-high heat until shimmering. Spoon about 3 tablespoons batter into the skillet for each cake. (You should be able to fry 4 cakes at one time.) Cook until golden brown, 4 to 5 minutes. Flip the cakes and cook for another 3 to 4 minutes, until golden. Transfer to a serving plate. Repeat with the remaining 1½ teaspoons of oil and batter. Serve warm topped with salsa.

TIP: *You can make your own millet flour by grinding 2 tablespoons millet in a clean spice grinder or blender.*

Serving Size 1 cake; Calories 106; Protein 3 g; Carbs 8 g; Dietary Fiber 1 g; Added Sugars 0 g; Total Fat 7 g; Sat Fat 1 g; Omega-3s 70 mg; Sodium 184 mg; Potassium 28 mg

SIMPLY COOKED QUINOA
Makes 3 cups (555 g)

Quinoa is a gluten-free whole grain that comes in three colors: white, red, and black. While some people believe quinoa is a rich source of protein, this is a misperception. Yes, quinoa provides slightly more protein than other whole grains, but it's lower in protein than other plant-based sources such as legumes. One definite benefit of quinoa is that it cooks more quickly than many other whole grains, usually requiring only 15 minutes.

2 cups (480 ml) water
1 cup (170 g) quinoa

1. Bring the water and quinoa to a boil in a medium saucepan. Reduce the heat to low, cover, and simmer until the water is absorbed, 15 to 20 minutes. Remove from the heat and allow to stand, covered, for 5 minutes. Fluff with a fork. The grains should be soft, not mushy, and separate easily.

2. Store in an airtight container in the refrigerator for up to 5 days. To freeze, package in ½- to 1-cup (95 to 185 g) portions in freezer bags. Press out as much air as you can, seal, label, and freeze for up to 4 months. Thaw in the refrigerator overnight or place in a bowl of warm water, massaging every few minutes to break up the grains.

Serving Size 3 cups (555 g); Calories 238; Protein 7 g; Carbs 34 g; Dietary Fiber 5 g; Added Sugars 0 g; Total Fat 8 g; Sat Fat 1 g; Omega-3s 380 mg; Sodium 339 mg; Potassium 279 mg

QUINOA & BLACK BEAN MEDLEY
Makes 4 servings

This recipe unites the benefits of quinoa—fiber and slow-release carbohydrates—with the plant-based protein power of pulses to create a salad that can work as well as a warm or cold side as it does a main dish. This medley also makes a wonderful filling for soft shell tacos or burritos, topped with Pico de Gallo (page 61).

1 cup (170 g) quinoa
2 cups (480 ml) water
One 15-ounce (425 g) can black beans, drained and rinsed
5 green onions, chopped
1 tomato, chopped
⅓ cup (5 g) chopped fresh cilantro
2 tablespoons extra virgin olive oil
Juice of 1 lime
2 garlic cloves, minced
2 teaspoons ground cumin
¼ teaspoon kosher salt
¼ teaspoon freshly ground black pepper

1. Combine the quinoa and water in a medium saucepan over medium heat. Bring to a boil, then reduce the heat to medium-low, cover, and cook until all the water has been absorbed, 10 to 12 minutes. Remove from the heat.

2. Add the beans, green onions, tomato, cilantro, oil, lime juice, garlic, cumin, salt, and pepper, and stir thoroughly. Serve immediately or refrigerate until cold.

Per Serving: Calories 282; Protein 12 g; Carbs 38 g; Dietary Fiber 12 g; Added Sugars 0 g; Total Fat 10 g; Sat Fat 1 g; Omega-3s 260 mg; Sodium 380 mg; Potassium 592 mg

SIMPLY COOKED SORGHUM

Makes 2½ cups (500 g)

Sorghum has a sweeter flavor than other whole grains. Here we add lemon juice to balance that sweetness. Cooked sorghum can be eaten alone as a side or used in recipes like our Savory Sorghum Porridge (page 229), a very flavorful accompaniment for lean pork chops.

- 1 cup (190 g) whole grain sorghum
- 6 cups (1.5 L) water
- 1 bay leaf
- Juice of ½ lemon
- ½ teaspoon kosher salt

1. Place the sorghum in a fine-mesh strainer and rinse under cold running water for 10 seconds, to remove any dust adhering to the grains.

2. Bring the water, sorghum, and bay leaf to a boil in a large pot. Reduce the heat to medium-low, cover, and gently simmer until the sorghum is chewy-tender, 50 to 60 minutes.

3. Drain off any excess water. Add the lemon juice and salt, stir, and serve warm. Store in an airtight container in the refrigerator for up to 1 week or in the freezer for up to 2 months.

Serving Size 1 cup (200 g); Calories 253; Protein 8 g; Carbs 56 g; Dietary Fiber 5 g; Added Sugars 0 g; Total Fat 3 g; Sat Fat 0 g; Omega-3s 50 mg; Sodium 188 mg; Potassium 289 mg

SAVORY SORGHUM PORRIDGE

Makes 4 servings

This savory side dish with a risotto-like consistency can be served with lean pork chops and broccoli rabe (aka rapini) or broccolini. Bitter broccoli rabe is a great counterbalance to the natural sweetness of the sorghum.

- 2 tablespoons extra virgin olive oil
- 1 large white onion, diced
- 2 garlic cloves, minced
- 2 teaspoons Italian Seasoning (page 34)
- ½ teaspoon red pepper flakes
- ½ teaspoon kosher salt
- 2½ cups (500 g) Simply Cooked Sorghum (page 229) or 2½ cups (425 g) Simply Cooked Farro (page 226)
- ½ cup (120 ml) Vegetable Broth (page 72)
- ½ cup (125 g) part-skim ricotta
- ½ cup (40 g) freshly grated Grana Padana, Parmigiano-Reggiano, or Parmesan
- Chopped fresh flat-leaf parsley

1. Heat the oil in a large sauté pan or skillet over medium heat. Add the onion, garlic, seasoning, red pepper flakes, and salt, and cook until the onions are very soft but not brown, 8 to 10 minutes.

2. Reduce the heat to medium-low. Add the sorghum and broth, stir, cover, and simmer for 10 to 12 minutes, until heated through.

3. Remove from the heat and stir in the ricotta and Grana Padana. Transfer to a serving dish, top with parsley, and serve.

Per Serving: Calories 510; Protein 18 g; Carbs 82 g; Dietary Fiber 8 g; Added Sugars 0 g; Total Fat 16 g; Sat Fat 5 g; Omega-3s 150 mg; Sodium 472 mg; Potassium 488 mg

SIMPLY COOKED BROWN RICE

Makes 3 cups (585 g)

Brown rice differs from white rice in taste and texture because brown rice kernels still have their germ and bran layer intact. The bran adds a nutty flavor and more than four times as much heart-healthy fiber as white rice, which is why brown rice takes a longer to cook. Cooked short-grain brown rice is sticky—it's perfect for eating with chopsticks. Long-grain brown rice is less starchy, and the cooked kernels separate easily. We use basmati, a long-grain rice that has a lovely aroma, in this recipe. So sit back, relax, and breathe deeply while the rice is cooking.

1½ cups (360 ml) water

1 cup (200 g) brown basmati rice

1 teaspoon extra virgin olive oil

¼ teaspoon kosher salt

1. Bring the water, rice, oil, and salt to a boil in a saucepan over high heat. Reduce the heat to low, cover, and simmer gently until the rice is soft and chewy and there are crater-like steam holes on the surface, 35 to 40 minutes.

2. Remove from the heat and let stand for 10 minutes, covered, to allow the rice to steam and absorb all the moisture. Fluff with a fork.

3. Store in an airtight container in the refrigerator for up to 5 days. To freeze, spread the rice out onto a rimmed baking sheet to cool quickly. Package ½- to 1-cup (100 to 195 g) portions in freezer bags. Press out as much air as you can, seal, label, and freeze for up to 6 months. Thaw in the refrigerator overnight, or place in a bowl of warm water, massaging every few minutes to break up the grains.

Serving Size 1 cup (195 g); Calories 236; Protein 6 g; Carbs 49 g; Dietary Fiber 3 g; Added Sugars 0 g; Total Fat 4 g; Sat Fat 0 g; Omega-3s 10 mg; Sodium 62 mg; Potassium 100 mg

BROWN RICE WITH PINE NUTS & ROASTED BUTTERNUT SQUASH

Makes 4 servings

This hearty, comforting side dish is perfect for a cool fall day. Serve with Roast Chicken with Lemon & Thyme (page 313) or Herb-Roasted Turkey Breast with Vegetables (page 317).

3 cups (420 g) diced butternut squash

1 white or yellow onion, sliced

2 tablespoons extra virgin olive oil

2 tablespoons minced fresh thyme

1½ cups (295 g) Simply Cooked Brown Rice (page 230)

⅓ cup (45 g) toasted pine nuts

Juice of 1 lemon

1. Preheat the oven to 400°F (200°C). Line a baking sheet with parchment paper.

2. Combine the squash, onion, oil, and thyme in a large bowl. Spread out the mixture in a single layer on the baking sheet and roast for 20 to 25 minutes, until the squash is fork-tender and brown on the edges.

3. Return the squash to the bowl, then stir in the rice. Add the pine nuts and lemon juice, and stir again.

4. Transfer to a serving bowl and serve warm or at room temperature.

Per Serving: Calories 451; Protein 9 g; Carbs 69 g; Dietary Fiber 6 g; Added Sugars 0 g; Total Fat 19 g; Sat Fat 2 g; Omega-3s 90 mg; Sodium 72 mg; Potassium 479 mg

MEDÍTERRANEAN RICE BAKE WITH EGGPLANT & TOMATOES

Makes 6 servings

This casserole can be the star of a meal or served as a side dish to baked fish or grilled shrimp. We like to pair it with our Sautéed Shrimp & Scallops (page 292).

Cooking spray

1½ cups (295 g) Simply Cooked Brown Rice (page 230)

6 cups (1,350 g) Creamy Eggplant with Tomatoes (page 277)

½ cup (40 g) freshly grated Parmesan

½ cup (75 g) crumbled feta

1 tablespoon extra virgin olive oil

1. Preheat the oven to 350°F (180°C). Line a 9 × 13-inch (23 × 33 cm) baking dish with parchment paper and spray with cooking spray.

2. Spoon the rice into the pan in an even layer. Top with the eggplant mixture. Sprinkle with the Parmesan and feta, and drizzle with the oil. Bake for 30 to 40 minutes, until the cheese is melted and starting to brown. Serve warm.

Per Serving: Calories 388; Protein 14 g; Carbs 50 g; Dietary Fiber 6 g; Added Sugars 0 g; Total Fat 18 g; Sat Fat 5 g; Omega-3s 100 mg; Sodium 296 mg; Potassium 540 mg

MOCK RISOTTO WITH ZUCCHINI

Makes 4 servings

This mock risotto uses precooked long-grain brown rice. That reduces the overall cooking time as well as the time spent adding liquid and stirring. Serve with Chicken & Chanterelles (page 305) or sautéed chicken breasts.

4 zucchini, trimmed and cubed

2 tablespoons extra virgin olive oil

2 cups (390 g) Simply Cooked Brown Rice (page 230)

1 cup (240 ml) Vegetable Broth (page 72) or Chicken Stock (page 70), plus more if needed

1 tablespoon red wine vinegar

½ cup (40 g) freshly grated Parmesan

1 teaspoon minced fresh rosemary

1. Combine the zucchini and oil in a medium saucepan over medium-high heat. Cook, stirring frequently, until the zucchini begins to brown and soften but does not stick to the pan, 6 to 8 minutes.

2. Stir in the rice, broth, and vinegar, then bring to a light simmer. Cover, reduce the heat to medium, and simmer gently for 10 minutes, stirring a few times, until thick and bubbly. Add more broth if necessary to keep a saucy yet thick consistency.

3. Remove from the heat, add the Parmesan and rosemary, stir to combine, and serve.

Per Serving: Calories 475; Protein 14 g; Carbs 77 g; Dietary Fiber 6 g; Added Sugars 0 g; Total Fat 16 g; Sat Fat 3 g; Omega-3s 200 mg; Sodium 285 mg; Potassium 532 mg

PERSIAN-INSPIRED RICE PILAF WITH CHERRIES & PISTACHIOS

Makes 8 servings

This pilaf offers tempting textures, alluring aromas, and fresh herbal tones of dill and mint. Serve with naan or Sheet Pan Tri-Tip Roast (page 328) for a classic Persian feast.

3 cups (585 g) Simply Cooked Brown Rice (page 230)

1 cup (120 g) dried cherries

⅔ cup (80 g) chopped toasted pistachios

2 tablespoons minced fresh dill

2 tablespoons minced fresh mint

¼ teaspoon ground cinnamon

Juice of 1 lemon

2 tablespoons extra virgin olive oil

Combine the rice, cherries, pistachios, dill, mint, and cinnamon in a large bowl. Transfer to a serving bowl and drizzle with the lemon juice and oil. Serve warm or at room temperature.

Per Serving: Calories 393; Protein 9 g; Carbs 67 g; Dietary Fiber 5 g; Added Sugars 0 g; Total Fat 12 g; Sat Fat 0 g; Omega-3s 60 mg; Sodium 69 mg; Potassium 186 mg

TOFU FRIED RICE

Makes 4 servings

With a crunchy exterior and a creamy interior, our Crispy Tofu Bites are well suited to the flavorful spices in this dish. The bright colors of the quickly cooked vegetables make a splendid-looking plate and offer an abundance of health-promoting nutrients!

2 tablespoons plus 1 teaspoon toasted sesame oil

2 large eggs

1 broccoli crown, cut into small florets

2 heads baby bok choy, finely chopped

2 carrots, thinly sliced

10 cremini mushrooms, coarsely chopped

4 or 5 radishes, trimmed and finely diced

3 garlic cloves, minced

2 tablespoons minced fresh ginger

2 tablespoons balsamic vinegar

1 teaspoon Chinese Five-Spice Blend (page 31)

1½ cups (370 g) Crispy Tofu Bites (page 250)

3 cups (585 g) Simply Cooked Brown Rice (page 230)

¼ cup (60 ml) Vegetable Broth (page 72)

2 tablespoons reduced-sodium teriyaki sauce

2 green onions, thinly sliced

2 tablespoons toasted sesame seeds

1. Heat 1 tablespoon of the oil in a large nonstick sauté pan or wok over medium heat. Whisk the eggs in a small bowl until lightly blended. When the oil shimmers, add the eggs. Use a slotted spatula to stir the eggs into small, gently cooked soft curds, less than a minute. Transfer to a medium bowl.

2. Return the pan to the heat, add 1 tablespoon of the oil, and increase the heat to medium-high. When the oil shimmers, add the broccoli, bok choy, carrots, mushrooms, radishes, garlic, and ginger. Stir the vegetables constantly until the bok choy and carrots begin to soften, the broccoli is bright green, the mushrooms begin to shrink, and the garlic and ginger are aromatic, about 2 minutes.

3. Stir in the vinegar and five-spice blend. Add the tofu and continue to stir-fry until the vegetables are tender-crisp and the liquid has evaporated, 1 to 2 minutes. Remove from the heat and transfer the mixture to the bowl with the eggs.

4. Reduce the heat to medium-low, return the pan to the heat, and add the remaining 1 tablespoon of oil, followed by the rice. Stir with the spatula to break up the rice, about 30 seconds. Add the broth, teriyaki sauce, vegetables, and eggs. Gently lift and toss, evenly distributing the ingredients throughout the pan. Stir-fry until heated through, 3 to 4 minutes. Divide among four plates, sprinkle each serving with one-quarter of the green onions and 1½ teaspoons sesame seeds, and serve hot.

Per Serving: Calories 445; Protein 24 g; Carbs 45 g; Dietary Fiber 12 g; Added Sugars 0 g; Total Fat 22 g; Sat Fat 3 g; Omega-3s 490 mg; Sodium 825 mg; Potassium 1,644 mg

VEGETABLE-ALMOND RICE WITH PARMESAN

Makes 6 servings

This recipe is easy to make and clean up after because it uses only one pan. It's a perfect dish to serve with the Spinach Salad with Honeycrisp Apples & Cheddar (page 148).

- 1 tablespoon extra virgin olive oil
- 1 white or yellow onion, finely chopped
- 2 celery stalks, thinly sliced
- 2 garlic cloves, minced
- 10 white mushrooms, thinly sliced
- 1 cup (200 g) brown basmati rice
- 2 cups (480 ml) Vegetable Broth (page 72) or Chicken Stock (page 70)
- 2 tablespoons chopped fresh thyme
- 1 teaspoon poultry seasoning
- ½ teaspoon freshly ground black pepper
- 1 cup (90 g) sliced almonds, toasted
- ½ cup (40 g) freshly grated Parmesan
- ½ cup (30 g) chopped fresh flat-leaf parsley

1. Heat the oil in a large skillet over medium heat. Add the onion, celery, and garlic, and sauté until the onion and celery have softened and the garlic is fragrant, about 2 minutes. Add the mushrooms and sauté until they begin to shrink and soften, about 3 minutes.

2. Stir in the rice and 1 cup (240 ml) of the broth. Bring to a boil over medium-high heat. Stir in the remaining 1 cup (240 ml) broth, the thyme, poultry seasoning, and pepper. Reduce the heat to medium-low to maintain a gentle simmer, cover, and cook until you see crater-like steam holes on the surface of the rice, 35 to 40 minutes.

3. Remove from the heat and let sit, covered, for 10 minutes to steam. The rice should be chewy, not crunchy nor mushy. Add the almonds, Parmesan, and parsley, using a fork to gently blend them in. Serve warm.

Per Serving: Calories 265; Protein 9 g; Carbs 32 g; Dietary Fiber 4 g; Added Sugars 0 g; Total Fat 13 g; Sat Fat 2 g; Omega-3s 30 mg; Sodium 142 mg; Potassium 276 mg

VEGETABLE FRIED RICE

Makes 4 servings

Need a short cut for getting this meal prepared more quickly? Feel free to use frozen carrots and peas and microwave them before adding to the other vegetables. Serve this with Sesame Chicken & Vegetable Foil Packs (page 315) for a fun and flavorful meal!

- 2 tablespoons plus 1 teaspoon peanut oil
- 2 large eggs
- 2 carrots, diced
- 2 celery stalks, thinly sliced on the diagonal
- 4 ounces (113 g) shiitake caps, cremini, or white mushrooms, coarsely chopped
- 2 garlic cloves, minced
- 2 tablespoons minced fresh ginger
- 2 tablespoons rice vinegar
- 3 cups (585 g) Simply Cooked Brown Rice (page 230)
- 1 cup (130 g) petite or baby green peas
- ½ cup (120 ml) Vegetable Broth (page 72)
- 3 tablespoons reduced-sodium soy sauce or tamari
- 1 teaspoon Chinese Five-Spice Blend (page 31)
- 2 green onions, thinly sliced
- ¼ cup (35 g) unsalted roasted peanuts

1. Heat 1 tablespoon of the oil in a large nonstick sauté pan or wok over medium heat. Whisk the eggs in a small bowl until lightly blended. When the oil shimmers, add the eggs. Use a slotted spatula to stir the eggs into small, gently cooked soft curds, less than a minute. Transfer to a medium bowl.

2. Return the pan to the heat, add 1 tablespoon oil, and increase the heat to medium-high. When the oil shimmers, add the carrots, celery, mushrooms, garlic, and ginger. Stir the vegetables constantly until the carrots and celery begin to soften and the mushrooms begin to shrink, about 2 minutes. Add the vinegar and toss until the vegetables are tender-crisp and the liquid has evaporated, 1 to 2 minutes. Remove from the heat and transfer the vegetables to the bowl with the eggs.

3. Reduce the heat to medium-low, return the pan to the heat, and add the remaining 1 tablespoon of oil, followed by the rice. Stir with the spatula to break up the rice, about 30 seconds. Add the peas, broth, soy sauce, and five-spice blend, and stir-fry for 1 minute.

4. Add the vegetables and eggs back to the pan and stir-fry until heated through, 2 to 3 minutes. Divide among four plates; sprinkle each serving with one-quarter of the green onions and 1 tablespoon of peanuts. Serve hot.

Per Serving: Calories 425; Protein 14 g; Carbs 53 g; Dietary Fiber 8 g; Added Sugars 0 g; Total Fat 18 g; Sat Fat 4 g; Omega-3s 50 mg; Sodium 710 mg; Potassium 460 mg

SIMPLY COOKED WILD RICE
Makes 4 cups (660 g)

If you've never tried wild rice, this recipe is a great way for you to experience its nutty flavor and chewy texture. After you've mastered this recipe, you can quickly prepare a variety of dishes like our Wild Rice & Chickpea Salad (page 171).

1 cup (160 g) wild rice

4 cups (960 ml) Vegetable Broth (page 72) or water

¼ teaspoon kosher salt

½ teaspoon freshly ground black pepper

1. Rinse the wild rice in a fine-mesh strainer or colander under running water to remove any grit. Drain.

2. Combine the wild rice, broth, salt, and pepper in a medium saucepan over medium-high heat. Bring to a boil, then reduce the heat to medium-low, cover, and simmer gently until the kernels split open, slightly curl on the ends, and are tender, 45 to 55 minutes.

3. Store in an airtight container in the refrigerator for up to 4 days. To freeze, package ½- to 1-cup (155 to 310 g) portions in freezer bags. Press out as much air as you can, seal, label, and freeze for up to 4 months. Thaw in the refrigerator overnight, or place in a bowl of warm water, massaging every few minutes to break up the grains.

Serving Size 1 cup (165 g); Calories 146; Protein 6 g; Carbs 30 g; Dietary Fiber 3 g; Added Sugars 0 g; Total Fat 1 g; Sat Fat 0 g; Omega-3s 120 mg; Sodium 60 mg; Potassium 177 mg

WILD RICE WITH MUSHROOMS, TARRAGON & PINE NUTS
Makes 4 servings

This is a great side dish to serve with pork chops, sautéed chicken breasts, or sautéed turkey breast cutlets. Add a vegetable side like our Citrus Glazed Carrots (page 265) to complete your meal.

1 tablespoon extra virgin olive oil

10 cremini or white mushrooms, sliced (2½ cups/225 g)

4 green onions, sliced

2 tablespoons minced fresh tarragon, rosemary, or thyme

4 cups (660 g) Simply Cooked Wild Rice

½ cup (70 g) toasted pine nuts

½ teaspoon freshly ground black pepper

1. Heat the oil in a large skillet or sauté pan over medium heat, then add the mushrooms and onions. Sauté until the mushrooms have released some liquid and the green onions have softened and the white parts have become translucent, 3 to 4 minutes.

2. Add the tarragon and sauté until wilted, 2 minutes.

3. Add the wild rice, warm or cold, stirring it in; reduce the heat to low, cover, and cook for 10 minutes to thoroughly heat the rice.

4. Stir in the pine nuts and pepper. Serve warm.

Per Serving: Calories 514; Protein 18 g; Carbs 78 g; Dietary Fiber 7 g; Added Sugars 0 g; Total Fat 17 g; Sat Fat 2 g; Omega-3s 320 mg; Sodium 148 mg; Potassium 733 mg

WILD RICE WITH SAUSAGE & SAGE

Makes 8 servings

This is Linda's traditional fall holiday dish and is the dish most often requested when the kids come home. It's easy to make and fills the house with the yummiest aroma of sage. She serves it with our Cranberry Sauce with Lime & Crystallized Ginger (page 54) and our Spinach Salad with Honeycrisp Apples & Cheddar (page 148).

Cooking spray

1 pound (454 g) bulk pork sausage with sage or uncooked Spicy Sage Breakfast Sausage (page 124)

1 large onion, diced

2 celery stalks, diced

4 cups (660 g) Simply Cooked Wild Rice (page 234)

1½ cups (360 ml) Béchamel (page 53)

1 tablespoon minced fresh sage leaves

Grated zest of 1 lemon

1 teaspoon Herb Blend for Poultry (page 34)

1. Preheat the oven to 350°F (180°C). Line a 9 × 13-inch (23 × 33 cm) baking dish with parchment paper. Spray with cooking spray.

2. Cook the sausage in a large skillet or sauté pan over medium heat until browned, 10 minutes, breaking the sausage into small pieces with a spatula as it cooks. Tilt the pan and spoon out and discard any excess fat. Add the onion and celery to the sausage and cook until the onion and celery have softened, another 10 minutes.

3. Stir in the wild rice, béchamel, sage, lemon zest, and poultry seasoning. Transfer to the baking dish and cover with foil. Bake for 30 to 40 minutes, until a digital food thermometer reads 165°F (75°C) when inserted in the center of the casserole. Serve hot. Store in an airtight container in the refrigerator for up to 4 days and reheat in the microwave, or in an airtight freezer- and oven-safe container in the freezer for up to 2 months and reheat in the oven.

Per Serving: Calories 362; Protein 16 g; Carbs 41 g; Dietary Fiber 4 g; Added Sugars 0 g; Total Fat 16 g; Sat Fat 5 g; Omega-3s 160 mg; Sodium 130 mg; Potassium 255 mg

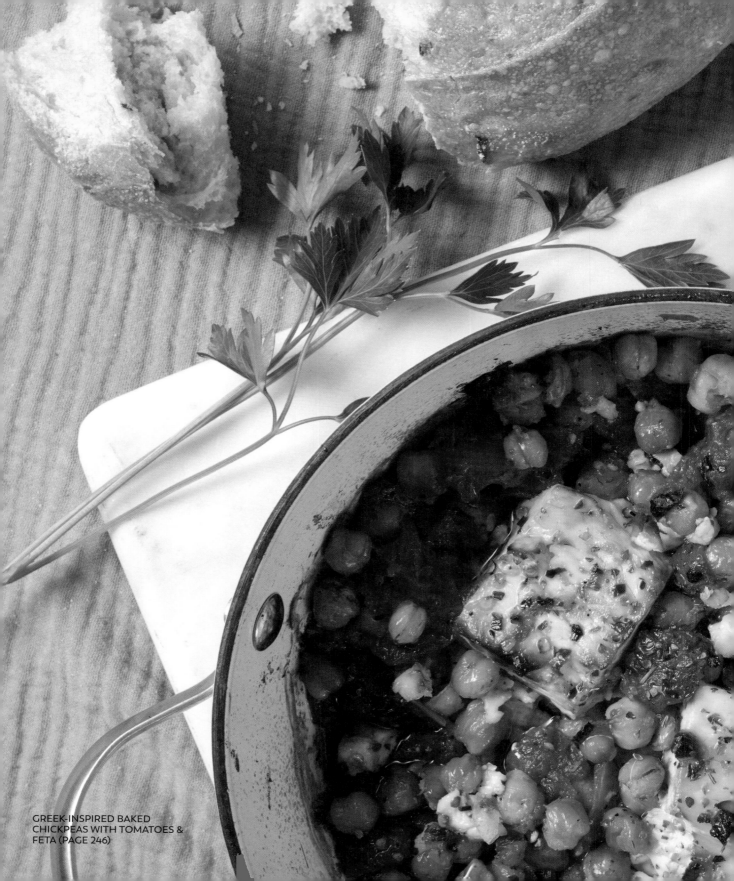

GREEK-INSPIRED BAKED
CHICKPEAS WITH TOMATOES &
FETA (PAGE 246)

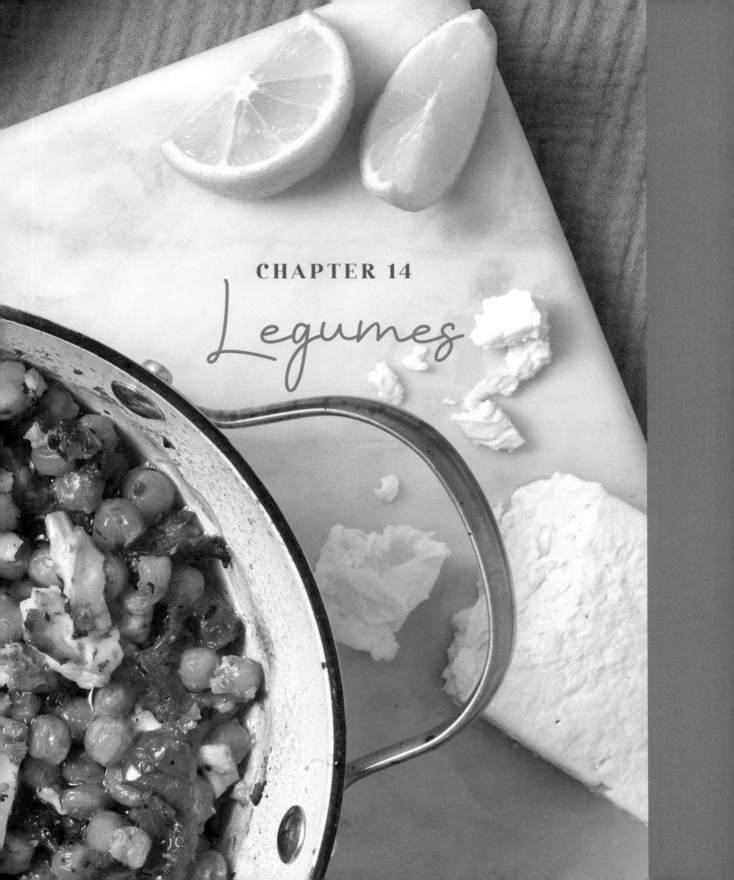

CHAPTER 14

Legumes

Legumes

Cooking with Pulses. 239

Beans

Simply Cooked Black Beans. 241

Simply Cooked White Beans 241

À la Heart Rice & Bean Bowls 242

Baked Beans with Maple Syrup 242

Baked Beans with Pomegranate
& Canadian Bacon 242

Red Beans & Rice 243

Refried Beans 243

Salmon & White Bean Bowls
with Lime & Dill. 244

Spicy Black Bean Chili 244

White Bean Salad with
Lemon & Rosemary 245

Chickpeas

Classic Hummus 245

Eastern Mediterranean Bowls
with Hummus & Tabbouleh 246

Greek-Inspired Baked Chickpeas
with Tomatoes & Feta 246

Lentils

Simply Cooked Lentils 247

Fragrant Warm Spiced Lentils. 247

East Indian–Inspired Lentil
& Chickpea Dal Bowls 248

Ginger Lentils. 249

Ginger Lentil & Brown Rice Bake. 249

Lentil-Fennel Lasagna. 249

Tofu

Crispy Tofu Bites 250

Tofu Italiano Bake. 251

egumes are a fascinating group of ingredients. They have many nutrition and health benefits (see Chapter 2) and are beneficial for farmers (they promote soil health and fertility), and there are many different types available. But the diversity of legumes and the associated terminology can make them seem a bit complicated.

The term "legume" refers to a plant family with three branches. The first branch includes crops like soybeans and peanuts that contain healthful oils. Soybeans and peanuts can be converted into many ingredients and products like soy milk, soy sauce, tempeh, peanut oil, and peanut flour. But in this chapter, we give you a few fun ways to cook with soybean curd (tofu), and in other chapters, we use peanuts in a myriad of ways—we use peanut butter in Peanut Sauce (page 56) and in the West African-Inspired Sweet Potato & Peanut Stew (page 84) and in Pork Lettuce Wraps (page 187).

The second branch includes fresh peas and beans. While they're technically legumes, most people think of them as vegetables. For this reason, we've included them in many other chapters: Vegetables, Pasta, Fruit & Vegetable Side Salads, and Entrée Salads.

The third branch, known as pulses, includes edible seeds that are harvested when the seed pod is dry. It includes beans, chickpeas, lentils, and split peas. These are sold dried, canned, and frozen (ready to heat and eat). Some pulses are converted into flours. And then, of course, there are endless products made with pulses, like refried beans, bean-based chips, soups, pastas, dips like hummus, and more! In this chapter, we've given you a wide variety of recipes for beans, chickpeas, and lentils.

All legumes have health-promoting properties, and they're all rich in dietary fiber. From immature, green soybeans (i.e., edamame) and peanut butter to lentils and hummus, cooking with and eating more legumes is a wonderful way to boost your fiber intake.

Cooking with Pulses

You can buy pulses—beans, chickpeas, lentils, and split peas—in their dry form, which will save you money, or you can buy them canned, which will save you time. Canned pulses are wonderful to have on hand for a quick, easy option, but they have added sodium. Draining and rinsing them can remove up to 35 percent of the added sodium. Dry pulses are virtually sodium free.

Soaking pulses prior to cooking is recommended, as it can speed up cooking time, but it's not required. There is no nutrient benefit to soaking, but it can reduce some of the fructooligosaccharides that can cause gas, though it doesn't remove these gas-causing carbs completely. While the gassiness may be unpleasant at times, it's a sign the good bacteria in your gut are doing good work!

There are four basic steps to follow when cooking pulses.

1. **Clean:** Beans, chickpeas, lentils, and split peas come out of the bag just like they came out of the field, so they need to be cleaned prior to cooking. It's important to sort through them to remove any twigs, small pebbles, or other items that have made their way into the bag after harvest. It's also good to remove any broken or cracked beans. We recommend pouring the pulses, 1 cup (227 g) at a time, into a pie plate so you can easily identify foreign matter and remove it with your fingers. Transfer the cleaned pulses to a strainer.

2. **Rinse:** Rinse the pulses under cold running water for 20 to 30 seconds to remove dust.

3. **Soak:** Split peas and lentils don't require soaking. For beans and chickpeas, there are four soaking methods. The two hot soak methods will produce the best results, but we offer the other methods to give you flexibility.

3a. Hot Soak: Place the pulses in a large pot. Add 5 cups (1.2 L) water for every cup (227 g) of pulses. Boil for 2 minutes. Turn the heat off and let stand for 4 hours. Drain off the soaking liquid.

3b. Hot Soak with Salt: This method introduces added sodium, but it also guarantees the softest, creamiest end product. Place the pulses in a large pot. Add 5 cups (1.2 L) water and ½ teaspoon kosher salt for every cup (227 g) of pulses. Boil for 2 minutes. Turn the heat off and let stand for 4 hours. Drain off the soaking liquid.

3c. Cold Soak: Place the pulses in a large pot. Cover with water at least 2 inches (5 cm) above top of the pulses. Soak for at least 8 hours or overnight. Drain off the soaking liquid.

3d. Quick Soak: Place your pulses in a large pot. Add 6 cups (1.4 L) water for every cup (227 g) pulses. Boil for 3 minutes. Turn the heat off and let stand for 1 hour. Drain off the soaking liquid.

4. Cook: Table 8 on this page provides guidance on stovetop cooking times for a wide variety of pulses. It's important to simmer pulses gently instead of boiling, which will cause them to break apart during the cooking process. Cooking times can range a bit, because the age and dryness of the pulses will have an impact on how long they take to fully hydrate and reach a desirable soft, creamy texture.

Other Tips for Cooking Pulses

- Use a large pot or Dutch oven; legumes expand greatly when cooked.
- Adding a teaspoon of vegetable oil (such as corn oil) to the cooking water can help prevent foaming.
- Don't add acidic ingredients like lemon juice, vinegar, or tomatoes to the cooking water until the beans are almost done, as acid slows the softening process.

- Use a pressure cooker or Instant Pot to cook pulses quickly; since they differ by manufacturer, refer to the manual for your model to get specific guidance.

Table 8: Cooking Pulses from Dry

Start with 1 pound (2 cups/454 g) of the pulse, prior to soaking.

PULSE	WATER	SIMMERING TIME	YIELD
Black beans	4 cups (1 L)	1–2 hours	4 cups (690 g)
Black-eyed peas (aka cowpeas)	4 cups (1 L)	1–2 hours	4 cups (660 g)
Cannellini beans (aka white kidney beans)	4 cups (1 L)	1–2 hours	4 cups (690 g)
Chickpeas (aka garbanzo beans)	6 cups (1.4 L)	1½–2 hours	4 cups (655 g)
Cranberry beans	4 cups (1 L)	1–2 hours	4 cups (710 g)
Fava beans	4 cups (1 L)	2–3 hours	4 cups (680 g)
Great Northern beans	4 cups (1 L)	2 hours	4 cups (700 g)
Kidney beans, dark or light red	4 cups (1 L)	1–2 hours	4 cups (690 g)
Lentils	5 cups (1.2 L)	20–40 minutes	4 cups (765 g)
Lima beans	4 cups (1 L)	1–2 hours	4 cups (735 g)
Navy beans	4 cups (1 L)	1–2 hours	4 cups (700 g)
Pink beans	4 cups (1 L)	1–2 hours	4 cups (675 g)
Small red beans	4 cups (1 L)	1–2 hours	4 cups (690 g)
Split peas	4 cups (1 L)	35–40 minutes	4 cups (785 g)

SIMPLY COOKED BLACK BEANS

Makes 6 cups (1,035 g)

This recipe is the base for our Spicy Black Bean Chili (page 244). You can always use canned beans to save some time, but cooking a batch of beans from dry allows you to package and freeze them for later use, making future meals a snap.

- 1 pound (2 cups/454 g) dry black beans, cleaned, rinsed, and soaked
- 1 white or yellow onion, halved
- 1½ teaspoons freshly ground black pepper
- 1 bay leaf
- 10 cups (2.4 L) water

1. Place the beans, onion, pepper, and bay leaf in a large stockpot, then add the water. Bring to a boil over high heat. Reduce the heat to a simmer and partially cover with a lid, allowing steam to escape. Cook until fork-tender, 3 to 4 hours. Add more water if the beans have absorbed most of the water but aren't fully cooked. When the beans are fork-tender and chewy but not mushy, remove from the heat, drain, and cool. Discard the onion and bay leaf.

2. Store in an airtight container in the refrigerator for up to 4 days. To freeze, divide into smaller portions and package 1- to 2-cup (175 to 350 g) portions in freezer bags. Press out as much air as you can, seal, label, and freeze for up to 4 months. Thaw in the refrigerator overnight or place in a bowl of warm water, massaging every few minutes to break up the beans.

Serving Size 1 cup (173 g); Calories 264; Protein 17 g; Carbs 49 g; Dietary Fiber 12 g; Added Sugars 0 g; Total Fat 1 g; Sat Fat 0 g; Omega-3s 210 mg; Sodium 4 mg; Potassium 1,147 mg

SIMPLY COOKED WHITE BEANS

Makes 3 cups (525 g)

If you have cooked white beans on hand, you can quickly make a very satisfying, nourishing meal like our Salmon & White Bean Bowls with Lime & Dill (page 244). Cooking the beans with a bay leaf intensifies the beans' natural flavor, and the mild acidity from the lemon brightens it.

- 4 cups (960 ml) water
- 8 ounces (1 cup/227 g) dried white beans (cannellini, navy, or Great Northern), cleaned, rinsed, and soaked
- 1 bay leaf
- 1 teaspoon freshly ground black pepper
- 2 tablespoons fresh lemon juice
- 1 tablespoon extra virgin olive oil

1. Place the water, beans, bay leaf, and pepper in a stockpot. Bring to a boil, cover partially with a lid, and reduce the heat to low to maintain a gentle simmer. Cook until the beans are fork-tender but not mushy, 60 to 70 minutes. (The cooking time will vary, and you may need to add more water during the cooking process.)

2. Drain any excess liquid, then stir in the lemon juice and oil. Serve.

3. Store in an airtight container in the refrigerator for up to 4 days. To freeze, divide into smaller portions and package 1- to 2-cup (175 to 350 g) portions in freezer bags. Press out as much air as you can, seal, label, and freeze for up to 4 months. Thaw in the refrigerator overnight or place in a bowl of warm water, massaging every few minutes to break up the beans.

Serving Size 1 cup (175 g); Calories 299; Protein 16 g; Carbs 46 g; Dietary Fiber 25 g; Added Sugars 0 g; Total Fat 5 g; Sat Fat 1 g; Omega-3s 40 mg; Sodium 13 mg; Potassium 1,060 mg

À LA HEART RICE & BEAN BOWLS

Makes 4 servings

Let's say you've made a few of our recipes earlier in the week. For a working lunch or dinner, pack the chili-rice blend in one container, the arugula in another, and the aïoli in a third. This enables you to heat the chili-rice blend, add the fresh arugula and top it with the sauce.

- 4 cups (1,110 g) Spicy Black Bean Chili (page 244), warmed
- 4 cups (780 g) Simply Cooked Brown Rice (page 230), warmed
- One 5 to 6-ounce (142 to 170 g) bag baby arugula, chopped, or 2 cups (300 g) roasted vegetables of your choice
- 1 cup (240 ml) Avocado Lime Cilantro Aïoli (page 44)
- ½ cup (80 g) chopped green onions
- ¼ cup (4 g) chopped cilantro

Divide the chili and rice among six bowls. Top each bowl with a handful of arugula, a dollop of aïoli, and a sprinkle of green onions and cilantro. Serve.

Serving Size 1 bowl; Calories 798; Protein 30 g; Carbs 149 g; Dietary Fiber 20 g; Added Sugars 0 g; Total Fat 14 g; Sat Fat 2 g; Omega-3s 380 mg; Sodium 181 mg; Potassium 1,405 mg

BAKED BEANS WITH MAPLE SYRUP

Makes 8 servings

Navy beans are traditional for baked beans, but you can use other dried white beans like cannellini beans (sometimes called white kidney beans), or great Northern beans for this recipe. We use turkey bacon, which has 60 percent less fat than regular bacon and only 130 mg of sodium per slice.

- 2 white or yellow onions, chopped
- 8 turkey bacon slices (120 g), cut into 8 pieces each
- 1 pound (2 cups/454 g) dried white beans, cleaned, rinsed, and soaked
- 5½ cups (1.3 L) water

- ¾ cup (180 ml) real maple syrup
- 2 tablespoons Dijon mustard
- 1 bay leaf
- 1 teaspoon hot sauce (such as Tabasco)
- 1 teaspoon white pepper
- ½ teaspoon kosher salt

1. Preheat the oven to 325°F (165°C).

2. Sauté the onions and bacon in a Dutch oven over medium-high heat until the onions are softened and translucent and the bacon is crisped, about 5 minutes. Drain any excess fat.

3. Add the beans, water, ½ cup (120 ml) of the maple syrup, the mustard, bay leaf, hot sauce, pepper, and salt. Bring to a boil. Cover and place in the oven. Bake for about 2½ hours, stirring every 45 minutes, until the beans have absorbed most of the water.

4. Uncover, stir in the remaining ¼ cup (60 ml) of maple syrup, and bake for 30 minutes or until the beans have thickened and are creamy yet tender. Remove and discard the bay leaf, then serve. Store in an airtight container in the refrigerator for up to 4 days. To freeze, package 1- to 2-cup (175 to 350 g) portions in freezer bags. Press out as much air as you can, seal, label, and freeze for up to 4 months. Thaw in the refrigerator.

Per Serving: Calories 205; Protein 8 g; Carbs 37 g; Dietary Fiber 6 g; Added Sugars 18 g; Total Fat 3 g; Sat Fat 1 g; Omega-3s 110 mg; Sodium 330 mg; Potassium 406 mg

BAKED BEANS WITH POMEGRANATE & CANADIAN BACON

Makes 8 servings

This is a unique, flavorful baked-bean dish; you can taste the pomegranate along with a little bit of heat in each bite. The beans cook up thick and bubbly and have an appealing deep red-brown hue from the sweet chili sauce.

- 2 teaspoons extra virgin olive oil
- 3 cups (525 g) Simply Cooked White Beans (page 241) or two 15-ounce (425 g) cans cannellini, great Northern, or navy beans, drained and rinsed

1 red onion, chopped

3.5 ounces (100 g) sliced or ¾ cup (105 g) cubed Canadian bacon

1 cup (240 ml) sweet red chile sauce

¾ cup (180 ml) 100% pomegranate juice

2 tablespoons honey

1 teaspoon Dijon mustard

1. Preheat the oven to 350°F (180°C). Brush the bottom of a 2-quart (2 L) or 8-inch (20 cm) square baking dish with oil.

2. Combine the beans, onion, and bacon in the baking dish. In a small bowl, whisk together the chili sauce, pomegranate juice, honey, and mustard. Pour over the bean mixture; mix well. Cover and bake for 30 minutes, until the beans are hot and bubbly, and a digital food thermometer reads 165°F (75°C. Serve hot.

3. Store in an airtight container in the refrigerator for up to 4 days. To freeze, divide and package in 1- to 2-cup (175 to 350 g) portions in freezer bags. Press out as much air as you can, seal, label, and freeze for up to 4 months. Thaw in the refrigerator overnight or place in a bowl of warm water, massaging every few minutes to break up the beans.

Per Serving: Calories 179; Protein 5 g; Carbs 33 g; Dietary Fiber 4 g; Added Sugars 4 g; Total Fat 3 g; Sat Fat 1 g; Omega-3s 20 mg; Sodium 614 mg; Potassium 277 mg

RED BEANS & RICE

Makes 6 servings

Red beans and rice is a Monday-night dish in Louisiana, appearing in homes and on restaurant menus throughout Creole country. This is a fast, easy recipe made with canned beans. If you can't find canned small red beans, use dark red kidney beans.

1 tablespoon extra virgin olive oil

1 white or yellow onion, diced

2 celery stalks, diced

1 green bell pepper, seeded and diced

Two 15-ounce (425 g) cans small red beans or dark red kidney beans, drained and rinsed

2 garlic cloves, minced

1 cup (240 ml) water

1 tablespoon Cajun Seasoning (page 30)

1 bay leaf

½ teaspoon freshly ground black pepper

6 cups (1,170 g) Simply Cooked Brown Rice (page 230), warmed

4 green onions, thinly sliced, optional

1. Heat the oil in a large sauté pan or Dutch oven over medium heat, then add the onion, celery, and bell pepper. Cover and cook the vegetables, stirring occasionally, until they soften, 15 to 20 minutes; don't let them brown.

2. Add the beans, water, garlic, seasoning, bay leaf, and pepper. Stir gently, cover again, and simmer for 10 minutes. Remove bay leaf prior to serving.

3. To serve, divide the rice among six bowls. Top with 1 cup (170 g) of the red bean mixture, and garnish with green onions if desired.

Per Serving: Calories 762; Protein 21 g; Carbs 153 g; Dietary Fiber 12 g; Added Sugars 3 g; Total Fat 13 g; Sat Fat 1 g; Omega-3s 50 mg; Sodium 280 mg; Potassium 205 mg

REFRIED BEANS

Makes 4 servings

While refried beans are typically made with pinto beans, you can use any bean you like in this recipe. The beans can be eaten as a side dish, as a dip with our Crispy Cajun Corn Chips (page 339), or use as the base to build a bean burrito or taco with Pico de Gallo (page 61) and Tomato Corn Salsa (page 62).

1 tablespoon extra virgin olive oil

½ red onion, finely chopped

2 jalapeño chiles, seeded and finely chopped

2 garlic cloves, finely chopped

1 tablespoon chili powder

One 15-ounce (425 g) can black, red, pinto, or kidney beans

½ cup (120 ml) liquid reserved from the can of beans

2 tablespoons chopped fresh cilantro

1. Heat the oil in a large skillet over medium high heat. Add the onion and sauté for 2 minutes. As onion begins to soften, add the jalapeños and garlic. Sauté until the jalapeños begin to soften and the onions begin to brown on the edges, about 1 minute. Reduce the heat to medium-low and stir in the chili powder.

2. Drain and rinse the beans, then stir them into the onion mixture. Add the reserved bean liquid. Cook, mashing the beans with a fork or potato masher until most (but not all) of the beans are mashed, the mixture has a somewhat smooth, thick texture, and most of the liquid has been absorbed, about 5 minutes. Remove from the heat, sprinkle cilantro on top, and serve.

Per Serving: Calories 186; Protein 10 g; Carbs 28 g; Dietary Fiber 10 g; Added Sugars 0 g; Total Fat 4 g; Sat Fat 1 g; Omega-3s 150 mg; Sodium 306 mg; Potassium 463 mg

SALMON & WHITE BEAN BOWLS WITH LIME & DILL

Makes 4 servings

Take simply cooked grains and beans and turn them into a fast, easy, one-bowl meal. Here we combine Simply Cooked White Beans and Simply Cooked Brown Rice with salmon. We love this bowl with our Citrusy Walnut Gremolata (page 63), but it's also great with Horseradish-Dijon Aïoli (page 44) or Cucumber-Dill Sauce (page 54).

Grated zest of 1 lime

4 tablespoons plus 1 teaspoon (2 g) minced fresh dill

⅛ teaspoon kosher salt

¼ teaspoon freshly ground black pepper

1 pound (454 g) fresh skin-on salmon fillet (1 whole or four 4-ounce/113 g fillets)

2 cups (350 g) Simply Cooked White Beans (page 241), warmed

2 cups (390 g) Simply Cooked Brown Rice (page 230), warmed

4 teaspoons extra virgin olive oil

4 teaspoons balsamic vinegar

One 3 to 6-ounce (85 to 170 g) bag microgreens or baby spring mix

4 tablespoons (25 g) Citrusy Walnut Gremolata (page 63)

1 lime, quartered

1. Preheat the oven to 400°F (200°C). Line a rimmed baking sheet with parchment paper.

2. Combine the lime zest, 3 tablespoons of the dill, the salt, and pepper in a small bowl. Place the salmon skin side down on the baking sheet and spread the mixture evenly over the fish. Bake for 15 minutes or until the salmon is opaque and flakes easily with a fork and a digital food thermometer reads 145°F (65°C) when inserted in the thickest part of the fillet. Remove from the oven and let rest for a few minutes.

3. Divide the beans and brown rice among four bowls. Drizzle each bowl with 1 teaspoon of the oil and 1 teaspoon of the balsamic vinegar. Break the roasted salmon into chunks using two forks. Divide evenly among the bowls, placing the salmon to one side and leaving the skin behind. Sprinkle 1 teaspoon of the remaining dill on top of each bowl. Add a handful of microgreens to the side opposite the salmon. Drizzle 1 teaspoon oil and 1 teaspoon balsamic vinegar over the greens in each bowl.

4. Top each bowl with 1 tablespoon gremolata. Add a lime wedge and serve.

Serving Size 1 bowl; Calories 723; Protein 36 g; Carbs 86 g; Dietary Fiber 11 g; Added Sugars 0 g; Total Fat 29 g; Sat Fat 5 g; Omega-3s 2,580 mg; Sodium 230 mg; Potassium 733 mg

SPICY BLACK BEAN CHILI

Makes 8 servings

This chili whips up in no time when made with our Simply Cooked Black Beans. Top the chili bowls with yogurt and Citrusy Walnut Gremolata. Yum!

2 tablespoons cumin seeds

2 tablespoons dried oregano

¼ cup (60 ml) extra virgin olive oil

2 yellow onions, finely chopped

1½ cups (225 g) finely chopped green bell pepper (about 2 peppers)

2 garlic cloves, minced

1½ tablespoons smoked paprika

1 teaspoon cayenne

6 cups (1,035 g) Simply Cooked Black Beans (page 241)

1 cup (240 ml) reduced-sodium Vegetable Broth (page 72)

½ cup (45 g) finely chopped fresh jalapeño chiles

Two 15-ounce (425 g) cans no-salt-added crushed tomatoes

1 cup (245 g) plain reduced-fat yogurt

½ cup (50 g) Citrusy Walnut Gremolata (page 63)

1. Place the cumin and oregano in a small dry skillet over medium heat. Swirl them around in the pan as they toast until fragrant, about 1 minute. Remove from the heat.

2. Heat the oil in a large stockpot or saucepan over medium heat. Add the onions, pepper, garlic, cayenne, paprika, and the toasted cumin and oregano. Cook, stirring occasionally, until the onions are soft, about 4 minutes.

3. Stir in the beans, broth, jalapeños, and tomatoes. Bring to a boil over high heat, then reduce to a simmer. Cook until the mixture has thickened and is hot and bubbling, about 20 minutes.

4. Divide the chili among bowls and top with yogurt and gremolata. Serve hot. Store in an airtight container in the refrigerator for up to 4 days. To freeze, package in 1- to 2-cup (175 to 350 g) portions in airtight freezer-safe containers and freeze for up to 4 months.

Per Serving: Calories 537; Protein 28 g; Carbs 85 g; Dietary Fiber 22 g; Added Sugars 0 g; Total Fat 11 g; Sat Fat 2 g; Omega-3s 560 mg; Sodium 84 mg; Potassium 2,157 mg

WHITE BEAN SALAD WITH LEMON & ROSEMARY

Makes 4 servings

You can use canned beans for this salad, but if you cook beans from dried, we recommend tossing the cooked beans with the dressing for this salad while they're still warm; they'll absorb more flavor from the dressing.

2 cups (350 g) Simply Cooked White Beans (page 241)

½ cup (80 g) minced sweet onion (such as Vidalia or Walla Walla)

1 ancho (dried poblano) chile, soaked in hot water (see Note), drained, and minced

3 tablespoons extra virgin olive oil

Grated zest of 1 lemon

2 tablespoons fresh lemon juice

3 tablespoons chopped fresh rosemary

1 garlic clove, minced

¼ teaspoon freshly ground black pepper

4 lettuce leaves, such as red leaf, Boston, or Bibb

1. Combine the beans, onion, chile, oil, lemon zest and juice, 2 tablespoons of the rosemary, the garlic, and pepper in a medium bowl. Cover and refrigerate for 2 hours, until well chilled.

2. Line four serving plates or bowls with lettuce leaves, spoon the bean salad on top, and sprinkle with the remaining 1 tablespoon rosemary.

NOTE: Rehydrating dried chiles is easy: Place the chile in a bowl, cover with hot water, and leave to soak for 10 to 15 minutes. When the chile is soft, drain off the water, remove the seeds and stem, and mince.

Per Serving: Calories 183; Protein 4 g; Carbs 15 g; Dietary Fiber 7 g; Added Sugars 0 g; Total Fat 12 g; Sat Fat 2 g; Omega-3s 100 mg; Sodium 9 mg; Potassium 391 mg

CLASSIC HUMMUS

Makes 2½ cups (480 g); 5 servings

This Middle Eastern dish consists of ground chickpeas, olive oil, garlic, lemon juice, and tahini (sesame paste). Hummus provides plant-based protein as well as dietary fiber, which has many health benefits including improving our heart health. We love to serve it with either fresh whole grain pita bread, cut into triangles, or with our Southwest Pita Chips.

One 15-ounce (425 g) can chickpeas, drained and rinsed

⅓ cup (80 g) sesame tahini

3 garlic cloves, halved

3 tablespoons fresh lemon juice

1 tablespoon hot water

½ cup (30 g) coarsely chopped fresh flat-leaf parsley

½ teaspoon chili powder

½ teaspoon ground cumin

3 tablespoons extra virgin olive oil, plus more for drizzling

⅛ teaspoon kosher salt

2 tablespoons toasted sesame seeds, optional

5 whole grain pita breads, cut into 6 wedges each, or Southwest Pita Chips (page 340), optional

1. Place the chickpeas, tahini, garlic, lemon juice, and water in a food processor or blender. Process to form a smooth, thick mixture.

2. Add ¼ cup (15 g) of the parsley, the chili powder, and cumin and process until blended. Add 3 tablespoons of the oil, 1 tablespoon at a time, streaming in if using a mixer or food processor with an opening in the cover, or adding between pulses if using a blender. Process until smooth and creamy, then add the salt. Process to combine.

3. To serve, place the hummus in a shallow bowl or in the middle of a platter, rim with the remaining ¼ cup (15 g) parsley, drizzle with the remaining 1 teaspoon oil. Sprinkle with the sesame seeds and surround with pita wedges, if using.

NOTE: Sesame tahini can go rancid quickly if stored at room temperature after opening. We recommend storing it in the refrigerator to maintain its fresh flavor.

Serving Size ½ cup (96 g); Calories 243; Protein 7 g; Carbs 17 g; Dietary Fiber 4 g; Added Sugars 0 g; Total Fat 18 g; Sat Fat 3 g; Omega-3s 150 mg; Sodium 146 mg; Potassium 184 mg

EASTERN MEDITERRANEAN BOWLS WITH HUMMUS & TABBOULEH

Makes 4 servings

This bowl brings together many ingredients commonly found in Mediterranean cuisines, including beans, seeds, whole grains, and yogurt, as well as fresh herbs, aromatics, and produce. We like to use fresh pita bread to soak up all the juices and flavor.

Hummus

Two 15-ounce (425 g) cans chickpeas, drained and rinsed

One 5.3-ounce (150 g) container plain Greek yogurt (about ⅔ cup)

½ cup (120 g) sesame tahini

¼ cup (15 g) chopped fresh flat-leaf parsley

3 tablespoons fresh lemon juice

2 garlic cloves, minced

1 teaspoon ground cumin

Bowls

2 cups (315 g) Simply Cooked Barley (page 223)

2 cups (400 g) Tabbouleh (page 225)

1 English cucumber, sliced

6 radishes, thinly sliced into half moons

1 lemon, quartered

½ cup (120 ml) balsamic vinegar

¼ cup (60 ml) extra virgin olive oil

4 whole wheat pita breads, cut into 6 wedges each

1. Place the chickpeas, yogurt, tahini, parsley, lemon juice, garlic, and cumin in a food processor or blender. Blend until smooth.

2. Divide the barley among four bowls. Add the hummus and tabbouleh on top of the barley, side by side. Top with the cucumber and radishes and add a lemon wedge. Splash each bowl with 2 tablespoons vinegar and 1 tablespoon oil. Enjoy with fresh pita bread.

Serving Size 1 bowl; Calories 887; Protein 27 g; Carbs 106 g; Dietary Fiber 18 g; Added Sugars 0 g; Total Fat 43 g; Sat Fat 6 g; Omega-3s 380 mg; Sodium 677 mg; Potassium 836 mg

GREEK-INSPIRED BAKED CHICKPEAS WITH TOMATOES & FETA

Makes 4 servings

This delicious recipe is very easy to prepare. Simply combine all of the ingredients, bake for 45 minutes, and dinner is ready. This dish can be enjoyed on its own or paired with roast chicken, grilled shrimp, or grilled lamb chops. Having a piece of hearty whole grain bread at the ready for sopping up the sauce is a wonderful way to enjoy every morsel.

Two 15-ounce (425 g) cans chickpeas, drained and rinsed

One 14.5-ounce (411 g) can diced tomatoes

4 ounces (113 g) crumbled feta

¼ cup (60 ml) extra virgin olive oil

2 tablespoons honey

1 tablespoon dried oregano

¼ teaspoon red pepper flakes

1 lemon, quartered, optional

1. Preheat the oven to 350°F (180°C).

2. Combine the chickpeas, tomatoes, feta, oil, honey, oregano, and red pepper flakes in an 8-inch (20 cm) square baking dish. Bake for 45 minutes, until much of the liquid has evaporated and some pieces of feta have started to brown.

3. Serve with lemon wedges on the side for an optional burst of bright acidity to balance the flavors.

Per Serving: Calories 409; Protein 12 g; Carbs 40 g; Dietary Fiber 9 g; Added Sugars 9 g; Total Fat 23 g; Sat Fat 6 g; Omega-3s 220 mg; Sodium 655 mg; Potassium 346 mg

SIMPLY COOKED LENTILS

Makes 2 cups (380 g)

Lentils are a favorite! They're inexpensive, shelf-stable, nutritious, filling, and very flavorful. Plus, they require no soaking prior to cooking. This Simply Cooked recipe is so tasty you may want to eat them right from the pot.

1 cup (190 g) dry brown or green lentils, cleaned and rinsed

2½ cups (600 ml) water

1 bay leaf

¼ teaspoon freshly ground black pepper

Juice of ½ lemon or ½ lime

1. Place the lentils, water, bay leaf, and pepper in a medium saucepan. Bring to a boil, cover partially with a lid, and reduce the heat to a gentle simmer. Cook until the lentils are tender but still intact, 20 to 30 minutes.

2. Remove from the heat, discard the bay leaf, and add the lemon juice.

3. Store in an airtight container in the refrigerator for up to 4 days. Freeze by dividing and packaging in 1-cup (190 g) portions in airtight freezer-safe containers or heavy-duty bags. Press out as much air as you can, seal, label, and freeze for up to 4 months. Thaw in the refrigerator overnight or place in a bowl of warm water, massaging every few minutes to break up the lentils.

Serving Size 1 cup (190 g); Calories 344; Protein 21 g; Carbs 61 g; Dietary Fiber 36 g; Added Sugars 0 g; Total Fat 1 g; Sat Fat 0 g; Omega-3s 0 mg; Sodium 12 mg; Potassium 919 mg

FRAGRANT WARM SPICED LENTILS

Makes 4 servings

You'll love the aromas generated by these lentils as they simmer. Top a bowl of these lentils with Greek yogurt and our Hot Mango Chutney (page 65) to create a fragrant, flavorful, and nutrient-rich meal.

1 cup (190 g) uncooked brown or green lentils, cleaned and rinsed

2½ cups (600 ml) water

1 cinnamon stick

3 green cardamom pods

1 whole clove

Juice of ½ lemon

2 tablespoons extra virgin olive oil

1. Combine the lentils, water, cinnamon, cardamom, and clove in a medium saucepan. Bring to a boil, cover partially with a lid, and reduce the heat to a gentle simmer. Cook until the lentils are tender but still intact, 20 to 30 minutes.

2. Remove and discard the cinnamon, cardamom, and clove. Stir in the lemon juice. Transfer to a serving bowl, drizzle with oil, and serve.

Per Serving: Calories 146; Protein 4 g; Carbs 10 g; Dietary Fiber 4 g; Added Sugars 0 g; Total Fat 10 g; Sat Fat 1 g; Omega-3s 220 mg; Sodium 104 mg; Potassium 178 mg

EAST INDIAN–INSPIRED LENTIL & CHICKPEA DAL BOWLS

Makes 8 servings

Dal refers both to dried legumes, typically lentils or chick-peas, and to the aromatic, comforting Indian dish of cooked legumes with fragrant spices. Usually, a dal recipe will have a tadka (tempering)—whole spices cooked in hot fat, either oil or ghee (clarified butter)—to flavor the dish.

Spinach-Lentil Dal

1 tablespoon extra virgin olive oil

1 teaspoon cumin seeds

1 teaspoon black or brown mustard seeds

½ teaspoon black cumin (nigella) seeds

1 cup (190 g) red lentils, cleaned, rinsed, and drained

1 teaspoon ground turmeric

¼ teaspoon ground fenugreek

5 cups (1.2 L) water

One 5- to 6-ounce (142 to 170 g) bag baby spinach leaves (about 4 cups)

Chana Dal

4 cups (960 ml) water

1 cup (200 g) chana dal (split chickpeas)

1 bay leaf

1 teaspoon ground turmeric

3 tablespoons extra virgin olive oil

¾ cup (160 g) minced onion (1 medium)

1 teaspoon cumin seeds

2 tomatoes, finely diced

1 tablespoon minced serrano chile

4 garlic cloves, minced

1 teaspoon finely chopped fresh ginger

1 teaspoon garam masala

¼ cup (4 g) finely chopped fresh cilantro

To Serve

3 cups (585 g) Simply Cooked Brown Rice (page 230), at room temperature or warm

1 cup (230 g) plain Greek yogurt

2 tablespoons fresh lime or lemon juice

2 limes or lemons, quartered

½ cup (8 g) finely chopped cilantro

4 whole wheat naan, cut into 6 wedges each

1. To prepare the spinach-lentil dal, start by making its tadka. Heat the oil, cumin seeds, mustard seeds, and black cumin seeds in a medium saucepan over medium heat. Cook, stirring continuously, until the spices sizzle and pop, about 45 seconds. Quickly add the lentils, turmeric, and fenugreek, stirring constantly for 30 seconds. Be careful, as the oil may splatter. Add the water and bring to a boil. Simmer until the lentils are completely cooked, tender but firm, 15 to 20 minutes.

2. Stir in the spinach, one handful at a time. Simmer until the spinach is fully wilted, 5 minutes, then remove from the heat and allow to cool to room temperature.

3. To prepare the chana dal, bring the water, chana dal, bay leaf, and turmeric to a boil in a medium saucepan. Reduce the heat to a simmer and cook until tender, 45 to 65 minutes.

4. While the chana dal cook, combine the oil, onions, and cumin seeds in a large sauté pan over medium heat. Cook until the onion is just starting to brown on the outside, about 2 minutes. Add the tomatoes, reduce the heat to medium low, cover, and cook until the tomatoes are soft, 6 to 7 minutes. Add the serrano, garlic, and ginger. Cook, stirring frequently, to create a paste, about 4 minutes. The contents of the pan should be sizzling, and the onions may stick a little, but don't let them burn. Add the garam masala and cook until fragrant, 1 minute.

5. When the chana dal are fully cooked, remove the bay leaf and stir in the tomato-onion paste and the cilantro. Let cool to room temperature.

6. To serve, divide the rice among eight bowls. Add a scoop of each dal on top of the rice, placing them side by side. Add 2 tablespoons of yogurt and a splash of lime juice to each, then sprinkle cilantro over the top. Add a lime wedge and a few pieces of naan to each bowl.

Serving Size 1 bowl; Calories 668; Protein 24 g; Carbs 109 g; Dietary Fiber 12 g; Added Sugars 3 g; Total Fat 18 g; Sat Fat 3 g; Omega-3s 140 mg; Sodium 557 mg; Potassium 512 mg

GINGER LENTILS

Makes 4 servings

Fresh ginger offers a lovely aroma as well as a bit of peppery heat, providing a counterbalance to the mild nutty flavor of lentils. These lentils are the star of our Ginger Lentil & Brown Rice Bake (see this page).

- 3 tablespoons extra virgin olive oil
- 2 teaspoons grated fresh ginger
- 1 green bell pepper, seeded and diced
- 3 or 4 green onions, chopped
- 3 cups (570 g) Simply Cooked Lentils (page 247)
- 2 tablespoons white wine vinegar

Heat the oil and ginger in a medium skillet over medium heat, stirring often, until the ginger is fragrant, 1 minute. Add the bell pepper and onions. Sauté until the peppers are crisp-tender, 2 minutes. Add the lentils and vinegar. Heat until the lentils are warmed through, about 5 minutes. Serve warm.

Per Serving: Calories 231; Protein 8 g; Carbs 25 g; Dietary Fiber 14 g; Added Sugars 0 g; Total Fat 11 g; Sat Fat 2 g; Omega-3s 80 mg; Sodium 8 mg; Potassium 427 mg

GINGER LENTIL & BROWN RICE BAKE

Makes 6 servings

This dish can be served as wonderful vegetarian entrée paired with our Watermelon, Grapefruit & Blueberry Salad (page 145) or served as an accompaniment to our Chicken Tikka Masala (page 309).

- Cooking spray
- 3 cups (585 g) Simply Cooked Brown Rice (page 230)
- 3 cups (600 g) Ginger Lentils (see this page)
- ½ cup (75 g) crumbled feta
- 1 tablespoon extra virgin olive oil
- ⅛ teaspoon kosher salt
- ½ teaspoon freshly ground black pepper

1. Preheat the oven to 350°F (180°C). Spray a 9-inch (23 cm) square baking dish with cooking spray.

2. Spread the rice on the bottom of the baking dish, top with the lentils, then the feta. Drizzle with oil, then sprinkle with salt and pepper. Cover with foil and bake for 20 minutes or until heated through.

3. Uncover and bake for another 10 minutes or until the dish is bubbling and the feta is starting to brown. Serve hot. Store in an airtight container in the refrigerator for up to 4 days. To freeze, store in an airtight freezer- and oven-safe container in the freezer for up to 4 months.

Per Serving: Calories 503; Protein 14 g; Carbs 82 g; Dietary Fiber 11 g; Added Sugars 0 g; Total Fat 16 g; Sat Fat 3 g; Omega-3s 100 mg; Sodium 223 mg; Potassium 219 mg

LENTIL-FENNEL LASAGNA

Makes 12 servings

Lentils take the place of meat in this comforting take on a classic layered pasta. The fresh fennel and fennel seeds provide a subtle licorice flavor typically found in Italian sausage. This vegetarian lasagna is just as good on the next day or two as it is on the day it's made.

- Cooking spray
- 1 large red onion, cut into large chunks
- 2 celery stalks, cut into large chunks
- 1 fennel bulb, trimmed and cut into large chunks
- ½ cup (60 ml) extra virgin olive oil
- 3 or 4 garlic cloves, minced
- ¼ cup (15 g) Italian Seasoning (page 34)
- 1 tablespoon fennel seeds
- 1 teaspoon red pepper flakes
- 1 teaspoon kosher salt
- One 28-ounce (794 g) can crushed tomatoes
- One 12-ounce (411 g) can tomato paste
- 2 cups (480 ml) water
- 5 cups (950 g) Simply Cooked Lentils (page 247)
- One 15-ounce (425 g) container part-skim ricotta
- One 16-ounce (454 g) box lasagna noodles
- ½ cup (40 g) freshly grated Parmesan
- Fresh basil leaves, optional

1. Preheat the oven to 350°F (180°C). Spray the bottom and sides of a 9 × 13-inch (23 × 33 cm) baking dish with cooking spray.

2. Place the onion, celery, and fennel in a food processor and process until finely shredded. Combine the shredded vegetables, oil, garlic, seasoning, fennel seeds, red pepper flakes, and salt in a large Dutch oven over medium heat. Cook, stirring often, until most of the moisture has evaporated, 12 to 15 minutes.

3. Stir in the tomatoes, tomato paste, and water. Reduce the heat to medium-low, cover, and simmer for 10 minutes.

4. Turn off the heat and stir in the lentils and ricotta.

5. Assemble the lasagna according to the guide below. Spread 2 cups (520 g) of the lentil sauce in the baking dish. Top with 5 lasagna noodles. Spoon 3 cups (780 g) of the sauce for the next layer, followed by 5 lasagna noodles. Continue layering until you've used up the sauce and noodles. The top layer (layer 9) should be sauce. Place the baking dish on a larger baking sheet and bake for 15 minutes.

6. Sprinkle with the Parmesan and bake for another 15 minutes or until a digital food thermometer reads 165°F (75°C). Store covered in the refrigerator for up to 3 days or in the freezer for up to 2 months.

Per Serving: Calories 387; Protein 17 g; Carbs 59 g; Dietary Fiber 14 g; Added Sugars 0 g; Total Fat 9 g; Sat Fat 3 g; Omega-3s 80 mg; Sodium 240 mg; Potassium 1,035 mg

Lentil-Fennel Lasagna Assembly Guide

LAYER	COMPONENT
1	2 cups (520 g) sauce
2	5 lasagna noodles
3	3 cups (780 g) sauce
4	5 lasagna noodles
5	3 cups (780 g) sauce
6	5 lasagna noodles
7	3 cups (780 g) sauce
8	5 lasagna noodles
9	3 cups (780 g) sauce
10	½ cup (40 g) Parmesan

CRISPY TOFU BITES

Makes 72 cubes (about 4 cups/625 g)

These tofu bites can be eaten right from the pan, added to stir-fried vegetables, or paired with a whole grain or greens salad bowl. We love making tacos with these tasty bites by adding them to warm corn tortillas, then filling with Wasabi-Ginger Coleslaw (page 155), drizzling with Honey-Ginger Dressing (page 50), and sprinkling with sesame seeds. Yum!

One 15.5- to 16-ounce (439 to 454 g) package extra firm tofu, drained, pressed, and patted dry (see Tip)

2 tablespoons reduced-sodium soy sauce

1 tablespoon rice vinegar

3 garlic cloves, finely minced

1 teaspoon brown sugar

1 teaspoon Chinese Five-Spice Blend (page 31)

¼ cup (40 g) cornstarch or whole wheat pastry flour

1½ cups (330 g) Garlic & Herb Bread Crumbs (page 33)

2 teaspoons extra virgin olive oil

1 teaspoon toasted sesame oil

¼ cup (12 g) sesame seeds

1. Using a twin pack of extra firm tofu, cut the tofu in half lengthwise, then cut each half lengthwise into 3 equal rows. Cut each row into 6 equal pieces (18 cubes total). Repeat the steps on the other half to make 36 cubes. Open the other twin pack and repeat the steps, for a total of 72 cubes. Gently prick the top and bottom of the tofu cubes with a fork to help it absorb the marinade. Arrange the tofu cubes in a single layer in a shallow glass baking dish. Whisk the soy sauce, vinegar, garlic, brown sugar, and five-spice blend in a small bowl. Spoon the marinade over the tofu, flip the pieces a couple of times, and marinate for 20 minutes.

2. Place the flour in a shallow bowl. Place the bread crumbs in a separate bowl. Transfer the tofu to a large plate with a slotted spatula. Leave the marinade in the baking dish.

3. Heat a large skillet on medium-high heat and add the olive and sesame oils. Heat the oil until it shimmers but doesn't smoke.

4. Dredge each tofu slice first in the flour to coat all sides, then dip in the marinade, then dredge in the bread crumbs. Place the slices immediately into the hot oil and sauté until golden brown, about 2 minutes. Gently flip the tofu slices and sauté until the tofu is golden brown on the second side, 1 minute. Sprinkle each serving with 1 tablespoon sesame seeds.

TIP: *Pressing your tofu before you start cooking helps remove any excess liquid to allow for better absorption of the marinade. This is an important step when pan-frying your tofu; it ensures a crisp exterior and a velvety compact interior. First, drain the water and gently remove the block of tofu from its packaging. Wrap the tofu in 3 to 4 sheets of paper towels and place on a rimmed plate. Place a flat cutting board on top of the tofu and weight it down with a heavy cookbook, a couple cans of vegetables, or a heavy pan, and let it "press" for 15 to 30 minutes. Then, drain any water from the plate, dispose of the towels, and dice or slice your tofu. If you are "pressed" for time, you can simply drain the water from the tofu packaging, dice or slice the tofu, and then blot or gently pat the pieces with a paper towel to dry. If you purchase super firm tofu, no pressing is required.*

Serving Size 1 cup (156 g); Calories 428; Protein 22 g; Carbs 43 g; Dietary Fiber 5 g; Added Sugars 1 g; Total Fat 20 g; Sat Fat 3 g; Omega-3s 80 mg; Sodium 698 mg; Potassium 98 mg

TOFU ITALIANO BAKE

Makes 8 servings

This delicious bake is often mistaken for lasagna when Linda brings it to potlucks. People are quite surprised that it has tofu, which shows how versatile tofu is, absorbing rich flavors from the spices and sauces yet imparting just the right texture to be mistaken for noodles. This recipe might just make you a tofu enthusiast!

- 2 teaspoons extra virgin olive oil
- Two 16-ounce (454 g) packages silken tofu, extra firm, blotted dry and diced
- 1½ cups (475 g) Simply Cooked Fresh Tomato Sauce (page 59)
- One 14.5-ounce (411 g) can petite diced tomatoes
- 1 onion, chopped
- 1 green or red bell pepper, seeded and chopped
- 3 large eggs
- ⅓ cup (40 g) all-purpose flour
- 4 garlic cloves, minced
- 3 tablespoons chopped fresh basil leaves
- ½ teaspoon ground nutmeg
- 16 ounces (4 cups/454 g) shredded part-skim mozzarella

1. Preheat the oven to 350°F (180°C). Line a 9 × 13-inch (23 × 33 cm) baking pan with foil, then brush with the oil.

2. Mix the tofu, tomato sauce, tomatoes, onion, bell pepper, eggs, flour, garlic, basil, and nutmeg in a large bowl. Spread half of the mixture into the baking pan. Top with 2 cups (227 g) of the mozzarella. Cover with the remaining tofu mixture, then cover the pan with foil. Bake for 40 minutes, or until hot and steamy. Uncover and sprinkle with the remaining 2 cups (227 g) mozzarella. Bake uncovered for another 10 minutes, until the cheese is melted and slightly brown and a digital food thermometer reads 165°F (75°C) when inserted in the center. Remove from the oven, tent with foil, and let rest for 10 minutes before cutting or serving. Serve hot.

3. Store in an airtight container in the refrigerator for up to 4 days and reheat in the microwave, or store in an airtight freezer- and oven-safe container in the freezer for up to 3 months and reheat in the oven.

Per Serving: Calories 317; Protein 23 g; Carbs 15 g; Dietary Fiber 3 g; Added Sugars 0 g; Total Fat 17 g; Sat Fat 8 g; Omega-3s 90 mg; Sodium 527 mg; Potassium 329 mg

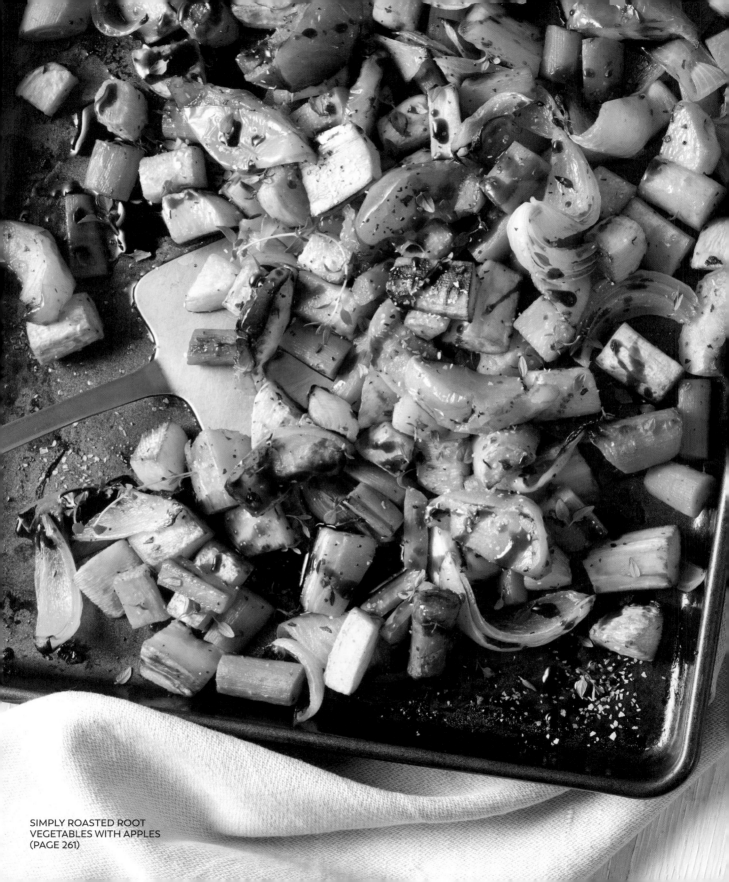

SIMPLY ROASTED ROOT
VEGETABLES WITH APPLES
(PAGE 261)

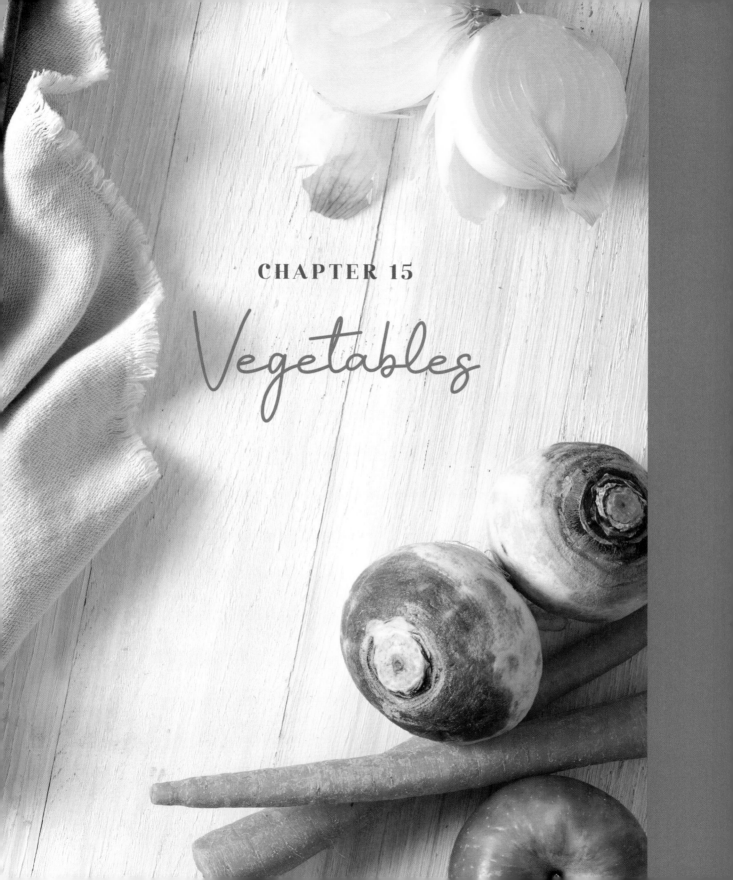

CHAPTER 15

Vegetables

Vegetables

Seasoning Vegetables 256

Simply Cooked Vegetables

Simply Roasted Butternut Squash 257

Simply Stewed Cabbage 257

Simply Roasted Carrots 257

Simply Roasted Cauliflower 258

Simply Roasted Garlic 258

Simply Roasted Green Beans 258

Simply Quick-Pickled Red Onions 259

Simply Roasted Peppers 259

Simply Spanish-Style Mashed
Potatoes 259

Simply Roasted Potatoes 260

Simply Smashed Potatoes 260

Simply Slow-Roasted Tomatoes 260

Simply Roasted Root Vegetables
with Apples 261

Simply Steamed Vegetable Medley 262

Simply Stir-Fried Vegetables 262

Simply Sautéed Zucchini 262

Seriously Seasoned Vegetables

Artichoke & Onions with
Lemon & Thyme 263

Asparagus with Sesame & Ginger 263

Citrus-Roasted Beets 264

Broccoli with Coriander & Tomatoes . . . 264

Maple-Roasted Brussels Sprouts 265

Tangy Sautéed Red Cabbage 265

Citrus-Glazed Carrots 265

Apricot & Sesame Roasted Carrots 266

Cardamom & Orange Roasted
Carrots 266

Fennel & Pear Roasted Carrots 266

Maple & Herb Roasted Carrots 267

Spicy Cauliflower Stir-Fry 267

Smoky Workaday Sweet Corn
& Pepper Sauté 268

Curiously Compatible Cucumbers
& Carrots 268

Smoky Roasted Mushrooms 269

Red Potato & Onion Roast with Cherry
Tomatoes & Kalamata Olives 269

Roasted Potatoes with Cinnamon 270

Rosemary Mashed Potatoes 270

Spicy Roasted Squash with
Tuscan-Style Glaze 271

Roasted Acorn Squash with
Allspice & Sage 271

Spaghetti Squash Sauté with
Black Olives & Feta 272

Savory Sweet Potato Fries 272

Roasted Sweet Potatoes
& Ginger-Spiced Apples 273

Fajita Vegetables 273

Quick-Pickled Vegetables 274

Savory Stuffed Vegetables

Garlicky Wild Rice & Mushroom–Stuffed
Acorn Squash 274

Bulgur-Stuffed Peppers 275

Mushroom & Spinach–Stuffed
Tomatoes 275

Curried Rice–Stuffed Tomatoes 276

Comforting Vegetable Casseroles

Cauliflower-Walnut Casserole 276

Creamy Eggplant with Tomatoes 277

Potato-Turnip Gratin 278

Vegetarian Shepherd's Pie 279

Flavor in food comes from two sources: ingredients and culinary techniques.

There are many factors that affect flavor in vegetables; quality is one of them. Quality is influenced by many factors, including

- the variety of vegetable (e.g., certain varieties of potatoes taste like butter even if no butter is added, and certain varieties of tomatoes taste sweeter than others);

- how and where the vegetable was grown (e.g., cruciferous vegetables like broccoli, cauliflower, and cabbage grown in colder climates taste sweeter);

- the environmental conditions a plant was exposed to during production (e.g., heat stress can cause some vegetables to produce more phytochemicals that have bitter flavors);

- storage conditions like temperature and humidity, as well as length of storage;

- the way the vegetable is processed (e.g., vegetables flash-frozen within hours of harvest retain "fresh-from-the-farm" flavors better than fresh vegetables that may take weeks to go from harvest to your kitchen).

Different vegetable cooking techniques bring out different flavors. This includes how a vegetable is cut, or if it isn't cut (e.g., minced garlic will have more intense flavor than coarsely chopped garlic) and if or how heat is applied (e.g., a roasted vegetable will develop caramelized flavors while a steamed vegetable will retain more "vegetal" flavors).

There are also many factors that influence how we perceive flavor in food. The classic saying "We eat with our eyes," refers to the impact of a food's visual appearance. A plate of brightly colored, beautifully cut, and artfully arranged assorted vegetables will likely be more appealing to most people than a pile of overcooked, dull, and mushy vegetables.

The next influence on our perception of flavor is aroma. Sensory scientists estimate that 80 percent of what we taste is perceived through our sense of smell. Most foods release more aromas when agitated or heated.

Textures in foods can also have an impact on our perception of flavor. For example, most people tend to prefer a creamy baked potato to a dry, crumbly one.

Some vegetables can be bitter, which is one reason many people say they don't like vegetables. But many ingredients and culinary techniques can tame these bitter flavors. Caramelizing bitter vegetables by roasting them is one method. Adding healthy fats like extra virgin olive oil is another.

All this sensory science boils down to one important point: If you don't like the flavor or texture of a vegetable prepared in one way, try another recipe, experiment with other culinary techniques, and continue this search until you find the ingredients, recipes, and techniques that are right for you. This is a much more effective way to get you and the people you cook for to eat more vegetables rather than finger wagging, cajoling, hiding vegetables in other foods, shaming, or game playing ("Finish your broccoli and you can have dessert!"). This is how Amy got her "I hate vegetables!" fiancé to become her vegetable-loving husband!

We organized the recipes in this chapter into a few categories.

- Simply Cooked recipes contain few ingredients and focus on a simple culinary technique. Some are perfect as a simple side dish, while others like Simply Roasted Garlic (page 258) and Simply Roasted Peppers (page 259) become ingredients for other recipes.

- Seriously Seasoned recipes focus on the use of ingredients like spices, herbs, aromatics, and acids like vinegars, as well as culinary techniques to enhance the flavor of the vegetables in the dish.

- Savory Stuffed recipes feature fillings made from vegetables, whole grains, or dairy. These recipes create individual servings that look beautiful on a plate as part of a meal.

- Comforting Vegetable Casseroles combine a variety of ingredients to create baked dishes that can be served as sides or main dishes, depending on the portion size.

Seasoning Vegetables

Here are some tips for spices, herbs, aromatics, and other ingredients that can add zest, zing, and flavors that sing to a variety of vegetables. Have fun finding your favorite combinations!

Table 9: Vegetable Seasoning Tips

VEGETABLE	SEASONING INGREDIENTS
Asparagus	Chervil, dill, garlic, lemon juice and zest, Dijon mustard, parsley, vinegar (red wine, tarragon)
Artichokes	Bay leaf, garlic, lemon juice and zest, mint, olive oil, onions, parsley, black pepper, thyme, tomatoes, vinegar (balsamic, red wine)
Beets	Basil, caraway seeds, chervil, chives, dill, garlic, honey, horseradish, lemon juice and zest, mint, black pepper, vinegar (balsamic, apple cider, tarragon)
Broccoli	Chiles, garlic, lemon juice and zest, ground mustard and mustard seeds, oregano, tarragon, thyme, vinegar (balsamic, red wine)
Brussels sprouts	Garlic, lemon juice, parsley, black pepper, thyme, vinegar (apple cider, white wine)
Cabbage	Apple cider, caraway seeds, celery seeds, garlic, ginger, Dijon mustard, ground mustard, black pepper, thyme, vinegar (champagne, apple cider, red wine, sherry, white wine)
Carrots	Chervil, chiles, cinnamon, coriander, cumin, dill, ginger, lemon juice, maple syrup, mint, orange juice, tarragon, thyme, white wine
Cauliflower	Cardamom, chili sauce, curry powder, dill, garlic, lemon juice and zest, mint, nutmeg, tarragon, thyme, vinegar (red wine, white wine)
Corn	Basil, bell peppers, cayenne, celery, chiles, chives, cilantro, dill, garlic, lime zest and juice, mushrooms
Green beans	Basil, cumin, dill, garlic, ginger, lemon juice, marjoram, onions, parsley, summer savory, tarragon, thyme, vinegar (red wine, white wine, rice, sherry)
Peas	Basil, bay leaf, celery, chives, dill, grassy extra virgin olive oil, garlic, lemon juice, mint, onions, parsley, black pepper, tarragon, thyme, champagne vinegar
Potatoes	Bay leaf, celery leaves, celery root, chives, garlic, grassy and peppery extra virgin olive oils, mushrooms, Dijon mustard, ground mustard, lemon juice, nutmeg, onions, parsley, black pepper, rosemary, sage, sorrel, thyme, vinegar (champagne, sherry, white wine)
Summer squash & zucchini	Basil, black pepper, chiles, chives, garlic, lemon juice and zest, marjoram, onions, oregano, parsley, sage, thyme, vinegar (balsamic, champagne, sherry, red wine, white wine)
Winter squash	Allspice, apple cider, cloves, coriander, cumin, garlic, ginger, maple syrup, nutmeg, onions, orange juice and zest, parsley, rosemary, sage, thyme
Tomatoes	Basil, bay leaf, bell peppers, chiles, chives, cilantro, fennel, garlic, lemon juice and zest, marjoram, onions, parsley, black pepper, thyme, vinegar (balsamic, raspberry, red wine, rice, sherry, tarragon, white wine)

SIMPLY ROASTED BUTTERNUT SQUASH

Makes 4 servings

Butternut squash is available year-round, fresh and frozen. When choosing fresh, select a squash that is heavy for its size. Cutting and peeling a squash can be challenging; if your local market sells precut squash, buy that to save time and effort.

> One 3-pound (1.4 kg) butternut squash, peeled and cut into 1-inch cubes
>
> 2 tablespoons extra virgin olive oil
>
> 2 tablespoons minced fresh thyme
>
> Freshly ground black pepper
>
> 2 tablespoons fresh lemon juice

1. Preheat the oven to 375°F (190°C). Line a baking sheet with foil or parchment paper.

2. Place the squash in a large bowl. Drizzle with oil, add the thyme, and toss to coat. Spread on the baking sheet in a single layer. Roast for 30 to 40 minutes, stirring occasionally, until fragrant and tender. Sprinkle with pepper, drizzle with lemon juice, and serve hot.

VARIATION: *Simply Roasted Acorn Squash*

This recipe also works well with acorn squash. To make 4 servings, buy 2 acorn squash, cut each squash in half vertically and scoop out the seeds. Place on a baking sheet cut side up and fill each half with 1½ teaspoons oil and 1½ teaspoons thyme. Roast for 50 to 60 minutes, until you can easily pierce the flesh with fork.

Per Serving: Calories 336; Protein 6 g; Carbs 71 g; Dietary Fiber 12 g; Added Sugars 0 g; Total Fat 8 g; Sat Fat 1 g; Omega-3s 210 mg; Sodium 24 mg; Potassium 2,127 mg

SIMPLY STEWED CABBAGE

Makes 6 servings

Green cabbage is hearty and delicious when stewed. Red cabbage can turn a bluish color when cooked, but the acid in the wine and tomatoes lessens this effect. You can save prep time by buying shredded cabbage.

> 2 tablespoons extra virgin olive oil
>
> 1 medium onion, chopped
>
> 1 green bell pepper, seeded and chopped
>
> 1 cup (100 g) thinly sliced celery (about 2 stalks)

> ½ cup (120 ml) dry white wine
>
> 3 cups (210 g) shredded green or red cabbage
>
> One 15-ounce (425 g) can no-salt-added diced tomatoes

Heat the oil in a large saucepan or skillet over medium heat. Add the onion, bell pepper, and celery. Sauté until the onion is translucent but not quite brown, 5 minutes. Add the wine and bring to a boil, about 1 minute. Add the cabbage, stirring until it has wilted some, about 5 minutes. Add the tomatoes and bring to a boil. Cover loosely, reduce the heat to medium-low, and simmer until the cabbage is tender, 12 to 15 minutes. Serve immediately.

Per Serving: Calories 94; Protein 1 g; Carbs 8 g; Dietary Fiber 3 g; Added Sugars 0 g; Total Fat 5 g; Sat Fat 1 g; Omega-3s 30 mg; Sodium 34 mg; Potassium 270 mg

SIMPLY ROASTED CARROTS

Makes 6 servings

Carrots are plentiful year-round, affordable, and have a long shelf life. We cut the carrot slices in half to shorten the roasting time and allow the natural sugars to caramelize. In this chapter, we offer three variations—Citrus-Glazed Carrots (page 265), Apricot & Sesame Roasted Carrots (page 266), and Cardamom & Orange Roasted Carrots (page 266).

> 2 pounds (907 g) carrots, halved lengthwise and sliced into ¼-inch-thick (6 mm) half-moons
>
> 2 tablespoons extra virgin olive oil
>
> ½ teaspoon freshly ground black pepper
>
> ¼ teaspoon kosher salt

1. Preheat the oven to 375°F (190°C). Line a rimmed baking sheet with parchment paper.

2. Combine the carrots, oil, pepper, and salt in a medium bowl. Toss well to coat. Spread the carrots in a single layer on the baking sheet. Roast for 20 to 25 minutes, until tender when pierced with a fork. Serve hot or cold. Store in an airtight container in the refrigerator for up to 5 days.

Per Serving: Calories 110; Protein 2 g; Carbs 16 g; Dietary Fiber 4 g; Added Sugars 0 g; Total Fat 5 g; Sat Fat 1 g; Omega-3s 30 mg; Sodium 109 mg; Potassium 3 mg

SIMPLY ROASTED CAULIFLOWER

Makes 4 servings

What could be easier than quickly trimming the leaves off the base of a whole head of cauliflower, placing the head on a baking sheet, and brushing it with an olive oil–spice blend before roasting, to create a stunning side dish for your next festive meal?

- 1 head cauliflower (1.5 to 2 pounds/680 to 907 g), trimmed
- 2 tablespoons extra virgin olive oil
- 1 tablespoon Habanero Spice Rub (page 33)
- ½ teaspoon kosher salt
- ½ teaspoon freshly ground black pepper
- 1 tablespoon butter, melted

1. Preheat the oven to 375°F (190°C).

2. Place the cauliflower stem end down in a baking dish or a cast-iron pan. Combine the oil, spice blend, salt, and pepper in a small bowl. Brush or spoon over the cauliflower. Bake for 60 to 75 minutes, until you can easily piece the cauliflower with a paring knife.

3. Transfer to a serving platter and drizzle with the butter.

Per Serving: Calories 130; Protein 3 g; Carbs 8 g; Dietary Fiber 3 g; Added Sugars 0 g; Total Fat 10 g; Sat Fat 3 g; Omega-3s 80 mg; Sodium 184 mg; Potassium 451 mg

SIMPLY ROASTED GARLIC

Makes 3 heads

When roasted, garlic becomes softer, sweeter, and spreadable. Roasted garlic cloves can be used in other recipes, like our Roasted Garlic Aïoli (page 45) or used as a simple spread for toasted baguettes.

- 3 heads garlic, unpeeled
- 3 teaspoons extra virgin olive oil

1. Preheat the oven to 350°F (180°C). Place a piece of foil at least 12 inches (30.5 cm) long on a baking sheet or pie plate.

2. Trim the top off each head of garlic, trimming enough to reveal most of the cloves. (Save any of the garlic tips you cut off to use in other recipes.)

3. Place the garlic, cut side up, on the foil. Drizzle each bulb with 1 teaspoon of the oil, focusing on getting as much oil on and in the bulbs as possible. Wrap the foil up and around the garlic. Fold the ends over each other to seal.

4. Roast for 55 to 70 minutes (depending on the size of the bulbs), until the cloves are golden brown and tender.

Serving Size 1 tablespoon; Calories 28; Protein 1 g; Carbs 4 g; Dietary Fiber 0 g; Added Sugars 0 g; Total Fat 1 g; Sat Fat 0 g; Omega-3s 10 mg; Sodium 2 mg; Potassium 47 mg

SIMPLY ROASTED GREEN BEANS

Makes 4 servings

These green beans are always received well by people who love finger foods, adults and kids alike! They can be eaten warm or at room temperature, and pair with everything from dishes like our Ginger Lentil & Brown Rice Bake (page 249) to chicken recipes like our Rosemary-Citrus Chicken (page 314).

- 1 pound (454 g) green beans, ends trimmed
- 2 tablespoons extra virgin olive oil
- 1 tablespoon Italian Seasoning (page 34)
- ¼ teaspoon kosher salt
- 1 lemon, quartered

1. Preheat the oven to 375°F (190°C).

2. Combine the green beans, oil, seasoning, and salt in bowl. Toss well to coat. Spread in a single layer on a rimmed baking sheet. Roast for 20 to 25 minutes, until some of the green beans begin to develop dark brown spots.

3. Transfer to a serving dish, garnish with the lemon wedges, and serve.

Per Serving: Calories 120; Protein 2 g; Carbs 10 g; Dietary Fiber 3 g; Added Sugars 1 g; Total Fat 8 g; Sat Fat 2 g; Omega-3s 60 mg; Sodium 378 mg; Potassium 179 mg

SIMPLY QUICK-PICKLED RED ONIONS

Makes 12 servings

Quick-pickled red onions are an easy way to add bright bursts of flavor to tacos or bowls. We feature these as a topping for the Spicy Shredded Beef Street Tacos (page 186). The pickling liquid will develop a beautiful pale pink hue, and the onions will take on the bright flavors of the lime juice and vinegar.

- 1 pound (454 g) red onions, halved across the "equator" and thinly sliced
- 1 Fresno, habanero, or serrano chile, halved lengthwise
- 2 cups (480 ml) white vinegar
- Juice of 4 limes
- ¼ teaspoon kosher salt

Combine the onions, chile, vinegar, lime juice, and salt in a large glass bowl. Cover and refrigerate for at least 2 hours. Store the onions in their pickling liquid in an airtight container in the refrigerator for up to 2 weeks.

Per Serving: Calories 44; Protein 0 g; Carbs 9 g; Dietary Fiber 1 g; Added Sugars 0 g; Total Fat 0 g; Sat Fat 0 g; Omega-3s 0 mg; Sodium 130 mg; Potassium 103 mg

SIMPLY ROASTED PEPPERS

Makes 4 peppers

This recipe works well with larger peppers, like bell peppers and poblano chiles. We feature simply roasted poblanos as a topping for the Southwestern Beef & Bean Burgers (page 180) and as the star ingredient for the Roasted Poblano Soup (page 81). Red bell peppers are featured in our Roasted Red Pepper Fettucine (page 212).

4 poblano chiles or red bell peppers

1. Place the top oven rack in the broiler so that it sits 3 to 5 inches (7.5 to 13 cm) from the broiler. Preheat the oven to 500°F (260°C). Line a rimmed baking sheet with foil. Use twice the length needed to cover the surface of the pan for wrapping the roasted peppers in the foil after roasting to steam the skins.

2. Place the peppers on the foil and roast for 12 to 20 minutes. Watch carefully for the skin to brown and blister or pull away from the flesh, but not to burn or dry out the peppers. Turn the peppers two or three times during roasting, as each side starts to turn dark brown.

3. Remove from the oven, wrap the foil up and around the peppers, and seal the edges as tightly as possible. Let sit at room temperature for 30 minutes.

4. Unwrap the foil and peel off the papery skin with your fingers or a dry paper towel. Pull out and discard the stems. There's no need to remove the seeds unless you don't like the texture.

5. Store in an airtight container in the refrigerator for up to 1 week.

Serving Size 1 pepper; Calories 13; Protein 1 g; Carbs 3 g; Dietary Fiber 1 g; Added Sugars 0 g; Total Fat 0 g; Sat Fat 0 g; Omega-3s 10 mg; Sodium 2 mg; Potassium 112 mg

SIMPLY SPANISH-STYLE MASHED POTATOES

Makes 6 servings

Home cooks around the Mediterranean use copious amounts of olive oil to make vegetables crave-worthy and delicious. This recipe shows how fresh, high-quality extra virgin olive oil can be used to make creamy mashed potatoes. Serve with Broiled Halibut with Pesto (page 284).

- 1.5 pounds (680 g) Yukon gold–type potatoes, quartered
- ½ cup (120 ml) extra virgin olive oil
- 1 teaspoon kosher salt
- ¼ to ½ cup (60 to 120 ml) reserved potato cooking water

1. Place the potatoes in a large pot; add just enough cold water to cover. Bring to a boil, then reduce the heat to medium-low and cook until the potatoes can be easily pierced with a fork, 20 to 25 minutes.

2. Drain off the cooking water, reserving at least ½ cup (120 ml).

3. Add the oil, salt, and ¼ cup (60 ml) of the cooking water. Mash well using a potato masher. Stir in more of the cooking water, if needed, to achieve a smooth, creamy consistency.

Per Serving: Calories 422; Protein 6 g; Carbs 63 g; Dietary Fiber 6 g; Added Sugars 0 g; Total Fat 19 g; Sat Fat 3 g; Omega-3s 130 mg; Sodium 266 mg; Potassium 475 mg

SIMPLY ROASTED POTATOES
Makes 4 servings

Potatoes are one of the most versatile—and most loved— vegetables. There are thousands of varieties of potatoes grown around the world, all differing in appearance, taste, texture, and nutrition properties, but every variety provides vitamin C, potassium, and fiber as well as other essential nutrients.

1.5 pounds (680 g) baby red-skin or Yukon gold potatoes, halved

3 tablespoons extra virgin olive oil

Freshly ground black pepper

3 thyme sprigs

3 tablespoons chopped fresh parsley

¼ teaspoon kosher salt

1. Preheat the oven to 375°F (190°C).

2. Toss the potatoes with the oil and pepper in a large bowl. Spread in a single layer on a rimmed baking sheet. Add the thyme sprigs on top. Roast, stirring after 15 to 20 minutes, until the potatoes are easily pierced with a fork, 30 to 45 minutes.

3. Sprinkle with parsley and salt; serve.

Per Serving: Calories 215; Protein 3 g; Carbs 27 g; Dietary Fiber 3 g; Added Sugars 0 g; Total Fat 11 g; Sat Fat 2 g; Omega-3s 100 mg; Sodium 79 mg; Potassium 792 mg

SIMPLY SMASHED POTATOES
Makes 4 servings

The technique of boiling then smashing and oven-roasting baby potatoes is a wonderful way to get the best of both worlds: a creamy interior with abundant surface area to create a crunchy exterior. These potatoes are wonderful drizzled with our Roasted Garlic Aïoli (page 45).

1.5 pounds (680 g) baby red-skin or Yukon gold potatoes

3 tablespoons extra virgin olive oil

1 teaspoon freshly ground black pepper

¼ cup (12 g) chopped fresh chives

¼ teaspoon kosher salt

1. Place the potatoes in a large stockpot and cover with plenty of water. Bring to a boil and cook until just tender, about 15 minutes.

2. Drain the potatoes, transfer to a large bowl, and let cool at room temperature for 15 minutes.

3. While the potatoes are cooling, preheat the oven to 375°F (190°C).

4. Toss the potatoes with the oil and pepper. Transfer the potatoes to a baking sheet. Use the bottom of a measuring cup or mug to gently press down on the potatoes until they are about ½ inch thick (13 mm).

5. Roast for 30 to 45 minutes, until the potatoes are crisp with darkened edges. Transfer to a serving platter, sprinkle with chives and salt, and serve.

Per Serving: Calories 216; Protein 3 g; Carbs 28 g; Dietary Fiber 3 g; Added Sugars 0 g; Total Fat 11 g; Sat Fat 2 g; Omega-3s 100 mg; Sodium 77 mg; Potassium 790 mg

SIMPLY SLOW-ROASTED TOMATOES
Makes 6 cups (1,100 g)

Slowly roasting tomatoes at a low temperature for five hours makes them candy-sweet! They make a wonderful eat-right-off-the-pan snack. You can add them to a quiche, frittata, or hot pasta.

16 ripe Roma (plum) tomatoes, quartered, or 60 to 80 cherry tomatoes, halved

¼ cup (60 ml) extra virgin olive oil

15 garlic cloves, thinly sliced

½ cup (12 g) chopped fresh basil, oregano, or thyme

½ teaspoon kosher salt

½ teaspoon freshly ground black pepper

1. Position the oven racks in the upper and lower thirds of the oven. Preheat the oven to 300°F (150°C). Line two rimmed baking sheets with parchment paper.

2. Place the tomatoes on the baking sheets, cut side up. Drizzle with the oil and sprinkle with the garlic and basil. Use your hands to massage the oil, garlic, and basil into the tomatoes.

3. Roast, one sheet per oven rack, 2 hours for Romas, or 1¼ hours for cherry tomatoes.

4. Season with salt and pepper, then switch the pans from top to bottom and front to back. Roast Romas for 2½ hours, cherry tomatoes for 1¼ hours, until the tomatoes are dehydrated, with the skins wrinkled and blackened in spots. Turn off the heat and leave the pans in the oven for 30 minutes.

5. Let cool completely before storing. Layer the tomatoes in a shallow airtight container with wax paper between the layers. Store in a cool, dark place at room temperature for up to 2 months. For longer storage, store in the refrigerator or freezer. You can also pack the tomatoes in an airtight jar, cover with olive oil, and store in the refrigerator. As you remove tomatoes, add more oil to cover the remaining tomatoes.

Serving Size 1 cup (183 g); Calories 121; Protein 2 g; Carbs 9 g; Dietary Fiber 2 g; Added Sugars 0 g; Total Fat 9 g; Sat Fat 1 g; Omega-3s 80 mg; Sodium 88 mg; Potassium 430 mg

SODIUM TIP: Using Diamond Crystal Kosher Salt will dramatically reduce the sodium in any recipe that uses kosher salt. This salt contains 50% less sodium per measure than regular kosher salt and 60% less than fine grain table salt.

SIMPLY ROASTED ROOT VEGETABLES WITH APPLES

Makes 6 servings

Roast any combination of root vegetables with apples and fresh herbs to bring out their natural sweetness and intensify their flavor. Serve with roast chicken, pork, or lamb. Top with Citrusy Walnut Gremolata (page 63).

3 turnips, peeled and cut into 1-inch (2.5 cm) cubes

4 carrots, cut into 1-inch (2.5 cm) cubes

4 parsnips, peeled and cut into 1-inch (2.5 cm) cubes

1 sweet yellow or white onion, cut into 8 wedges

2 Honeycrisp, Gala, or Fuji apples, cored and sliced

2 tablespoons extra virgin olive oil

2 tablespoons balsamic vinegar

1 teaspoon minced fresh rosemary

1 teaspoon minced fresh sage

2 tablespoons minced fresh thyme

1 teaspoon freshly ground black pepper

¼ teaspoon kosher salt

1. Heat oven to 400°F (200°C). Line a large rimmed baking sheet with parchment paper.

2. Toss the turnips, carrots, parsnips, onion, and apples in a large bowl with the oil, 1 tablespoon of the vinegar, the rosemary, sage, and 1 tablespoon of the thyme. Arrange in a single layer on the baking sheet. Roast for 20 to 25 minutes.

3. Stir or flip the vegetables to prevent sticking. Roast for 20 minutes, or until the vegetables are tender and slightly caramelized.

4. Drizzle with the remaining 1 tablespoon vinegar and the remaining 1 tablespoon of thyme, sprinkle with pepper and salt, and serve hot. Store in an airtight container in the refrigerator for up to 4 days. Enjoy cold or hot. Reheat in the microwave in 30-second increments on HIGH until hot.

Per Serving: Calories 151; Protein 2 g; Carbs 26 g; Dietary Fiber 6 g; Added Sugars 0 g; Total Fat 5 g; Sat Fat 1 g; Omega-3s 60 mg; Sodium 95 mg; Potassium 487 mg

SIMPLY STEAMED VEGETABLE MEDLEY

Makes 4 servings

These stovetop-steamed vegetables—finished with olive oil, lemon juice, and herbs—are an easy side to pair with meat, chicken, fish, or pasta dishes.

- 2 cups (215 g) cauliflower florets (about 1 small head)
- 1 cup (120 g) diagonally sliced carrots
- 1 medium red onion, sliced into rings
- 1 cup (70 g) sliced white or cremini mushrooms
- 2 tablespoons extra virgin olive oil
- 1 tablespoon fresh lemon juice
- 1½ tablespoons chopped fresh basil
- 1½ tablespoons chopped fresh marjoram

1. Place the cauliflower, carrots, and onion in a steamer basket inside a 4-quart (3.8 L) saucepan with a lid. Add water to just below the bottom of the basket. Cover, bring to a boil, and steam the vegetables until they begin to soften, about 10 minutes.

2. Add the mushrooms and steam until the vegetables are crisp-tender, 5 minutes.

3. Whisk the oil, lemon juice, basil, and marjoram together in a large bowl. Add the vegetables and toss to coat. Serve.

Per Serving: Calories 106; Protein 2 g; Carbs 9 g; Dietary Fiber 2 g; Added Sugars 0 g; Total Fat 7 g; Sat Fat 1 g; Omega-3s 70 mg; Sodium 34 mg; Potassium 281 mg

SIMPLY STIR-FRIED VEGETABLES

Makes 6 servings

The term "stir-fry" implies high heat and constant stirring. It's important to have all the ingredients prepared and nearby for quick and easy cooking. If your wok or skillet can't accommodate all the vegetables, stir-fry in two batches. For spicier vegetables, add ½ teaspoon red pepper flakes when you add the garlic and ginger.

- 2 tablespoons reduced-sodium soy sauce or tamari
- 2 tablespoons water
- 2 teaspoons cornstarch
- 2 tablespoons peanut oil
- 3 garlic cloves, minced
- 1 teaspoon finely grated fresh ginger
- 8 green onions, sliced
- 1 cup (120 g) thinly sliced carrots
- 2 cups (180 g) bite-size fresh broccoli or cauliflower florets
- 1 pound (454 g) bok choy, thinly sliced diagonally
- 1 tablespoon toasted sesame oil
- ½ teaspoon freshly ground black pepper
- ¼ cup (4 g) chopped fresh cilantro

1. Combine the soy sauce, water, and cornstarch in a small bowl. Stir to form a slurry.

2. Heat the peanut oil in a wok or large skillet over high heat until shimmering. Add the garlic and ginger and stir fry until fragrant, about 15 seconds.

3. Add the green onions and stir-fry for 1 minute.

4. Add the carrots and stir-fry for 1 minute.

5. Add the broccoli or cauliflower and stir-fry until bright in color and beginning to soften, 2 minutes.

6. Add the bok choy and stir-fry until the vegetables begin to char in spots and are crisp-tender, about 2 minutes. Stir in the cornstarch slurry and stir-fry until it thickens and coats the vegetables, about 3 minutes. Remove from the heat and drizzle with sesame oil. Stir in the pepper, then sprinkle with cilantro. Serve immediately.

Per Serving: Calories 105; Protein 3 g; Carbs 9 g; Dietary Fiber 3 g; Added Sugars 0 g; Total Fat 7 g; Sat Fat 1 g; Omega-3s 90 mg; Sodium 268 mg; Potassium 366 mg

SIMPLY SAUTÉED ZUCCHINI

Makes 6 servings

When shopping for this recipe, either in your home garden or at your local market, select smaller zucchini as they are more tender, have very thin (edible) skins, and contain small or no seeds. Cooking zucchini brings out its sweeter side. Fresh herbs like basil, marjoram, and thyme accentuate zucchini's mild flavor.

3 tablespoons extra virgin olive oil

3 garlic cloves, thinly sliced

6 small zucchini, trimmed and thinly sliced

1 tablespoon chopped fresh basil

1 tablespoon chopped fresh thyme

1 teaspoon ground marjoram

⅓ cup (20 g) chopped fresh parsley

1 tablespoon balsamic or red wine vinegar

¼ teaspoon freshly ground black pepper

1. Place the oil and garlic in a cold, large skillet. Turn on the heat to medium and heat until the garlic begins to sizzle, about 2 minutes.

2. Stir in the zucchini, basil, thyme, and marjoram. Cook, stirring as the zucchini softens, until fork-tender, creamy, and brown in spots, 15 minutes.

3. Remove from the heat. Add the parsley, toss to mix, then splash in the vinegar. Add pepper to finish. Serve hot.

Per Serving: Calories 90; Protein 2 g; Carbs 5 g; Dietary Fiber 1 g; Added Sugars 0 g; Total Fat 7 g; Sat Fat 1 g; Omega-3s 130 mg; Sodium 12 mg; Potassium 341 mg

ARTICHOKE & ONIONS WITH LEMON & THYME

Makes 4 servings

When we eat artichokes, we're eating flowers. Using frozen artichoke hearts to make this recipe is an easy, approachable way to cook with this unique vegetable. Serve with roast chicken and your favorite potato side dish.

One 12-ounce (340 g) bag frozen artichoke hearts

2 tablespoons extra virgin olive oil

2 tablespoons fresh lemon juice

¼ teaspoon kosher salt

½ teaspoon freshly ground black pepper

1 onion, cut into 10 wedges

6 tablespoons (15 g) chopped fresh thyme

1. Adjust an oven rack to the middle position. Preheat the oven to 425°F (220°C). Line a rimmed baking sheet with parchment paper.

2. Open the bag of artichoke hearts and add 1 tablespoon of the oil and 1 tablespoon of the lemon juice. Tightly close the bag and shake to coat the artichokes. Spread them in a single layer on the baking sheet. Sprinkle with salt and pepper. Roast for 10 minutes.

3. Stir and add the onion wedges. Drizzle with the remaining 1 tablespoon of oil and sprinkle with 4 tablespoons of the thyme. Roast for 15 to 20 minutes, until the artichokes have begun to crisp and brown and the onion has softened and begun to char.

4. Transfer to a serving plate. Drizzle with the remaining 1 tablespoon lemon juice, sprinkle with the remaining 2 tablespoons (5 g) thyme, and serve.

Per Serving: Calories 121; Protein 3 g; Carbs 13 g; Dietary Fiber 6 g; Added Sugars 0 g; Total Fat 7 g; Sat Fat 1 g; Omega-3s 100 mg; Sodium 99 mg; Potassium 303 mg

ASPARAGUS WITH SESAME & GINGER

Makes 4 servings

Asparagus is best when it is tender-crisp. Roasting it in the oven creates tasty charred spots on the skin while leaving the center bright green and crunchy. To trim asparagus, break or cut it where the stalk becomes fibrous. Discard or—better yet—compost the trimmings, because they are too pungent to use in a stock.

2 pounds (907 g) fresh asparagus, trimmed

1 tablespoon extra virgin olive oil

1 tablespoon sesame seeds, toasted

2 teaspoons reduced-sodium soy sauce

1 teaspoon toasted sesame oil

1 teaspoon rice vinegar

1 garlic clove, minced

¼ teaspoon ground ginger

1. Preheat the oven to 400°F (200°C). Line a rimmed baking sheet with parchment paper.

2. Spread the asparagus spears in a single layer on the baking sheet. Drizzle with the oil. Roast for 8 minutes, until the asparagus starts to turn dark green.

3. Combine the sesame seeds, soy sauce, sesame oil, vinegar, garlic, and ginger in a small bowl. Drizzle over the asparagus, rubbing it into the stalks by turning and rolling them gently from side to side. Roast for 5 minutes, or until the stalks are tender-crisp. Serve immediately.

Per Serving: Calories 103; Protein 6 g; Carbs 10 g; Dietary Fiber 5 g; Added Sugars 0 g; Total Fat 6 g; Sat Fat 1 g; Omega-3s 60 mg; Sodium 102 mg; Potassium 479 mg

CITRUS-ROASTED BEETS
Makes 4 servings

Beets, celery, and parsley contain a compound called sodium nitrate that gets converted to nitric oxide in our bodies. Nitric oxide relaxes our arteries, reducing blood pressure and increasing blood flow throughout the body. Beets definitely promote heart health! Roasting beets makes them sweeter; the addition of citrus adds bright flavor and mild acidity to offset the beets' natural sweetness.

- 3 tablespoons walnut oil
- 2 tablespoons minced fresh thyme
- ½ teaspoon freshly ground black pepper
- 1 pound (454 g) beets, trimmed, peeled, and cubed
- 2 cups (460 g) grapefruit or orange segments (see Tip)
- Juice of 1 lemon
- Grated zest of 1 orange

1. Preheat the oven to 375°F (190°C). Line a rimmed baking sheet with parchment paper.

2. Combine 2 tablespoons of the oil, the thyme, and pepper in a medium bowl. Add the beets and toss to combine. Add 1 cup (230 g) of the grapefruit sections and gently toss. Spread in a single layer on the baking sheet and roast for 20 to 30 minutes, until the beets are tender when pierced with a fork.

3. Transfer to a serving bowl. Add the remaining grapefruit sections, the lemon juice, orange zest, and the remaining 1 tablespoon oil. Toss well and serve.

TIP: *You can buy citrus segments in the refrigerated section of most grocery stores, but you can also segment whole grapefruit or oranges for this recipe. You'll need approximately 2 grapefruits or 3 oranges to get 2 cups segments. We recommend cutting supremes from whole fruit: Use a sharp knife to peel the fruit and remove*

all the white pith, then cut the segments out from the membranes that divide them. The membranes can become bitter when roasted.

Per Serving: Calories 202; Protein 2 g; Carbs 22 g; Dietary Fiber 7 g; Added Sugars 0 g; Total Fat 13 g; Sat Fat 2 g; Omega-3s 1,180 mg; Sodium 225 mg; Potassium 193 mg

BROCCOLI WITH CORIANDER & TOMATOES
Makes 4 servings

Use a hot pan to sear the broccoli, as it heightens its flavor, helps retain its bright green color, and leaves its crunchy texture intact. The gently cooked tomatoes add bright color and natural sweetness. Turn this colorful side dish into a complete meal by tossing the cooked vegetables with penne pasta and a bit of freshly grated Parmesan.

- 4 cups (285 g) fresh broccoli florets, chopped into bite-size pieces
- 2 tablespoons extra virgin olive oil
- 1 teaspoon ground coriander
- 10 ounces (283 g) cherry tomatoes, halved
- 2 garlic cloves, chopped
- Grated zest of 1 lemon
- ¼ teaspoon freshly ground black pepper

1. Heat a large sauté pan or skillet over high heat for 1 minute. Add the broccoli, 1 tablespoon of the oil, and the coriander. Reduce the heat to medium-high and sauté until the broccoli is tender and bright green, 5 minutes.

2. Reduce the heat to medium, then add the remaining 1 tablespoon of oil, followed by the tomatoes and garlic. Cook until the tomatoes are warmed through and the skins begin to wrinkle, about 2 minutes. Stir in the lemon zest and pepper and serve immediately.

Per Serving: Calories 103; Protein 2 g; Carbs 8 g; Dietary Fiber 4 g; Added Sugars 0 g; Total Fat 8 g; Sat Fat 1 g; Omega-3s 140 mg; Sodium 33 mg; Potassium 381 mg

MAPLE-ROASTED BRUSSELS SPROUTS

Makes 6 servings

Brussels sprouts resemble miniature cabbages; they're a cruciferous vegetable, closely related to cauliflower and kale. Many people who think they don't love Brussels sprouts change their minds quickly when a little sweetness from an ingredient like maple syrup is added. This recipe is a perfect side dish to serve with Fresh Herb–Roasted Turkey Breast (page 317) and Rosemary Mashed Potatoes (page 270).

- 1.5 pounds (680 g) Brussels sprouts, trimmed and halved
- 2 tablespoons apple cider vinegar
- 1 tablespoon extra virgin olive oil
- 1 tablespoon minced fresh thyme
- ¼ teaspoon freshly ground black pepper
- 2 tablespoons real maple syrup
- 2 tablespoons Smoky Pecan Bits (page 173), optional

1. Preheat the oven to 375°F (190°C). Line a rimmed baking sheet with parchment paper.

2. Combine the Brussels sprouts, vinegar, oil, thyme, and pepper in a medium bowl. Spread in a single layer on the baking sheet. Roast for 15 minutes or until slightly charred.

3. Drizzle with the maple syrup, then roast for 2 minutes to caramelize.

4. Transfer to a serving dish, top with pecans, if desired, and serve.

Per Serving: Calories 95; Protein 4 g; Carbs 14 g; Dietary Fiber 4 g; Added Sugars 4 g; Total Fat 3 g; Sat Fat 0 g; Omega-3s 30 mg; Sodium 20 mg; Potassium 436 mg

TANGY SAUTÉED RED CABBAGE

Makes 6 servings

Red cabbage can turn an unexpected blue color when cooked. To retain the red color, add an acid like vinegar or fresh lemon juice. To save time, you can buy shredded red cabbage. Serve with Fresh Herb & Honey Batter Bread (page 102) and Simply Cooked Pork Tenderloin (page 332) for a casual, comforting meal.

- ½ cup (120 ml) apple cider vinegar
- 2 tablespoons sugar
- 1 teaspoon whole cloves or caraway seeds
- 1 onion, chopped
- ½ cup (120 ml) water
- 1 head red cabbage, shredded

1. Combine the vinegar, sugar, and cloves in a small saucepan. Bring to a boil, then reduce the heat and simmer until the mixture is reduced and has the consistency of syrup, about 6 minutes. Remove and discard the cloves. (If you use caraway seeds, you can leave them in.)

2. Add the onion and water; simmer until the onion has softened, 5 minutes.

3. Place the cabbage in a large skillet over medium heat and pour over the onion mixture. Cook until the cabbage is hot, wilted, and crisp-tender, 5 to 6 minutes. Serve.

Per Serving: Calories 81; Protein 3 g; Carbs 19 g; Dietary Fiber 4 g; Added Sugars 4 g; Total Fat 0 g; Sat Fat 0 g; Omega-3s 90 mg; Sodium 52 mg; Potassium 481 mg

CITRUS-GLAZED CARROTS

Makes 4 servings

Use fresh whole carrots for this recipe. Baby carrots may be uniform in size, but they tend to be less flavorful. If your local market sells pre-cut rainbow carrots, try those. They offer great flavor and gorgeous color. Note that this recipe calls for orange zest as well as fresh orange juice. Be sure to zest the orange before juicing it.

- 1 tablespoon extra virgin olive oil
- 1 pound (454 g) carrots, sliced diagonally ½ inch thick (13 mm)
- ½ cup (120 ml) fresh orange juice
- ¼ cup (60 ml) water
- 2 tablespoons chopped fresh basil or oregano
- 1 tablespoon honey
- 1 garlic clove, minced
- ½ teaspoon freshly ground black pepper
- 2 tablespoons chopped fresh parsley
- 1 tablespoon finely grated orange zest

1. Heat the oil in a large skillet over medium heat. Add the carrots, cover, and cook, stirring occasionally, until softened, 10 minutes.

2. Add the orange juice, water, basil, honey, garlic, and pepper. Cook, uncovered, until the carrots are fork-tender and the liquid has reduced to a thin syrup, about 10 minutes.

3. Transfer to a serving bowl, sprinkle with the parsley and orange zest, and serve.

Per Serving: Calories 115; Protein 2 g; Carbs 20 g; Dietary Fiber 3 g; Added Sugars 4 g; Total Fat 4 g; Sat Fat 1 g; Omega-3s 30 mg; Sodium 60 mg; Potassium 85 mg

APRICOT & SESAME ROASTED CARROTS

Makes 6 servings

Apricots add additional sweetness while sesame oil adds nuttiness to roasted carrots. This is a great dish to serve with Pork Fried Rice (page 332).

- 2 pounds (907 g) carrots, sliced into ¼-inch (6 mm) half-moons
- 2 tablespoons extra virgin olive oil
- ½ teaspoon freshly ground black pepper
- ¼ teaspoon kosher salt
- ½ cup (65 g) chopped dried apricots
- 2 teaspoons toasted sesame oil
- 1 teaspoon toasted sesame seeds

1. Preheat the oven to 375°F (190°C). Line a rimmed baking sheet with parchment paper.

2. Combine the carrots, oil, pepper, and salt in a medium bowl. Toss well to coat. Spread the carrots on the baking sheet in a single layer. Roast for 20 to 25 minutes, until tender when pierced with a fork.

3. Transfer to a serving bowl. Add the apricots, sesame oil, and sesame seeds and toss to combine. Serve. Store in an airtight container in the refrigerator for up to 4 days. Enjoy cold or hot. Reheat in the microwave in 30-second increments on HIGH until hot.

Per Serving: Calories 153; Protein 2 g; Carbs 22 g; Dietary Fiber 5 g; Added Sugars 0 g; Total Fat 7 g; Sat Fat 1 g; Omega-3s 40 mg; Sodium 79 mg; Potassium 130 mg

CARDAMOM & ORANGE ROASTED CARROTS

Makes 6 servings

Cardamom loves to be paired with citrus, and both ingredients pair perfectly with carrots in this recipe. Serve with Honey-Ginger Chicken & Apples (page 312) and Simply Cooked Farro (page 226) for a nourishing and memorable meal.

- 2 pounds (907 g) carrots, sliced into ¼-inch (6 mm) half-moons
- 2 tablespoons extra virgin olive oil
- ½ teaspoon freshly ground black pepper
- ¼ teaspoon kosher salt
- ½ teaspoon ground cardamom
- Juice and grated zest of 1 orange

1. Preheat the oven to 375°F (190°C). Line a rimmed baking sheet with parchment paper.

2. Combine the carrots, oil, pepper, salt, cardamom, and orange juice in a medium bowl. Toss well to coat. Spread the carrots on the baking sheet in a single layer. Roast for 20 to 25 minutes, until tender when pierced with a fork.

3. Transfer to a serving dish, sprinkle the orange zest on top, and serve.

Per Serving: Calories 117; Protein 2 g; Carbs 17 g; Dietary Fiber 4 g; Added Sugars 0 g; Total Fat 5 g; Sat Fat 1 g; Omega-3s 30 mg; Sodium 109 mg; Potassium 29 mg

FENNEL & PEAR ROASTED CARROTS

Makes 6 servings

Fennel has a mild licorice flavor that complements the sweetness of the carrots and pears so well. We like to serve this dish with the Turkey Tenderloins with Spinach Pesto & Pistachios (page 319) for an elegant and memorable meal.

- 2 pounds (907 g) carrots, sliced into ¼-inch (6 mm) half-moons
- 2 fennel bulbs, trimmed and thinly sliced vertically,
- 2 tablespoons chopped fennel fronds
- 2 tablespoons extra virgin olive oil

½ teaspoon freshly ground black pepper

¼ teaspoon kosher salt

2 Bosc pears, cored and coarsely chopped

1. Preheat the oven to 375°F (190°C). Line a rimmed baking sheet with parchment paper.

2. Combine the carrots, fennel bulbs, oil, pepper, and salt in a medium bowl. Toss well to coat. Spread the vegetables on the baking sheet in a single layer. Roast for 15 minutes.

3. Add the pears and roast for 10 minutes, until the carrots are tender when pierced with a fork.

4. Transfer to a serving bowl, top with the fennel fronds, and serve warm. Store in an airtight container in the refrigerator for up to 4 days. Enjoy cold or hot. Reheat in the microwave in 30-second increments on HIGH until hot.

Per Serving: Calories 174; Protein 3 g; Carbs 31 g; Dietary Fiber 8 g; Added Sugars 0 g; Total Fat 5 g; Sat Fat 1 g; Omega-3s 30 mg; Sodium 150 mg; Potassium 398 mg

MAPLE & HERB ROASTED CARROTS
Makes 6 servings

There are endless ways to pair roast carrots with spices, herbs, and aromatics. In this recipe, we combine fresh herbs and maple syrup to play up the sweetness of the carrots. Serve this with Smoky Workaday Pork Tenderloin (page 333) and Rosemary Mashed Potatoes (page 270).

2 pounds (907 g) carrots, sliced into ¼-inch (6 mm) half-moons

2 tablespoons extra virgin olive oil

1 tablespoon chopped fresh thyme

1 teaspoon chopped fresh rosemary

½ teaspoon freshly ground black pepper

¼ teaspoon kosher salt

1 tablespoon real maple syrup

1. Preheat the oven to 375°F (190°C). Line a rimmed baking sheet with parchment paper.

2. Combine the carrots, oil, thyme, rosemary, pepper, and salt in a medium bowl. Toss well to coat. Spread the carrots on the baking sheet in a single

layer. Roast for 20 to 25 minutes, until tender when pierced with a fork.

3. Transfer to a serving bowl, toss with the maple syrup, and serve. Store in an airtight container in the refrigerator for up to 4 days. Enjoy cold or hot. Reheat in the microwave in 30-second increments on HIGH until hot.

Per Serving: Calories 160; Protein 2 g; Carbs 18 g; Dietary Fiber 4 g; Added Sugars 2 g; Total Fat 5 g; Sat Fat 1 g; Omega-3s 40 mg; Sodium 109 mg; Potassium 13 mg

SPICY CAULIFLOWER STIR-FRY
Makes 4 servings

This spicy stir-fry uses cauliflower, carrots, and leeks, but you could use any combination of vegetables you love. Consider adding marinated but not yet cooked Crispy Tofu Bites (page 250) or shrimp, then serving with Simply Cooked Brown Rice (page 230) or Simply Cooked Millet (page 227) to complete your meal.

½ cup (120 ml) Vegetable Broth (page 72)

1 tablespoon cornstarch

1 tablespoon grated lemon zest

2 tablespoons fresh lemon juice

1 tablespoon reduced-sodium soy sauce or tamari

2 tablespoons extra virgin olive oil

4 garlic cloves, minced

2 teaspoons minced fresh ginger

¼ teaspoon red pepper flakes

2 cups (215 g) cauliflower florets, cut into bite-size pieces

2 carrots, cut into matchsticks

2 leeks, cleaned (see Tip, page 79) and thinly sliced

Freshly ground black pepper

1. Stir together the broth, cornstarch, lemon zest, lemon juice, and soy sauce in a small bowl.

2. Heat the oil in a wok or large skillet over medium-high heat. Add the garlic, ginger, and red pepper flakes. Stir-fry until fragrant, about 30 seconds. Add the cauliflower and stir-fry for 2 minutes. Add the carrots and stir-fry for 2 minutes. Add the zucchini and stir-fry for 2 minutes. The

vegetables will be crisp-tender.

3. Stir in the broth mixture and bring to a simmer, cover, and cook for 1 minute. Uncover and cook until the sauce thickens, about 2 minutes. Serve immediately with pepper to taste.

TIP: If you'd like to add tofu or shrimp to this recipe, add them at the end of Step 2 and stir-fry for about 2 minutes before adding the broth mixture in Step 3. Cook the shrimp just long enough that they start to change color. They will continue to cook in Step 3.

Per Serving: Calories 139; Protein 3 g; Carbs 17 g; Dietary Fiber 3 g; Added Sugars 0 g; Total Fat 7 g; Sat Fat 1 g; Omega-3s 100 mg; Sodium 190 mg; Potassium 284 mg

SMOKY WORKADAY SWEET CORN & PEPPER SAUTÉ
Makes 4 servings

This simple sauté of both fresh and frozen vegetables pairs well with grilled or smoked meats. It can also be served as fajita vegetables, paired with grilled shrimp or chicken. If you have a cast-iron pan, you can create a beautiful char on the peppers that adds a slightly bitter yet appealing contrast to their sweetness.

1 pound (454 g) mini sweet bell peppers (about 16), stems removed, halved lengthwise

1 white or red onion, sliced

2 tablespoons extra virgin olive oil

1 cup (165 g) frozen white or yellow corn kernels, thawed

1 tablespoon Smoky Workaday Seasoning (page 37)

¼ cup (4 g) chopped fresh cilantro or parsley, optional

1. Combine the peppers, onion, and oil in a large skillet or sauté pan over medium-high heat. Sauté until the onions and peppers start to soften, about 10 minutes.

2. Add the corn and seasoning, reduce the heat to medium, and cook until the corn is heated through, about 10 minutes.

3. Transfer to a serving bowl, top with the cilantro, if desired, and serve.

Per Serving: Calories 148; Protein 3 g; Carbs 17 g; Dietary Fiber 4 g; Added Sugars 0 g; Total Fat 8 g; Sat Fat 1 g; Omega-3s 80 mg; Sodium 7 mg; Potassium 290 mg

CURIOUSLY COMPATIBLE CUCUMBERS & CARROTS
Makes 6 servings

This is an unusual and unbelievably delicious vegetable combination. These two veggies bring out the best in each other. This recipe is a great way to use up surplus cucumbers when you have too many on hand or just want to switch things up a bit.

3 cucumbers, partially peeled, seeded, and sliced into ½-inch (6 mm) half-moons

1 teaspoon kosher salt

2 carrots, cut into 1½-inch-long (4 cm) matchsticks

Boiling water

2 tablespoons butter or plant-based spread

1 green onion, finely chopped

¼ teaspoon ground cumin

Freshly ground black pepper

2 tablespoons chopped fresh cilantro

1. Place the cucumber slices in a colander over a rimmed baking sheet or in the sink. Sprinkle with the salt, toss, and let sit for 30 minutes to allow any excess water to drain.

2. Rinse well and pat dry with paper towels.

3. Place the carrots in a medium saucepan and add enough boiling water to cover. Cook over medium heat until the carrots have just begun to soften, about 4 minutes.

4. Add the cucumbers and cook until just heated through, about 1 minute more. Drain well.

5. Melt the butter in a large skillet over medium heat. Add the green onions and cook until softened, stirring frequently, 3 to 5 minutes.

6. Add the carrots and cucumbers and sprinkle with the cumin and pepper. Cook, stirring occasionally, until the flavors have had time to blend, the vegetables are hot, and the cucumbers still retain their crunch, about 2 minutes.

7. Sprinkle with cilantro and serve hot or at room temperature. Store in an airtight container in the refrigerator for up to 4 days. Enjoy cold or hot. Reheat in the microwave in 15-second increments on HIGH until hot.

Per Serving: Calories 39; Protein 2 g; Carbs 6 g; Dietary Fiber 2 g; Added Sugars 0 g; Total Fat 1 g; Sat Fat 0.5 g; Omega-3s 10 mg; Sodium 180 mg; Potassium 221 mg

SMOKY ROASTED MUSHROOMS

Makes 4 servings

This recipe can be made with a variety of mixed mushrooms (white, cremini, portobello, shiitake, and oyster, to name a few), or you can use just one variety. Doubling the recipe to make a large batch allows you to save some to add to scrambled eggs, grain or lentil bowls, soups, or salads.

- 1 pound (454 g) fresh mushrooms, cleaned, trimmed, and cut into bite-size pieces
- 2 tablespoons extra virgin olive oil
- ¼ teaspoon kosher salt
- ½ teaspoon freshly ground black pepper
- 1 tablespoon butter or plant-based spread
- ½ cup (80 g) finely chopped shallots
- 3 garlic cloves, thinly sliced
- 1 teaspoon smoked paprika
- ¾ cup (45 g) chopped fresh parsley
- 1 tablespoon chopped fresh marjoram or thyme

1. Preheat the oven to 375°F (190°C). Line a large baking sheet with parchment paper.

2. Toss the mushrooms with 1 tablespoon of the oil in a medium bowl. Spread on the baking sheet, then sprinkle with salt and pepper. Roast for 20 to 30 minutes, until the mushrooms are tender and browned.

3. Heat the remaining 1 tablespoon of oil and the butter in a medium skillet over medium-high heat. Add the shallots, garlic, and paprika. Sauté until the shallot and garlic are softened, 2 to 3 minutes.

4. Add the mushrooms, parsley, and marjoram, toss well, and serve. Store in an airtight container in the refrigerator for up to 3 days. Enjoy cold or hot. Reheat either in the microwave in 15-second increments on HIGH until hot or in a small skillet over medium-high heat with a little olive oil, sautéing until hot.

Per Serving: Calories 138; Protein 3 g; Carbs 9 g; Dietary Fiber 2 g; Added Sugars 0 g; Total Fat 10 g; Sat Fat 3 g; Omega-3s 70 mg; Sodium 87 mg; Potassium 627 mg

RED POTATO & ONION ROAST WITH CHERRY TOMATOES & KALAMATA OLIVES

Makes 6 servings

Dijon mustard and olives bring bold flavor to this vegetable side. Serve with baked fish or grilled chicken breasts.

- Cooking spray
- 1.5 pounds (680 g) small red-skin potatoes, quartered
- 2 red onions, cut into ¼-inch-thick (6 mm) wedges
- 2 tablespoons extra virgin olive oil
- 1 tablespoon plus 1 teaspoon Dijon mustard
- 1 tablespoon finely chopped fresh thyme
- 1 garlic clove, finely minced
- Grated zest of 1 lemon
- ½ teaspoon freshly ground black pepper
- 2 cups (300 g) cherry tomatoes, halved
- ½ cup (70 g) pitted kalamata olives, halved

1. Preheat the oven to 425°F (220°C). Line a large rimmed baking pan with foil and spray with cooking spray.

2. Place the potatoes and onions in large bowl. Whisk together the oil, mustard, thyme, garlic, lemon zest, and pepper in a small bowl; reserve 2 tablespoons to use later. Pour the remaining mixture over the potatoes and onions and stir to coat.

3. Spread the potatoes and onions in a single layer on the baking sheet. Roast for 30 minutes.

4. Flip or stir the vegetables. Add the tomatoes and olives. Spoon the remaining oil-mustard mixture over the vegetables. Roast for 10 to 15 minutes, until the potatoes are tender, the onions are crisped and browned on the edges, and the tomato skins are wrinkled and browned in spots.

5. Transfer to a serving bowl or platter and serve warm. Store in an airtight container in the refrigerator for up to 5 days. Enjoy cold or hot. Reheat either in the microwave in 30-second increments on HIGH until hot or in a skillet over medium-high heat with a little olive oil, sautéing until hot.

Per Serving: Calories 108; Protein 1 g; Carbs 9 g; Dietary Fiber 2 g; Added Sugars 0 g; Total Fat 7 g; Sat Fat 1 g; Omega-3s 40 mg; Sodium 249 mg; Potassium 239 mg

ROASTED POTATOES WITH CINNAMON

Makes 4 servings

Cinnamon adds a warm, alluring aroma and sweet, spiced flavor to roasted potatoes. Serve these with Lamb Chops with Cilantro-Mint Pesto (page 46) and Dilly Cucumber Salad (page 152).

1.5 pounds (680 g) baby red-skin or Yukon gold potatoes, halved

6 garlic cloves, halved

3 tablespoons extra virgin olive oil

Four 3-inch (7.5 cm) cinnamon sticks

½ teaspoon freshly ground black pepper

½ teaspoon kosher salt

1. Preheat the oven to 375°F (190°C).

2. Toss the potatoes and garlic with the oil and pepper in a large bowl. Spread in a single layer on a rimmed baking sheet. Place the cinnamon sticks among the potatoes. Roast for about 15 minutes, then stir. Continue roasting for 15 to 20 minutes (30 to 35 minutes total), until the potatoes are beginning to brown.

3. Increase the oven temperature to 400°F (200°C) and roast for 10 minutes, until the potatoes are crispy, brown, and easily pierced with a fork.

4. Sprinkle with salt and discard the cinnamon sticks. Serve warm.

Per Serving: Calories 222; Protein 4 g; Carbs 29 g; Dietary Fiber 3 g; Added Sugars 0 g; Total Fat 11 g; Sat Fat 2 g; Omega-3s 100 mg; Sodium 148 mg; Potassium 798 mg

ROSEMARY MASHED POTATOES

Makes 6 servings

This recipe uses a steeping technique to infuse rosemary flavor into the milk and produce a faint rosemary flavor in the final dish. Your guests will take their first bite and say, "Mmm . . . what is that?" Serve these aromatic mashed potatoes with Simply Cooked Pork Tenderloin (page 332) and Citrus-Glazed Carrots (page 265).

2 pounds (907 g) Yukon gold–type potatoes, quartered

1 cup (240 ml) milk

1 tablespoon dry rosemary leaves

2 tablespoons extra virgin olive oil

½ teaspoon kosher salt

½ teaspoon freshly ground black pepper

1. Place the potatoes in a large pot; add just enough cold water to cover. Bring to a boil, then reduce the heat to medium-low. Simmer for 20 to 25 minutes, until the potatoes can be easily pierced with a fork.

2. When the potatoes are about half done, heat the milk and rosemary in a small saucepan over low heat until tiny bubbles appear on the surface at the edge of the pan. Infuse the milk for about 10 minutes. Strain the milk to remove the rosemary.

3. Drain the water from the potatoes and add the rosemary-infused milk, oil, salt, and pepper. Mash well. Serve immediately.

Per Serving: Calories 175; Protein 4 g; Carbs 30 g; Dietary Fiber 3 g; Added Sugars 0 g; Total Fat 6 g; Sat Fat 1 g; Omega-3s 40 mg; Sodium 142 mg; Potassium 73 mg

SPICY ROASTED SQUASH WITH TUSCAN-STYLE GLAZE

Makes 4 to 6 servings

This dish is a festive alternative to simple roasted squash or mashed sweet potatoes. Consider using pumpkin or any other winter squash like acorn, buttercup, or turban, butternut, Hubbard, kabocha, or Golden Nugget. Orange sweet potatoes, purple sweet potatoes, and white-fleshed sweet potatoes also work well.

- 6 cups (695 g) peeled, seeded, cubed pumpkin or winter squash (about 2 pounds/907 g), or sweet potatoes (about 3 pounds/1.4 kg)
- 2 tablespoons extra virgin olive oil
- 6 garlic cloves, minced
- 1 tablespoon chopped fresh rosemary, plus 4 sprigs
- ½ teaspoon red pepper flakes
- ½ teaspoon freshly ground black pepper
- 1 cup (240 ml) dry light-bodied red wine (such as Chianti or Pinot Noir)
- 1 tablespoon butter or plant-based spread
- 1 tablespoon honey
- 1 teaspoon minced fresh ginger
- ¼ teaspoon kosher salt

1. Preheat the oven to 400°F (200°C). Line a large, rimmed baking sheet with foil or parchment paper.

2. Place the squash into a large bowl. Drizzle with the oil. Add the garlic, chopped rosemary, red pepper flakes, and pepper, and toss to coat. Spread the squash in a single layer on the baking sheet, then top with 2 of the rosemary sprigs. Roast for 10 minutes.

3. Flip the squash cubes with a spatula. Continue roasting for 10 to 15 minutes, until the cubes have browned edges and can be pierced with a fork.

4. While the squash is roasting, simmer the wine in a small saucepan over medium heat for 15 minutes or until the liquid is reduced to ½ cup (120 ml). Whisk in the butter, honey, and ginger. Cook until thickened, stirring continuously, 3 to 4 minutes.

5. Transfer the squash to a serving bowl or leave it on the baking sheet, if preferred. Drizzle the glaze over the squash and gently toss to coat. Top with salt and the remaining 2 rosemary sprigs. Serve hot.

NOTE: *When choosing a wine to cook with, it's important to choose a great-quality wine. Never spend your money on something marketed as "cooking wine"; only cook with wine you'd want to drink.*

Per Serving: Calories 168; Protein 2 g; Carbs 15 g; Dietary Fiber 1 g; Added Sugars 3 g; Total Fat 8 g; Sat Fat 2 g; Omega-3s 60 mg; Sodium 60 mg; Potassium 562 mg

ROASTED ACORN SQUASH WITH ALLSPICE & SAGE

Makes 4 servings

Squash and sage are a classic flavor pairing. The sage deepens the savory flavors of the squash, and the allspice and cinnamon bolster the squash's natural sweetness. Serve this simple side dish with Simply Cooked Pork Tenderloin (page 332) and a whole grain like Simply Cooked Farro (page 226).

- 1 acorn squash
- 1 tablespoon extra virgin olive oil
- 1 tablespoon finely chopped fresh sage
- 1 tablespoon apple cider vinegar
- ½ teaspoon ground allspice
- ¼ teaspoon ground cinnamon

1. Preheat the oven to 375°F (190°C). Line a large rimmed baking sheet with parchment paper.

2. Remove and discard the stem and ¼ inch (6 mm) from the bottom of the squash. Halve the squash lengthwise and scoop out the seeds and membrane. Cut each squash half crosswise into four 1-inch-thick (2.5 cm) slices.

3. Whisk together the oil, sage, vinegar, allspice, and cinnamon in large shallow dish. Add the squash and toss to coat. Arrange the squash on the baking sheet. Drizzle any remaining oil mixture over the slices.

4. Roast for 30 minutes, or until fork-tender. Serve warm.

Per Serving: Calories 76; Protein 1 g; Carbs 12 g; Dietary Fiber 2 g; Added Sugars 0 g; Total Fat 4 g; Sat Fat 1 g; Omega-3s 50 mg; Sodium 3 mg; Potassium 379 mg

SPAGHETTI SQUASH SAUTÉ WITH BLACK OLIVES & FETA
Makes 4 servings

This Greek-inspired dish uses spaghetti squash in place of the more traditional eggplant. Olives and feta round out the Greek flavor profile. Feta, whether made from sheep's or cow's milk, provides a briny tanginess, offering a satisfying flavor contrast to the sweetness of the squash.

1 spaghetti squash
2 tablespoons extra virgin olive oil
8 green onions, chopped
3 garlic cloves, minced
1 tablespoon chopped fresh oregano
½ cup (30 g) chopped fresh parsley
1 tablespoon fresh lemon juice
½ cup (70 g) sliced pitted kalamata or black olives
½ cup (75 g) crumbled feta
Freshly ground black pepper

1. Pierce all sides of the squash several times with a fork. Microwave on a large microwave-safe plate on HIGH for 10 to 12 minutes, until slightly soft when squeezed. Let stand for 10 minutes to cool.

2. Halve the squash lengthwise and remove the seeds. With a fork, shred the squash into spaghetti-like strands.

3. Heat the oil in a large skillet over medium-high heat. Cook the green onions and garlic, stirring constantly, until aromatic and just starting to brown, about 3 minutes. Stir in the oregano and the squash, and cook until heated through, 3 to 5 minutes.

4. Add the parsley, sprinkle with lemon juice, and toss using two forks. Add the olives and feta, and toss again. Top with black pepper and serve hot.

Per Serving: Calories 267; Protein 6 g; Carbs 28 g; Dietary Fiber 6 g; Added Sugars 0 g; Total Fat 17 g; Sat Fat 4 g; Omega-3s 550 mg; Sodium 479 mg; Potassium 506 mg

SAVORY SWEET POTATO FRIES
Makes 4 servings

Did you know that sweet potatoes aren't actually potatoes? Sweet potatoes are members of the morning glory plant family, while potatoes are part of the nightshade family. Both are nutrient-rich vegetable choices, and both come in a wide variety of sizes, shapes, and colors. We like to use dark orange sweet potatoes in this recipe for their gorgeous color and vitamin A (beta-carotene) content. These fries are great served with Avocado Lemon Dill Aïoli (page 43) or Chimichurri (page 54).

3 tablespoons extra virgin olive oil
1 teaspoon ground cumin
1 teaspoon ground thyme
½ teaspoon freshly ground black pepper
4 medium sweet potatoes, peeled (if desired) and cut lengthwise into ½-inch (13 mm) strips
3 tablespoons chopped fresh flat-leaf parsley
¼ teaspoon kosher salt

1. Preheat the oven to 400°F (200°C). Line two baking sheets with foil or parchment paper.

2. Whisk together the oil, cumin, thyme, and pepper in a large bowl. Add the sweet potatoes and toss to coat. Spread in a single layer on the baking sheets and bake for 15 minutes.

3. Flip the fries and bake for 10 to 15 minutes, until golden brown and fork-tender.

4. Sprinkle with the parsley and salt, and serve hot.

VARIATION: *Spiced Sweet Potato Fries*
Replace the cumin, thyme, and black pepper with 1 teaspoon ground cinnamon, 1 teaspoon ground nutmeg, and ½ teaspoon ground ginger. Place one 3-inch (7.5 cm) cinnamon stick on each of the baking sheets before baking. Serve with Raspberry-Chipotle Sauce (page 57), apple butter, or your favorite dipping sauce.

Per Serving: Calories 229; Protein 2 g; Carbs 34 g; Dietary Fiber 4 g; Added Sugars 0 g; Total Fat 11 g; Sat Fat 1 g; Omega-3s 80 mg; Sodium 94 mg; Potassium 23 mg

ROASTED SWEET POTATOES & GINGER-SPICED APPLES

Makes 6 servings

Apples and sweet potatoes are a terrific duo that bring fall flavors to the table. This dish pairs well with the Smoked Tri-Tip (page 329). The Savory Roasted Mixed Nuts add crunch and intensify the flavors of the spiced apples and creamy sweet potatoes.

3 medium sweet potatoes, peeled and sliced in ½-inch medallions

1 tablespoon extra virgin olive oil

3 tart apples (McIntosh, Jonathan, Cortland, or Braeburn), cored and sliced

¾ cup (180 ml) fresh orange juice

1 teaspoon ground cinnamon

1 teaspoon grated fresh ginger

½ teaspoon ground allspice

½ teaspoon ground nutmeg

1 tablespoon grated orange zest

6 tablespoons chopped nuts from Savory Roasted Mixed Nuts (page 347)

1. Preheat the oven to 375°F (190°C). Line a large rimmed baking sheet with foil or parchment paper.

2. Place the sweet potatoes on the baking sheet and drizzle with the oil. Roast for 30 to 40 minutes, until crisp-tender.

3. Heat the apples, orange juice, cinnamon, ginger, allspice, and nutmeg in a large skillet over medium-high heat. Cover and cook until the apples soften, 3 to 5 minutes. Uncover, reduce the heat, and simmer until the apples are fragrant, moist, and fork-tender, 2 to 3 minutes.

4. Gently mix in the sweet potatoes and orange zest. Heat for 1 to 2 minutes. Serve with 1 tablespoon Savory Roasted Mixed Nuts sprinkled over each serving.

Per Serving: Calories 201; Protein 3 g; Carbs 35 g; Dietary Fiber 5 g; Added Sugars 0 g; Total Fat 7 g; Sat Fat 1 g; Omega-3s 80 mg; Sodium 28 mg; Potassium 216 mg

FAJITA VEGETABLES

Makes 6 servings

This colorful mixture of sautéed vegetables is the perfect accompaniment for tortillas filled with Crispy Tofu Bites (page 250) or your favorite grilled meat, poultry, or seafood. Cooking these vegetables ahead of time and warming them up right before serving is a great way to get dinner on the table in minutes.

¼ cup (60 ml) Beef Stock (page 69) or Vegetable Broth (page 72)

2 teaspoons cornstarch

2 tablespoons peanut or extra virgin olive oil

3 garlic cloves, minced

1 white onion, thinly sliced

1 green bell pepper, seeded and thinly sliced

1 red bell pepper, seeded and thinly sliced

1 orange bell pepper, seeded and thinly sliced

1 yellow bell pepper, seeded and thinly sliced

1 teaspoon ground cumin

1 teaspoon dried oregano

1 teaspoon red pepper flakes

½ teaspoon freshly ground black pepper

½ cup (8 g) chopped fresh cilantro

1. Stir together the broth and cornstarch in a small bowl to form a slurry.

2. Heat the oil in a wok or large skillet over high heat until shimmering. Add the garlic and stir-fry until fragrant, about 15 seconds.

3. Reduce the heat to medium-high, then add the onion, the green, red, orange, and yellow bell peppers, and the cumin, oregano, red pepper flakes, and black pepper. Stir-fry until the peppers start to soften, 5 to 6 minutes.

4. Reduce the heat to low, add the slurry, and cook until the sauce starts to thicken, 1 to 2 minutes.

5. Remove from the heat, add the cilantro, and serve. Store in an airtight container in the refrigerator for up to 4 days.

Per Serving: Calories 81; Protein 2 g; Carbs 9 g; Dietary Fiber 2 g; Added Sugars 0 g; Total Fat 5 g; Sat Fat 1 g; Omega-3s 10 mg; Sodium 21 mg; Potassium 264 mg

QUICK-PICKLED VEGETABLES

Makes 3 cups (1,400 g)

Pickling vegetables is much easier than it sounds. With this recipe you can pickle any vegetable that appeals to you. Remember, the thinner you cut the vegetable, the more quickly it will pickle. Serve as a topping on Beef & Mushroom Burgers (page 178) or as an accompaniment to Seafood Trio Rolls (page 294).

- 3 cups (350 g) thinly sliced vegetables, such as asparagus, carrots, cauliflower, cucumbers, bell peppers, green beans, radishes, kohlrabi, and rutabaga
- ¼ cup (40 g) thinly sliced red onion, slices separated
- 2 garlic cloves, peeled
- 1 teaspoon coriander seeds
- ½ teaspoon dill seeds
- ¼ teaspoon black peppercorns
- 2 cups (480 ml) cold water
- 1 cup (240 ml) white vinegar or apple cider vinegar
- 1 tablespoon kosher salt
- 2 teaspoons sugar
- 1 bay leaf

1. Place the vegetables in a large, heat-proof bowl. Add the garlic, coriander seeds, dill seeds, and peppercorns.

2. Combine the water, vinegar, salt, sugar, and bay leaf in a medium saucepan. Bring to a boil over medium heat, stirring until the sugar and salt have dissolved, 2 minutes. Discard the bay leaf.

3. Pour the brine over the vegetables. Stir to make sure all the vegetables are covered. Cover loosely and let cool to room temperature, about 30 minutes.

4. Transfer to a clean container or a large glass jar and cover, making sure the brine is completely covering the vegetables. Refrigerate for at least 2 hours before serving. Store in an airtight container in the refrigerator for up to 2 weeks.

Serving Size 3 cups (1,400 g); Calories 99; Protein 2 g; Carbs 25 g; Dietary Fiber 4 g; Added Sugars 3 g; Total Fat 0 g; Sat Fat 0 g; Omega-3s 0 mg; Sodium 360 mg; Potassium 481 mg

GARLICKY WILD RICE & MUSHROOM–STUFFED ACORN SQUASH

Makes 4 servings

This super flavorful stuffed squash is easy to make. If wild rice isn't handy, consider substituting an equal amount of cooked farro or quinoa. So delicious!

- 2 acorn squash, halved lengthwise and seeded
- 2 tablespoons extra virgin olive oil
- ¼ teaspoon freshly ground black pepper
- ¼ teaspoon kosher salt
- 1½ cups (105 g) chopped mushrooms (of choice)
- 1 celery stalk, chopped
- 1 shallot, chopped
- 3 garlic cloves, minced
- 1 tablespoon chopped fresh sage
- 1 tablespoon chopped fresh thyme
- ½ teaspoon ground nutmeg
- 1½ cups (250 g) Simply Cooked Wild Rice (page 234)
- 4 tablespoons chopped, toasted walnuts or dried cranberries
- 4 tablespoons chopped fresh parsley

1. Preheat the oven to 400°F (200°C). Line a baking sheet with foil or parchment paper.

2. Place the squash cut side up on the baking sheet and brush with 1 tablespoon of the oil. Sprinkle with the salt and pepper. Turn the squash cut side down and roast for 30 minutes, or until softened.

3. Heat the remaining 1 tablespoon oil in a large skillet over medium-high heat. Add the mushrooms, celery, shallots, and garlic. Sauté until the shallots are softened and translucent, the celery is tender, and the mushrooms have released their liquid, about 5 minutes. Add the sage, thyme, nutmeg, and wild rice and mix well.

4. Turn the squash cut side up. Fill each squash half with the vegetable–wild rice mixture. Bake for 15 to 20 minutes, until the squash is heated through and the filling is bubbly.

5. Sprinkle each squash with 1 tablespoon each of walnuts and parsley. Serve warm.

Per Serving: Calories 260; Protein 6 g; Carbs 36 g; Dietary Fiber 5 g; Added Sugars 0 g; Total Fat 13 g; Sat Fat 2 g; Omega-3s 830 mg; Sodium 124 mg; Potassium 1,000 mg

BULGUR-STUFFED PEPPERS

Makes 4 servings

Stuffed bell peppers (green, orange, red, or yellow) make for a quick and easy weeknight entrée with any of the Simply Cooked whole grains in chapter 13. Here, we use Simply Cooked Bulgur. Once you've made this meal-in-a-pepper, you'll be inspired to stuff peppers with other whole grains such as millet, sorghum, or brown rice.

- 2 bell peppers, halved lengthwise, stems, seeds, and membranes removed
- 2 tablespoons water
- 1 tablespoon extra virgin olive oil
- ½ cup (80 g) chopped onion
- ½ cup (35 g) chopped mushrooms (of choice)
- 8 cherry tomatoes, halved, or 1 medium tomato, chopped
- 3 garlic cloves, chopped
- 2 tablespoons chopped fresh tarragon or thyme
- ¼ teaspoon freshly ground black pepper
- 1 tablespoon balsamic vinegar
- 2 cups (365 g) Simply Cooked Bulgur (page 224)
- 4 tablespoons freshly grated Parmesan
- 4 tablespoons pine nuts
- 4 tarragon or thyme sprigs

1. Preheat the oven to 350°F (180°C).

2. Place the bell peppers cut side down on a microwave-safe dish, add the water, and cover loosely. Microwave on HIGH until slightly softened, about 3 minutes. Place the peppers cut side up in a single layer in an 8-inch (20 cm) square baking dish.

3. Heat the oil in a large skillet over medium heat. Add the onion and sauté until just starting to soften, 1 minute. Add the mushrooms, tomatoes, garlic, tarragon, and black pepper. Sauté until the onion is translucent, the mushrooms have reduced, and the tomato skins are wrinkled, 3 to 4 minutes. Remove from the heat, then stir in the vinegar and bulgur.

4. Fill each pepper half with one-fourth of the vegetable-bulgur mixture. Cover and bake for 15 minutes.

5. Uncover and sprinkle the pepper halves with 1 tablespoon each of Parmesan and pine nuts. Bake for 10 minutes, until the pine nuts are toasted, the filling is hot, and the peppers are tender. Garnish with a tarragon sprig prior to serving.

Per Serving: Calories 236; Protein 6 g; Carbs 25 g; Dietary Fiber 4 g; Added Sugars 0 g; Total Fat 13 g; Sat Fat 2 g; Omega-3s 60 mg; Sodium 115 mg; Potassium 369 mg

MUSHROOM & SPINACH–STUFFED TOMATOES

Makes 4 servings

These light yet flavorful mushrooms pair well with Italian-inspired dishes like our Mock Risotto with Zucchini (page 231), Roasted Red Pepper Fettucine (page 212) or Tuscan-Inspired Pork (page 333).

- 4 round tomatoes, cored, insides scooped out
- 1 tablespoon extra virgin olive oil
- 6 ounces (170 g) coarsely chopped white or cremini mushrooms
- ½ cup (80 g) minced sweet onion (such as Vidalia or Walla Walla)
- 3 garlic cloves, minced
- 6 cups (180 g) fresh baby spinach leaves, chopped
- 1 tablespoon Italian Seasoning (page 34)
- 1 tablespoon grated lemon zest
- 1 teaspoon ground nutmeg
- ¾ cup (45 g) panko bread crumbs, toasted
- ½ cup (55 g) Garlic & Herb Bread Crumbs (page 33)

1. Preheat the oven to 350°F (180°C). Line an 8-inch (20 cm) square baking dish with foil or parchment paper and place the tomatoes in the dish.

2. Heat the oil in a large skillet over medium-low heat. Cook the mushrooms, onion, and garlic, stirring constantly, until the mushrooms start to soften, the onions are translucent, and the garlic is fragrant, 5 to 7 minutes. Stir in the spinach and cook until it's wilted, 4 to 6 minutes. Stir in the seasoning, lemon zest, nutmeg, and panko.

3. Divide the filling among the tomato shells. Bake for 20 to 30 minutes, until hot and bubbly.

4. Spoon 2 tablespoons of the bread crumbs over each stuffed tomato. Return to the oven for 5 to 7 minutes, until the topping is crispy and golden brown.

Per Serving: Calories 168; Protein 7 g; Carbs 25 g; Dietary Fiber 4 g; Added Sugars 0 g; Total Fat 6 g; Sat Fat 1 g; Omega-3s 50 mg; Sodium 153 mg; Potassium 548 mg

CURRIED RICE–STUFFED TOMATOES

Makes 4 servings

These tomatoes are a fun side dish to serve with a meal featuring Indian-inspired dishes like Chicken Tikka Masala (page 309), Chicken Tandoori Skewers (page 307), or Cucumber Raita (page 63).

4 round tomatoes, cored, insides scooped out

¼ teaspoon kosher salt

¼ teaspoon freshly ground black pepper

1 tablespoon extra virgin olive oil

¼ cup (40 g) minced shallots

2 garlic cloves, minced

1 tablespoon grated lemon zest

1 teaspoon Curry Powder (page 32)

½ teaspoon ground cumin

½ teaspoon smoked paprika

¼ teaspoon red pepper flakes

2 cups (390 g) Simply Cooked Brown Rice (page 230)

Juice of 1 lemon

4 tablespoons chopped fresh cilantro

4 teaspoons pine nuts, toasted

1. Preheat the oven to 350°F (180°C). Line an 8-inch (20 cm) square baking dish with foil or parchment paper and place the tomatoes into the dish. Sprinkle the inside of each tomato lightly with the salt and pepper.

2. Heat the oil in large skillet over medium heat for 1 minute. Add the shallot and garlic and sauté until the garlic just starts to brown, 2 minutes. Stir in the lemon zest, curry powder, cumin, and paprika, and cook until the spices are fragrant, 1 minute. Stir in the rice and lemon juice.

3. Stuff each tomato with ½ cup (115 g) of the rice mixture. Bake for 15 to 20 minutes, until hot and steamy.

4. Top each tomato with 1 tablespoon chopped cilantro and 1 teaspoon pine nuts, and serve.

Per Serving: Calories 423; Protein 10 g; Carbs 79 g; Dietary Fiber 7 g; Added Sugars 0 g; Total Fat 11 g; Sat Fat 1 g; Omega-3s 50 mg; Sodium 145 mg; Potassium 382 mg

CAULIFLOWER-WALNUT CASSEROLE

Makes 6 servings

This casserole garners rave reviews every time! Our built-in shortcut is to use frozen cauliflower florets—no cleaning, cutting, or chopping required. We roast the cauliflower first, but you could use steam-in-bag cauliflower to save even more time.

6 cups (640 g) frozen cauliflower florets, thawed

Cooking spray

Two 5.3-ounce (150 g) containers plain Greek yogurt (about ⅔ cup each)

1 cup (115 g) shredded medium cheddar

½ cup (40 g) freshly grated Parmesan or Gruyère

1 tablespoon reduced-sodium chicken or vegetable broth

1 tablespoon Dijon mustard

1 teaspoon ground cumin

¾ cup (90 g) chopped walnuts

½ cup (30 g) panko bread crumbs

2 tablespoons butter or plant-based spread

⅓ cup (20 g) chopped fresh flat-leaf parsley or cilantro

¼ teaspoon white pepper

1. Preheat the oven to 450°F (230°C). Line a large rimmed baking sheet with parchment paper.

2. Spread the cauliflower florets on the baking sheet in a single layer. Spray generously with the cooking spray. Roast for 15 minutes.

3. Flip the florets, and spray again with cooking spray. Roast for 10 minutes, until the cauliflower has browned, crispy edges.

4. Spray a 9 × 13-inch (23 × 33 cm) baking dish with cooking spray. Transfer the cauliflower to the baking dish. Leave the oven on.

5. Mix the yogurt, cheddar, Parmesan, chicken broth, mustard, and cumin in a medium bowl. Spoon over the cauliflower.

6. Combine the walnuts, bread crumbs, and butter in a small skillet over medium-low heat. Cook, stirring occasionally, until the bread crumbs start to brown and the walnuts are toasted, about 2 minutes. Sprinkle over the cauliflower.

7. Bake for about 20 minutes, until the casserole is bubbly and hot. Sprinkle with the parsley and pepper, and serve hot. Store in an airtight container in the refrigerator for up to 4 days. Either reheat individual servings in the microwave in 15-second increments on HIGH until hot or place the casserole in an oven-safe baking dish, cover, and reheat at 350°F (180°C) for 40 minutes or until heated through and a digital food thermometer reads 165°F (75°C).

Per Serving: Calories 305; Protein 14 g; Carbs 14 g; Dietary Fiber 4 g; Added Sugars 0 g; Total Fat 23 g; Sat Fat 8 g; Omega-3s 1,510 mg; Sodium 395 mg; Potassium 361 mg

CREAMY EGGPLANT WITH TOMATOES

Makes 4 servings

Slowly cooking eggplant creates a desirable creamy and soft base for this recipe, similar to mashed potatoes. Tomatoes provide a subtle sweetness, pine nuts add a bit of gentle crunch, and a dollop of yogurt, added just before serving, gives this dish a range of varying tastes, textures, and temperatures. This recipe is integral to the Mediterranean Rice Bake with Eggplant and Tomatoes (page 231).

1 tablespoon extra virgin olive oil

1 shallot, chopped

1 green bell pepper, seeded and chopped

3 garlic cloves, minced

3 large tomatoes, diced

1 medium eggplant, trimmed, peeled, and cubed

2 tablespoons thinly sliced fresh basil

1 tablespoon fresh lemon juice

½ teaspoon freshly ground black pepper

One 5.3-ounce (150 g) container plain Greek yogurt (about ⅔ cup)

¼ cup (35 g) pine nuts, toasted

1. Heat the oil in a Dutch oven or large skillet over medium heat. Sauté the shallot, bell pepper, and garlic until fragrant, about 4 minutes.

2. Stir in the tomatoes. Cover; cook until the tomatoes have started to break down, 5 minutes. Mash the tomatoes with the back of a spoon.

3. Add the eggplant and stir to coat. Cover; cook over medium-low heat, stirring occasionally, until the eggplant is soft, and some of the excess liquid is released to concentrate the flavors, 20 to 25 minutes.

4. Stir in the basil, lemon juice, and black pepper. Serve with yogurt and pine nuts on the side.

Per Serving: Calories 182; Protein 8 g; Carbs 17 g; Dietary Fiber 6 g; Added Sugars 0 g; Total Fat 11 g; Sat Fat 2 g; Omega-3s 50 mg; Sodium 22 mg; Potassium 692 mg

POTATO-TURNIP GRATIN

Makes 6 servings

This dish is flavored with Emmental, a hard yellow Swiss cheese that melts easily and imparts fruity, earthy, and nutty flavors to the creamy turnips and potatoes. We top it off with Garlic & Herb Bread Crumbs, which further enhance the flavors.

Cooking spray

1 pound (454 g) russet potatoes, cut into ¼-inch (6 mm) slices

1 pound (454 g) white turnips, cut into ¼-inch (6 mm) slices

1 cup (240 ml) milk, plus more if needed

1 leek, cleaned (see Tip, page 79) and chopped

2 tablespoons butter or plant-based spread, melted

3 tablespoons all-purpose flour

½ cup (55 g) shredded Emmental or Gruyère

1 teaspoon ground sage or 1 tablespoon chopped fresh sage

1 teaspoon ground thyme or 1 tablespoon chopped fresh thyme

½ teaspoon white pepper

¼ teaspoon kosher salt

⅔ cup (145 g) Garlic & Herb Bread Crumbs (page 33)

1. Preheat the oven to 375°F (190°C). Spray a 7 × 11-inch (18 × 28 cm) baking dish with cooking spray.

2. Bring 1 inch (2.5 cm) of water to a boil in a medium saucepan. Add the potatoes and turnips. Cover and simmer until slightly softened but not fork-tender, 5 to 8 minutes.

3. Drain, saving ½ cup (120 ml) of the cooking water. If you don't have enough water, add milk to the water to make ½ cup (120 ml). Spread the turnips and potatoes across the baking dish. Evenly distribute the leeks over the top.

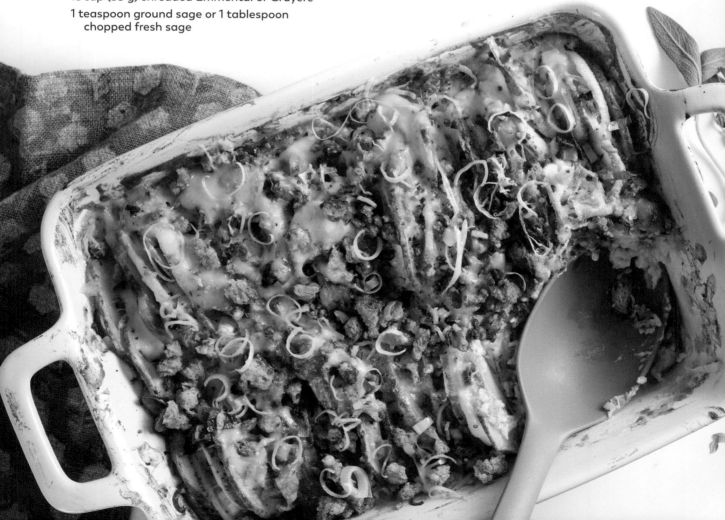

4. Melt the butter in a small saucepan over medium-high heat. Gradually whisk in the flour. When well blended and paste-like, slowly add the reserved water, whisking constantly. Slowly add 1 cup (240 ml) milk and cook until thick, 5 to 7 minutes. Remove from the heat and whisk in the Emmental, sage, thyme, pepper, and salt until the cheese has melted.

5. Pour the cheese sauce over the vegetables, then sprinkle the bread crumbs over the top. Bake for 20 to 25 minutes, until the vegetables are fork-tender and the topping is golden brown. Serve immediately. Store in an airtight container in the refrigerator for up to 4 days. Reheat individual servings either in the microwave in 15-second increments on HIGH until hot or place the gratin in an oven-safe baking dish, cover, and reheat at 350°F (180°C) for 40 minutes or until heated through and a digital food thermometer reads 165°F (75°C).

Per Serving: Calories 263; Protein 10 g; Carbs 35 g; Dietary Fiber 4 g; Added Sugars 0 g; Total Fat 10 g; Sat Fat 5 g; Omega-3s 100 mg; Sodium 270 mg; Potassium 581 mg

VEGETARIAN SHEPHERD'S PIE

Makes 6 servings

This all-vegetable version of a traditional shepherd's pie is just as warm and filling as the meaty original. We've shortened the time in the kitchen by preparing the vegetables in one pot on the stove, then placing the pot in the oven to finish cooking.

4 cups (915 g) Simply Spanish-Style Mashed Potatoes (page 259)

⅔ cup (150 g) plain Greek yogurt

½ cup (25 g) chopped fresh chives

¾ cup (45 g) chopped fresh parsley

2 tablespoons extra virgin olive oil

1½ cups (240 g) chopped onion (about 1 large onion)

2 garlic cloves, minced

2 medium eggplants, peeled and cubed

1 red bell pepper, seeded and finely chopped

1 celery stalk, finely chopped

One 14.5-ounce (411 g) can diced tomatoes

1½ tablespoons Italian Seasoning (page 34)

½ cup (55 g) shredded sharp cheddar

1 tablespoon apple cider vinegar

1. Preheat the oven to 350ºF (180ºC).

2. Mix the potatoes with the yogurt, chives, and ½ cup (30 g) of the parsley in a medium bowl until just combined. Do not overmix.

3. Heat the oil in a Dutch oven over medium heat. Sauté the onions and garlic until just softened, about 3 minutes. Add the eggplant, pepper, and celery. Cover and cook, stirring occasionally, until the eggplant is softened but not sticking to the pan, 6 to 8 minutes.

4. Increase the heat to medium-high. Stir in the tomatoes and seasoning and cook until the liquid is simmering, about 5 minutes. Add the cheddar and vinegar, and cook until the vegetables are heated through, the mixture is fragrant, and the cheese is melted, 5 minutes.

5. Top with the mashed potato mixture to form a crust. Bake for 25 to 30 minutes, until the pie is bubbling around the edges and potatoes are brown in spots. Sprinkle the remaining ¼ cup (15 g) parsley over the top just before serving.

Per Serving: Calories 362; Protein 11 g; Carbs 47 g; Dietary Fiber 10 g; Added Sugars 0 g; Total Fat 17 g; Sat Fat 4 g; Omega-3s 140 mg; Sodium 206 mg; Potassium 696 mg

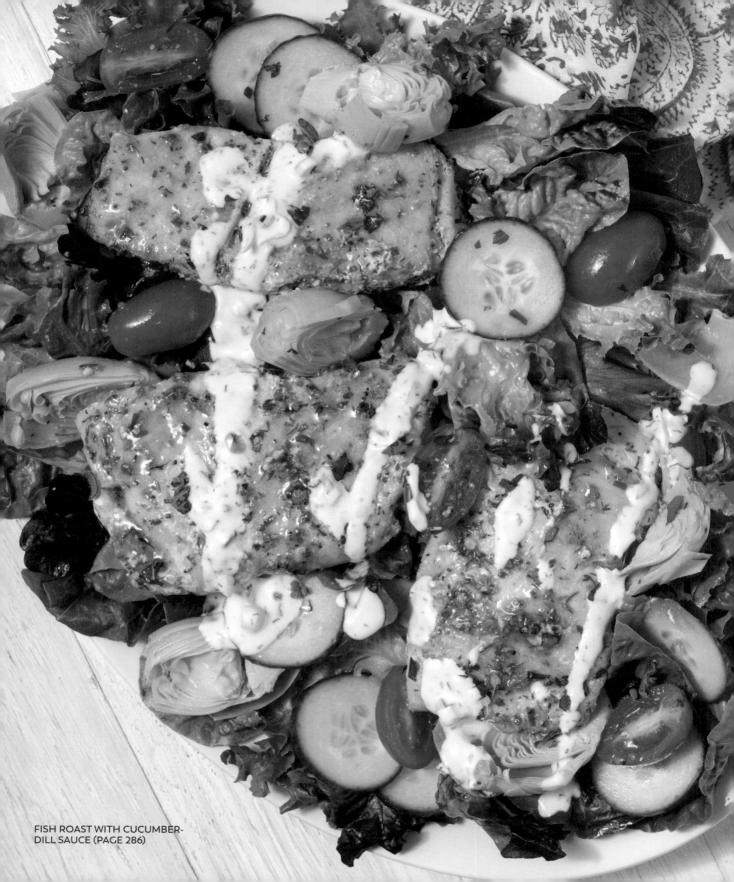

FISH ROAST WITH CUCUMBER-
DILL SAUCE (PAGE 286)

CHAPTER 16

Fish & Shellfish

Fish & Shellfish

Fish Flavor Pairings 283

Broiled Halibut with Pesto 284

Clams in Chorizo Tomato
Saffron Broth 284

Coconut Fish Curry 285

Crispy Fish Sticks 286

Fish Roast with Cucumber-Dill Sauce . . 286

Gingery Mackerel with
Lemon & Garlic 287

Mediterranean Tilapia en Papillote 287

Mini Crab Cakes 289

Miso-Glazed Scallops 289

Mussels in Coconut-Lemongrass
Broth 290

Pan-Seared Crispy Catfish 290

Roasted Almond-Crusted Snapper 291

Roasted Balsamic-Glazed Salmon 291

Roasted Salmon with Honey
Walnut Lemon Sauce 292

Sautéed Shrimp and Scallops 292

Scallops en Papillote with Shallots,
Edamame & Bell Pepper 293

Seafood Trio Rolls 294

Sesame Shrimp en Papillote 294

Sheet Pan Fish & Vegetable Bake 295

Shrimp Curry 296

Shrimp Fried Rice 296

Shrimp Jambalaya 297

Simply Broiled Salmon 298

Smoky Seared Salmon for One 298

Summer Lake Bake 299

White Fish with Fennel & Leeks 299

Eating more fish and shellfish is another great way to add essential nutrients to your diet, especially omega-3 fatty acids. While many people think of fatty fish like salmon and tuna, omega-3s are found in all fish and shellfish in varying amounts. Experts at the Seafood Nutrition Partnership, a nonprofit organization, urge adults to consume least 8 ounces (227 grams) of fish and shellfish per week. Their website (seafoodnutrition.org) provides valuable information about making smart seafood choices. It also includes guidance on mercury, which is only a concern for pregnant people who should avoid "The Big 7" (shark, tilefish from the Gulf of Mexico, swordfish, king mackerel, orange roughy, marlin, and bigeye tuna).

We've worked diligently to include recipes for as many species of fish and types of shellfish as possible, knowing that names vary by region. We've also kept sustainable seafood fishing and farming practices in mind, focusing on the species that are least likely to be overfished. And as in all other recipe chapters, we've included recipes that draw their culinary inspiration from food cultures around the world.

We've included many salmon and shrimp recipes because we know they are popular options for many—we also love their flavor and texture. But we encourage you to venture beyond these two proteins by trying other recipes in this chapter. For flavor inspiration, refer to our fish flavor pairing table on this page.

We also focused on a wide variety of cooking techniques, including three en papillote recipes. "En papillote" is the French term for cooking in a paper packet, typically made of parchment paper, or sometimes foil. This moist-heat cooking method is forgiving; it makes it difficult to overcook fish. It's also a fun way to present food to guests because everyone gets their own individually wrapped gift of goodness.

If you're striving to increase your seafood intake, focus on trying one new recipe from this chapter every week for a few months to find the ones that work for you. Most of our recipes work for various types of seafood, and other ingredients like aromatics or vegetables can be varied to create different flavor profiles. So go forth, cast a line, and "fish" for some new inspiration in this chapter!

Table 10: Fish Flavor Pairings

FISH	NUT	CITRUS	AROMATIC OR VEGETABLE	OTHER FLAVORING INGREDIENT
Cod or haddock	Pine nuts	Lemon	Potatoes	Parsley
Flounder	Almonds	Lemon	Sweet onion (e.g., Vidalia or Walla Walla)	White wine
Grouper	Almonds	Lemon	Tomatoes	Sesame seeds
Halibut	Almonds	Lemon	Garlic	Balsamic vinegar
	Hazelnuts	Lemon	Shallots	Parsley
Trout	Pine nuts or almonds	Lemon	Parsley	Sherry vinegar

BROILED HALIBUT WITH PESTO

Makes 4 servings

This recipe is a quick and easy dinner option. Topping fish with a sauce like pesto adds flavor and helps keep the fish moist while broiling. Basil Pesto may seem like the most obvious choice, but Cilantro Pesto (page 46) and Spinach Pesto (page 46) also work well. This recipe calls for halibut, but we encourage you to choose a firm, white fish (such as cod, flounder, haddock, pollack, walleye, or whiting) that best suits your budget and preferences. Serve broiled fish on a bed of Simply Cooked whole grains (see chapter 13), like brown rice, couscous, farro, or millet.

- 1 teaspoon extra virgin olive oil
- 1 pound (454 g) halibut fillets or steaks, patted dry
- ½ teaspoon white pepper
- ½ cup (125 g) Basil Pesto (page 45), plus more for serving

1. Place an oven rack within 4 to 5 inches (10 to 13 cm) of the broiler heat source and heat the broiler on HIGH. Oil the bottom of a 7 × 11-inch (18 × 28 cm) flameproof baking dish.

2. Place the fish in the baking dish and sprinkle over the white pepper. Top each piece of fish with a generous spoonful of pesto.

3. Broil for 10 minutes per inch (2.5 cm) of thickness, until the digital thermometer reads 145°F (65°C) when inserted in the center of the thickest fillet; the fish should be opaque and flake easily with a fork. Serve hot, with additional pesto on the side.

Per Serving: Calories 251; Protein 24 g; Carbs 2 g; Dietary Fiber 1 g; Added Sugars 0 g; Total Fat 16 g; Sat Fat 3 g; Omega-3s 680 mg; Sodium 232 mg; Potassium 557 mg

CLAMS IN CHORIZO TOMATO SAFFRON BROTH

Makes 2 servings

Clams and other bivalves like mussels are amazing creatures, working tirelessly to filter water in oceans and other bodies of water around the world. They are also nutrition powerhouses, packed with heart health–promoting omega-3 fatty acids and many other essential nutrients. This recipe, with smoky chorizo and saffron, draws its culinary inspiration from Spain. Serve with a crusty bread like our Whole Wheat French Baguettes (page 114) for dipping in the savory sauce.

- 2 pounds (907 g) fresh clams or mussels, such as little neck clams or blue mussels
- 2 tablespoons kosher salt
- 8 ounces (227 g) starchy potatoes (such as russet), peeled and cut into ½-inch (13 mm) cubes
- 2 tablespoons extra virgin olive oil
- 1 shallot, diced
- 4 to 6 garlic cloves, minced
- ½ teaspoon smoked paprika
- ¼ teaspoon red pepper flakes
- 3 ounces (85 g) fully cooked chicken chorizo sausage, quartered lengthwise and diced
- 2 cups (360 g) diced fresh tomatoes
- ¼ teaspoon saffron threads
- 1 tablespoon butter
- Crusty bread for serving

1. Wash each clam under cold running water to remove dirt and sand, and then place in a colander inside a large glass or plastic bowl. Cover the clams with water, add the salt, and let sit for 30 minutes to give them time to purge any additional sand.

2. Place the potatoes in a saucepan, cover with cold water, and place over high heat. Bring to a boil, then reduce the heat to medium. Cover and cook until the potatoes are tender but not falling apart, 8 minutes. Drain.

3. Heat the oil in a large, deep sauté pan or skillet over medium-high heat. Add the shallot, garlic, paprika, and red pepper flakes. Sauté until the shallots are soft and the garlic is fragrant, 4 to 5 minutes. If the pan gets dry and the mixture starts to stick to the bottom, add 1 or 2 tablespoons water. Add the chorizo and cook until some fat starts to render out, 4 to 5 minutes. Stir in the tomatoes and saffron and cook until they start to soften and release their liquid, 4 to 5 minutes.

4. Pull the colander from the water and rinse the clams under cold running water to remove any salt on the shells. Add the clams to the pan. Cover and steam the clams until all of them have opened, 6 to 10 minutes. (This timing will largely depend on the size of the clams; smaller clams will cook and open more quickly.) If a few clams refuse to open, remove and discard them.

5. Reduce the heat to low, add the potatoes and butter, and let the butter melt into the broth, 1 to 2 minutes. Serve in large shallow bowls with bread on the side for dipping.

Per Serving: Calories 485; Protein 29; Carbs 39 g; Dietary Fiber 4 g; Added Sugars 0 g; Total Fat 24 g; Sat Fat 7 g; Omega-3s 285 mg; Sodium 340 mg; Potassium 1,050 mg

COCONUT FISH CURRY

Makes 4 servings

This delicate, savory curry pairs well with a flaky white fish like tilapia, but catfish, red snapper, pollack, and flounder also work well. This dish has a bold flavor, and makes a fragrant and mouthwatering presentation when served over Simply Cooked Brown Rice, sprinkled with lime juice, cilantro, and chopped cashews.

- 1 pound (454 g) fresh tilapia fillets, cut into 3-inch (7.5 cm) pieces
- 2 teaspoons ground turmeric or Curry Powder (page 32)
- ¼ teaspoon kosher salt
- ¼ teaspoon freshly ground black pepper
- 2 shallots, halved
- 4 garlic cloves, halved
- One 2-inch (5 cm) piece ginger, peeled, halved lengthwise
- 1 serrano chile, halved lengthwise
- 2 tablespoons extra virgin olive oil
- 1 teaspoon mustard seeds
- 1 bay leaf, crushed

- 2 teaspoons chili powder
- ½ teaspoon ground cumin
- 1 teaspoon water
- One 15-ounce (425 g) can no-salt-added petite diced tomatoes or 2 cups (360 g) diced fresh tomatoes
- One 13.5-ounce (383 ml) can light coconut milk
- 2 cups (390 g) Simply Cooked Brown Rice (page 230), warmed
- 4 tablespoons fresh lime juice
- 4 tablespoons minced fresh cilantro
- 4 tablespoons chopped cashews, optional

1. Place the tilapia in a shallow baking dish. Sprinkle with 1 teaspoon of the turmeric and the salt and pepper. Work the seasonings into the fish with your fingers.

2. Combine the shallots, garlic, ginger, and serrano in the food processor and pulse to a fine paste.

3. Combine 1 tablespoon of the oil, the mustard seeds, and the bay leaf in a large skillet over medium-high heat. Stir until the mustard seeds start popping and the mustard and bay leaf become fragrant, about 1 minute. Add the remaining 1 tablespoon of oil and the shallot-garlic paste, lower the heat to medium, and cook until the paste is aromatic and any liquid has evaporated, about 3 minutes.

4. Stir together the chili powder, the remaining 1 teaspoon turmeric, the cumin, and the water in a small bowl, then add to the pan. Continue to stir until the mixture is hot and just barely sticks to the skillet, 1 minute.

5. Slowly stir in the tomatoes and coconut milk. Bring to a gentle simmer. Lay the fish on top of the curry. Reduce the heat to medium-low, partially cover the skillet with a lid, and simmer gently for 15 to 20 minutes, until the curry is thick, hot, and bubbling.

6. Divide the rice among four shallow bowls and ladle on the fish and curry. Sprinkle each bowl with 1 tablespoon each lime juice, cilantro, and cashews, if using. Serve hot.

Per Serving: Calories 632; Protein 33 g; Carbs 88 g; Dietary Fiber 8 g; Added Sugars 0 g; Total Fat 20 g; Sat Fat 6 g; Omega-3s 240 mg; Sodium 282 mg; Potassium 715 mg

CRISPY FISH STICKS

Makes 4 servings

These fish sticks are crunchy on the outside and moist and tender on the inside. Serve with Savory Sweet Potato Fries (page 272), and Chipotle Aïoli (page 44) or Roasted Garlic Aïoli (page 45) as dipping sauces.

- 1 pound (454 g) firm white fish (such as cod, haddock, or pollack)
- ½ cup (60 g) whole wheat pastry flour
- 2 tablespoons yellow cornmeal
- 1 tablespoon Seafood Seasoning (page 37)
- 1 teaspoon smoked paprika
- 1 large egg
- 1 tablespoon water
- ¾ cup (165 g) Garlic & Herb Bread Crumbs (page 33)
- 1 tablespoon extra virgin olive oil

1. Cut the fish into 1 × 3-inch (2.5 × 7.5 cm) strips to make fish sticks or 1-inch (2.5 cm) chunks to make nuggets.

2. Preheat the oven to 400°F (200°C). Line a baking sheet with parchment paper.

3. Set out three shallow bowls or pie plates. Combine the flour, cornmeal, seasoning, and paprika in one bowl. Beat the egg and water in the second bowl. Place the bread crumbs in the third bowl.

4. Dredge the fish in the flour mixture, dip it into the egg, and then thoroughly coat it with bread crumbs, pressing the bread crumbs into the fish gently but firmly. Place the fish on the baking sheet. Brush or drizzle with the oil.

5. Bake for 6 minutes. Flip the pieces and bake for 4 to 6 minutes, until the fish flakes easily with a fork. If you're making nuggets, bake for a total of 5 to 7 minutes, flipping after about 3 minutes. Serve hot.

Per Serving: Calories 332; Protein 28 g; Carbs 31 g; Dietary Fiber 4 g; Added Sugars 0 g; Total Fat 10 g; Sat Fat 2 g; Omega-3s 300 mg; Sodium 279 mg; Potassium 532 mg

FISH ROAST WITH CUCUMBER-DILL SAUCE

Makes 4 servings

This recipe makes an excellent bowl meal. Start with baby greens, then add the roasted fish, cucumber slices, artichoke hearts, and halved grape tomatoes. Top with Cucumber-Dill Sauce, a squeeze of fresh lemon, and a sprinkle of cilantro. It's also great served over a bed of Simply Cooked whole grains (see chapter 13) or Simply Spanish-Style Mashed Potatoes (page 259).

- 1 teaspoon extra virgin olive oil
- Four 4-ounce (113 g) fillets (halibut, mahi mahi, or hake)
- 2 tablespoons fresh lemon juice
- 1 tablespoon Seafood Seasoning (page 37)
- ¼ teaspoon kosher salt
- 1 cup (400 g) Cucumber-Dill Sauce (page 54) for serving

1. Preheat the oven to 400°F (200°C). Lightly oil a 9-inch (23 cm) square baking dish.

2. Place the fish in the baking dish and sprinkle with lemon juice, seasoning, and salt. Bake for 10 to 12 minutes, until the fish is firm, no longer translucent, and a digital food thermometer reads 145°F (65°C) when inserted in the thickest part of the fillets.

3. Remove the fillets from the dish and discard any liquid. Serve hot, with the sauce alongside.

Per Serving: Calories 211; Protein 8 g; Carbs 5 g; Dietary Fiber 1 g; Added Sugars 0 g; Total Fat 18 g; Sat Fat 4 g; Omega-3s 1,090 mg; Sodium 217 mg; Potassium 162 mg

GINGERY MACKEREL WITH LEMON & GARLIC

Makes 4 servings

Mackerel is an environmentally sustainable and affordable fatty fish that is packed with omega-3s. It may become a family favorite because it's easy to prepare and it pairs well with ingredients commonly on hand, such as ginger, garlic, lemon, and parsley. Serve this with Cucumber Raita (page 63) and Potato Dinner Rolls (page 112).

- Four 4-ounce (113 g) Atlantic mackerel fillets
- 2 tablespoons finely chopped or grated fresh ginger
- 2 tablespoons fresh lemon juice
- 2 tablespoons chopped fresh parsley, plus more for serving
- 1 tablespoon Dijon mustard
- 1 tablespoon peanut or toasted sesame oil
- 2 garlic cloves, minced
- ¼ teaspoon kosher salt
- ¼ teaspoon freshly ground black pepper
- 1 lemon, cut into wedges

1. Adjust the top oven rack to the highest position, about 4 inches (10 cm) from the broiler heat source. Heat the broiler on HIGH. Line the broiler pan with parchment paper.

2. Arrange the fillets on the pan. Combine the ginger, lemon juice, parsley, mustard, oil, garlic, salt, and pepper in a small bowl, then brush the mixture evenly over the tops and sides of the fillets.

3. Broil for 4 to 5 minutes on each side, flipping the fish once, until it flakes easily with a fork and a digital food thermometer reads 145°F (65°C) when inserted in the side of the fillet. Serve with the lemon wedges and chopped parsley.

Per Serving: Calories 102; Protein 6 g; Carbs 3 g; Dietary Fiber 1 g; Added Sugars 0 g; Total Fat 7 g; Sat Fat 2 g; Omega-3s 700 mg; Sodium 163 mg; Potassium 134 mg

MEDITERRANEAN TILAPIA EN PAPILLOTE

Makes 4 servings

Cooking in parchment paper packets (en papillote, in French) is an easy way to cook fish perfectly every time. Consider serving with our Lentil & Brown Rice Salad with Fresh Thyme (page 170), with Wine-Poached Pears (page 354) for dessert.

- Four 4-ounce (113 g) tilapia fillets
- 1 teaspoon dried or ground oregano
- ¼ teaspoon freshly ground black pepper
- 2 zucchini, trimmed and thinly sliced
- 2 tomatoes, cut into 4 slices each
- 1 green or red bell pepper, sliced into 8 rings
- 8 pitted green olives, halved
- 1½ lemons, cut into 12 thin slices
- ¼ cup (60 ml) red wine vinegar

1. Preheat the oven to 400°F (200°C). Sprinkle one side of the fish fillets with the oregano and pepper.

2. Cut four 15 × 18-inch (38 × 45.5 cm) rectangles of parchment paper. Fold in half lengthwise, making a sharp crease; cut the edges at angles to resemble a heart. Working one at a time, open a parchment heart and place 3 slices zucchini, 2 slices tomato, and 2 bell pepper rings on one side, near the crease. Place a fish fillet on top of the vegetables, then add 4 olive halves and 3 lemon slices. Sprinkle over 1 tablespoon vinegar. Fold the other half of the parchment over the fish and vegetables, aligning the edges. Close by making small rolling folds from the edge to the filling, going around on all three sides. (This makes a tight seal to trap the steam.) Repeat to make three more packets. Place the packets in a single layer on a baking sheet.

3. Bake for 15 to 20 minutes, until the packets are puffed and starting to brown on top. Serve in the packets, but be sure to open carefully; the packets will release very hot steam!

Per Serving: Calories 81; Protein 8 g; Carbs 9 g; Dietary Fiber 3 g; Added Sugars 0 g; Total Fat 2 g; Sat Fat 0 g; Omega-3s 110 mg; Sodium 134 mg; Potassium 583 mg

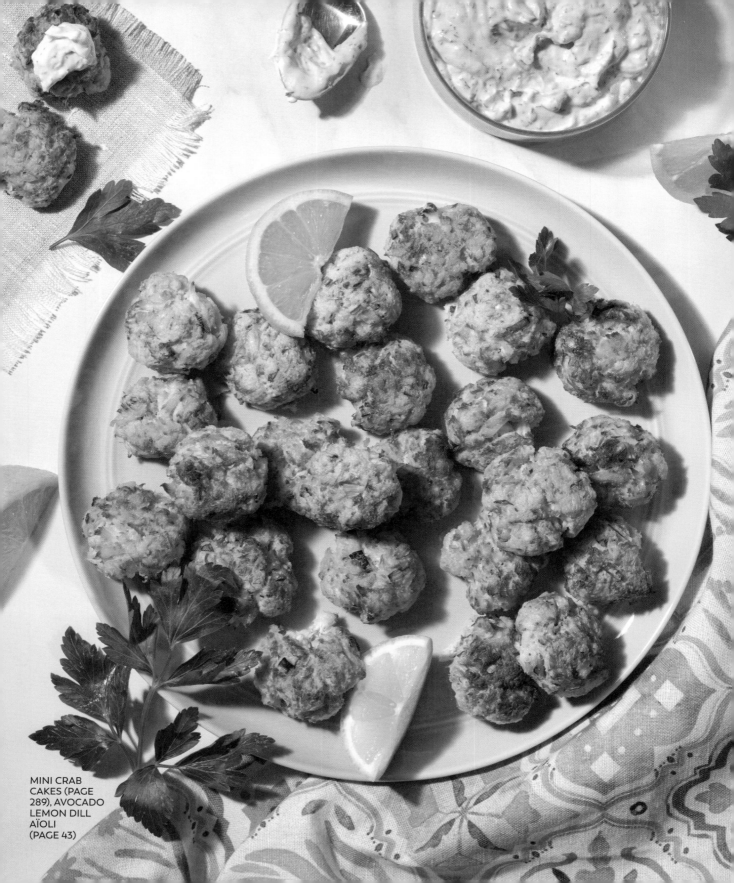

MINI CRAB
CAKES (PAGE
289), AVOCADO
LEMON DILL
AÏOLI
(PAGE 43)

MINI CRAB CAKES

Makes 36 mini crab cakes

Crab is perceived as a luxury food by some and too much work by others. To keep the cost down and the effort easy, we chose to use convenient ready-to-use canned lump crab meat and to make the crab cakes bite-size. Serve with Creamy Dill Dressing (page 49) and Avocado Lemon Dill Aïoli (page 43).

⅔ cup (150 g) plain Greek yogurt

2 teaspoons Seafood Seasoning (page 37)

1 teaspoon Dijon mustard

1 teaspoon prepared horseradish

1 teaspoon Worcestershire sauce

4 green onions, chopped

1 large egg, well beaten

2 tablespoons chopped fresh parsley

2 teaspoons fresh lemon juice

Two 6-ounce (170 g) cans lump crab meat, drained, liquid reserved

⅔ cup (40 g) panko bread crumbs

Freshly cracked black pepper

1. Preheat the oven to 400°F (200°C). Line a large rimmed baking sheet with parchment paper.

2. Whisk together the yogurt, seasoning, mustard, horseradish, and Worcestershire in a medium bowl. Stir in the green onions, egg, parsley, and lemon juice. Fold in the crab, bread crumbs, and pepper. The mixture should be moist yet firm enough to hold its shape when compressed into a ball. If it seems too dry, add the reserved canning liquid 1 tablespoon at a time.

3. Scoop out the mixture with a tablespoon, then shape into a ball using your hands. Place the balls on the baking sheet. (You should have 36 balls.) Press the balls slightly to flatten.

4. Bake for 18 to 20 minutes, until light to golden brown and a digital food thermometer reads 145°F (65°C).

5. Set the baking sheet on a wire rack to cool for 5 minutes. Transfer the crab cakes to a serving platter. Serve hot.

Serving Size 3 cakes; Calories 41; Protein 4 g; Carbs 4 g; Dietary Fiber 0 g; Added Sugars 0 g; Total Fat 1 g; Sat Fat 0 g; Omega-3s 10 mg; Sodium 110 mg; Potassium 53 mg

MISO-GLAZED SCALLOPS

Makes 4 servings as an entrée; 8 servings as an appetizer

Getting a perfect sear on a scallop can be challenging—the scallops need to be very dry and the pan needs to be very hot. Brushing on miso and broiling the scallops after searing them creates amazing flavor and a gorgeous brown crust. .

1 pound (454 g) 10/20 count sea scallops

1 tablespoon extra virgin olive oil

1 tablespoon butter or plant-based spread

2 tablespoons white (shiro) miso, plus more if needed

Grated zest and juice of 1 lime

1. Line a large plate or baking sheet with paper towels. Place the scallops on the paper towels to absorb any surface water. Place another paper towel on top of the scallops and press down to dry.

2. Place the top oven rack in the highest position under the broiler heat source. Heat the broiler on HIGH.

3. Heat a large oven-safe sauté pan, skillet, or cast-iron skillet over high heat for 3 minutes. Add the oil and butter. When the butter has completely melted and the mixture is sizzling, add the scallops. Sear the scallops on one side until they develop a brown crust around the edges, 3 to 4 minutes. Turn off the heat, flip the scallops, and baste by tilting the pan and spooning over the oil-butter mixture. Brush the top of each scallop with about ¼ teaspoon of the miso. The exact amount of miso you'll use depends on the number of scallops you cook.

4. Place the pan under the broiler for 2 to 3 minutes, until the miso glaze has developed dark brown spots.

5. Sprinkle the scallops with lime zest and juice. Serve warm.

Per Serving (entrée): Calories 153; Protein 15 g; Carbs 6 g; Dietary Fiber 1 g; Added Sugars 0 g; Total Fat 7 g; Sat Fat 3 g; Omega-3s 190 mg; Sodium 788 mg; Potassium 255 mg

MUSSELS IN COCONUT-LEMONGRASS BROTH

Makes 4 servings

There are so many types of mussels; use the ones most available and/or familiar to you for this recipe, which is inspired by the coconut milk–based curries of Thailand. Serve with steamed rice or a crusty bread.

1 tablespoon extra virgin olive oil

1 red onion, thinly sliced

Four 4-inch (10 cm) pieces fresh lemongrass (white part only)

2 tablespoons grated or finely minced ginger

1 or 2 serrano chiles, minced

3 to 4 garlic cloves, minced

2 cups (480 ml) Fish Broth (page 71) or Shrimp Stock (page 71)

1 tablespoon honey or palm sugar

1 tablespoon reduced-sodium soy sauce

2 cups (480 ml) lite coconut milk

1 pound (454 g) frozen fully cooked or fresh mussels in the shell

2 green onions, sliced

½ cup (8 g) chopped fresh cilantro leaves

1 lime, quartered

1. Heat the oil in a large Dutch oven over medium-high heat. Add the red onion and sauté until softened, about 5 minutes.

2. Set the lemongrass on a cutting board and use the dull side of a chef's knife or a meat tenderizer to pound it a bit. (This breaks up the cells and allows the lemongrass to release more of its flavor.) Add the lemongrass, ginger, chiles, and garlic to the red onion and sauté until the mixture becomes aromatic and the garlic has softened, 4 to 5 minutes. Stir in the stock, honey, and soy sauce, reduce the heat to low, and simmer for 15 minutes for the flavors to develop.

3. Add the coconut milk, and increase the heat to medium-high. When the mixture is bubbling gently, add the mussels and cook until all of them have opened, 5 to 7 minutes. Remove and discard any unopened mussels. (Mussels that open just a wee bit can be pried open and safely eaten.)

4. Divide the mussels and broth among four large bowls and top each bowl with green onions and cilantro. Serve lime wedges on the side.

Per Serving: Calories 450; Protein 18 g; Carbs 20 g; Dietary Fiber 4 g; Added Sugars 4 g; Total Fat 35 g; Sat Fat 16 g; Omega-3s 685 mg; Sodium 590 mg; Potassium 670 mg

PAN-SEARED CRISPY CATFISH

Makes 4 servings

Chipotle chiles are dried smoked jalapeños; they are sold on their own or in a tomato-vinegar adobo sauce. We use dried chipotles as part of the dry coating to dredge the fish in this recipe, but you can also use chipotle chile powder. To adjust the heat level in this recipe, reduce or increase the number of chiles.

¼ cup (30 g) whole wheat pastry flour

1 teaspoon smoked paprika

¼ teaspoon kosher salt

¼ teaspoon freshly ground black pepper

1 large egg

1 tablespoon water

¼ cup (30 g) finely ground whole grain yellow cornmeal

2 chipotle chiles, seeded and finely chopped, or 1 tablespoon ground chipotle chile

2 tablespoons panko bread crumbs

2 tablespoons freshly grated Parmesan

2 tablespoons extra virgin olive oil

1 pound (454 g) fresh or thawed frozen catfish fillets (see Tip)

1 lime, halved

¼ cup (4 g) chopped fresh cilantro leaves

1. Set out three shallow bowls or pie plates. Combine the flour, paprika, salt, and pepper in one bowl. Whisk together the egg and water in the second bowl. Combine the cornmeal, chipotles, bread crumbs, and Parmesan in the third bowl.

2. Heat the oil in a large skillet over medium heat. As the oil heats, first dredge each fillet in the flour, then dip in the egg mixture, then dredge in the cornmeal mixture until evenly coated. When the oil is hot, place the fillets in the skillet.

3. Cook the fillets for 4 to 5 minutes per side, turning once, until they are golden brown, the fish flakes easily with a fork, and a digital food thermometer reads 145°F (65°C) when inserted in the thickest part of a fillet.

4. Place the fillets on a serving platter, squeeze the ½ lime over them, and sprinkle on the cilantro. Cut the remaining ½ lime into 4 wedges and serve with the fillets.

TIP: *This recipe can also be made with tilapia, flounder, or grouper.*

Per Serving: Calories 327; Protein 25 g; Carbs 17 g; Dietary Fiber 3 g; Added Sugars 0 g; Total Fat 17 g; Sat Fat 3 g; Omega-3s 300 mg; Sodium 582 mg; Potassium 496 mg

ROASTED ALMOND-CRUSTED SNAPPER

Makes 4 servings

Our Savory Nut Crumb Topping, when made with almonds and lemon zest, is the perfect crispy crust for a mild fish like snapper. To make this with another fish such as cod, tilapia, or pollack, refer to the Fish Flavor Pairings chart on page 283. This dish pairs well with roasted vegetables, such as the Red Potato & Onion Roast with Cherry Tomatoes & Kalamata Olives (page 269) or a salad, such as Cherry Tomato Caprese Salad (page 150).

- 1 tablespoon extra virgin olive oil
- 1 pound (454 g) firm snapper fillet, whole or cut into 4 portions
- 2 teaspoons Seafood Seasoning (page 37)
- 1 cup (235 g) Savory Nut Crumb Topping (page 36)
- ½ teaspoon white pepper
- 1 lemon, quartered, optional

1. Preheat the oven to 400°F (200°C). Line a large rimmed baking sheet with parchment paper.

2. Place the snapper skin side down on the baking sheet (the skin will separate very easily once the fish is roasted). Brush the top with oil, sprinkle evenly with the seasoning, then coat with the nut crumb topping, pressing in gently to help it adhere.

3. Bake for 8 to 10 minutes, until the fish is opaque

and flakes easily, and a digital food thermometer reads 145°F (65°C) when inserted in the side of the fillet.

4. Sprinkle with the pepper and serve with lemon wedges, if desired.

Per Serving: Calories 417; Protein 34 g; Carbs 19 g; Dietary Fiber 4 g; Added Sugars 0 g; Total Fat 23 g; Sat Fat 3 g; Omega-3s 410 mg; Sodium 385 mg; Potassium 787 mg

ROASTED BALSAMIC-GLAZED SALMON

Makes 4 servings

The acid in balsamic vinegar is a flavor enhancer; it pairs well with roasted vegetables, fresh berries, and fish, as in this recipe. When reduced, it becomes a thick, syrupy glaze.

- 1 tablespoon extra virgin olive oil
- 2 shallots, finely diced
- 4 garlic cloves, minced
- ¼ cup (60 ml) balsamic vinegar
- 3 tablespoons dry white wine (such as Chenin Blanc, Pinot Gris, or Pinot Grigio)
- 1 tablespoon Dijon mustard
- 1 tablespoon honey
- One 1-pound (454 g) or four 4-ounce (113 g) salmon fillets, fresh or thawed frozen, skin-on or skinless, patted dry
- 3 tablespoons finely chopped fresh basil

1. Preheat the oven to 400°F (200°C). Line a small rimmed baking sheet with parchment paper.

2. Heat the oil in a small saucepan over medium-high heat. Sauté the shallots until softened, 2 to 3 minutes. Add the garlic and sauté until fragrant, about 1 minute. Stir in the vinegar, wine, mustard, and honey. Bring to a boil, then reduce the heat to medium-low and simmer until the glaze has reduced and is slightly thickened, 3 to 4 minutes.

3. Place the fillets on the baking sheet. Brush with the glaze and sprinkle with the basil. Bake for 15 to 20 minutes, until the salmon is opaque and flakes easily with a fork, and a digital food thermometer reads 145°F (65°C) when inserted in the thickest part of the fillet. Brush with more glaze, if desired, but be sure to use a clean brush. Serve warm.

Per Serving: Calories 296; Protein 23 g; Carbs 11 g; Dietary Fiber 1 g; Added Sugars 4 g; Total Fat 15 g; Sat Fat 4 g; Omega-3s 2,340 mg; Sodium 151 mg; Potassium 553 mg

ROASTED SALMON WITH HONEY WALNUT LEMON SAUCE

Makes 4 servings

Oven-roasting salmon is an easy way to perfectly cook it, then top with a sauce like this Honey Lemon Walnut sauce as an elegant way to add bright bursts of flavor to the fatty, rich salmon. The sauce also works well on sautéed or grilled shrimp.

- One 16- to 24-ounce (454 to 680 g) whole skin-on salmon fillet
- ½ cup (60 g) finely minced raw walnuts
- 1 teaspoon extra virgin olive oil
- Grated zest and juice of 1 lemon
- ¼ cup (85 g) honey
- ⅛ teaspoon kosher salt
- Lemon slices, optional
- Chopped fresh flat-leaf parsley, optional

1. Preheat the oven to 375°F (190°C). Place the salmon on a large rimmed baking sheet, skin side down.

2. Roast for 14 to 18 minutes, until the flesh has turned to pale pink and a digital food thermometer reads 145°F (65°C).

3. Heat the walnuts, oil, lemon zest and juice, honey, and salt in a small saucepan over medium-high heat. Once the sauce starts bubbling rapidly, cook for another 30 seconds, then remove immediately from the heat. Overcooking the sauce will turn it from a light sauce to a sticky, candied mix in a matter of moments.

4. Place the salmon on a serving dish or platter, spoon over the sauce, and garnish with lemon slices and chopped parsley, and serve hot.

NOTE: *If you struggle with the decision to buy wild versus farmed salmon, rest assured that both are great choices for getting more beneficial omega-3 fatty acids. But farmed salmon contains far higher levels. Why? Wild fish must work hard to find their food, while farmed salmon are contained in pens, often in ocean water near the shore, where they are fed. The farmed salmon become fattier than their wild cousins, and therefore contain more fatty acids, including omega-3s.*

Per Serving: Calories 419; Protein 28 g; Carbs 21 g; Dietary Fiber 1 g; Added Sugars 17 g; Total Fat 25 g; Sat Fat 5 g; Omega-3s 2,670 mg; Sodium 86 mg; Potassium 541 mg

SAUTÉED SHRIMP & SCALLOPS

Makes 4 servings

Scallops and shrimp are extremely lean protein sources that are very tender when cooked properly. Sauté them at relatively high heat with a little oil for a very short time to retain their creamy, firm textures and to prevent them from drying out.

- 1 pound (454 g) fresh or thawed frozen sea scallops, rinsed and patted dry
- 12 ounces (340 g) jumbo fresh or thawed frozen shrimp (16/20 count), peeled and deveined, rinsed, and patted dry
- 4 tablespoons (60 ml) fresh lime juice
- 1 tablespoon Seafood Seasoning (page 37)
- ⅛ teaspoon kosher salt
- ¼ teaspoon freshly ground black pepper
- 3 tablespoons extra virgin olive oil
- 2 garlic cloves, minced
- 3 carrots, cut lengthwise into thin strips
- 1 bell pepper, seeded and cut into thin strips
- 3 shallots, thinly sliced
- 2 cups (140 g) chanterelle mushrooms or sliced shiitake mushroom caps
- 2 garlic cloves, minced
- ¼ cup (60 ml) dry white wine (such as Sauvignon Blanc, Chardonnay, Chenin Blanc, or Riesling)
- 3 tablespoons Sour Cream Crème Fraîche (page 361)
- 2 teaspoons grated lime zest
- 2 teaspoons chopped fresh thyme or ½ teaspoon dried thyme
- ¼ cup (15 g) chopped fresh parsley

1. Place the scallops and shrimp on a large platter or plate. Rub with 2 tablespoons of the lime juice, the seasoning, salt, and pepper. Let stand at room temperature for 30 minutes.

2. Heat a heavy skillet over medium-high heat. When a drop of water rolls around the pan, the pan is ready, 2 to 3 minutes. Remove the skillet from the heat and add 2 tablespoons of the oil. Swirl to coat the bottom of the skillet, and return the skillet to medium-high heat. Add the shrimp and scallops and sauté until the shrimp are pink and the scallops are opaque, 2 minutes on the first side, flipping and cooking for about 2 minutes on the other side. Transfer the shrimp and scallops to a warm plate.

3. Pour the remaining 1 tablespoon oil into the hot pan and return it to medium-high heat. Add the carrots, bell pepper, and shallots, and sauté until the vegetables are brighter and starting to soften, 2 to 3 minutes. Add the mushrooms and garlic and sauté until the vegetables are crisp-tender and the garlic is fragrant, 2 to 3 minutes.

4. Reduce the heat to medium-low and stir in the wine, crème fraîche, lime zest, and thyme. Continue to heat until the sauce is hot and creamy, 2 minutes.

5. Spoon the vegetables and sauce onto a serving platter or four individual plates, top with the shrimp and scallops, sprinkle with parsley, and serve hot.

Per Serving: Calories 338; Protein 29 g; Carbs 22 g; Dietary Fiber 5 g; Added Sugars 0 g; Total Fat 14 g; Sat Fat 3 g; Omega-3s 230 mg; Sodium 886 mg; Potassium 773 mg

SCALLOPS EN PAPILLOTE WITH SHALLOTS, EDAMAME & BELL PEPPER

Makes 4 servings

Serve these packets with pasta like our Creamy Spinach Lasagna (page 208) or Roasted Red Pepper Fettucine (page 212) and your favorite salad.

¼ cup (60 ml) dry white wine (Riesling, Chardonnay, or Chablis)

3 tablespoons finely chopped fresh thyme

2 tablespoons extra virgin olive oil

2 tablespoons vinegar (champagne, white balsamic, or white wine)

Grated zest of 1 lemon

¼ teaspoon white pepper

1 cup thinly sliced shallots

1 orange or yellow bell pepper, seeded and thinly sliced

One 12-ounce bag (340 g) frozen edamame (green soybeans) in the pod, thawed and patted dry

1 pound (454 g) sea scallops, fresh or thawed frozen

¼ teaspoon cayenne

¼ cup (60 ml) fresh lemon juice

¼ cup (15 g) chopped fresh parsley

1. Preheat the oven to 400°F (200°C).

2. Whisk together the wine, thyme, oil, vinegar, lemon zest, and white pepper in a small bowl.

3. To make the parchment packets, cut four 15 × 18-inch (38 × 45.5 cm) rectangles of parchment paper. Fold in half lengthwise, making a sharp crease; cut the edges at angles to resemble a heart. Working with one at a time, open the parchment and place one-quarter of the shallots, bell pepper, edamame, and scallops on one side, near the crease. Drizzle with one-quarter of the dressing (about 2 tablespoons) and sprinkle with cayenne. Fold the other half of the parchment over the scallop-edamame mixture, aligning the edges. Close by making small, rolling folds from the edge to the filling, going around on all 3 sides. (This makes a tight seal to trap the steam.) Repeat to form three more packets.

4. Place the packets in a single layer on a baking sheet. Bake for 15 to 20 minutes, until the packets are puffed and starting to brown on top.

5. Carefully cut a hole in the top of each packet. Sprinkle lemon juice and parsley into the packets. Serve in the packets.

Per Serving: Calories 297; Protein 25 g; Carbs 22 g; Dietary Fiber 6 g; Added Sugars 0 g; Total Fat 12 g; Sat Fat 1 g; Omega-3s 180 mg; Sodium 459 mg; Potassium 942 mg

SEAFOOD TRIO ROLLS

Makes 4 servings

This elegant yet easy dish starts with sole, a flat-bodied firm fish with a mild, sweet flavor, which is then stuffed with shrimp and crab. Serve with Greek Orzo Salad with Spinach & Tomatoes (page 209) and a glass of white wine for a light, flavorful meal.

1 teaspoon extra virgin olive oil

Four 4-ounce (113 g) sole fillets

3 teaspoons Seafood Seasoning (page 37)

⅔ cup (150 g) plain Greek yogurt

¼ cup (25 g) minced celery

¼ cup (40 g) thinly sliced green onions

¼ cup (15 g) chopped fresh parsley

2 tablespoons chopped fresh chives

8 ounces (227 g) cooked peeled shrimp, chopped

4 ounces (113 g) flaked crab meat

½ cup (120 ml) dry white wine (such Chenin Blanc or Pinot Grigio)

1. Preheat the oven to 375°F (190°C). Coat a 7 × 11-inch (18 × 28 cm) baking dish with oil. Place the fish in the dish and sprinkle with 1 teaspoon of the seasoning.

2. Mix the yogurt, celery, green onions, parsley, 1 tablespoon of the chives, and the remaining 2 teaspoons of seasoning in a medium bowl. Gently fold in the shrimp and crab.

3. Equally divide the filling among the fillets and spread on one end. Roll up each fillet and secure with toothpicks. Pour the wine around the fish. Bake for about 20 minutes, until the fish is cooked through,

flaky, and opaque. If the fish is browning too fast, cover with foil.

4. Transfer the rolls to a serving plate and remove the toothpicks. Spoon the cooking liquid over the top. Sprinkle with the remaining 1 tablespoon chives and serve.

Serving Size 1 roll; Calories 181; Protein 18 g; Carbs 8 g; Dietary Fiber 1 g; Added Sugars 3 g; Total Fat 6 g; Sat Fat 3 g; Omega-3s 100 mg; Sodium 624 mg; Potassium 202 mg

SESAME SHRIMP EN PAPILLOTE

Makes 4 servings

This recipe differs from our other two en papillote recipes—this one includes pasta in the packets. The cooked pasta absorbs flavors from other ingredients during baking, intensifying its deliciousness. Serve with Radish & Cabbage Slaw (page 153) or Wasabi-Ginger Coleslaw (page 155) to complete the meal.

8 ounces (227 g) angel hair pasta, cooked al dente and drained (2 cups/480 ml)

4 asparagus spears, trimmed and cut into 1-inch (2.5 cm) lengths

½ red onion, thinly sliced

3 garlic cloves, minced

1 tablespoon minced fresh ginger

¼ teaspoon white pepper

1 pound (454 g) raw jumbo 21/25 shrimp, peeled and deveined

2 tablespoons rice vinegar

2 tablespoons sesame seeds

4 teaspoons toasted sesame oil

¼ cup (15 g) chopped fresh parsley

1 lemon, quartered

1. Preheat the oven to 400°F (200°C). Cut four 18-inch (45.5 cm) rectangles of parchment paper. Fold in half lengthwise, making a sharp crease; cut the edges at angles to resemble a heart.

2. Toss together the pasta, asparagus, onion, garlic, and ginger in a large bowl. Mix the shrimp, vinegar, and sesame seeds in a medium bowl.

3. Working one at a time, place one-quarter of the pasta mixture on one side, near the crease. Top with one-quarter of the shrimp mixture. Fold the other half of parchment over the filling, aligning the edges. Close by making small, rolling folds from the edge to the filling, going around on all three sides. (This makes a tight seal to trap the steam.) Repeat to make three more packets.

4. Place the packets in a single layer on a baking sheet and bake for 15 to 20 minutes until the packets are puffed and starting to brown on top.

5. Carefully cut a hole in the top of each packet. Drizzle 1 teaspoon sesame oil and sprinkle 1 tablespoon parsley into each packet. Serve with lemon wedges.

Per Serving: Calories 225; Protein 20 g; Carbs 19 g; Dietary Fiber 2 g; Added Sugars 0 g; Total Fat 8 g; Sat Fat 1 g; Omega-3s 30 mg; Sodium 505 mg; Potassium 275 mg

SHEET PAN FISH & VEGETABLE BAKE

Makes 4 servings

The secret to cooking fish and vegetables together on a baking sheet is to give the vegetables a head start. Adding the fish halfway through their roasting time ensures the fish doesn't dry out. Serve with a whole grain and a bowl of Citrusy Walnut Gremolata (page 148).

- Four 4-ounce (113 g) fillets tilapia, red snapper, catfish, trout, or walleye
- 2 tablespoons extra virgin olive oil
- 1 teaspoon ground coriander
- ¼ teaspoon kosher salt
- ¼ teaspoon freshly ground black pepper
- 4 Roma (plum) tomatoes, quartered
- 2 cups (140 g) sliced white mushrooms
- 2 cups (240 g) thinly sliced shallots
- 2 tablespoons fresh lemon juice
- 1 teaspoon fennel seeds
- 2 tablespoons white wine vinegar
- 4 thyme sprigs

1. Preheat the oven to 425°F (220°C). Line the bottom and two sides of a 9 × 13-inch (23 × 33 cm) baking dish with parchment paper.

2. Drizzle the fillets with 1 tablespoon of the oil and sprinkle with the coriander, salt, and pepper.

3. Combine the remaining 1 tablespoon of the oil and the tomatoes, mushrooms, shallots, 1 tablespoon of the lemon juice, and fennel seeds in a large bowl. Spread evenly in the baking dish. Pour any juices that remain in the bowl over the vegetables. Roast for 15 minutes, until the vegetables begin to soften, brighten in color, and release some liquid.

4. Gently stir or flip the vegetables. Place the fillets on top. Sprinkle with the remaining 1 tablespoon lemon juice and the vinegar and place the thyme sprigs on top. Roast for 15 minutes or until the fillets are flaky and opaque and a digital thermometer reads 145°F (65°C) when inserted in the side of a fillet. Serve hot.

Per Serving: Calories 160; Protein 9 g; Carbs 16 g; Dietary Fiber 3 g; Added Sugars 0 g; Total Fat 8 g; Sat Fat 1 g; Omega-3s 80 mg; Sodium 75 mg; Potassium 604 mg

SHRIMP CURRY

Makes 4 servings

This rich, aromatic curry, inspired by the seafood gravy dishes of Southern India, is made with an aromatic vegetable- and spice-infused base. Servie over Simply Cooked Millet (page 227) or Simply Cooked Brown Rice (page 230) and pair with Cucumber Raita (page 63).

2 tablespoons extra virgin olive oil

1 tablespoon black mustard seeds

1 tablespoon cumin seeds

2 teaspoons ground turmeric

½ cup (120 ml) water

Juice of 1 lemon

1 red onion, thinly sliced

1 to 2 serrano chiles, minced

2 tablespoons minced fresh ginger

3 cups (540 g) diced fresh red tomatoes

2 garlic cloves, minced

2 cups (480 ml) coconut milk

1 pound (454 g) 41/50 shrimp, peeled and deveined, tails removed

Chopped fresh cilantro

1. Heat the oil, mustard seeds, cumin seeds, and turmeric in a Dutch oven over medium heat. Sauté until the mustard seeds start to pop, 2 to 3 minutes.

2. Add the water, lemon juice, onion, serranos, and ginger. Cook until the onions start to soften, 6 to 8 minutes.

3. Stir in the tomatoes and garlic. Reduce the heat to medium-low, cover, and simmer until the tomatoes have softened and released their juices, 8 to 10 minutes.

4. Add the coconut milk and increase the heat to medium-high. Once the curry is gently bubbling on the surface, add the shrimp, stir, reduce the heat to low, and gently poach the shrimp until they start to change color, 2 to 3 minutes. Watch the shrimp closely; turn off the heat as soon as all the shrimp have started to change color. The heat of the curry will continue cooking the shrimp even after you remove the pan from the heat.

5. Top with cilantro and serve.

TIPS: Save the shrimp shells and tails to make Shrimp Stock (page 71). They can be frozen in an airtight container for up to 2 months.

To make this a make-ahead meal, prepare it up to adding the coconut milk in step 4, then refrigerate the sauce for up to 24 hours. Before serving, reheat the sauce and add the shrimp. (Shrimp don't reheat well; they tend to get tough.)

Per Serving: Calories 225; Protein 18 g; Carbs 13 g; Dietary Fiber 2 g; Added Sugars 3 g; Total Fat 11 g; Sat Fat 4 g; Omega-3s 240 mg; Sodium 677 mg; Potassium 579 mg

SHRIMP FRIED RICE

Makes 4 servings

We suggest using individually quick frozen (IQF) fully cooked shrimp for this quick and easy fried rice. Shrimp are sold by the number of shrimp in a pound; the smaller the number, the bigger the shrimp. For this recipe, we suggest either using whole medium shrimp (31 to 40 per pound/62 to 80 per kilo), or larger shrimp (16 to 20 per pound/32 to 40 per kilo), cut in half.

2 tablespoons plus 1 teaspoon peanut oil

2 large eggs

2 carrots, thinly sliced

8 ounces (227 g) sugar snap peas, trimmed, halved diagonally

4 ounces (113 g) shiitake mushroom caps or chanterelle mushrooms, sliced

2 garlic cloves, minced

2 tablespoons rice vinegar

¼ teaspoon red pepper flakes

1 pound (454 g) cooked peeled shrimp, thawed if frozen, tails removed, and halved if large

3 cups (585 g) Simply Cooked Brown Rice (page 230)

¼ cup (60 ml) Fish Broth (page 71) or Dashi Broth (page 70)

3 tablespoons sweet red chile sauce

2 green onions, thinly sliced

¼ cup (25 g) sliced almonds, toasted

2 tablespoons fresh lemon juice

1. Heat 1 teaspoon of the oil in a large nonstick sauté pan or wok over medium heat. Whisk the eggs in a small bowl until lightly blended. When the oil shimmers, add the eggs. Use a slotted spatula to stir the eggs into small, gently cooked soft curds, less than a minute. Transfer to a medium bowl.

2. Return the pan to the heat, add 1 tablespoon oil, and increase the heat to medium-high. When the oil shimmers, add the carrots, snap peas, mushrooms, and garlic. Stir continuously until the carrots and snap peas are bright in color and beginning to soften, the mushrooms begin to shrink, and the garlic is aromatic, about 2 minutes.

3. Stir in the vinegar and red pepper flakes. Add the shrimp and toss until the vegetables are crisp-tender and the liquid has evaporated, 1 to 2 minutes. Transfer to the bowl with the eggs.

4. Reduce the heat to medium-low, return the pan to the heat, add the remaining 1 tablespoon oil, followed by the rice. Use the spatula to break up the rice for about 30 seconds. Add the broth and chili sauce, and return the vegetables, shrimp, and eggs to the pan. Gently toss to mix. Cook until heated through, 3 to 4 minutes. Divide among four plates or shallow bowls and sprinkle with the green onions, almonds, and a splash of lemon juice. Serve hot.

Per Serving: Calories 510; Protein 38 g; Carbs 57 g; Dietary Fiber 6 g; Added Sugars 0 g; Total Fat 16 g; Sat Fat 3 g; Omega-3s 90 mg; Sodium 550 mg; Potassium 840 mg

SHRIMP JAMBALAYA

Makes 6 servings

Jambalaya can be Creole or Cajun. Both are rice based and use the trio of onion, celery, and bell pepper as the base, but Cajun jambalaya includes tomatoes and Creole doesn't. Both cultures consider jambalaya a favorite comfort dish that is often passed down from older generations within a family; recipes vary from kitchen to kitchen. Our recipe is tomato-based, which leans it toward Cajun. We omit the traditional smoked sausage and simply use shrimp in this crave-worthy, one-pot meal.

- 2 tablespoons extra virgin olive oil
- 1 yellow onion, chopped
- 2 green or red bell peppers, seeded and chopped
- 2 celery stalks, chopped
- 3 garlic cloves, minced

- 8 ounces (227 g) white or cremini mushrooms, sliced
- 5 or 6 Roma (plum) tomatoes, diced
- One 6-ounce (170 g) can tomato paste
- 2 cups (480 ml) Shrimp Stock (page 71) or Fish Broth (page 71), plus more if needed
- 2 tablespoons Cajun Seasoning (page 30)
- 2 bay leaves
- 3 cups (585 g) Simply Cooked Brown Rice (page 230)
- 1 pound (454 g) raw shrimp, peeled and deveined
- ⅓ cup (20 g) chopped fresh flat-leaf parsley
- ½ teaspoon freshly ground black pepper
- 2 tablespoons fresh lemon juice
- 6 green onions, chopped, optional

1. Heat the oil in a large saucepan or Dutch oven over medium-high heat. Add the onion, bell pepper, and celery, and sauté until the onion is translucent and the celery and bell peppers start to become tender, about 4 minutes. Add the garlic and mushrooms. Sauté until the garlic is aromatic and the mushrooms begin to shrink and release their juices, about 3 minutes.

2. Add the tomatoes and tomato paste, followed by the stock, seasoning, and bay leaves. Bring to a gentle boil. Reduce the heat to medium-low, cover, and simmer until the vegetables are tender, 10 minutes.

3. Stir in the rice and shrimp. Cover and simmer for 3 to 4 minutes, until the shrimp are pink and thoroughly cooked Add more stock for a thinner consistency; for a thicker consistency, uncover, reduce the heat to low, and gently simmer until some of the liquid has evaporated. The dish is done when a digital food thermometer reads 165°F (75°C) when inserted in the center of the saucepan.

4. Remove the bay leaves, stir in the parsley and black pepper, and sprinkle with the lemon juice. Offer green onions as a topping. Serve hot.

Per Serving: Calories 501; Protein 22 g; Carbs 85 g; Dietary Fiber 7 g; Added Sugars 0 g; Total Fat 11 g; Sat Fat 1 g; Omega-3s 160 mg; Sodium 585 mg; Potassium 504 mg

SIMPLY BROILED SALMON

Makes 4 servings

There's no quicker, easier way to prepare this salmon than simply seasoning and broiling it. Serve with Avocado Lemon Dill Aïoli (page 43) and a tomato-based dish such as the Broccoli with Coriander & Tomatoes (page 264).

- Four 4-ounce (113 g) fresh or thawed frozen skin-on salmon fillets
- Freshly ground black pepper
- 3 tablespoons finely chopped fresh dill
- 2 tablespoons lemon juice
- 2 tablespoons extra virgin olive oil
- ⅛ teaspoon kosher salt
- ¼ cup (15 g) chopped fresh parsley
- 1 lemon, cut into wedges

1. Adjust an oven rack to the highest position, about 4 inches (10 cm) from the broiler heat source. Heat the broiler to HIGH. Line a large rimmed baking sheet with foil.

2. Remove the skin from the salmon and season both sides with pepper. Combine the dill, lemon juice, oil, and salt in a small bowl. Place the salmon on the baking sheet skin side down and drizzle with half of the dill mixture. Broil for 3 to 5 minutes.

3. Flip the salmon and broil for 3 to 5 minutes, until the fish is opaque and flakes easily with a fork and a digital food thermometer reads 145°F (65°C) when inserted in the thickest part of a fillet. Drizzle with the remaining dill mixture, sprinkle with the parsley, and serve with lemon wedges.

Per Serving: Calories 273; Protein 23 g; Carbs 2 g; Dietary Fiber 1 g; Added Sugars 0 g; Total Fat 19 g; Sat Fat 5 g; Omega-3s 2,910 mg; Sodium 116 mg; Potassium 497 mg

SMOKY SEARED SALMON FOR ONE

Makes 1 serving

If you're cooking for one, this recipe is perfect for you. It also works well if you're cooking for a crowd—just use 1 tablespoon of rub for each salmon fillet. The secret to perfectly cooked salmon is to start with a cold pan and cook over medium heat, to slowly render the fat from the skin and create a crispy skin with silky smooth fish. Finishing in the oven ensures the salmon doesn't get overcooked. This salmon pairs well with Smoky Workaday Sweet Corn & Pepper Sauté (page 268).

- 1 tablespoon Salmon Rub (page 36)
- One 4- to 6-ounce (113 to 170 g) skin-on salmon fillet
- 1 teaspoon butter, melted
- 1 teaspoon extra virgin olive oil

1. Preheat the oven to 375°F (190°C).

2. Massage the rub into the flesh of the fillet with your fingertips. If the fillet is thick, rub the seasoning on the sides as well.

3. Place the butter and oil in a cold oven-safe non-stick pan (a well-seasoned cast-iron pan works well). Place the salmon in the pan, skin side down.

4. Turn the heat to medium and cook until the fat renders out of the skin and the bottom ¼ inch (6 mm) of the salmon starts to turn pale pink, 8 to 10 minutes. Use a teaspoon to occasionally baste the top of the salmon with the fat in the pan.

5. Transfer the pan to the oven and roast for 5 to 6 minutes, until all the flesh has turned a pale pinkish white and a digital food thermometer reads 145°F (65°C) when inserted in the thickest part of the fillet. Serve hot.

Per Serving: Calories 335; Protein 28 g; Carbs 2 g; Dietary Fiber 0 g; Added Sugars 1 g; Total Fat 23 g; Sat Fat 7 g; Omega-3s 2,910 mg; Sodium 162 mg; Potassium 573 mg

SUMMER LAKE BAKE

Makes 4 servings

Whether you're relaxing at home, vacationing at the lake, or enjoying R&R on the ocean shore, plan on this easy catch-of-the-day, quick-fix meal. Serve with steamed baby potatoes, a fresh green salad, and one of our juicy salsas (pages 61 to 63) for a summer vacation meal that may quickly become part of your family tradition.

- 1 tablespoon plus 2 teaspoons extra virgin olive oil
- 1 pound (454 g) walleye, rockfish, trout, sunfish, perch, striped bass, or "catch-of-the-day" fillets
- 2 teaspoons fresh lemon juice
- ¼ teaspoon kosher salt
- ¼ teaspoon freshly ground black pepper
- 2 large tomatoes, sliced
- 1 bell pepper, sliced into rings and seeded
- 1½ cups (250 g) fresh or frozen corn kernels
- ⅔ cup (145 g) Garlic & Herb Bread Crumbs (page 33)
- 2 teaspoons chopped fresh basil
- 1 teaspoon dried oregano
- Chopped fresh parsley
- Lemon wedges

1. Preheat the oven to 350°F (180°C). Coat a 9-inch (23 cm) square baking dish with 2 teaspoons of the oil.

2. Place the fish in the baking dish, skin side down. Sprinkle with the lemon juice, salt, and pepper. Layer the tomato and bell pepper slices over the fish, and top with the corn. Combine the bread crumbs, basil, and oregano in a small bowl. Spread over the corn. Drizzle with the remaining 1 tablespoon oil.

3. Bake for 20 minutes or until the fish is opaque and flaky and a digital food thermometer reads 145°F (65°C) when inserted into the side of the thickest fillet in the center of the baking dish. Serve hot with parsley and lemon wedges.

Per Serving: Calories 334; Protein 28 g; Carbs 26 g; Dietary Fiber 3 g; Added Sugars 2 g; Total Fat 11 g; Sat Fat 2 g; Omega-3s 440 mg; Sodium 456 mg; Potassium 759 mg

WHITE FISH WITH FENNEL & LEEKS

Makes 4 servings

Select a firm, thick white fish for this recipe—delicate and thin-bodied fish will not stand up as well to the strong fennel flavor. Pair with Orzo with Peas & Parmesan (page 210) and one of our fruit salads with citrus (see chapter 8).

- 3 teaspoons extra virgin olive oil
- Four 4-ounce (113 g) firm white fish fillets, such as cod, halibut, monkfish, or sea bass
- 2 cups (175 g) thinly sliced fennel bulbs, fronds reserved and chopped, for garnish
- 1 cup (90 g) chopped cleaned leeks (see Tip, page 79), white and light green parts only
- ½ teaspoon white pepper
- 1 tablespoon Seafood Seasoning (page 37)
- ½ cup (120 ml) half-and-half
- ¼ cup (20 g) shredded Parmesan
- 1 teaspoon grated lemon zest
- 1 lemon, halved

1. Preheat the oven to 425°F (220°C). Lightly oil a 7 × 11-inch (18 × 28 cm) baking dish with 1 teaspoon of the oil.

2. Layer the fennel and leeks in the baking dish, drizzle with the remaining 2 teaspoons oil, and sprinkle with pepper. Bake for 15 minutes, until the vegetables just begin to soften and deepen in color.

3. Add the fish fillets in a single layer. Sprinkle with the seasoning and drizzle the half-and-half over the top. Cover loosely with foil and bake for 8 minutes.

4. Sprinkle with the Parmesan and lemon zest, and bake covered for 4 to 6 minutes, until the fillets are no longer translucent, the cheese is melted, and the vegetables are softened. The fillets are cooked when a digital food thermometer reads 145°F (65°C) when inserted in the thickest part. Add a squeeze of lemon, top with fennel fronds, and serve hot.

Per Serving: Calories 146; Protein 9 g; Carbs 12 g; Dietary Fiber 2 g; Added Sugars 0 g; Total Fat 7 g; Sat Fat 2 g; Omega-3s 290 mg; Sodium 172 mg; Potassium 452 mg

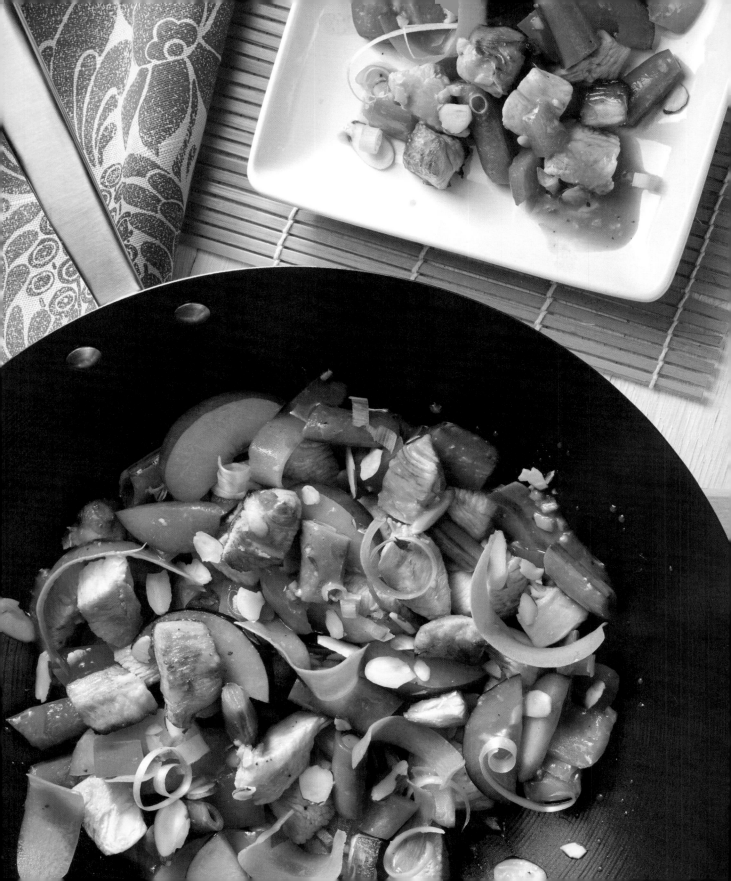

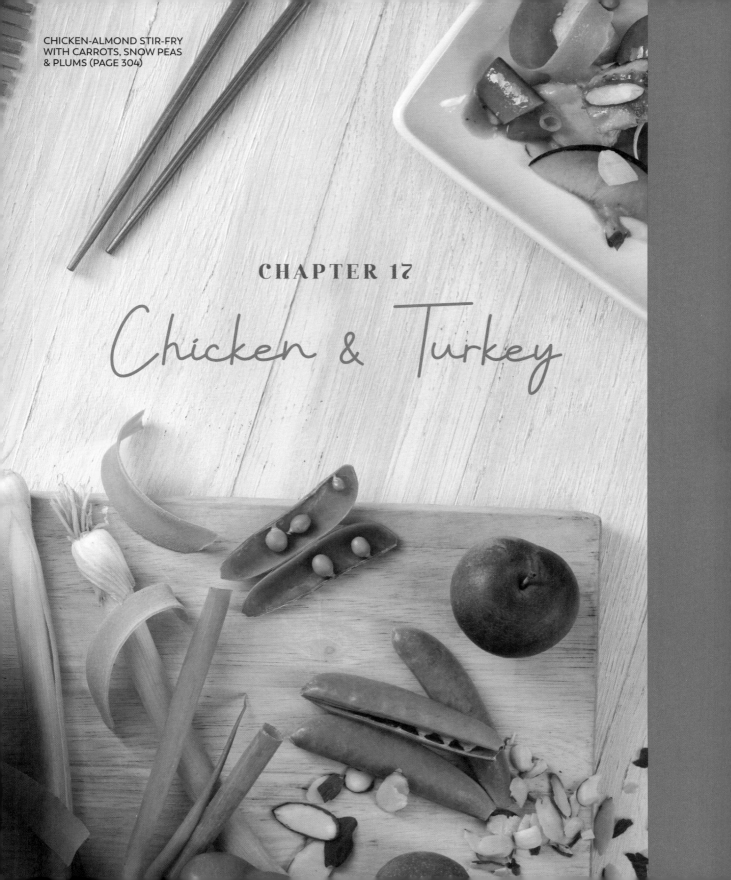

CHICKEN-ALMOND STIR-FRY
WITH CARROTS, SNOW PEAS
& PLUMS (PAGE 304)

CHAPTER 17

Chicken & Turkey

Chicken & Turkey

Chicken

Almond-Crusted Chicken Strips 303

Breaded Chicken Tenders with Herbs . . 304

Chicken-Almond Stir-Fry
with Carrots, Snow Peas & Plums 304

Chicken & Chanterelles 305

Chicken Enchiladas. 306

Chicken Fried Rice. 306

Chicken Tandoori Skewers 307

Chicken Teriyaki with Soba
Noodles & Cashews 308

Chicken Tikka Masala 309

Chicken with Artichokes & Capers 309

Crispy Almond Chicken Bowl 310

Crispy Chicken Nuggets 310

Curry-Glazed Chicken 311

Habanero Chicken Wings 311

Honey-Ginger Chicken & Apples 312

Lemon Chicken with Smoked Paprika . . 312

Moroccan-Inspired Chicken &
Couscous. 313

Roast Chicken with Lemon & Thyme . . . 313

Rosemary-Citrus Chicken 314

Rosemary-Garlic Chicken Wings 315

Sesame Chicken & Vegetable
Foil Packs 315

Sheet Pan Chicken, Broccoli &
Red Peppers. 316

Zesty Chicken Bites 316

Turkey

Herb-Roasted Turkey Breast
with Vegetables 317

Turkey Jambalaya. 318

Turkey & Squash Couscous
with Apricots & Peanuts 318

Turkey Tenderloins with
Spinach Pesto & Pistachios 319

Chicken and turkey are wonderful protein sources for heart-healthy dietary patterns. They are very versatile and work well with the flavor profiles of so many world cuisines, from Asia and Latin America to the Mediterranean. They also pair well with other heart-health promoting ingredients like whole grains, legumes, and vegetables.

We created a wide range of recipes—quick recipes for busy weeknights using no prep, quick-cooking cuts like chicken tenders, and leisurely recipes like roast chicken and turkey that provide ample leftovers for future meals. We've even provided two options for baked chicken wings for all the wing lovers out there. (It's okay to admit it; we love wings, too!)

At your local grocery store, you'll see many choices for chicken and turkey, including whole birds raw or fully cooked; popular cuts like boneless, skinless breasts and thighs; and large money-saving family packs. There are also frozen options. When you buy fresh poultry, refrigerate and use it within three days. You can store frozen poultry in the freezer for up to six months, ensuring you'll always have a lean protein option on hand.

We love cooking poultry with the skin on to keep the meat moist and juicy. If you enjoy eating the skin occasionally, don't despair: Most of the fat in chicken and turkey skin is unsaturated.

Finally, when cooking chicken or turkey, it's important to cook them to a temperature that ensures bacteria and other microorganisms that cause food-borne illness are destroyed. Use a digital food thermometer to make sure that the meat is cooked all the way through. Whether whole, cut up, or ground, chicken or turkey should be cooked to an internal temperature of 165°F (75°C).

ALMOND-CRUSTED CHICKEN STRIPS

Makes 6 servings

These chicken strips are enjoyed by both adults and kids. We make the Savory Nut Crumb Topping with almonds for this recipe. Serve these tender crunchy strips with Chipotle Aïoli (page 44). You can also use them in Chicken Fried Rice (page 310) or the Crispy Almond Chicken Bowl (page 310).

⅔ cup (160 ml) cultured buttermilk

1 large egg

2 tablespoons reduced-sodium Worcestershire sauce

2 garlic cloves, minced

1.5 pounds (680 g) boneless, skinless chicken breasts or chicken tenderloins, cut into 12 strips

1 teaspoon paprika

½ teaspoon freshly ground black pepper

1 cup (235 g) almonds from Savory Nut Crumb Topping (page 36)

2 tablespoons minced fresh rosemary

1. Preheat the oven to 400°F (200°C). Line a large rimmed baking sheet with parchment paper.

2. Whisk together the buttermilk, egg, Worcestershire sauce, and garlic in a medium bowl. Season the chicken with paprika and pepper. Combine the nut crumb topping and rosemary in a large bowl. Dip the chicken in the buttermilk mixture, then dredge in the nut crumb topping to coat. Place on the baking sheet.

3. Bake for about 30 minutes, until the chicken is plump and the breading is golden brown. The chicken is cooked when a digital food thermometer reads 165°F (75°C) when inserted in the thickest part.

4. Let the chicken rest for 5 minutes on the baking sheet, then serve. Store in an airtight container in the refrigerator for up to 3 days.

Per Serving: Calories 342; Protein 35 g; Carbs 15 g; Dietary Fiber 3 g; Added Sugars 0 g; Total Fat 16 g; Sat Fat 3 g; Omega-3s 50 mg; Sodium 367 mg; Potassium 636 mg

BREADED CHICKEN TENDERS WITH HERBS

Makes 4 servings

Chicken tenders are a meal you can get on the table in less than a half hour. They cook up quickly and need very little preparation because they're already so tender (hence the name!). Serve with Pico de Gallo (page 61), Horseradish-Dijon Aïoli (page 44), or Plum Sauce (page 57).

1 pound (454 g) chicken tenders

Freshly ground black pepper

½ cup (120 ml) buttermilk

¾ cup (45 g) panko bread crumbs

¼ cup (15 g) fresh parsley, finely chopped

2 tablespoons minced fresh rosemary

2 garlic cloves, crushed or finely minced

1 teaspoon ground mustard

Cooking spray

1. Preheat the oven to 375°F (190°C). Line a baking sheet with foil or parchment paper.

2. Cut the chicken into strips, then lightly sprinkle with pepper. Pour the buttermilk into a shallow bowl. Combine the bread crumbs, parsley, rosemary, garlic, and mustard in a medium bowl.

3. Dip the chicken in the buttermilk, then roll in the bread crumb mixture, coating well. (For a thicker breading, roll the chicken first in the bread crumb mixture, then dip in the buttermilk and roll again in the bread crumb mixture.)

4. Place the chicken on the baking sheet and spray with cooking spray. Bake for 18 to 20 minutes, until the crust is brown and a digital food thermometer reads 165°F (75°C) when inserted in the thickest part. Serve hot. Store in an airtight container in the refrigerator for up to 3 days. To reheat, preheat the oven to 350°F (180°C). Place the chicken tenders on a wire rack set on a baking sheet and bake at 350°F (180°C) for 10 minutes or until heated through.

Per Serving: Calories 170; Protein 28; Carbs 10 g; Dietary Fiber 1 g; Added Sugars 0 g; Total Fat 3 g; Sat Fat 0 g; Omega-3s 30 mg; Sodium 160 mg; Potassium 95 mg

CHICKEN-ALMOND STIR-FRY WITH CARROTS, SNOW PEAS & PLUMS

Makes 4 servings

Plums add a subtle sweetness and juiciness to this stir-fry. Serve over soba (buckwheat) or cellophane (bean thread) noodles, steamed basmati rice, or our Simply Cooked Quinoa (page 228).

3 tablespoons Chicken Stock (page 70) or reduced-sodium chicken broth, plus more if needed

3 tablespoons plum, apple, or pineapple juice

2 tablespoons reduced-sodium soy sauce

2 tablespoons white wine

3 garlic cloves, finely chopped

2 teaspoons finely grated ginger

1 tablespoon cornstarch

1 pound (454 g) boneless, skinless chicken breasts, cubed

2 tablespoons toasted sesame or peanut oil

3 carrots, peeled and thinly sliced

6 ounces (170 g) snow peas or sugar snap peas, trimmed and halved

1 red bell pepper, seeded and coarsely chopped

6 green onions, thinly sliced

3 fresh plums, halved, pitted, and thinly sliced

½ cup (45 g) slivered almonds, toasted

Freshly ground black pepper

1. Whisk together the stock, juice, soy sauce, wine, garlic, and ginger in a medium bowl. Slowly whisk in the cornstarch. Stir in the chicken cubes and cover. Marinate in the refrigerator for 30 minutes. Occasionally stir and lift the chicken pieces with a slotted spatula to coat all sides.

2. Heat 1 tablespoon of the oil in a wok or heavy skillet over medium-high heat. When the oil is shimmering, add the chicken using a slotted spatula; reserve the marinade. Stir-fry until opaque and light to dark brown in spots, 2 to 3 minutes.

3. Add the remaining 1 tablespoon oil, the carrots, snow peas, and bell pepper. Stir-fry until the vegetables begin to soften, about 2 minutes.

4. Add the marinade. Cook until the sauce is thickened and smooth, the vegetables are bright in color, and the garlic and ginger are fragrant, 2 to 3 minutes. For a thinner consistency, add more chicken stock, 1 tablespoon at a time.

5. Add the plums, green onions, and slivered almonds. Stir-fry to gently heat the plums and to incorporate the green onions and almonds, 1 minute.

6. The stir-fry is ready to serve when a digital food thermometer reads 165°F (75°C) when inserted in a few of the chicken cubes. Add black pepper and serve hot.

Per Serving: Calories 363; Protein 32 g; Carbs 22 g; Dietary Fiber 6 g; Added Sugars 0 g; Total Fat 16 g; Sat Fat 2 g; Omega-3s 70 mg; Sodium 383 mg; Potassium 845 mg

CHICKEN & CHANTERELLES

Makes 4 servings

Chanterelle mushrooms have a tender texture, a wavy top, and a golden-brown to orange-yellow color. They stand out! And they hold their own, remaining firm after cooking. Here we've paired them with tender chicken in a creamy and flavorful sauce to allow their peppery, fruity flavors to come through. Serve with Simply Cooked Farro (page 226) or Rosemary Mashed Potatoes (page 270).

  1 pound (454 g) boneless, skinless chicken breasts
  1 tablespoon extra virgin olive oil
  1 green onion, chopped
  2 garlic cloves, minced
  2 tablespoons chopped fresh marjoram
  4 thyme sprigs
  ½ cup (120 ml) dry white wine
  8 ounces (227 g) chanterelle mushrooms (see Note)
  1 teaspoon fresh lemon juice
  2 tablespoons half-and-half
  ¼ teaspoon kosher salt
  Freshly ground black pepper

1. Heat the oil in a heavy-bottomed sauté pan or Dutch oven over medium-high heat. Sear the chicken breasts until brown and crisp but not cooked through, about 3 minutes per side. Transfer to a plate.

2. Reduce the heat to medium and add the green onion, garlic, marjoram, and thyme; sauté until fragrant, 1 minute. Deglaze the pan with the wine and use a spoon to loosen up any stuck bits on the pan.

3. Return the chicken to the pan along with any juices that have accumulated. Add the mushrooms. Bring to a boil, partially cover, and reduce the heat to low to bring to a gentle simmer. Cook about 15 minutes, until a digital food thermometer reads 165°F (75°C) when inserted in the thickest part of a chicken breast, the mushrooms are tender, and the liquid has reduced by more than half. Stir in the half-and-half, salt, and pepper to taste and serve.

NOTE: *Washing mushrooms with water is not recommended because mushrooms absorb water, changing their texture and diminishing their flavor. It's best to clean chanterelles and other mushrooms by brushing them with a damp kitchen towel to remove any dirt or dust.*

Per Serving: Calories 223; Protein 27 g; Carbs 7 g; Dietary Fiber 2 g; Added Sugars 0 g; Total Fat 7 g; Sat Fat 1 g; Omega-3s 50 mg; Sodium 113 mg; Potassium 728 mg

CHICKEN ENCHILADAS

Makes 6 servings

This recipe makes six generous enchiladas with chipotle chiles and pinto beans. By using reduced-sodium canned products, we can use our favorite Cotija, a salty aged cheese that adds a creaminess to the filling.

One 15.5-ounce (439 g) can pinto beans, drained, rinsed, and mashed

¾ cup (120 g) finely chopped onion

½ cup (8 g) chopped fresh cilantro

2 or 3 chipotles in adobo sauce, chopped

2 to 4 tablespoons of the adobo sauce

Grated zest and juice of 1 lime

One 14.5-ounce (411 g) can no-salt-added petite diced tomatoes

1½ cups (475 g) Simply Cooked Fresh Tomato Sauce (page 59)

1 tablespoon Adobo Seasoning (page 30)

Six 8-inch (20 cm) whole wheat tortillas

12 ounces (340 g) meat from Roast Chicken with Lemon & Thyme (page 313), shredded

4 ounces (113 g) Cotija, crumbled

8 green onions, chopped

1 lime, cut into wedges

1. Preheat the oven to 350°F (180°C). Line a 13 × 9-inch (33 × 23 cm) baking pan with foil.

2. Combine the beans, onion, ¼ cup (4 g) of the cilantro, the chipotles, and lime zest in a medium bowl. Mix the tomatoes, tomato sauce, adobo sauce, and adobo seasoning in a separate medium bowl. Ladle and spread 1½ cups (420 g) of the tomato mixture over the bottom of the baking pan.

3. Heat the tortillas, one at a time, in a skillet over medium-high heat for 10 to 15 seconds. Flip and heat for 5 to 10 seconds. As each is done, transfer to a plate. Tent with foil to keep warm.

4. To assemble the enchiladas, lay out a tortilla on a work surface. Coat the top of the tortilla with 2 tablespoons of the remaining tomato sauce mixture. Add one-sixth each of the shredded chicken and bean mixtures, then sprinkle with 4 teaspoons of the cheese. Roll up the tortilla and place it seam side down in the baking pan. Repeat with the remaining tortillas, sauce, fillings, and cheese. Spoon the remaining tomato sauce over the enchiladas in the pan.

5. Cover and bake for 30 to 40 minutes, until the enchiladas are thoroughly heated, the mixture is bubbly, and most of the tomato sauce on top has been absorbed. A digital food thermometer should read 165°F (75°C) when inserted in the center of the dish.

6. Plate the enchiladas. Spoon over the tomato sauce from the pan and top with the remaining ¼ cup cilantro and green onions. Sprinkle with the lime juice and place a lime wedge on each plate.

Per Serving: Calories 395; Protein 28 g; Carbs 37 g; Dietary Fiber 6 g; Added Sugars 0 g; Total Fat 15 g; Sat Fat 6 g; Omega-3s 200 mg; Sodium 700 mg; Potassium 635 mg

CHICKEN FRIED RICE

Makes 4 servings

If you have Simply Cooked Brown Rice and Roast Chicken with Lemon & Thyme on hand, this recipe is quick to assemble. Add fresh vegetables from your produce drawer, a small bag of frozen peas from the freezer, and dinner is on the table in under 30 minutes.

2 tablespoons plus 1 teaspoon toasted sesame oil

2 large eggs

2 carrots, diced

1 red onion, chopped

1 cup (70 g) finely chopped napa cabbage or bok choy

4 ounces (113 g) thinly sliced cremini mushrooms

3 garlic cloves, minced

2 tablespoons rice vinegar

1½ cups (190 g) meat from Roast Chicken with Lemon & Thyme (page 313)

2 cups (390 g) Simply Cooked Brown Rice (page 230), cold

¼ cup (60 ml) Chicken Stock (page 70) or reduced-sodium chicken broth

1 cup (135 g) frozen green peas, partially thawed

2 tablespoons reduced-sodium soy sauce or
  tamari

2 teaspoons grated fresh ginger

¼ cup (25 g) sliced almonds, toasted

2 green onions, thinly sliced

1 tablespoon plus 1 teaspoon fresh lemon juice

1. Heat 1 teaspoon of the oil in a large nonstick sauté pan or wok over medium heat. Whisk the eggs in a small bowl until lightly blended. When the oil shimmers, add the eggs. Use a slotted spatula to stir the eggs into small, gently cooked soft curds, less than 1 minute. Transfer to a medium bowl.

2. Return the pan to the heat, add 1 tablespoon oil, and increase the heat to medium-high. When the oil is shimmering, add the carrots, red onion, cabbage, mushrooms, and garlic. Stir-fry until the carrots, onion, and cabbage begin to soften, the mushrooms begin to shrink, and the garlic is aromatic, about 2 minutes. Add the vinegar and continue to stir-fry until the vegetables are crisp-tender and the liquid has evaporated, 1 to 2 minutes. Transfer the vegetables to the bowl with the eggs.

3. Reduce the heat to medium-low, return the pan to the heat, and add the remaining 1 tablespoon oil, followed by the chicken and rice. Use the spatula to stir the chicken and rice until the rice is broken up and everything is slightly heated, about 1 minute. Add the stock and peas, stir, and cook for 1 minute. Stir in the soy sauce and ginger.

4. Return the vegetables and eggs to the pan and stir everything together. Continue to cook until heated through, 2 to 3 minutes. Plate immediately and top each serving with a tablespoon of almonds, a tablespoon of green onions, and a teaspoon of lemon juice. Serve hot.

TIP: *Zesty Chicken Bites (page 316) work well in this recipe, but we recommend omitting the added ginger.*

Per Serving: Calories 631; Protein 30 g; Carbs 86 g; Dietary Fiber 9 g; Added Sugars 0 g; Total Fat 11 g; Sat Fat 3 g; Omega-3s 150 mg; Sodium 633 mg; Potassium 495 mg

CHICKEN TANDOORI SKEWERS

Makes 8 to 12 skewers

Traditional tandoori chicken, a featured dish of Punjabi cuisine, is cooked in a large clay oven called a tandoor, which perfectly sears the chicken without overcooking it. In this recipe, we sought to imitate this process without the use of a tandoor by broiling skewers of marinated chicken in the oven. The result is an easy-to-clean-up dish with perfectly charred tender chunks of chicken and bell pepper. Serve with basmati rice, Cucumber & Tomato Salad (page 152) and Tzatziki (page 60).

One 5.3-ounce (150 g) plain Greek yogurt
  (about ⅔ cup)

1 tablespoon fresh lemon juice

4 garlic cloves, crushed

1 tablespoon ground coriander

1 tablespoon grated fresh ginger

1 teaspoon chili powder

1 teaspoon ground cumin

1 teaspoon ground turmeric

¼ teaspoon ground cardamom

2 pounds (907 g) boneless, skinless chicken
  thighs or breasts, cut into 2-inch (5 cm)
  pieces

2 red bell peppers, seeded and cut into 1-inch
  (2.5 cm) squares

¼ cup (60 ml) extra virgin olive oil

1. Combine the yogurt, lemon juice, garlic, coriander, ginger, chili powder, cumin, turmeric, and cardamom in a large bowl. Add the chicken and use your hands to massage the marinade into each piece. Cover, place in the refrigerator, and marinate for at least 2 hours or overnight.

2. If using bamboo skewers, soak them in warm water for 30 minutes.

3. Thread alternating pieces of chicken and bell pepper onto 8 to 12 skewers.

4. To cook on a grill, heat the grill to medium-high heat for 10 to 15 minutes. Brush the pieces of chicken and bell pepper with the oil. Grill the skewers over medium-high heat, for 4 to 5 minutes on each side, turning occasionally until the vegetables are blistered, the chicken is golden brown, and a digital food thermometer reads 165°F (75°C) when inserted through a few chicken cubes (not touching a metal skewer), 8 to 10 minutes total.

5. **To cook on the stovetop,** add 2 tablespoons of oil to a large skillet on medium-high heat. When the oil is hot and shimmering, but not smoking, add the skewers to the skillet. Pan-sear the skewers, for 4 to 5 minutes on each side, turning occasionally until chicken is golden brown, vegetables are crisp-tender, and a digital food thermometer reads 165°F (75°C) when inserted through a few chicken cubes (not touching a metal skewer) 10 to 12 minutes total. Place the fully cooked skewers in a baking dish and place in a warm oven (200°F/95°C) if doing the skewers in two batches. Add the remaining 2 tablespoons oil to the skillet and prepare the next batch as in Step Serve warm.

Serving Size 1 skewer; Calories 228; Protein 26 g; Carbs 4 g; Dietary Fiber 1 g; Added Sugars 0 g; Total Fat 12 g; Sat Fat 2 g; Omega-3s 60 mg; Sodium 117 mg; Potassium 115 mg

CHICKEN TERIYAKI WITH SOBA NOODLES & CASHEWS
Makes 4 servings

Soba noodles are thin noodles made from buckwheat flour and have a slightly nutty, earthy flavor. Some versions also contain wheat flour, but we encourage you to try those made from 100 percent buckwheat. We think you'll enjoy their unique flavor in this dish.

6 ounces (170 g) soba noodles

¼ cup (60 ml) rice wine, sake, or white wine

3 tablespoons reduced-sodium soy sauce

2 tablespoons rice vinegar

1 tablespoon honey

2 garlic cloves, minced

1 teaspoon grated fresh ginger

¼ teaspoon red pepper flakes

2 tablespoons toasted sesame or peanut oil

12 ounces (340 g) chicken tenders or boneless, skinless chicken breast, cut into bite-size pieces

1 large orange or red bell pepper, seeded and cut into thin strips

8 Brussels sprouts, trimmed and thinly sliced

8 ounces (227 g), shiitake mushroom caps or white mushrooms, quartered

4 green onions, thinly sliced diagonally

½ cup (70 g) roasted cashews

1. Cook the soba noodles according to package directions. Set aside and keep warm.

2. Whisk together the wine, soy sauce, vinegar, honey, garlic, ginger, and red pepper flakes in a small bowl.

3. Heat 1 tablespoon of the oil in a large sauté pan or wok over medium heat. When the oil is shimmering, add the chicken and sauté until opaque, firm, and golden brown, about 4 minutes. Transfer the chicken to a medium bowl with a slotted spoon.

4. Return the pan to the heat, adjust to medium-high, and add the remaining 1 tablespoon oil. When the oil is hot, add the bell pepper and Brussels sprouts and stir-fry for 1 minute. Add the mushrooms and stir-fry until the mushrooms have softened and the other vegetables are slightly browned on the edges and crisp-tender, 2 to 3 minutes.

5. Add the chicken back to the pan along with the sauce. Reduce the heat to medium. Cook, stirring occasionally, until the chicken is thoroughly heated through and the sauce coats everything, 1 to 2 minutes.

6. Spoon the chicken and vegetables mixture over the soba noodles. Top with green onions and cashews. Serve hot.

Per Serving: Calories 562; Protein 25 g; Carbs 51 g; Dietary Fiber 5 g; Added Sugars 4 g; Total Fat 29 g; Sat Fat 5 g; Omega-3s 660 mg; Sodium 750 mg; Potassium 722 mg

CHICKEN TIKKA MASALA

Makes 4 servings

While many believe this is a classic Indian dish, chicken tikka masala was actually created by a chef in Great Britain. This nontraditional version uses curry powder instead of garam masala, incorporates diced tomatoes to create a chunkier consistency, and includes peanut butter for creamy richness. To make a vegetarian version, substitute 2 cups (305 g) canned chickpeas, drained and rinsed, for the chicken. Serve with Simply Cooked Brown Rice (page 230) for a very aromatic, satisfying meal that can be made in 30 minutes or less.

- 1 red onion, thinly sliced
- 1 tablespoon peanut oil
- ¼ teaspoon kosher salt
- 1 tablespoon Curry Powder (page 32) or store-bought curry powder
- ¼ cup (60 ml) water
- One 15-ounce (425 g) can diced tomatoes
- 2 tablespoons minced fresh ginger
- 1 serrano chile, minced
- 2 garlic cloves, minced
- 1 pound (454 g) chicken tenders, cut into bite-size pieces
- ¼ cup (65 g) creamy or crunchy peanut butter
- One 5.3-ounce (150 g) container plain Greek yogurt (about ⅔ cup)

1. Combine the onions, oil, and salt in a saucepan over medium high heat. Sauté until the onions start to brown, 10 minutes.

2. Add the curry powder and sauté for 1 minute. Stir in the water. Reduce the heat to medium and add the tomatoes and their liquid, the ginger, serrano, and garlic. Stir, cover, and bring to a simmer. Once the mixture is bubbling, add the chicken, stir, and cover. Cook, stirring occasionally, until the chicken has turned from pink to white, 10 minutes.

3. Reduce the heat to low. Stir the peanut butter and yogurt together in a small dish, then add to the mixture. Cook for another 1 to 2 minutes to warm through. Serve.

Per Serving: Calories 568; Protein 29 g; Carbs 37 g; Dietary Fiber 5 g; Added Sugars 1 g; Total Fat 34 g; Sat Fat 8 g; Omega-3s 810 mg; Sodium 758 mg; Potassium 732 mg

CHICKEN WITH ARTICHOKES & CAPERS

Makes 4 servings

Many people mistakenly believe capers are green peppercorns, but they are actually immature flower buds, pickled or preserved in brine. We recommend buying capers the size of a baby green pea or smaller; the smaller the caper, the more delicate the texture and better the flavor. Typically sold in 2- to 3.5-ounce (57 to 100 g) jars, capers are shelf stable until opened; after opening, store them in the refrigerator.

- 2 tablespoons extra virgin olive oil
- 1 pound (454 g) boneless, skinless chicken breasts, thinly sliced
- 1 small fennel bulb, trimmed and thinly sliced
- 4 garlic cloves, minced
- One 9-ounce (255 g) package frozen artichoke hearts, thawed, halved if large
- One 14.5-ounce (411 g) can no-salt-added petite diced tomatoes
- 1 cup (315 g) Simply Cooked Fresh Tomato Sauce (page 59)
- 1 tablespoon chopped fresh basil
- 1 tablespoon capers, drained
- 1 tablespoon chopped fresh oregano
- 1 tablespoon chopped fresh thyme
- 1 tablespoon balsamic vinegar
- ½ teaspoon red pepper flakes
- ¼ teaspoon freshly ground black pepper
- 8 ounces (227 g) whole grain vermicelli
- ½ cup (40 g) freshly grated Parmesan
- ½ cup (30 g) minced fresh parsley

1. Bring a large pot of water to a boil.

2. Heat 1 tablespoon of the oil in a large skillet over medium-high heat. Add the chicken and cook until lightly browned, about 3 minutes. Add the fennel and garlic and sauté until the fennel starts to soften and the garlic is aromatic, 1 to 2 minutes. Add the artichoke hearts and cook until the artichokes are starting to brown on the edges, about 2 minutes.

3. Stir in the tomatoes and tomato sauce. Reduce the heat to medium-low, then stir in the basil, capers, oregano, thyme, vinegar, red pepper flakes, and black pepper. Simmer, stirring occasionally, to blend the flavors and thicken the sauce, 4 to 6 minutes.

4. Cook the vermicelli in the boiling water according to package directions. Drain when the pasta is al dente, reserving ⅓ cup (80 ml) of the pasta water. Return the vermicelli to the pot and add the remaining 1 tablespoon oil, the reserved pasta water, ¼ cup (20 g) of the Parmesan, and ¼ cup (15 g) of the parsley. Mix well.

5. Using tongs, divide the vermicelli among the four shallow bowls or plates. Stir the sauce and chicken, then ladle over the top. Sprinkle each plate with the remaining Parmesan and parsley. Serve hot.

Per Serving: Calories 557; Protein 38 g; Carbs 71 g; Dietary Fiber 9 g; Added Sugars 0 g; Total Fat 13 g; Sat Fat 3 g; Omega-3s 110 mg; Sodium 596 mg; Potassium 1,241 mg

CRISPY ALMOND CHICKEN BOWL

Makes 4 servings

This bowl combines a few of our other recipes. While we provide tips for what to combine based on complementary flavor profiles, the final decision is up to you. Use roasted vegetables, add some beans, or try a different sauce. Have fun creating a bowl that inspires you!

- 4 cups (620 g) Simply Steamed Couscous or Simply Cooked Quinoa, Brown Rice, or Wild Rice (pages 205, 228, 230, or 234)
- 12 Almond-Crusted Chicken Strips (page 291)
- 4 cups (140 g) mixed greens
- ½ cup (200 g) Cucumber-Dill Sauce (page 54)
- ¼ cup (15 g) fresh flat-leaf parsley, chopped
- 4 lemon wedges, optional

Divide the whole grains among four bowls. Top each with 3 chicken strips, 1 cup (35 g) greens, 2 tablespoons sauce, and 1 tablespoon parsley. Add a lemon wedge to each bowl, if desired, and serve.

Per Serving: Calories 787; Protein 59 g; Carbs 57 g; Dietary Fiber 10 g; Added Sugars 0 g; Total Fat 36 g; Sat Fat 6 g; Omega-3s 640 mg; Sodium 690 mg; Potassium 1,078 mg

CRISPY CHICKEN NUGGETS

Makes 4 servings

Use chicken breasts or thighs to make these flavorful chicken nuggets that are perfectly juicy on the inside and crunchy on the outside. We use our À la Heart House Dressing as the liquid before rolling the chicken in the bread crumbs. The dressing also makes a great dipping sauce.

- 1 pound (454 g) boneless, skinless chicken breasts or thighs, trimmed and cut into 1½-inch (4 cm) pieces
- ½ cup (120 ml) À la Heart House Dressing (page 47)
- ½ cup (110 g) Garlic & Herb Bread Crumbs (page 33)
- ½ cup (30 g) panko bread crumbs
- ¼ cup (20 g) freshly grated Parmesan
- 1 tablespoon Italian Seasoning (page 34)
- ⅛ teaspoon kosher salt
- 1 teaspoon freshly ground black pepper

1. Preheat the oven to 375°F (190°C). Line a rimmed baking pan with parchment paper.

2. Pour the dressing into a shallow bowl or pie plate. In a separate shallow bowl, combine the garlic bread crumbs and panko bread crumbs, the Parmesan, seasoning, salt, and pepper.

3. Dip the chicken in the dressing; shake off any extra. Roll in the bread crumb mixture, coating all sides. Place on the pan.

4. Bake for 30 to 35 minutes, until the coating is crispy and golden brown, and a digital food thermometer reads 165°F (75°C) when inserted in the largest nuggets. Serve warm.

TIP: *It's fun to offer a variety of dipping sauces for these nuggets. Try a trio of our À la Heart House Dressing (page 47), Plum Sauce (page 57), and Homestyle Barbecue Sauce (page 55).*

Per Serving: Calories 264; Protein 31 g; Carbs 17 g; Dietary Fiber 2 g; Added Sugars 0 g; Total Fat 7 g; Sat Fat 2 g; Omega-3s 50 mg; Sodium 326 mg; Potassium 439 mg

CURRY-GLAZED CHICKEN

Makes 4 servings

Curry powder combines both savory and sweet spices, giving this dish a depth of flavor while adding pep and brightness. Try our Curry Powder, a mild blend made with cumin, turmeric, coriander, ginger, and cayenne. If you prefer more heat, add red pepper flakes or a chopped jalapeño to the glaze.

- 1 pound (454 g) boneless, skinless chicken breasts or thighs
- 2 tablespoons extra virgin olive oil
- 2 tablespoons honey
- 2 tablespoons fresh lemon juice
- 1 tablespoon Curry Powder (page 32)
- 1 tablespoon Dijon mustard

1. Preheat the oven to 375°F (190°C). Line an 11 × 7-inch (28 × 18 cm) baking dish with parchment paper or foil.

2. Cut the chicken breasts or thighs in half or into 4 to 6 equal pieces. Whisk together the oil, honey, lemon juice, curry powder, and mustard in a large bowl. Add the chicken and turn to coat.

3. Arrange the chicken in the baking dish in a single layer. Pour over any remaining glaze. Cover with foil. Bake for 20 minutes.

4. Remove the foil and bake for 15 to 20 minutes, until the chicken is sticky, bubbling, and brown, and a digital food thermometer reads 165°F (75°C) when inserted in the thickest part. Remove from the oven, tent the chicken with the foil, and let rest for 10 minutes. Serve hot.

TIP: *The glaze used in this recipe also works well over oven-roasted vegetables, such as our Simply Roasted Root Vegetables with Apples (page 261).*

Per Serving: Calories 241; Protein 26 g; Carbs 10 g; Dietary Fiber 1 g; Added Sugars 9 g; Total Fat 10 g; Sat Fat 2 g; Omega-3s 70 mg; Sodium 142 mg; Potassium 401 mg

HABANERO CHICKEN WINGS

Makes 10 to 12 wings

If you love Buffalo wings, give these a try! The heat from the habanero builds slowly and intensifies quickly. To cool the heat a bit, try dipping these in our À la Heart House Dressing (page 47), which is similar to ranch.

- 1 pound (454 g) whole chicken wings (10 to 12 wings)
- 1 tablespoon Habanero Spice Rub (page 33)
- 1 tablespoon extra virgin olive oil
- ¼ teaspoon habanero powder
- ¼ teaspoon kosher salt

1. Preheat the oven to 425°F (220°C). Place a wire rack on a rimmed baking sheet.

2. Place the wings in a large bowl. Sprinkle with 1½ teaspoons of the habanero spice rub and toss to coat. Sprinkle with the remaining 1½ teaspoons rub and toss again. Arrange the wings on the wire rack about 1 inch (2.5 cm) apart. Bake for 20 minutes.

3. Flip the wings and bake for 20 minutes, until they are dark brown and crispy.

4. Combine the oil, habanero powder, and salt in a clean large bowl. Add the wings and toss well to coat. Place on a serving platter and enjoy!

TIP: *The longer the wings sit in the oil, the hotter they become. If you're serving these to a group of people who may "graze" on them slowly, cut back on or eliminate the habanero powder.*

Serving Size 3 to 4 wings; Calories 337; Protein 27 g; Carbs 1 g; Dietary Fiber 0 g; Added Sugars 0 g; Total Fat 24 g; Sat Fat 6 g; Omega-3s 210 mg; Sodium 183 mg; Potassium 298 mg

HONEY-GINGER CHICKEN & APPLES

Makes 4 servings

Enjoy this fragrant and succulent dish with Cardamom & Orange Roasted Carrots (page 266) and Simply Cooked Farro (page 226).

- 4 teaspoons peanut or toasted sesame oil
- 1 pound (454 g) boneless, skinless chicken breast, cut into long, narrow strips
- ½ cup (120 ml) Chicken Stock (page 70) or reduced-sodium chicken broth
- ½ cup (120 ml) white wine
- 1 green onion, thinly sliced
- 2 garlic cloves, finely minced
- 2 teaspoons grated fresh ginger
- 1 bay leaf
- 1 cinnamon stick
- 2 tart apples (such as Granny Smith, Braeburn, or Jonathan)
- ½ teaspoon ground cardamom
- 1 tablespoon honey

1. Preheat the oven to 350°F (180°C). Oil an 11 × 7-inch (28 × 18 cm) baking dish with 2 teaspoons of the oil.

2. Place the chicken in a single layer in the baking dish. Whisk together the stock, wine, the remaining 2 teaspoons oil, the green onion, garlic, ginger, and bay leaf in a small bowl. Add the cinnamon stick. Pour the mixture over the chicken and use your hands to massage the marinade into the chicken. Let marinate while you prepare the apples.

3. Core and slice the apples; place the slices in a medium bowl. Sprinkle with the cardamom and stir gently to coat.

4. Layer the apples on top of the chicken and drizzle with the honey.

5. Bake for 40 minutes, until the honey and marinade form a nice caramelized crust on the bottom of the chicken and the apples are tender. The chicken is fully cooked when a digital food thermometer reads 165°F (75°C). Serve hot.

Per Serving: Calories 269; Protein 26 g; Carbs 19 g; Dietary Fiber 2 g; Added Sugars 4 g; Total Fat 8 g; Sat Fat 1 g; Omega-3s 20 mg; Sodium 55 mg; Potassium 523 mg

LEMON CHICKEN WITH SMOKED PAPRIKA

Makes 4 servings

Smoked paprika is made from peppers that are smoked and dried over oak fires. We add a bit of honey in this recipe to deepen its savoriness. Serve over Simply Cooked Barley (page 223) or Simply Steamed Couscous (page 205), with steamed green peas on the side.

- 3 tablespoons fresh lemon juice
- 3 tablespoons extra virgin olive oil
- 2 tablespoons chopped fresh thyme
- 2 garlic cloves, minced
- 2 teaspoons honey
- 2 teaspoons dried oregano
- 2 teaspoons smoked paprika
- 1 pound (454 g) boneless, skinless chicken breasts, each piece cut into 4 to 8 strips or chunks

1. Preheat the oven to 375°F (190°C). Line a rimmed baking pan with parchment paper or foil.

2. Combine the lemon juice, oil, thyme, garlic, honey, oregano, and paprika in a bowl. Add the chicken and stir well to coat. Transfer to the baking pan.

3. Bake for 30 to 40 minutes, until the outside of the chicken is a golden red-brown color, the bottom of the pan is sizzling, and a digital thermometer reads 165°F (75°C) when inserted in the thickest part of the chicken. Serve immediately.

Per Serving: Calories 252; Protein 26 g; Carbs 5 g; Dietary Fiber 1 g; Added Sugars 3 g; Total Fat 14 g; Sat Fat 2 g; Omega-3s 100 mg; Sodium 53 mg; Potassium 439 mg

MOROCCAN-INSPIRED CHICKEN & COUSCOUS

Makes 6 servings

Couscous is the traditional accompaniment to tagine, a North African stew made with meat, vegetables, dried fruit, and spices. This version combines couscous with chicken, zucchini, dried apricots, raisins, and our Moroccan-Style Seasoning to provide the right balance of sweet and hot in this fragrant, comforting dish.

1 pound (454 g) boneless, skinless chicken thighs, each cut into 4 to 6 pieces

3 teaspoons Moroccan-Style Seasoning (page 35)

1 teaspoon paprika

2 tablespoons extra virgin olive oil

1 yellow onion, sliced

4 garlic cloves, minced

3 zucchini, trimmed and sliced

½ cup (65 g) chopped dried apricots

½ cup (80 g) raisins

1½ cups (360 ml) Chicken Stock (page 70) or reduced-sodium chicken broth

3 cups (470 g) Simply Steamed Couscous (page 205)

¾ cup (100 g) sliced pitted green olives

Grated zest and juice of 1 lemon

½ cup (70 g) slivered almonds, toasted

½ cup (8 g) chopped fresh cilantro

1. Rub the chicken with 2 teaspoons of the seasoning and the paprika in a shallow dish. Cover and refrigerate for 2 hours.

2. Heat the oil in a Dutch oven over medium-high heat. Add the onion and garlic and sauté until softened, 3 to 4 minutes. Add the chicken. Cook, stirring constantly, until the chicken begins to turn opaque and the edges begin to brown, 5 minutes.

3. Reduce the heat to medium. Add the apricots, raisins, zucchini, and remaining 1 teaspoon seasoning. Cook, stirring occasionally, until everything is fragrant and starting to soften, 2 to 3 minutes. Stir in the stock and cover. Simmer over medium-low heat until heated thoroughly, 10 minutes.

4. Uncover the pan and stir in the couscous. Cook until the chicken is tender and the couscous has absorbed the liquid, 10 minutes. If some liquid remains, continue to cook until the liquid has evaporated.

5. Remove from the heat. Add the olives, then stir in lemon zest and juice. Top with the almonds and cilantro. Serve hot.

Per Serving: Calories 370; Protein 23 g; Carbs 32 g; Dietary Fiber 7 g; Added Sugars 0 g; Total Fat 18 g; Sat Fat 2 g; Omega-3s 120 mg; Sodium 364 mg; Potassium 531 mg

ROAST CHICKEN WITH LEMON & THYME

Makes 12 servings

Whole chickens of any size would work well for this recipe, in which the chicken is roasted surrounded by vegetables. Leftover chicken can be used to make Chicken Enchiladas (page 306) or Chicken Fried Rice (page 306).

Cooking spray

One 4- to 6-pound (1.8 to 2.7 kg) whole chicken, giblets & neck removed

2 tablespoons extra virgin olive oil

1 tablespoon butter or plant-based spread, melted

1 teaspoon grated lemon zest

1 tablespoon fresh lemon juice

2 garlic cloves, minced

1 teaspoon poultry seasoning

1 teaspoon coarsely chopped fresh rosemary or sage leaves

1 teaspoon chopped fresh thyme

½ teaspoon white pepper

4 fresh thyme sprigs

2 onions, cut into 8 wedges each

3 carrots, cut into 2-inch (5 cm) pieces

2 celery stalks, cut into 2-inch (5 cm) pieces

6 to 8 small red-skin potatoes (2 pounds/ 907 g total), halved

¾ cup (180 ml) Chicken Stock (page 70) or reduced-sodium chicken broth

1. Place an oven rack in the lowest position. Preheat the oven to 375°F (190°C). Line a rimmed baking sheet or roasting pan with foil. Insert a roasting rack and spray it with cooking spray. Place the chicken on the rack.

2. Whisk together 1 tablespoon of the oil, the butter, lemon zest and juice, garlic, poultry seasoning, rosemary, thyme, and ¼ teaspoon of the pepper. Using your hands or a pastry brush, rub some of the mixture all around the chicken cavity. Rub the mixture into the skin all over and under the breast skin, gently lifting the skin and taking care not to tear it. Place a thyme sprig between the flesh and the skin on either side of the breastbone. Turn the chicken breast up and tuck the wing tips underneath.

3. Toss the onions, carrots, celery, and potatoes with the remaining 1 tablespoon oil and the remaining ¼ teaspoon pepper in a large bowl. Arrange the vegetables and remaining 2 thyme sprigs around the chicken. Pour the stock over the vegetables.

4. Roast for 60 to 75 minutes, until a digital food thermometer reads 165°F (75°C) when inserted in the thickest part of a thigh (not touching bone). The legs should lift easily when twisted and the vegetables should pierce easily with a fork.

5. Tent the pan with foil and let the chicken stand for 10 to 15 minutes for easier carving. Serve warm.

TIP: *Check the chicken after roasting for 60 minutes. If the chicken breast is getting overly browned, cover the top of the chicken with foil for the last 15 minutes of roasting.*

Per Serving: Calories 510; Protein 37 g; Carbs 20 g; Dietary Fiber 3 g; Added Sugars 0 g; Total Fat 31 g; Sat Fat 9 g; Omega-3s 370 mg; Sodium 173 mg; Potassium 819 mg

ROSEMARY-CITRUS CHICKEN
Makes 4 servings

This recipe requires little preparation yet yields a beautiful result. We use whole herbs, and sandwich the chicken between citrus slices and rosemary sprigs, allowing the flavor and fragrance of lemon, orange, and rosemary to infuse into the chicken while it roasts. Serve with Lentil & Mixed Greens with Goat Cheese (page 314) or Curried Rice–Stuffed Tomatoes (page 276), or add Simply Roasted Root Vegetables with Apples (page 261).

1 pound (454 g) boneless, skinless chicken breasts, halved if large

2 oranges, thinly cut into round slices

2 lemons, thinly cut into round slices

4 rosemary sprigs

¼ cup (60 ml) extra virgin olive oil

1 teaspoon paprika

½ teaspoon poultry seasoning

Freshly ground black pepper

1. Preheat the oven to 350°F (180°C). Line an 7 × 11-inch (18 × 28 cm) baking dish with parchment paper or foil.

2. Layer three-quarters of the orange and lemon slices in the baking dish. Place 2 rosemary sprigs on top, then drizzle over 1 teaspoon of the oil. Place the chicken on top and season with the paprika, poultry seasoning, and pepper. Place the remaining 2 rosemary sprigs on top of the chicken, then top with the remaining citrus. Drizzle with the remaining oil.

3. Cover the pan with foil and bake for 40 minutes, until the citrus is soft, the oil sizzles on the bottom of the pan, and a digital food thermometer reads 165°F (75°C) when inserted in the thickest part of the chicken. Use the citrus and rosemary as a garnish or discard. Serve warm.

TIP: *Keep the peel on the oranges and lemons. It contains aromatic oils that will help flavor the chicken along with the fruit juices and herbs.*

Per Serving: Calories 310; Protein 27 g; Carbs 12 g; Dietary Fiber 3 g; Added Sugars 0 g; Total Fat 17 g; Sat Fat 3 g; Omega-3s 130 mg; Sodium 53 mg; Potassium 553 mg

ROSEMARY-GARLIC CHICKEN WINGS

Makes 10 to 12 wings

If you love dipping your wings in sauce, try our Tzatziki (page 60).

1½ teaspoons dried rosemary

1½ teaspoons garlic powder

1 pound (454 g) chicken wings (10 to 12 wings)

1 tablespoon extra virgin olive oil

1 tablespoon finely minced garlic

1 tablespoon minced fresh rosemary

¼ teaspoon kosher salt

1. Preheat the oven to 425°F (220°C). Place a wire rack on a rimmed baking sheet.

2. Combine the dried rosemary and garlic powder, using a mortar and pestle or spice grinder; grind to a fine powder.

3. Place the wings in a large bowl. Sprinkle with 1½ teaspoons of the rosemary-garlic powder and toss to coat. Sprinkle with the remaining powder, then toss again. Arrange the wings on the wire rack about 1 inch (2.5 cm) apart. Bake for 20 minutes.

4. Flip the wings and bake for 20 minutes, until they are dark brown and crispy.

5. Combine the oil, garlic, fresh rosemary, and salt in a clean large bowl. Add the wings and toss well to coat. Transfer to a serving platter and enjoy!

Serving Size 3 to 4 wings; Calories 294; Protein 23 g; Carbs 2 g; Dietary Fiber 0 g; Added Sugars 0 g; Total Fat 21 g; Sat Fat 5 g; Omega-3s 190 mg; Sodium 164 mg; Potassium 277 mg

SESAME CHICKEN & VEGETABLE FOIL PACKS

Makes 4 servings

It's easy to create crisp-tender vegetables and juicy, flavorful chicken in individual foil packs. When the thighs are marinating, use the time to prepare the vegetables. The marinade also serves as the sauce to add moisture and flavor as the foil packs bake.

Marinated Chicken

4 boneless, skinless chicken thighs (about 1 pound/454 g)

2 tablespoons toasted sesame oil

2 tablespoons reduced-sodium soy sauce

1 tablespoon water

2 green onions, thinly sliced

1 tablespoon black sesame seeds

1 teaspoon grated fresh ginger

1 garlic clove, minced

¼ teaspoon red pepper flakes

Foil Packs

Cooking spray

4 Yukon gold potatoes, sliced

1 head cauliflower, cut into small florets

4 shallots, sliced

4 garlic cloves, quartered

Freshly cracked black pepper

4 teaspoons black sesame seeds

4 teaspoons toasted sesame oil

¼ cup (15 g) chopped fresh parsley

1 lemon, quartered

1. Place the chicken in a shallow baking dish. Whisk together the 2 tablespoons oil, soy sauce, water, green onions, sesame seeds, ginger, garlic, and red pepper flakes in a small bowl. Pour the marinade over the chicken and turn to coat well. Cover and refrigerate for 1 hour, turning after 30 minutes.

2. Preheat the oven to 350°F (180°C). Cut four 12 × 18-inch (30.5 × 45.5 cm) pieces of foil and spray the centers with cooking spray.

3. Evenly distribute the potatoes among the pieces of foil. Distribute the cauliflower and shallots over the potatoes. Place a chicken thigh on top of each pack, reserving the marinade. Distribute the garlic among the packs and add cracked pepper to each.

4. Bring the foil sides up around the filling. Spoon 1 tablespoon of the reserved marinade, then sprinkle 1 teaspoon of the sesame seeds and drizzle 1 teaspoon of the oil over each. Seal each pack by folding two opposite ends of the foil over the filling. Bring the other two sides together, joining in the center of the pack. Fold the edge of the foil over twice to make a tightly closed pack. Place on a baking sheet.

5. Bake for 50 to 60 minutes, until the vegetables are fork-tender and a digital food thermometer reads 165°F (75°C). The foil packs will be hot and release steam; open carefully to avoid burns. Sprinkle each pack with 1 tablespoon chopped parsley and a squeeze of lemon juice. Serve hot.

TIP: *Add more color to your foil packs by using orange, purple, or green cauliflower.*

Per Serving: Calories 377; Protein 30 g; Carbs 29 g; Dietary Fiber 6 g; Added Sugars 0 g; Total Fat 19 g; Sat Fat 3 g; Omega-3s 60 mg; Sodium 455 mg; Potassium 703 mg

SHEET PAN CHICKEN, BROCCOLI & RED PEPPERS

Makes 4 servings

The flavors of this garlic-ginger chicken with Smoky Workaday Seasoning pair well with similar seasonings on the vegetables. Serve with a green salad or coleslaw, or over Simply Cooked Brown Rice (page 230).

- 1 pound (454 g) boneless, skinless chicken thighs, cut into 1½-inch (4 cm) cubes
- ⅓ cup (80 ml) dry white wine
- ¼ cup (60 ml) reduced-sodium teriyaki sauce
- 2 teaspoons grated fresh ginger
- 2 garlic cloves, minced
- 1 broccoli crown, cut into florets and stems
- 2 medium red bell peppers, seeded and thinly sliced
- 2 medium white onions, sliced into rings
- 2 tablespoons toasted sesame oil
- 1 tablespoon Smoky Workaday Seasoning (page 37)
- Freshly ground black pepper

1. Place chicken in a single layer in a small baking dish. Whisk together the wine, teriyaki sauce, ginger, and garlic in a small bowl. Pour the marinade over the chicken, stir well to coat, and cover. Marinate in the refrigerator for 2 hours. Occasionally stir and lift the chicken pieces with a slotted spatula to coat all sides.

2. Preheat the oven to 400°F (200°C). Line a rimmed baking sheet with parchment paper or foil.

3. Place the broccoli, bell peppers, and onions in a large bowl. Drizzle with 1 tablespoon of the oil and sprinkle with the seasoning. Stir to coat. Spread the vegetables in a single layer on the baking sheet. Add the chicken on top. Spoon any remaining marinade over the top.

4. Roast for 30 minutes or until the vegetables are brown in spots and fork-tender. Stir and flip the vegetables and chicken; return to the oven for 10 minutes if further roasting is required. The chicken is cooked when a digital food thermometer reads 165°F (75°C) when inserted through two or three cubes.

5. Drizzle with the remaining 1 tablespoon oil and sprinkle with 4 to 5 grinds of black pepper. Serve warm.

TIP: *Chicken breasts also work well in this recipe, but not tenders; they're too thin.*

Per Serving: Calories 302; Protein 29 g; Carbs 19 g; Dietary Fiber 5 g; Added Sugars 0 g; Total Fat 12 g; Sat Fat 2 g; Omega-3s 190 mg; Sodium 461 mg; Potassium 615 mg

ZESTY CHICKEN BITES

Makes 4 servings

You can use either chicken breasts or thighs to make these spicy chicken nuggets that are great with a dipping sauce or in a bowl with one of our Simply Cooked whole grains (see chapter 13). They pair well with our Homestyle Barbecue Sauce (page 55) and our Cucumber-Dill Sauce (page 54).

- 3 tablespoons extra virgin olive oil
- 3 tablespoons apple cider vinegar
- 2 garlic cloves, finely minced
- 1 teaspoon smoked paprika

1 teaspoon minced fresh ginger

½ teaspoon ground cumin

¼ teaspoon freshly ground black pepper

⅛ teaspoon kosher salt

1 pound (454 g) boneless, skinless chicken breasts or thighs, trimmed and cut into 1½-inch (4 cm) pieces

1. Preheat the oven to 375°F (190°C), or position an oven rack 4 to 5 inches (10 to 12.5 cm) from the broiler heat source and heat the broiler on HIGH. Line a rimmed baking sheet with foil.

2. Whisk together the oil, vinegar, garlic, paprika, ginger, cumin, pepper, and salt in a medium bowl. Reserve 2 tablespoons of the marinade. Add the chicken to the remaining marinade and stir to coat. Spread the chicken in a single layer on the baking sheet.

3. Bake for 30 to 35 minutes or broil for 15 to 20 minutes, flipping once, until the nuggets are tender and no longer pink and a digital food thermometer reads 165°F (75°C) when inserted in the center of a few nuggets.

4. Drizzle with the reserved dressing and serve hot.

Per Serving: Calories 236; Protein 26 g; Carbs 1 g; Dietary Fiber 0 g; Added Sugars 0 g; Total Fat 14 g; Sat Fat 2 g; Omega-3s 90 mg; Sodium 76 mg; Potassium 402 mg

HERB-ROASTED TURKEY BREAST WITH VEGETABLES

Makes 12 servings

There are times you just don't need or want to purchase and roast an entire turkey; the smaller turkey breast will do. You can retain the moisture and boost the flavor by adding an herb rub and then roasting with vegetables, fruit, and stock. Roasting a turkey breast will provide for several meals. Remaining turkey can be frozen and stored to make enchiladas, sandwiches (delicious with the Fresh Cranberry Citrus Pear Relish, page 64) or Turkey-Vegetable Soup (page 84).

One 6-pound (2.7 kg) skin-on whole turkey breast

2 tablespoons extra virgin olive oil

4 tablespoons (10 g) Herb Blend for Poultry (page 34)

1 pound (454 g) baby red-skin potatoes, quartered

2 cups (245 g) baby carrots, halved lengthwise, or about 9 ounces (255 g) parsnips, trimmed, halved crosswise, then into sticks

2 cups (320 g) pearl onions, halved

1 apple, cored and cut into 8 wedges

3 garlic cloves, quartered

¼ teaspoon kosher salt

¼ teaspoon freshly ground black pepper

1 cup (240 ml) Chicken Stock (page 70) or reduced-sodium chicken broth

1. Place an oven rack in the lowest position. Preheat the oven to 350°F (180°C). Line a rimmed baking sheet or roasting pan with foil. Insert a roasting rack.

2. Brush the turkey with 1 tablespoon of the oil. Massage 3 tablespoons of the herb blend into the turkey, under the skin flap, sides, and underside. Turn the turkey skin side up on the roasting rack. Roast for 20 minutes.

3. Combine the potatoes, carrots, onions, apples, and garlic with the remaining 1 tablespoon oil and the remaining 1 tablespoon herb rub, the salt, and pepper in a large bowl.

4. Remove the pan from the oven, arrange the vegetables and fruit around the turkey, and pour the stock over the vegetables. Return to the oven.

5. Roast for 60 to 80 minutes more, until the turkey is golden to dark brown and a digital food thermometer reads 165°F (75°C) when inserted in the thickest part of the breast (not touching bone). If the turkey is getting overly brown after an hour of cooking, cover loosely with foil.

6. Remove from the oven. Tent the turkey and let stand for 20 to 30 minutes to allow the juices to settle and make carving easier.

7. Transfer the turkey to a cutting board and carve the meat from the bones. Serve with the vegetables and fruit from the pan. Store leftover turkey separate from any remaining vegetables and fruit in an airtight container in the refrigerator for up to 3 days. To freeze, carve the turkey breast in uniform slices. Wrap in wax paper or plastic wrap and place in an airtight freezer-safe container. To reheat, preheat the oven to 325°F (165°C). Remove the turkey from the refrigerator and place on the counter for up to 30 minutes to bring to room temperature. Place on a foil-lined baking dish, add a small amount of chicken stock or broth to moisten, and seal the foil around the turkey. Bake for 20 minutes, until heated through.

VARIATION: Fresh Herb–Roasted Turkey Breast
Replace the herb rub with fresh herbs: 1 tablespoon chopped marjoram, 1 tablespoon chopped rosemary, 1 tablespoon chopped sage, and 1 tablespoon chopped thyme.

Per Serving: Calories 208; Protein 25 g; Carbs 14 g; Dietary Fiber 2 g; Added Sugars 0 g; Total Fat 6 g; Sat Fat 2 g; Omega-3s 30 mg; Sodium 395 mg; Potassium 293 mg

TURKEY JAMBALAYA

Makes 4 servings

This spicy, filling one-dish meal is easy to prepare and loaded with vegetables and fresh herbs. Cajun cuisine typically features paprika, cayenne, garlic powder, oregano, thyme, and black pepper. Our Cajun Seasoning is on the milder side, so we've added red pepper flakes for a bit more heat. You could also add a jalapeño or two and top with our Cajun-Spiced Peanuts.

1 tablespoon extra virgin olive oil

1 onion, chopped

1 bell pepper, seeded and chopped

2 celery stalks, chopped

3 garlic cloves, minced

One 14.5-ounce (411 g) can no-salt-added petite diced tomatoes

½ cup (120 ml) Chicken Stock (page 70) or reduced-sodium chicken broth

6 ounces (170 g) cooked lean ground turkey (about 1 cup)

6 ounces (170 g) cooked lean turkey sausage (about 4 links), casings discarded, crumbled, and cooked

¼ cup (65 g) no-salt-added tomato paste

1 bay leaf

2 tablespoons chopped fresh basil

1 tablespoon Cajun Seasoning (page 30)

¼ teaspoon red pepper flakes

1 cup (190 g) uncooked brown rice

½ cup (30 g) chopped fresh curly parsley

½ cup (80 g) Cajun-Spiced Peanuts (page 345)

Freshly ground black pepper

1. Heat the oil in a large skillet over medium-high heat. Add the onion, bell pepper, celery, and garlic. Sauté until the vegetables begin to soften and the garlic is fragrant, about 3 minutes.

2. Stir in the tomatoes and their juices, the chicken stock, ground turkey, turkey sausage, tomato paste, bay leaf, basil, seasoning, and red pepper flakes. Add the rice and bring to a boil. Reduce the heat to medium-low, cover, and simmer about 10 minutes, until the rice is tender and a digital food thermometer reads 165°F (75°C) when inserted in the center of the skillet.

3. Serve hot from the pan. Sprinkle parsley and peanuts over each serving along with a couple grinds of pepper.

Per Serving: Calories 331; Protein 25 g; Carbs 19 g; Dietary Fiber 5 g; Added Sugars 0 g; Total Fat 18 g; Sat Fat 3 g; Omega-3s 1 40 mg; Sodium 381 mg; Potassium 722 mg

TURKEY & SQUASH COUSCOUS WITH APRICOTS & PEANUTS

Makes 4 servings

This North African–inspired dish offers tempting spicy, sweet, and smoky flavors. The squash lends creaminess, which complements the seasoned turkey bites beautifully. Briny olives and crunchy peanuts added at the end provide texture and flavor.

2 tablespoons extra virgin olive oil

2 teaspoons ground cumin

2 teaspoons finely grated ginger

1 teaspoon smoked paprika

1 teaspoon ground turmeric

½ teaspoon ground allspice

1 pound (454 g) boneless, skinless turkey breast or turkey tenderloins, cut into bite-size pieces

1½ cups (240 g) chopped onion (1 large onion)

3 garlic cloves, minced

2 cups (480 ml) reduced-sodium chicken broth

2 cups (280 g) cubed peeled, seeded acorn or butternut squash

6 dried apricot halves, chopped

½ cup (70 g) pitted kalamata olives, halved

½ cup (75 g) roasted, unsalted peanuts

Grated zest and juice of 1 lemon

3 cups (470 g) Simply Steamed Couscous (page 205), warmed

Freshly ground black pepper

1. Whisk together 1 tablespoon of the oil, the cumin, ginger, paprika, turmeric, and allspice in a large bowl. Add the turkey and stir to coat. Marinate for 20 minutes at room temperature, stirring after 10 minutes.

2. Heat the remaining 1 tablespoon oil in a Dutch oven or large skillet over medium heat for 1 minute. When the oil is hot, add the onion and garlic. Cook, stirring occasionally, until the onion is translucent and the garlic is fragrant, 3 to 4 minutes. Stir in the turkey and marinade. Cook until the turkey is white and opaque and the spices are aromatic, about 3 minutes.

3. Add the stock, squash, and apricots and bring to a boil. Cover, reduce the heat to medium-low, and simmer until the squash is tender, the liquid has reduced, and the mixture is thickened, 10 to 15 minutes. Remove from the heat when a digital food thermometer reads 165°F (75°C) when inserted in the center of a few turkey pieces.

4. Fold in the olives, peanuts, and lemon zest. Divide the couscous among four shallow bowls and top with the turkey mixture. Sprinkle with the lemon juice and black pepper to taste and serve hot.

Per Serving: Calories 536; Protein 37 g; Carbs 41 g; Dietary Fiber 7 g; Added Sugars 1 g; Total Fat 25 g; Sat Fat 3 g; Omega-3s 90 mg; Sodium 630 mg; Potassium 548 mg

TURKEY TENDERLOINS WITH SPINACH PESTO & PISTACHIOS

Makes 4 servings

In place of the traditional Florentine filling of fresh spinach, we use our easy-to-apply Spinach Pesto to stuff these turkey tenderloins. Serve with orzo and our Mixed Greens & Mushroom Salad (page 153).

4 turkey tenderloins (about 1 pound/454 g total)

½ cup (130 g) Spinach Pesto (page 46)

1 large egg white

1 tablespoon water

1 cup (220 g) Garlic & Herb Bread Crumbs (page 33)

½ cup (60 g) finely chopped pistachios or pine nuts

¼ cup (15 g) finely chopped fresh parsley

2 teaspoons Italian Seasoning (page 34)

4 teaspoons extra virgin olive oil

Freshly ground black pepper

1. Preheat the oven to 350°F (180°C). Line a rimmed baking sheet with parchment paper.

2. One at a time, place the tenderloins in between two sheets of plastic wrap or wax paper. Use a meat mallet to gently pound and flatten each tenderloin so they are equal in thickness.

3. Spread 2 tablespoons of the pesto down the center of each tenderloin. Roll the tenderloins and secure the seam with a toothpick.

4. Whisk the egg white until frothy in a shallow bowl or pie plate. Add the water and whisk to combine. Combine the bread crumbs, pistachios, parsley, and seasoning in a separate shallow bowl or pie plate.

5. Dip each tenderloin first in the egg white mixture, then roll it in the bread crumb mixture and press the crumbs into the tenderloin. Place seam side down on the baking sheet. Repeat with the remaining tenderloins. Drizzle each with 1 teaspoon of oil.

6. Bake for 35 to 40 minutes, until the tenderloins are brown and crispy on the outside and a digital food thermometer reads 165°F (75°C) Serve hot.

Per Serving: Calories 511; Protein 40 g; Carbs 27 g; Dietary Fiber 5 g; Added Sugars 0 g; Total Fat 28 g; Sat Fat 4 g; Omega-3s 160 mg; Sodium 476 mg; Potassium 267 mg

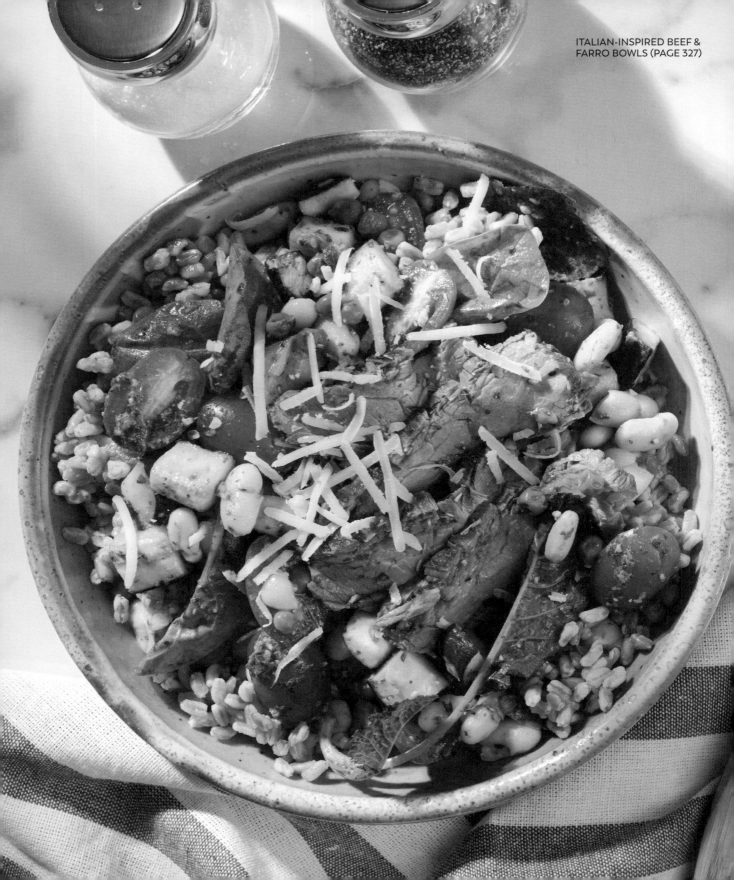

ITALIAN-INSPIRED BEEF &
FARRO BOWLS (PAGE 327)

CHAPTER 18

Beef, Pork & Lamb

Beef, Pork & Lamb

Food Safety & Quality Guidelines for
Cooking Beef, Veal, Lamb & Pork 323

Beef

Beef & Vegetable Kabobs 324

Beef & Vegetable Stir-Fry 324

Classic Beef Stroganoff............... 325

Easy Weeknight Ground
Beef Stroganoff..................... 325

French-Style Beef Stew 326

Greek-Flavor Beef & Barley Bowls 326

Italian-Inspired Beef & Farro Bowls 327

Quebec City Shepherd's Pie
(Pâté Chinois) 328

Sheet Pan Tri-Tip Roast.............. 328

Smoked Tri-Tip..................... 329

Spanish-Style Beef & Brown
Rice Bowls......................... 330

Swedish Meatballs 330

Pork

Pork Chops with Caraway Rice 331

Pork Chops with Pesto 331

Pork Fried Rice..................... 332

Simply Cooked Pork Tenderloin 332

Smoky Workaday Pork Tenderloin 333

Tuscan-Inspired Pork 333

Lamb

Lamb Chops with Cilantro-Mint
Pesto 333

Lamb & Rice-Stuffed Bell Peppers 334

South African Lamb Pie (Bobotie) 335

Many people who love red meat often express guilt or doubt about how much or how often they can eat it while still promoting heart health. We discussed the role of red meat in healthful diets in chapter 1 and how to choose lean cuts of red meat in chapter 2.

As we developed our red meat recipes, we focused not only on using lean cuts but also on portion sizes. You'll notice that most of these recipes feature 3 ounces (85 g) or less per serving and that we emphasize serving beef, pork, and lamb dishes with other health-promoting foods like whole grains, legumes, and vegetables.

Our red meat recipes are inspired by food cultures around the globe—from Asia and the Mediterranean to Latin America and Africa, as well as regional cuisines of the United States.

Finally, our recipes also feature a variety of cooking techniques, including sautéing, braising, baking, and grilling. If you've realized you may be in a rut in terms of the types of protein you're eating and how you're cooking them, we encourage you to try these recipes. Variety, after all, is the spice of life!

Food Safety & Quality Guidelines for Cooking Beef, Veal, Lamb & Pork

Beef, Veal & Lamb Steaks & Chops

From a food safety perspective, beef, veal, and lamb steaks and chops are safe to eat when cooked to at least 145°F (65°C). Larger cuts of meat will increase in temperature up to 5°F (2.8°C) after being removed from the heat source; this is called carryover cooking. The best way to determine degree of doneness is to use a digital food thermometer. For the most accurate reading, insert the thermometer horizontally into the side of the steak or chop in the thickest section, being careful not to hit fat or bone.

Cooking to medium-rare produces a tender, juicy steak; cooking much beyond this can compromise tenderness, especially for lean cuts of beef. Allowing steaks and chops to rest for 3 minutes prior to cutting and eating helps maintain juiciness. Marinating lean cuts of meat can help improve juiciness, especially if your desired degree of doneness is greater than medium-rare.

Table 11: Beef, Veal & Lamb Steaks & Chops Doneness

Rare	135°F (55°C)	Cool red center
Medium-rare	145°F (65°C)	Warm red center
Medium	160°F (70°C)	Warm pink center
Medium-well	165°F (75°C)	Slightly pink center
Well	170°F (77°C)	No pink

Beef Roasts

A roast or other whole-muscle cut of beef is safe to eat when cooked to an internal temperature of at least 145°F (65°C). To maintain juiciness, allow the roast to rest for at least 3 minutes prior to cutting or carving.

Pork Chops, Tenderloin & Roasts

Whole cuts of pork can be safely consumed at 145°F (65°C). Allow to rest for at least 3 minutes prior to cutting or carving.

Ground Beef, Lamb & Pork

To ensure food safety, ground beef, lamb, and pork must be cooked to at least 160°F (70°C).

BEEF & VEGETABLE KABOBS

Makes 6 servings

Kabobs are a traditional way of presenting and serving meat in many countries where charcoal or hard wood is a common fuel source. Yes, you can use a gas grill to make these; you'll just get a slightly different flavor—less smoky but still delicious. There are endless ways to serve kabobs or skewers, but we love to pair them with whole wheat pita bread. Tzatziki (page 60) is a perfect sauce to pair with this recipe.

- 2 tablespoons fresh lemon juice
- 2 tablespoons extra virgin olive oil
- 1 teaspoon dried oregano
- 1 bay leaf
- Freshly ground black pepper
- 1.5 pounds (680 g) round steak or sirloin tip, trimmed and cut into 1.5-inch (4 cm) cubes
- 12 large white or cremini mushrooms
- 2 tomatoes, quartered, or 8 cherry tomatoes
- 1 red bell pepper, seeded and cut into 1.5-inch (4 cm) squares
- 1 green bell pepper, seeded and cut into 1.5-inch (4 cm) squares
- 1 red onion, cut into eighths

1. Combine the lemon juice, oil, oregano, bay leaf, and pepper in a medium bowl. Stir in the beef, cover, and marinate in the refrigerator, stirring occasionally, for at least 3 hours.

2. If you're using bamboo skewers, soak them in warm water for 30 minutes. Heat a charcoal grill to medium-hot for direct cooking. Lightly oil the grill grate.

3. Thread the beef cubes onto skewers, alternating with the mushrooms, tomatoes, peppers, and onions. Grill the kabobs, turning once per side, for 3 minutes per side for medium-rare (to 145°F/65°C) or until the meat reaches your desired doneness (see Table 11, page 323). Serve warm.

Per Serving: Calories 212; Protein 28 g; Carbs 7 g; Dietary Fiber 2 g; Added Sugars 0 g; Total Fat 8 g; Sat Fat 2 g; Omega-3s 50 mg; Sodium 67 mg; Potassium 678 mg

BEEF & VEGETABLE STIR-FRY

Makes 6 servings

Stir-frying is a quick and easy way to get dinner on the table. Be sure to do all your prep ahead of time; once you start cooking, you'll need to constantly stir the ingredients as you add them so they cook evenly. Serve with rice, or over lo mein (wheat) or soba (buckwheat) noodles.

- ¼ cup (60 ml) reduced-sodium soy sauce
- 1 tablespoon cornstarch
- 1 pound (454 g) beef sirloin tip, cut into ¼-inch-thick (6 mm) slices (see Tip)
- Water
- 2 tablespoons peanut oil
- 2 green onions, thinly sliced
- 1 tablespoon grated or finely minced fresh ginger
- 2 garlic cloves, minced
- 1 cup (70 g) small fresh broccoli florets or chopped bok choy
- 1 carrot or celery stalk, sliced
- 1 green or red bell pepper, seeded and diced
- 4 ounces (113 g) snow peas or cremini mushrooms, sliced

1. Mix the soy sauce and cornstarch in a medium bowl. Add the meat and toss to coat it thoroughly. Marinate for 30 minutes.

2. Drain the marinade into a liquid measuring cup and add enough water to make 1 cup (240 ml). Leave the beef in the bowl.

3. Heat a wok or large skillet over high heat for 30 seconds. Swirl in 1 tablespoon of the oil and heat for 30 seconds. Add the green onions, ginger, and garlic, and stir-fry until the garlic is fragrant, 30 seconds. Add the beef and stir-fry until it begins to brown, 2 minutes.

4. Transfer the meat from the wok to a clean bowl. Pour the remaining 1 tablespoon of oil into the wok, swirl to distribute it evenly, and heat for 30 seconds. Add the broccoli, carrot, and pepper, and stir-fry until the vegetables begin to soften and brighten in color, 2 minutes.

5. Add the snow peas. Return the beef to the wok, along with any juices. Stir-fry until the beef is browned and the vegetables are crisp-tender, 2 to 3 minutes.

6. Push the vegetables and beef to the side of the wok. Pour the marinade mixture into the center and stir for 1 to 2 minutes, until thickened. Stir in the beef and vegetables, cook for 15 seconds, and serve.

NOTE: *Raw beef is easier to slice thin if placed in the freezer for 30 minutes prior to slicing.*

Per Serving: Calories 192; Protein 18 g; Carbs 7 g; Dietary Fiber 2 g; Added Sugars 0 g; Total Fat 10 g; Sat Fat 2 g; Omega-3s 40 mg; Sodium 443 mg; Potassium 415 mg

CLASSIC BEEF STROGANOFF

Makes 4 servings

Food historians trace this dish's origin to nineteenth-century Russia. Some recipes call for beef cubes, but we recommend thinly slicing the beef to make the cooking process quicker. Serve over egg noodles and pair with a green salad or your favorite green vegetable.

- 3 tablespoons all-purpose flour
- 1½ teaspoons paprika
- 1 pound (454 g) top sirloin steak, thinly sliced (see Note, page 325)
- 1 tablespoon peanut or canola oil
- 8 ounces (113 g) white mushrooms, sliced
- 1 white or yellow onion, diced
- 2 garlic cloves, minced
- ½ teaspoon freshly ground black pepper
- ½ cup (120 ml) dry white wine (such as Chenin Blanc, Pinot Gris, or Pinot Grigio)
- ¾ cup (170 g) plain Greek yogurt or light sour cream
- 1 teaspoon sodium-free beef bouillon granules (such as HerbOx)
- ½ cup (30 g) chopped fresh parsley or dill, optional

1. Combine the flour and paprika in a medium bowl. Add the steak and toss to coat.

2. Heat the oil in a large skillet or Dutch oven over high heat. Add the steak, mushrooms, onion, garlic, and pepper, and cook until the steak is no longer pink, 7 to 8 minutes.

3. Stir in the wine, yogurt, and bouillon. Bring to a boil for 1 minute, stirring constantly. Reduce the heat to low, cover, and simmer until the sauce thickens, 12 to 15 minutes. Serve.

Per Serving: Calories 143; Protein 5 g; Carbs 14 g; Dietary Fiber 1 g; Added Sugars 0 g; Total Fat 8 g; Sat Fat 3 g; Omega-3s 10 mg; Sodium 128 mg; Potassium 288 mg

EASY WEEKNIGHT GROUND BEEF STROGANOFF

Makes 8 servings

Stroganoff is one of those creamy, comforting foods that can soothe the soul after a long workday. This version comes together easily. Buy presliced mushrooms to save a step. Serve hot over egg noodles with a green vegetable.

- 2 pounds (907 g) 93% lean ground beef
- 2 white onions, chopped
- 8 ounces (227 g) white mushrooms, sliced
- 2 garlic cloves, minced
- ¼ cup (30 g) all-purpose flour
- 1½ cups (345 g) plain Greek yogurt
- 1 cup (240 ml) water
- 3 tablespoons tomato paste
- 2 teaspoons sodium-free granulated beef bouillon (such as Herb-Ox)
- ¼ teaspoon kosher salt
- ¼ teaspoon freshly ground black pepper

1. Brown the beef in a large skillet or Dutch oven over medium-high heat for 10 minutes, stirring occasionally to break up large chunks.

2. Add the onions, mushrooms, and garlic. Cook, stirring occasionally, until the onions are soft, 10 minutes.

3. Add the flour and stir well, scraping to remove any bits stuck to the pan. Stir in the yogurt, water, tomato paste, bouillon, salt, and pepper. Cover and simmer over low heat until thickened, hot, and bubbling, 25 to 30 minutes. The stroganoff is ready when a digital food thermometer reads 165°F (75°C).

Per Serving: Calories 239; Protein 29 g; Carbs 9 g; Dietary Fiber 1 g; Added Sugars 0 g; Total Fat 9 g; Sat Fat 4 g; Omega-3s 50 mg; Sodium 218 mg; Potassium 635 mg

FRENCH-STYLE BEEF STEW

Makes 6 servings

French home cooks have long appreciated the flavor and texture benefits of slowly braising lean or tough cuts of beef in red wine with abundant vegetables. This is an exceptionally comforting dish to have slowly simmering on the stovetop on cold winter days. Serve with rustic whole grain bread.

1 tablespoon extra virgin olive oil

1 pound (454 g) top round steak or London broil, trimmed and cut into 2-inch (5 cm) cubes

1 tablespoon all-purpose flour

4 cups (1 L) Beef Stock (page 69)

One 15-ounce (425 g) can no-salt-added diced tomatoes

8 ounces (113 g) white or cremini mushrooms, sliced

1 yellow onion, diced

3 carrots, sliced

1 green bell pepper, seeded and cut into 1-inch (2.5 cm) squares

1 cup (240 ml) red wine (such as Cabernet Sauvignon)

3 garlic cloves, minced

½ teaspoon freshly ground black pepper

1 teaspoon dried thyme

1 pound (454 g) small red-skin potatoes, halved

1. Heat the oil in a Dutch oven over high heat. Add the beef and sprinkle with the flour. Cook, stirring often, to sear the beef on all sides, 5 to 6 minutes.

2. Reduce the heat to low. Stir in the stock, tomatoes, mushrooms, onion, carrots, bell pepper, wine, garlic, pepper, and thyme. Simmer until the beef is very tender, 2 to 3 hours, stirring occasionally.

3. About 30 minutes prior to serving, add the potatoes. Cover and cook until you can easily pierce the largest potato half with a paring knife. Serve warm. Store covered in the refrigerator for up to 3 days or in the freezer for up to 2 months.

Per Serving: Calories 277; Protein 24 g; Carbs 27 g; Dietary Fiber 4 g; Added Sugars 0 g; Total Fat 5 g; Sat Fat 1 g; Omega-3s 30 mg; Sodium 389 mg; Potassium 1,198 mg

GREEK-FLAVOR BEEF & BARLEY BOWLS

Makes 4 servings

This is the perfect meal for a warm summer day. Tzatziki, a classic Greek cucumber and yogurt sauce, adds an appealing fragrance and flavor. You can also top the bowls with skordalia, a thick sauce made with potatoes, bread, nuts, aromatics, and oil. Tzatziki is better in warm weather, while skordalia is perfect for cooler temperatures. You can prepare everything you need for these delicious bowls a day or two in advance—including marinating and cooking the beef—and put together a quick and easy meal in minutes.

Marinated Beef

1 pound (454 g) flank steak, sliced across the grain into ¼ × 3-inch (6 mm × 7.5 cm) strips

1½ tablespoons extra virgin olive oil

Grated zest and juice of 1 lemon

3 garlic cloves, minced

1 teaspoon minced fresh oregano or ½ teaspoon dried oregano

¼ teaspoon kosher salt

¼ teaspoon freshly ground black pepper

Bowls

3 cups (470 g) Simply Cooked Barley (page 223)

1 English cucumber, ends trimmed, halved lengthwise, thinly sliced

One 15-ounce (425 g) can Great Northern or navy beans, drained and rinsed

1 cup (160 g) frozen lima beans, microwaved for 3 minutes

1 cup (150 g) grape tomatoes, halved

2 cups (425 g) Tzatziki (page 60) or Skordalia (page 59)

½ cup (70 g) pitted kalamata olives, chopped

¼ cup (40 g) minced red onion

2 ounces (57 g) feta, crumbled

1. Combine the steak, oil, lemon zest and juice, garlic, oregano, salt, and pepper in a medium bowl. Stir to coat, cover, and place in the refrigerator to marinate for 4 to 24 hours. Stir occasionally.

2. Place a large sauté pan or skillet over high heat. When it's hot, add the beef and cook for 4 to 5 minutes.

Stir minimally to get a good sear. Use a digital food thermometer to ensure the beef has reached a minimum temperature of 145°F (65°C). Remove from the heat and set aside.

3. To make the bowls, divide the barley among four shallow bowls. Add the cucumber slices, navy beans, lima beans, and tomatoes, followed by the beef. Top each bowl with ½ cup (105 g) tzatziki. Garnish with olives, onions, and feta.

NOTE: Draining and rinsing canned beans can remove up to 35 percent of the sodium added during the canning process.

Serving Size 1 bowl; Calories 685; Protein 49 g; Carbs 79 g; Dietary Fiber 14 g; Added Sugars 0 g; Total Fat 20 g; Sat Fat 7 g; Omega-3s 235 mg; Sodium 950; Potassium 1,440 mg

ITALIAN-INSPIRED BEEF & FARRO BOWLS

Makes 4 servings

With a little advance prep, you can enjoy these Italian-flavored whole grain and lean beef bowls—packed with vegetables in the Mediterranean tradition—in a matter of minutes. Just prepare all ingredients ahead of time. Want to save even more time? Buy quick-cooking farro and a prepared pesto.

Marinated Beef

1 pound (454 g) flank steak, sliced across the grain into ¼ × 3-inch (6 mm × 7.5 cm) strips

1½ tablespoons extra virgin olive oil

1½ tablespoons red wine vinegar

1 tablespoon fresh rosemary leaves, minced or 1 teaspoon ground dried rosemary

3 garlic cloves, minced

¼ teaspoon kosher salt

¼ teaspoon freshly ground black pepper

Roasted Zucchini

2 zucchini, trimmed and diced

1 tablespoon extra virgin olive oil

½ teaspoon Italian Seasoning (page 34)

¼ teaspoon kosher salt

Bowls

One 15-ounce (425 g) can white kidney or cannellini beans, drained and rinsed

2 cups (60 g) fresh baby spinach leaves

1 cup (135 g) frozen green peas, microwaved on HIGH for 2 minutes

1 cup (150 g) grape tomatoes, halved

½ cup (125 g) Basil Pesto (page 45)

2½ cups (425 g) Simply Cooked Farro (page 226)

¼ cup (20 g) shredded Parmesan

1. Combine the steak, oil, vinegar, rosemary, salt, and pepper in a medium bowl. Stir, cover, and place in the refrigerator to marinate for 4 to 24 hours. Stir occasionally.

2. Preheat the oven to 375°F (190°C). Line a baking sheet with parchment paper.

3. Place the zucchini in a small bowl and toss with the oil, seasoning, and salt. Spread evenly on the baking sheet. Roast for 15 minutes, until golden brown, then transfer to a large bowl.

4. While the zucchini is roasting, place a large sauté pan or skillet over high heat. When it's hot, add the beef and marinade and cook for 4 to 5 minutes total. Stir minimally to get a good sear. Use a digital food thermometer to ensure the beef has reached a minimum temperature of 145°F (65°C). Transfer to a plate.

5. Transfer to a large bowl and let cool to room temperature. (If preparing in advance, store in a covered container in the refrigerator.)

6. Add the beans, spinach, peas, tomatoes, and pesto to the zucchini and stir to coat. Divide the farro among four bowls. Top with the beef, vegetables, and Parmesan.

Serving Size 1 bowl; Calories 780; Protein 45 g; Carbs 69 g; Dietary Fiber 15 g; Added Sugars 0 g; Total Fat 36 g; Sat Fat 9 g; Omega-3s 645 mg; Sodium 910 mg; Potassium 1,325 mg

QUEBEC CITY SHEPHERD'S PIE (PÂTÉ CHINOIS)

Makes 6 servings

Amy loves watching Andrew Zimmern's Delicious Destinations. *She was inspired to create this recipe after watching an episode filmed in Quebec City that featured Pâté Chinois, an iconic home-cooked comfort food classic. The dish was developed by Chinese immigrants living in Quebec in the 1880s, who were likely adapting recipes for British shepherd's pie.*

- 1.5 pounds (680 g) 93% lean ground beef
- 1 white or yellow onion, diced
- ½ teaspoon kosher salt
- 1 teaspoon freshly ground black pepper
- 2 cups (330 g) frozen corn kernels
- ¼ cup (60 ml) milk
- 4 cups (915 g) mashed potatoes (see Tip)
- 1 cup (115 g) shredded part-skim mozzarella

1. Preheat the oven to 350°F (180°C).

2. Brown the beef in a large skillet over medium heat for 10 minutes, stirring occasionally to break up large chunks.

3. While the beef is cooking, heat the corn in the microwave for 3 minutes.

4. When the beef is nearly fully cooked and only a little pink remains, stir in the onions, salt, and pepper. Reduce the heat to low, cover, and cook until the onions are soft, 10 to 12 minutes.

5. Spread the beef-onion mixture in an 8-inch (20 cm) or 9-inch (23 cm) square baking dish. Cover with half of the corn (about 1 cup/115 g).

6. Combine the rest of the corn and the milk in a blender or food processor and process until smooth. Pour over the top of the corn.

7. Combine the mashed potatoes and mozzarella in a medium bowl and spoon on top of the casserole. Use a spatula or large spoon to smooth out the potatoes.

8. Bake for 45 minutes or until the top is golden brown and a digital food thermometer reads 165°F (75°C) when inserted into the center of the pie. Serve warm.

TIP: *You can save some time and effort by using instant mashed potatoes, which are dehydrated cooked potatoes. We recommend a plain version (like Idahoan Original) that doesn't include any added flavorings or sodium.*

Per Serving: Calories 455; Protein 34 g; Carbs 36 g; Dietary Fiber 5 g; Added Sugars 0 g; Total Fat 20 g; Sat Fat 10 g; Omega-3s 200 mg; Sodium 742 mg; Potassium 1,035 mg

SHEET PAN TRI-TIP ROAST

Makes 12 servings

A tri-tip beef roast comes from the bottom sirloin cut and is lean, tender, and rich in juicy, beefy flavor. It can be roasted slowly in a low-heat oven, roasted very quickly at a high temperature with vegetables, or smoked (try our Smoked Tri-Tip on page 329). Serve the roasted vegetables and beef with Persian Fresh Herb Mix (page 35) on the side. Adding a fresh, green salad—and perhaps a glass of Zinfandel or Syrah—completes this meal.

- 4 tablespoons (15 g) Herb Blend for Beef (page 34)
- 1 tablespoon extra virgin olive oil
- 1 teaspoon freshly ground black pepper
- 4 medium Yukon gold–type potatoes, quartered, or 8 small red-skin potatoes, halved
- 2 white onions, cut into thin wedges
- 3 garlic cloves, minced
- One 3-pound (1.4 kg) tri-tip or bottom sirloin beef roast

1. Preheat the oven to 425°F (220°C). Line a large rimmed baking sheet with foil.

2. Combine 2 tablespoons of the herb blend, the oil, and ½ teaspoon of the pepper in a large bowl. Add the potatoes and onions and toss to coat. Spread in a single layer on the prepared baking sheet. Roast for 15 minutes.

3. Combine the remaining 2 tablespoons herb rub, the garlic, and the remaining ½ teaspoon pepper in a small bowl. Rub and press the mixture into the roast on all sides.

4. Remove the baking sheet from the oven, stir the vegetables, and move them to the outer edges. Place a roasting rack in the middle of the pan, place the roast on the rack, and return the baking sheet to the oven. Roast for about 30 to 35 minutes, then start checking the roast's temperature with a digital food thermometer.

5. Remove the roast when the thermometer reads 140°F (60°C) for medium-rare (the roast will have a warm red center) or 155°F (70°C) for medium (a warm pink center). Carryover cooking will increase the final temperature by 5°F (2.8°C). Transfer the roast to a cutting board, tent with foil, and let rest for 5 to 10 minutes. If the potatoes and onions are not fork-tender, return them to the oven for 10 minutes.

6. Thinly slice the roast against the grain and serve. Store covered in the refrigerator for up to 3 days.

TIP: *We're very fond of cooking enough beef to use for future meals. This supports smaller serving sizes of red meat, saves time in the kitchen, and stretches food budgets. Set aside enough sliced roast beef to make a sandwich the next day and Classic Beef Stroganoff (page 325) perhaps on the weekend.*

Per Serving: Calories 234; Protein 32 g; Carbs 2 g; Dietary Fiber 1 g; Added Sugars 0 g; Total Fat 11 g; Sat Fat 4 g; Omega-3s 50 mg; Sodium 67 mg; Potassium 440 mg

1. Combine the garlic powder, paprika, pepper, rosemary, cayenne, onion powder, and salt in a small bowl. Place the roast in a baking pan. Generously rub with the dry rub. Cover with plastic wrap and refrigerate for 4 to 12 hours.

2. Heat a pellet smoker to 225°F (105°C).

3. Smoke the roast with the cover closed for 2 hours, or until a digital food thermometer reads 140°F (60°C) when inserted into the thickest part of the roast.

4. Transfer the roast to a cutting board, tent with foil, and allow to rest for 10 to 15 minutes. The residual cooking heat will increase the temperature to 145ºF (65°C) and allow the juices to redistribute, resulting in tender medium-rare tri-tip. Store covered in the refrigerator for up to 3 days.

TIP: *Use leftovers to create flavorful barbecue sandwiches or "loaded" baked potatoes. Chop the meat into small cubes and heat with Homestyle Barbecue Sauce (page 55) or Rhubarbecue Sauce (page 58).*

Per Serving: Calories 217; Protein 31 g; Carbs 1 g; Dietary Fiber 0 g; Added Sugars 0 g; Total Fat 10 g; Sat Fat 4 g; Omega-3s 30 mg; Sodium 143 mg; Potassium 422 mg

SMOKED TRI-TIP

Makes 12 servings

This recipe was created for pellet smokers that can be set at specific temperatures. The dry rub releases the most amazing rosemary aroma when the meat is smoked. The cayenne adds a bit of heat, which we love, but if you prefer less spice, cut back to ½ teaspoon or omit it all together. Serve with corn on the cob or Simply Smashed Potatoes (page 260), a favorite vegetable salad, and fresh fruit for dessert.

- 2 teaspoons garlic powder
- 2 teaspoons smoked paprika
- 2 teaspoons freshly ground black pepper
- 2 teaspoons finely minced fresh rosemary
- 1 teaspoon cayenne
- 1 teaspoon onion powder
- 1 teaspoon kosher salt
- One 3-pound (1.4 kg) tri-tip beef roast

SODIUM TIP: Using Diamond Crystal Kosher Salt will dramatically reduce the sodium in any recipe that uses kosher salt. This salt contains 50% less sodium per measure than regular kosher salt and 60% less than fine grain table salt.

SPANISH-STYLE BEEF & BROWN RICE BOWLS

Makes 4 servings

A popular saying in the foodservice industry is "sauce is boss," which refers to the power of a great sauce to make us fall in love with food. In Spain, a boss sauce is Romesco. Romesco gets its alluring smoky flavor from roasted tomatoes and red bell peppers as well as smoked paprika. It's so delicious with beef!

Marinated Beef

1 pound (454 g) flank steak, sliced across the grain into ¼ × 3-inch (6 mm × 7.5 cm) strips

1½ tablespoons extra virgin olive oil

1½ tablespoons red wine vinegar

1 teaspoon Spanish smoked paprika

¼ teaspoon kosher salt

¼ teaspoon freshly ground black pepper

Bowls

3 cups (585 g) Simply Cooked Brown Rice (page 230)

One 15-ounce (425 g) can dark red kidney beans, drained and rinsed

One 15-ounce (425 g) can chickpeas, drained and rinsed

1 cup (175 g) fresh baby spinach leaves

1 cup (150 g) grape tomatoes, halved

1 cup (175 g) Romesco Sauce (page 58)

4 ounces (113 g) Manchego, grated

1. Combine the steak, oil, vinegar, paprika, salt, and pepper in a medium bowl. Stir, cover, and place in the refrigerator to marinate for 4 to 24 hours. Stir occasionally.

2. Place a large sauté pan or skillet over high heat. When it's hot, add the beef and marinade and cook for 4 to 5 minutes total. Stir minimally to get a good sear. Use a digital food thermometer to ensure the beef has reached a minimum temperature of 145°F (65°C). Remove from the heat.

3. Divide the rice among four bowls. Add the kidney beans, chickpeas, spinach, and tomatoes. Top with the beef, then the Romesco. Garnish with Manchego.

Serving Size 1 bowl; Calories 785; Protein 49 g; Carbs 72 g; Dietary Fiber 16 g; Added Sugars 0 g; Total Fat 33 g; Sat Fat 13 g; Omega-3s 154 mg; Sodium 830 mg; Potassium 1,225 mg

SWEDISH MEATBALLS

Makes 10 servings

Meatballs with mashed potatoes and gravy is the ultimate comfort food. The secret to making Swedish meatballs is using high-quality meat and finely minced onion, thoroughly mixing the ingredients, and using a light hand to form the meatballs. Serve with Simply Spanish-Style Mashed Potatoes (page 259).

1 white or yellow onion, minced

1 tablespoon water

1.5 pounds (680 g) 93% lean ground beef

8 ounces (227 g) lean ground pork

2 cups (180 g) whole wheat bread crumbs

½ teaspoon ground cloves

½ teaspoon kosher salt

¼ teaspoon ground allspice

3 tablespoons all-purpose flour

2 cups (480 ml) milk

1½ tablespoons sodium-free granulated beef bouillon (such as Herb-Ox)

1. Preheat the oven to 350°F (180°C).

2. Simmer the onions and water in a covered saucepan over medium high until the onions are soft, 10 minutes. Transfer to a large bowl and allow to cool for 10 minutes.

3. Add the beef, pork, bread crumbs, cloves, salt, and allspice to the onion and mix thoroughly but gently. Form into 30 medium balls about 1 inch (2.5 cm) in diameter.

4. Brown the meatballs in a nonstick skillet over medium-high heat, then transfer to a baking dish. Whisk the flour into the pan drippings in the skillet. Cook over medium heat for 1 minute, then whisk in the milk and bouillon until smooth. Reduce the heat to low and cook until thickened, 10 minutes.

5. Pour the gravy over the meatballs. Bake for 45 minutes or until a digital food thermometer reads 160°F (70°C) when inserted in the center of a few meatballs. Serve immediately. Store leftovers covered in the refrigerator for up to 2 days or in the freezer for up to 2 months.

Per Serving: Calories 285; Protein 24 g; Carbs 19 g; Dietary Fiber 2 g; Added Sugars 0 g; Total Fat 13 g; Sat Fat 5 g; Omega-3s 30 mg; Sodium 335 mg; Potassium 415 mg

PORK CHOPS WITH CARAWAY RICE

Makes 4 servings

Pork and caraway is a classic flavor pairing. Serve this dish with your favorite green vegetable, sauerkraut, or our Spinach Salad with Honeycrisp Apples & Cheddar (page 148).

1 tablespoon extra virgin olive oil

2 celery stalks, diced

1 white or yellow onion, diced

2½ cups (600 ml) water

1¼ cups (230 g) uncooked long-grain brown rice

2 teaspoons caraway seeds

¼ teaspoon kosher salt

Four 6-ounce (170 g) bone-in pork loin chops, trimmed

1. Preheat the oven to 350°F (180°C).

2. Heat the oil in a saucepan or skillet over medium-high heat. Sauté the celery and onion, stirring frequently, until softened, 5 minutes. Stir in the water, rice, caraway seeds, and salt. Bring to a boil, reduce the heat to low, and cover. Simmer until the liquid is absorbed, 35 to 40 minutes. Fluff the rice with a fork, then cover and set aside until ready to serve.

3. While the rice cooks, place an oven-safe skillet over medium-high heat and sear the pork chops on each side for 2 minutes.

4. Transfer the skillet to the oven and roast for 10 to 12 minutes, until a digital food thermometer reads 145°F (65°F) when inserted in the thickest chop (not touching bone).

5. Divide the rice and pork chops among four plates or shallow bowls and serve.

Per Serving: Calories 200; Protein 13 g; Carbs 18 g; Dietary Fiber 2 g; Added Sugars 0 g; Total Fat 8 g; Sat Fat 2 g; Omega-3s 50 mg; Sodium 107 mg; Potassium 230 mg

PORK CHOPS WITH PESTO

Makes 4 servings

This is an exceptionally easy weeknight dinner recipe, especially if you've made the pesto ahead of time. The key to keeping lean pork moist and juicy is to use the restaurant chef's trick of searing the meat on the stovetop and then finishing the cooking in the oven. Serve with Simply Roasted Root Vegetables with Apples (page 261).

Four 4-ounce (113 g) boneless center-cut pork loin chops

2 teaspoons extra virgin olive oil

½ cup (125 g) Basil Pesto (page 45)

1. Preheat the oven to 350°F (180°C).

2. Heat an oven-safe skillet over medium-high heat for 1 minute. Add the oil. When the oil is shimmering, add the pork chops. Sear on each side for 2 minutes.

3. Transfer the skillet to the oven and roast for 10 to 12 minutes, until a digital food thermometer reads 145°F (65°F) when inserted into the center of the thickest chop. Serve with pesto on the side.

Per Serving: Calories 197; Protein 8 g; Carbs 2 g; Dietary Fiber 1 g; Added Sugars 0 g; Total Fat 18 g; Sat Fat 4 g; Omega-3s 460 mg; Sodium 200 mg; Potassium 190 mg

PORK FRIED RICE

Makes 4 servings

This fried rice comes together very easily with Simply Cooked Brown Rice and thinly sliced or cubed cooked pork from the Simply Cooked Pork Tenderloin. Add whatever fresh vegetables you have on hand and peas from the freezer, and dinner is on the table in under 30 minutes. Serve with Plum Sauce (page 57).

2 tablespoons plus 1 teaspoon peanut oil

2 large eggs

2 cups (140 g) finely chopped napa cabbage, bok choy, or Chinese white cabbage

2 carrots, diced

4 ounces (113 g) white or cremini mushrooms, chopped

3 garlic cloves, minced

2 tablespoons red wine vinegar

8 ounces (227 g) diced Simply Cooked Pork Tenderloin (page 332)

3 cups (585 g) Simply Cooked Brown Rice (page 230)

2 teaspoons Chinese Five-Spice Blend (page 31)

1 cup (145 g) petite or baby peas, thawed and drained if frozen

¼ cup (60 ml) Beef Stock (page 69) or Chicken Stock (page 70)

2 tablespoons reduced-sodium soy sauce or tamari

2 teaspoons finely chopped fresh ginger

2 green onions, thinly sliced

¼ cup (35 g) chopped roasted peanuts

1. Heat 1 teaspoon of the oil in a large nonstick sauté pan or wok over medium heat. Whisk the eggs in a small bowl until lightly blended. When the oil shimmers, add the eggs and stir into small, gently cooked soft curds, less than a minute. Transfer to a medium bowl.

2. Return the pan to the heat, add 1 tablespoon of the oil, and increase the heat to medium-high. Add the cabbage, carrots, mushrooms, and garlic. Stir-fry until the cabbage and carrots begin to soften and the mushrooms start to shrink, about 2 minutes. Add the vinegar and continue to stir-fry until the vegetables are crisp-tender and the liquid has evaporated, 1 to

2 minutes. Transfer the vegetables to the bowl with the eggs.

3. Return the pan to the heat, add the remaining 1 tablespoon oil, and reduce the heat to medium-low. Add the pork, rice, and five-spice blend. Use a spatula to stir and break up the rice, about 1 minute. Add the peas and stock and continue to stir for 1 minute. Add the soy sauce and ginger and stir fry for 1 minute.

4. Return the vegetables and eggs to the pan. Stir-fry until heated through, 2 to 3 minutes. Transfer to a serving platter, sprinkle with green onions and peanuts, and serve.

Per Serving: Calories 430; Protein 26 g; Carbs 43 g; Dietary Fiber 7 g; Added Sugars 0 g; Total Fat 18 g; Sat Fat 4 g; Omega-3s 95 mg; Sodium 615 mg; Potassium 970 mg

SIMPLY COOKED PORK TENDERLOIN

Makes 4 servings

This tenderloin finishes cooking quickly in the oven, so you can have dinner on the table in no time—especially if you pair it with Simply Cooked Farro (page 226) from the fridge and your favorite microwave-in-the-bag veggies.

1 teaspoon salt-free seasoning blend (of choice; see Tip)

½ teaspoon kosher salt

½ teaspoon freshly ground black pepper

1 tablespoon extra virgin olive oil

One 1-pound (454 g) pork tenderloin, trimmed and patted dry

1. Preheat the oven to 375°F (190°C).

2. Combine the seasoning, salt, and pepper in a small bowl. Sprinkle over the pork on all sides.

3. Heat the oil in a large oven-safe skillet over medium-high heat for 1 minute. If the pork is longer than your skillet is wide, cut it in half.

4. Add the pork to the skillet and sear to develop a dark crust, 1 to 2 minutes. Repeat as needed to sear on all sides.

5. Transfer the skillet to the oven and roast for 23 to 35 minutes, until a digital food thermometer reads

145°F (65°C) when inserted in the thickest part of the tenderloin. Remove from the oven and let the rest for 2 to 3 minutes, then slice and serve. Store covered in the refrigerator for up to 3 days.

TIP: *Choose a seasoning that pairs well with other foods you'll be serving with the pork. For example, if you'll be pairing the pork with farro, our Italian Seasoning (page 34) would work well. Or if you are making a meal with Southwestern flavors, use our Southwest Seasoning (page 37).*

Per Serving: Calories 158; Protein 24 g; Carbs 1 g; Dietary Fiber 0 g; Added Sugars 0 g; Total Fat 6 g; Sat Fat 1 g; Omega-3s 40 mg; Sodium 177 mg; Potassium 469 mg

SMOKY WORKADAY PORK TENDERLOIN

Makes 4 servings

This is a simple, approachable dinner option for a busy weeknight. Serve with Simply Smashed Potatoes (page 260) or a baked sweet potato for a simple, satisfying meal.

One 1-pound (454 g) pork tenderloin

2 tablespoons Smoky Workaday Seasoning (page 37)

1 tablespoon whole grain mustard

1 tablespoon brown sugar or honey

1. Preheat the oven to 350°F (180°C). Place the pork on a rimmed baking sheet.

2. Combine the seasoning, mustard, and sugar in a small bowl. Use a knife to spread the mixture on the top and sides of the pork, as if you're frosting a cake.

3. Roast for 20 to 25 minutes, until a digital meat thermometer reads 145°F (65°C) when inserted in the thickest part of the tenderloin.

4. Remove from the oven, cover with foil, and allow the tenderloin to rest for 5 minutes before slicing. Slice into ½-inch-thick (13 mm) pieces and serve.

Per Serving: Calories 143; Protein 24 g; Carbs 4 g; Dietary Fiber 0 g; Added Sugars 3 g; Total Fat 3 g; Sat Fat 1 g; Omega-3s 10 mg; Sodium 122 mg; Potassium 480 mg

TUSCAN-INSPIRED PORK

Makes 4 servings

This recipe is a play on porchetta, the slowly roasted pork dish found throughout central Italy. This fast-cooking version, perfect for a busy weeknight dinner, can be served with our Simply Cooked Farro (page 226) or Farro with Roasted Grapes (page 226) and steamed broccoli or broccolini for a complete meal.

2 tablespoons extra virgin olive oil

4 garlic cloves, crushed

One 1-pound (454 g) pork tenderloin, cut into 1-inch (2.5 cm) cubes

1 tablespoon fennel seeds

1 tablespoon minced fresh rosemary

½ teaspoon kosher salt

½ teaspoon freshly ground black pepper

Heat the oil and garlic in a large sauté pan over medium-high heat. Sauté until the garlic starts to brown on the edges, 2 minutes. Add the pork and fennel seeds and sauté until the pork is light brown on all sides, 5 to 6 minutes. Reduce the heat to low. Add the rosemary, salt, and pepper, stir, and cook 1 to 2 minutes, until a digital food thermometer reads 145°F (65°C) when inserted in a few cubes of pork. Remove from the heat and serve.

Per Serving: Calories 198; Protein 24 g; Carbs 2 g; Dietary Fiber 1 g; Added Sugars 0 g; Total Fat 10 g; Sat Fat 2 g; Omega-3s 60 mg; Sodium 179 mg; Potassium 498 mg

LAMB CHOPS WITH CILANTRO-MINT PESTO

Makes 4 servings

This is a contemporary take on lamb with mint jelly. Serve with Simply Steamed Couscous (page 205), a simple mixed greens salad with Herbed Red Wine Vinaigrette (page 50) for a festive and healthy dinner that can be on the table in less than 30 minutes!

Four 4-ounce (113 g) lamb loin chops

¼ teaspoon kosher salt

¼ teaspoon freshly ground black pepper

¼ cup (50 g) Cilantro-Mint Pesto (page 46)

1. Sprinkle the lamb chops with the salt and pepper. Heat a sauté or grill pan over medium-high heat. Sear the lamb chops for 5 to 7 minutes on each side, until a digital meat thermometer reads 145°F (65°C) when inserted sideways into the center of the thickest chop (not touching bone).

2. Transfer the chops to serving plates and let rest for 3 minutes. Top each chop with a generous 1 tablespoon of pesto and serve.

Per Serving: Calories 156; Protein 8 g; Carbs 1 g; Dietary Fiber 0 g; Added Sugars 0 g; Total Fat 13 g; Sat Fat 3 g; Omega-3s 470 mg; Sodium 99 mg; Potassium 128 mg

LAMB & RICE–STUFFED BELL PEPPERS

Makes 4 servings

Stuffed peppers are a fun way to combine all the components of a complete meal into one dish. If you can't find ground lamb, feel free to use ground beef. Green bell peppers are usually the least expensive option, but yellow, red, and orange peppers are typically a bit sweeter and retain their vibrant color after baking. Using a variety of peppers creates a beautiful presentation.

Stuffed Peppers

1 pound (454 g) ground lamb

2 cups (390 g) Simply Cooked Brown Rice (page 230)

1 cup (180 g) diced fresh tomatoes

2 garlic cloves, minced

Juice of 1 lemon

1 teaspoon dried oregano

1 teaspoon kosher salt

¼ teaspoon freshly ground black pepper

4 bell peppers, stems removed, halved from top to bottom, seeded

2 ounces (57 g) feta, crumbled

Fresh Tomato Sauce

2 cups (360 g) diced fresh tomatoes (about 2 tomatoes)

¼ cup (60 ml) extra virgin olive oil

2 garlic cloves, minced

½ teaspoon dried oregano

½ teaspoon kosher salt

1. Preheat the oven to 350°F (180°C).

2. To make the peppers, combine the lamb, rice, tomatoes, garlic, lemon juice, oregano, salt, and black pepper in a bowl. Spoon ½ cup (130 g) of the filling into each pepper half. Place the pepper halves in a 9 × 13-inch (23 × 33 cm) baking dish.

3. Bake for 60 minutes. Top each pepper half with feta. Bake for 15 minutes or until the feta starts to brown and a digital food thermometer reads 160°F (70°C) when inserted in the center of a pepper half.

4. While the peppers bake, make the fresh tomato sauce. Cook the tomatoes, oil, garlic, oregano, and salt in a saucepan over medium-low heat until the tomatoes start to break down and the garlic becomes soft, 15 to 20 minutes.

5. Spoon the sauce over the peppers prior to serving or offer the sauce on the side.

Per Serving: Calories 861; Protein 33 g; Carbs 85 g; Dietary Fiber 9 g; Added Sugars 0 g; Total Fat 47 g; Sat Fat 16 g; Omega-3s 530 mg; Sodium 669 mg; Potassium 613 mg

SOUTH AFRICAN LAMB PIE (BOBOTIE)

Makes 8 servings

There are endless variations for this South African layered casserole with spiced ground meat on the bottom and an egg custard on top. Leftover bobotie reheats beautifully in the microwave; Amy has been known to eat it for breakfast the next morning. We like to serve it with Mixed Fruit with Yogurt-Cardamom Dressing (page 52) for a complete meal.

2 tablespoons extra virgin olive oil

2 yellow onions, finely chopped

2 garlic cloves, minced

1 tablespoon Curry Powder (page 32)

1 slice day-old bread

1 cup (240 ml) milk

1.5 pounds (680 g) ground lamb

Lemon zest and juice of 1 lemon

4 eggs

½ cup (45 g) slivered almonds

½ cup (80 g) raisins

3 tablespoons Hot Mango Chutney (page 65)

1 tablespoon brown or granulated sugar

½ teaspoon freshly ground black pepper

½ teaspoon ground turmeric

1. Preheat the oven to 350°F (180°C).

2. Heat the oil in a sauté pan over medium heat. Sauté the onion and garlic until the onions are soft, 8 minutes. Add the curry powder and cook until the curry powder is fragrant, 2 minutes. Remove from the heat.

3. Soak the bread in the milk for 5 minutes in a medium bowl. Squeeze the bread dry, reserving the milk in the bowl. Using your hands, thoroughly mix the onion mixture, bread, lamb, lemon zest and juice, 1 egg, the almonds, raisins, chutney, sugar, pepper, and turmeric in a large bowl. Spread the mixture in a 7 × 11-inch (18 × 28 cm) baking dish. Bake for 30 minutes.

4. Beat the remaining 3 eggs with the reserved milk and pour over the meat. Bake for 15 to 20 minutes, until the custard is set, the top is golden, and a digital food thermometer reads 165°F (75°C) when inserted in the center. Serve warm. Store covered in the refrigerator for up to 3 days or in the freezer for up to 2 months. Thaw frozen leftovers in the refrigerator before reheating in the microwave.

Per Serving: Calories 403; Protein 21 g; Carbs 21 g; Dietary Fiber 2 g; Added Sugars 0 g; Total Fat 27 g; Sat Fat 10 g; Omega-3s 340 mg; Sodium 229 mg; Potassium 230 mg

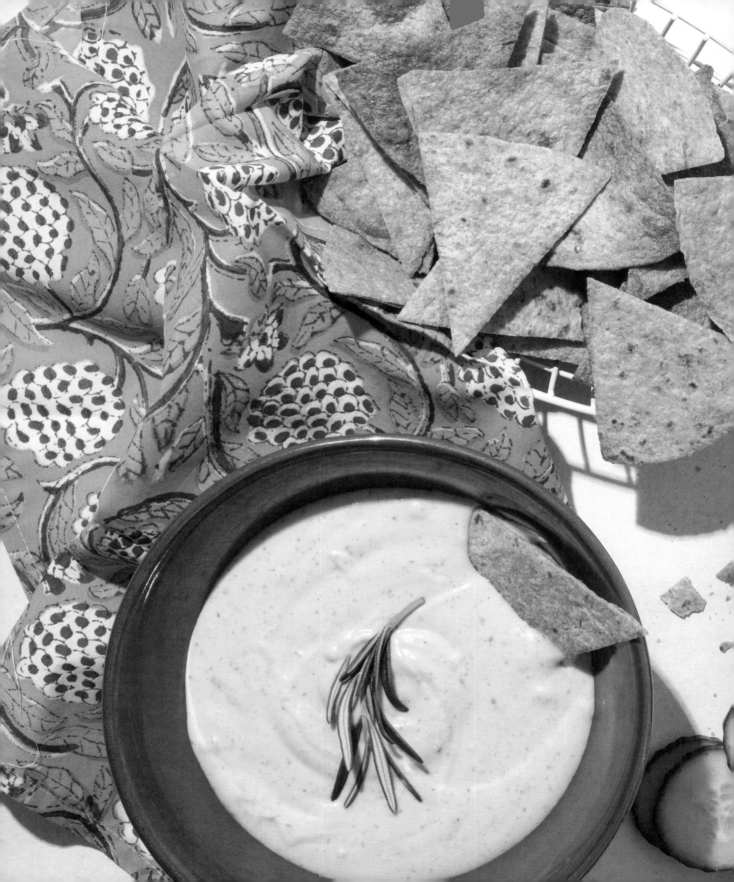

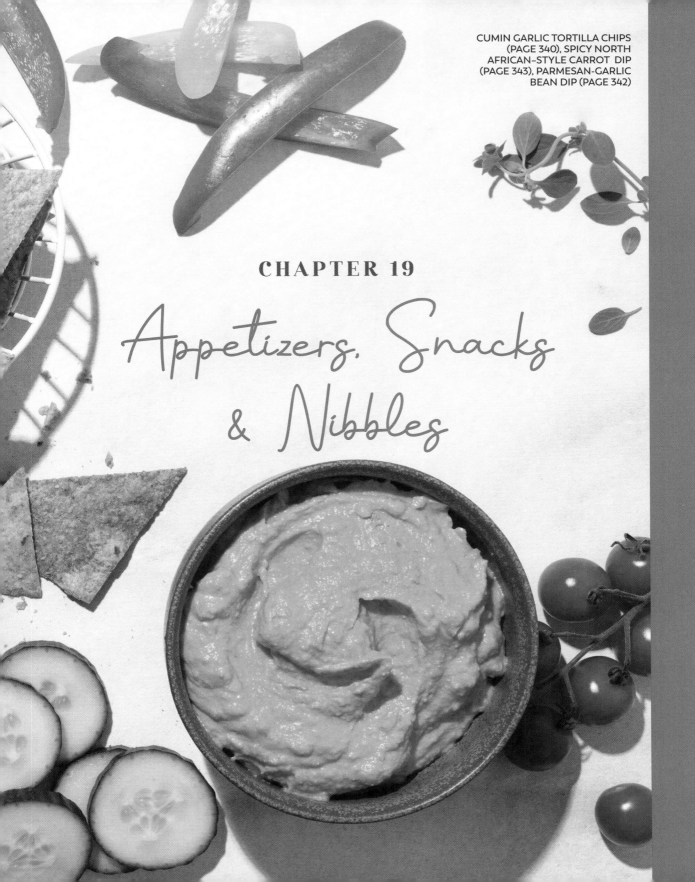

CUMIN GARLIC TORTILLA CHIPS
(PAGE 340), SPICY NORTH
AFRICAN–STYLE CARROT DIP
(PAGE 343), PARMESAN-GARLIC
BEAN DIP (PAGE 342)

CHAPTER 19

Appetizers, Snacks
& Nibbles

Appetizers, Snacks & Nibbles

Chips & Crisps

Crispy Cajun Corn Chips 339

Cumin-Garlic Tortilla Chips. 340

Kale Chips. 340

Southwest Pita Chips 340

Wonton Crisps 341

Dips & Spreads

Baked Ricotta 341

Creamy Curry-Cashew Dip. 342

Edamame-Pea Pesto Spread. 342

Parmesan-Garlic Bean Dip. 342

Spicy North African–Style Carrot Dip . . 343

Tomato Jam. 343

Nibbles & Nuts

Brown Bag Popcorn
with Herb Seasonings 344

Oven-Roasted Seasoned Popcorn 344

Cajun-Spiced Peanuts 345

Curry-Roasted Cashews 346

Moroccan-Spiced Almonds. 346

Pumpkin Spice Pecans. 346

Savory Roasted Mixed Nuts. 347

Smoky Roasted Edamame. 347

We had so much fun developing recipes for this chapter. We all love crunchy, crispy chips paired with creamy dips, so the first two sections feature a variety of crunchy items to pair with the dips and spreads in the second section. They can also be paired with recipes that appear in other chapters, like the salsas in chapter 4. We love snacking on Southwest Pita Chips (page 340) with Spicy North African–Style Carrot Dip (page 343) and Wonton Crisps (page 341) with Edamame-Pea Pesto Spread (page 342) as a dip.

Many of these recipes can be go-to sources of inspiration for entertaining, too. Imagine a share board with a variety of the chips, dips, spiced nuts, and small bunches of grapes that invites people to nibble and nosh. And we guarantee if you offer guests Baked Ricotta (page 341) with whole grain crostini or crackers at your next gathering, they'll ask you for the recipe!

The third section is packed with nuts and nibbles, where you can explore some new flavor combinations like the Savory Roasted Mixed Nuts (page 347), which combines the savory herbs rosemary and thyme with the heat of cayenne and the subtle sweetness of maple syrup. And just as in other chapters, we focused on using mostly plant-based ingredients. You'll find whole grains, vegetables, legumes, and sources of healthy fats like extra virgin olive oil and nuts. You'll also find that most of the recipes in this chapter are very simple, requiring little effort while delivering a big flavor and enjoyment payoff!

CRISPY CAJUN CORN CHIPS

Makes 6 servings

Small street taco tortillas are great for this recipe—when the tortillas are quartered, each chip is the perfect size for a single scoop of dip or salsa. Serve these alongside Chicken Chili Verde (page 85), with Refried Beans (page 243) and Avocado Salsa (page 61).

Fifteen 4½-inch (11.5 cm) white or yellow soft corn tortillas

2 tablespoons extra virgin olive oil

1 tablespoon Cajun Seasoning (page 30)

1. Preheat the oven to 300°F (150°C). Line a large rimmed baking sheet with parchment paper.

2. Stack 5 tortillas, then cut them in quarters. Repeat with the remaining tortillas to create 60 chips.

3. Whisk together the oil and seasoning in a small bowl. Lightly brush on both sides of each chip. Arrange the chips in a single layer on the baking sheet. Bake for 8 minutes.

4. Flip the chips over, brush with any remaining oil, and rotate the tray from back to front. Bake for another 6 minutes or until chips are crisp and light to golden brown.

5. Cool on the baking sheet on a wire rack. Enjoy immediately or store in an airtight container for up to 5 days.

TIP: To make tortilla strips to sprinkle on bowls, salads, or soups, cut the tortillas in half. then cut each half into ¼-inch-wide (6 mm) strips.

Serving Size 10 chips; Calories 145; Protein 3 g; Carbs 21 g; Dietary Fiber 3 g; Added Sugars 0 g; Total Fat 6 g; Sat Fat 1 g; Omega-3s 51 mg; Sodium 20 mg; Potassium 90 mg

CUMIN-GARLIC TORTILLA CHIPS

Makes 6 servings

These chips are a bit thicker than ones made with corn tortillas. They can be served with soups and stews, or paired with dips. Try them with Pico de Gallo (page 61) or Spicy North African–Style Carrot Dip (page 343).

> Ten 6-inch (15 cm) whole wheat flour tortillas
> 2 tablespoons extra virgin olive oil
> 2 teaspoons ground cumin
> 1 teaspoon garlic powder

1. Preheat the oven to 300°F (150°C). Line a large rimmed baking sheet with parchment paper.

2. Stack 5 tortillas, cut them in half, and then cut each half in thirds so each tortilla creates 6 chips. Repeat with the remaining tortillas

3. Whisk together the oil, cumin, and garlic powder in a small bowl. Lightly brush the oil on both sides of each chip. Arrange the chips in a single layer on the baking sheet. Bake for 8 minutes.

4. Flip the chips over, brush with any remaining oil, and rotate the tray from back to front. Bake for 6 minutes or until the chips are crisp and light to golden brown.

5. Cool on the baking sheet on a wire rack. Enjoy immediately or store in an airtight container for up to 5 days.

Serving Size 10 chips; Calories 222; Protein 5 g; Carbs 33 g; Dietary Fiber 4 g; Added Sugars 0 g; Total Fat 8 g; Sat Fat 2 g; Omega-3s 30 mg; Sodium 202 mg; Potassium 24 mg

KALE CHIPS

Makes 4 servings

These chips are difficult to keep around, as they walk off the pan almost by themselves! This recipe works well for all varieties of kale and you can use many different seasonings, including Moroccan-Style Seasoning (page 35), Cajun Seasoning (page 30), or Taco Seasoning (page 38).

> 1 tablespoon extra virgin olive oil
> 1 tablespoon Habanero Spice Rub (page 33)

> 1 to 2 bunches kale, heavy stems removed, leaves torn in 4-inch (10 cm) pieces
> ¼ teaspoon kosher salt

1. Preheat the oven to 250°F (120°C). Position the racks in the middle and lower third of the oven. Line two large rimmed baking sheets with parchment paper.

2. Whisk together the oil and spice rub in a small bowl. Place the kale in a large bowl, pour in the oil, and use your hands to massage the oil into the leaves. (Don't be tempted to add more oil, or your chips won't crisp.)

3. Arrange the kale in a single layer on the baking sheets. Sprinkle with the salt. Bake for 8 minutes

4. Switch the positions of the pans and rotate each from back to front. Bake for 15 to 20 minutes, until the leaves feel dry and crispy to the touch.

5. Cool on the baking sheets on wire racks. Enjoy immediately or store in an airtight container for up to 3 days. Do not freeze.

Per Serving: Calories 91; Protein 5 g; Carbs 11 g; Dietary Fiber 4 g; Added Sugars 0 g; Total Fat 5 g; Sat Fat 1 g; Omega-3s 230 mg; Sodium 90 mg; Potassium 564 mg

SOUTHWEST PITA CHIPS

Makes 6 servings

These chips make good scoops for Classic Hummus (page 245) or Spicy North African–Style Carrot Dip (page 343).

> Six 6-inch (15 cm) whole wheat pita pockets
> 2 tablespoons plus 1 teaspoon extra virgin olive oil
> 1 tablespoon Southwest Seasoning (page 37)

1. Adjust an oven rack to the center position. Preheat the oven to 350°F (180°C). Place a large wire rack on a large rimmed baking sheet; brush the rack with 1 tablespoon of the oil.

2. With kitchen shears or a sharp knife, separate each pita along the edges into 2 thin rounds. Cut each round into quarters. Arrange the pieces smooth side down in a single layer on the wire rack.

3. Whisk the remaining 2 tablespoons oil and the seasoning in a small bowl. Brush the oil on the pita pieces. Bake for 12 to 14 minutes, until crisp and golden.

4. Remove from the oven and let cool. Enjoy immediately or store in an airtight container for up to 5 days.

Serving Size 8 chips; Calories 191; Protein 6 g; Carbs 27 g; Dietary Fiber 4 g; Added Sugars 0 g; Total Fat 8 g; Sat Fat 1 g; Omega-3s 40 mg; Sodium 231 mg; Potassium 150 mg

WONTON CRISPS

Makes 6 servings

These chips can be made savory or sweet. They're a fun addition to a share board with fruits, vegetables, and a variety of dips and salsas including Stone Fruit Salsa (page 62). Change out the Cinnamon Spice Mix for Rustic Herb Seasoning (page 36) to create a completely different flavor to pair with a dip like the Parmesan-Garlic Bean Dip (page 342).

30 wonton wrappers

2 tablespoons extra virgin olive oil

1 tablespoon Cinnamon Spice Mix (page 31)

1. Preheat the oven to 300°F (150°C). Line a large rimmed baking sheet with parchment paper.

2. Stack 5 wonton wrappers. Cut the stack diagonally in half. Repeat with the remaining wrappers.

3. Whisk the oil and spice mix in a small bowl. Brush the oil on both sides of the wrapper halves. Arrange wrappers in a single layer so edges don't overlap. Bake for 10 to 12 minutes, until the wrappers become crisp and golden brown.

4. Cool to room temperature on the baking sheet on a wire rack. Enjoy immediately or store in an airtight container for up to 5 days.

Serving Size 10 crisps; Calories 159; Protein 4 g; Carbs 24 g; Dietary Fiber 1 g; Added Sugars 0 g; Total Fat 5 g; Sat Fat 1 g; Omega-3s 50 mg; Sodium 229 mg; Potassium 35 mg

BAKED RICOTTA

Makes 2 cups (450 g)

This is an easy, elegant appetizer you can serve with whole wheat crostini, whole grain crackers, or plain pita chips. It can be mixed ahead of time, refrigerated, and then baked when you're nearly ready to serve. Don't be surprised if family and friends request the recipe; it's a hit at parties at Amy's home!

One 15-ounce (425 g) container part-skim ricotta

3 tablespoons extra virgin olive oil

1 teaspoon red pepper flakes

1 teaspoon minced fresh rosemary

½ teaspoon kosher salt

½ teaspoon freshly ground black pepper

1. Preheat the oven to 400°F (200°C).

2. Combine the ricotta, 2 tablespoons of the oil, the red pepper flakes, rosemary, salt, and pepper in a small bowl.

3. Transfer to a small ceramic baking dish, about 4 × 8 inches (10 × 20 cm) or into eight small oven-safe ramekins to create individual 2-ounce (57 g) portions. Drizzle the top with the remaining 1 tablespoon oil.

4. Bake for 25 minutes if using one pan, or 18 to 20 minutes if using ramekins, until the edges are bubbling and starting to brown. Serve warm. Store in an airtight container in the refrigerator for up to 3 days. Reheat in the microwave.

Serving Size ⅓ cup (75 g); Calories 162; Protein 8 g; Carbs 4 g; Dietary Fiber 0 g; Added Sugars 0 g; Total Fat 13 g; Sat Fat 4 g; Omega-3s 100 mg; Sodium 148 mg; Potassium 98 mg

CREAMY CURRY-CASHEW DIP

Makes 1⅔ cups (525 g)

This sweet dip perfectly pairs with slices of crisp apples, firm Bosc pears, or pineapple spears. It's also a great spread for thin, crispy crackers made with dried nuts and fruit. We feature our Curry Powder, but you can use a store-bought curry blend.

- 2 tablespoons Curry Powder (page 32) or store-bought curry powder
- One 15-ounce (425 g) can pear halves in 100% juice, drained, juice reserved
- 1 cup (135 g) roasted, salted cashew halves and pieces

1. Toast the curry powder in a small sauté pan or skillet over medium heat for 45 seconds to 1 minute. Stir constantly with a wooden spoon to keep it from overtoasting.

2. Combine the pears, cashews, and curry powder in a food processor or blender. Puree until smooth. Add 1 to 2 tablespoons of the reserved pear juice to achieve the desired consistency. (Save the rest of the pear juice to add to a smoothie or oatmeal.) Serve at room temperature. Store in an airtight container in the refrigerator for up to 10 days.

Serving Size ⅓ cup (105 g); Calories 176; Protein 6 g; Carbs 12 g; Dietary Fiber 3 g; Added Sugars 0 g; Total Fat 13 g; Sat Fat 3 g; Omega-3s 60 mg; Sodium 249 mg; Potassium 310 mg

EDAMAME-PEA PESTO SPREAD

Makes 2 cups (395 g)

This beautiful, aromatic green spread pairs well with raw veggies like sliced cucumbers, jicama sticks, and bell pepper strips. It's also a wonderful spread for whole wheat crostini. If you want to pair a glass of wine with this appetizer, a citrusy, herbaceous Sauvignon Blanc from the Marlborough region of New Zealand is a fitting option.

- 1 cup (150 g) frozen shelled edamame (immature, green soybeans), thawed
- 1 cup (130 g) frozen petite or baby green peas, thawed
- ½ cup (15 g) chopped fresh mint leaves
- ¼ cup (60 ml) extra virgin olive oil
- 2 teaspoons grated lemon zest
- 2 tablespoons fresh lemon juice
- 1 garlic clove, minced
- ¼ teaspoon kosher salt

Combine the edamame, peas, mint, oil, lemon zest and juice, garlic, and salt in a food processor. Process until the mixture is thick and mostly smooth. Serve. Store in an airtight container in the refrigerator for up to 1 week (see Tip).

TIP: *If you plan on storing this for more than a day, wait to add the lemon zest until right before serving, as the lemon zest will continue to infuse into the spread as it sits, intensifying the lemon flavor.*

Serving Size ½ cup (100 g); Calories 214; Protein 6 g; Carbs 10 g; Dietary Fiber 3 g; Added Sugars 0 g; Total Fat 17 g; Sat Fat 2 g; Omega-3s 120 mg; Sodium 103 mg; Potassium 282 mg

PARMESAN-GARLIC BEAN DIP

Makes 2 cups (560 g)

This delicious dip comes together in minutes in a food processor. Set it out with a variety of whole grain pita chips and raw veggies for an easy appetizer or snack.

- One 15.5-ounce (439 g) can cannellini beans, drained and rinsed
- ½ cup (40 g) freshly grated Parmesan
- ⅓ cup (80 ml) extra virgin olive oil
- 2 garlic cloves, chopped
- 1 teaspoon Italian Seasoning (page 34)
- 1 teaspoon red wine vinegar
- Pinch of red pepper flakes
- Water, if needed

Combine the beans, Parmesan, oil, garlic, seasoning, vinegar, and pepper flakes in a food processor. Blend until smooth. Add a tablespoon or two of water if the dip is too thick. Serve immediately at room temperature or store in an airtight container in the refrigerator for up to 1 week.

Serving Size ¼ cup (70 g); Calories 159; Protein 5 g; Carbs 10 g; Dietary Fiber 4 g; Added Sugars 0 g; Total Fat 11 g; Sat Fat 2 g; Omega-3s 80 mg; Sodium 175 mg; Potassium 20 mg

SPICY NORTH AFRICAN–STYLE CARROT DIP

Makes 3 cups (750 g)

This dip gets its creaminess from pureed cooked carrots, extra virgin olive oil, and ground almonds, and its spicy, lingering heat from harissa, a Tunisian chili paste. Use as a dip with raw veggies or a spread for whole grain crostini or crackers. It's also great as a sauce for whole grain penne pasta topped with a bit of mild, creamy goat cheese.

4 cups (490 g) diced carrots (about 4 to 8 carrots)

½ cup (70 g) unsalted roasted almonds

½ cup (120 ml) extra virgin olive oil

2 tablespoons harissa

2 tablespoons fresh lemon juice

1 teaspoon ground cumin

½ teaspoon ground coriander

½ teaspoon kosher salt

1. Place the carrots in a saucepan, cover with water, and cook over medium-high heat until very soft, 15 to 20 minutes. Drain off the cooking water and let the carrots cool to room temperature.

2. Combine the carrots, almonds, oil, harissa, lemon juice, cumin, coriander, and salt in a blender or food processor and blend until smooth. Serve at room temperature. Store in an airtight container in the refrigerator for up to 1 week.

Serving Size ½ cup (125 g); Calories 283; Protein 4 g; Carbs 12 g; Dietary Fiber 4 g; Added Sugars 0 g; Total Fat 25 g; Sat Fat 3 g; Omega-3s 130 mg; Sodium 180 mg; Potassium 29 mg

TOMATO JAM

Makes 1½ cups (340 g)

Tomato jam is a savory spread that loves to be paired with cheese. You can create an easy, elegant appetizer by serving this with Brie and a whole grain baguette, or your favorite cheese and whole grain crackers. Try it with our Very Veggie Grilled Cheese Sandwiches (page 182).

One 28-ounce (794 g) can diced tomatoes in juice, drained

½ cup (170 g) honey

1 tablespoon balsamic vinegar

½ teaspoon freshly ground black pepper

¼ teaspoon ground cloves

1. Combine the tomatoes, honey, vinegar, pepper, and cloves in a medium saucepan. Cook over medium-low heat, stirring occasionally, until the mixture becomes thick, jammy, and dark purple in color, 30 to 40 minutes.

2. Remove from the heat and cool to room temperature. Serve. Store in the refrigerator in an airtight container for up to 1 month.

Serving Size 2 tablespoons; Calories 61; Protein 1 g; Carbs 15 g; Dietary Fiber 1 g; Added Sugars 12 g; Total Fat 0 g; Sat Fat 0 g; Omega-3s 0 mg; Sodium 9 mg; Potassium 136 mg

BROWN BAG POPCORN WITH HERB SEASONINGS

Makes 1 serving

Popcorn is a whole grain food that is full of fiber, with satisfying crunch. Here we provide directions for popping the popcorn in a brown paper lunch bag without butter or oil. Then we add toppings directly to the bag and shake everything up! Offer a popcorn bar at your next gathering: Provide a bag for each of your guests and let them add their favorite flavorings.

2 tablespoons yellow or white popcorn kernels

Italian Garlic

1 teaspoon garlic powder

1 teaspoon Italian Seasoning (page 34)

1 tablespoon freshly grated Parmesan

⅛ teaspoon kosher salt

Rosemary-Parmesan

1 tablespoon freshly grated Parmesan

1 tablespoon chopped fresh rosemary or
   1 teaspoon crushed dried rosemary

⅛ teaspoon kosher salt

Smokin' Hot

½ cup (65 g) Smoky Roasted Edamame
   (page 347)

1 teaspoon chili powder

¼ teaspoon red pepper flakes

⅛ teaspoon kosher salt

1. Pour the kernels into a brown paper lunch bag with a flat bottom, measuring 5 ⅛ × 3 ⅛ × 10 ⅝ inches (13 × 8 × 26.5 cm). Close the bag by folding the top over twice.

2. Mix your choice of seasonings together in a small bowl.

3. Place the bag upright in the middle of the turntable and microwave on HIGH for 1 minute and 10 seconds. Once the popping slows and a few seconds pass between pops, stop the microwave so as not to burn the popcorn. Let the bag sit for a few seconds to allow all the kernels to pop.

4. Open the bag and immediately sprinkle the seasonings over the popcorn. Refold the top of the bag to retain the heat and shake to distribute the seasoning.

Enjoy straight from the bag or empty into a serving bowl.

TIP: Exact microwave timing will vary depending on the type and age of the kernels and your microwave's power. If using more kernels, you will need to microwave for longer (see Table 12, on this page).

Per Serving (Italian Garlic Popcorn): Calories 110; Protein 5 g; Carbs 22 g; Dietary Fiber 4 g; Added Sugars 0 g; Total Fat 2 g; Sat Fat 1 g; Omega-3s 6 mg; Sodium 390 mg; Potassium 40 mg

Table 12: Brown Bag Popcorn Yields

Yield is dependent on the number of kernels that do or don't pop. One serving is 3 cups (25 g).

UNPOPPED KERNELS	POPPING TIME	POPPED YIELD	SERVINGS
2 tablespoons	70 seconds	3 to 4 cups (25 to 30 g)	1
¼ cup (55 g)	1½ minutes	6 to 8 cups (50 to 65 g)	2
⅓ cup (70 g)	1½ to 2 minutes	10 to 12 cups (80 to 95 g)	4
½ cup (110 g)*	2½ minutes	14 to 16 cups (110 to 130 g)	5

*This is the maximum amount to add to a lunch-size bag; the popped kernels will completely fill the bag.

OVEN-ROASTED SEASONED POPCORN

Makes 4 servings

If you're expecting a crowd or nestling in to watch movies with friends, here are two versions of larger batches of popcorn. They are made with a small amount of oil and butter and specially seasoned, then roasted in the oven for a short time at a low temperature. We think you'll be pleased with the results.

12 cups (95 g) popped popcorn
   (from ⅓ cup/70 g popcorn kernels)

Five-Spice

1 tablespoon butter or plant-based spread

1 tablespoon toasted sesame oil

1 tablespoon Chinese Five-Spice Blend (page 31)

1 tablespoon grated or finely minced fresh ginger

2 teaspoons reduced-sodium soy sauce

1 teaspoon rice vinegar

⅛ teaspoon kosher salt

¾ teaspoon red pepper flakes

Southwest Chili-Lime

1 tablespoon butter or plant-based spread

1 tablespoon extra virgin olive oil

1 tablespoon chili powder

1 teaspoon ground cumin

1 tablespoon grated lime zest

¼ teaspoon kosher salt

3 tablespoons freshly grated Parmesan

1 tablespoon fresh lime juice

1. Preheat the oven to 300°F (150°C). Line a large rimmed baking sheet with parchment paper.

2. Transfer the popped corn into a very large bowl. Choose your seasoning blend. Combine the butter and oil in a small microwave-proof bowl and microwave on MEDIUM for 20 seconds to melt the butter.

3. To make the five-spice popcorn, add the spice blend, ginger, soy sauce, vinegar, and salt to the melted butter. Drizzle over the popcorn and toss to combine.

4. To make the chili-lime popcorn, add the chili powder, cumin, lime zest, and salt to the melted butter. Drizzle over the popcorn, toss well, and sprinkle with the Parmesan and lime juice.

5. Spread the popcorn on the baking sheet. Roast for 15 to 20 minutes, until the popcorn is warm and the seasonings have adhered to the popcorn.

6. Remove from the oven. If making the five-spice popcorn, sprinkle with the red pepper flakes. Serve immediately. Store in an airtight container at room temperature for up to 1 month.

Per Serving (Five-Spice Seasoned Popcorn): Calories 115; Protein 2 g; Carbs 14 g; Dietary Fiber 3 g; Added Sugars 0 g; Total Fat 7 g; Sat Fat 2 g; Omega-3s 15 mg; Sodium 210 mg; Potassium 125 mg

CAJUN-SPICED PEANUTS

Makes 8 servings

These nuts offer a smoky, savory, spicy kick that will keep you coming back for more. Enjoy as a snack, add to a bowl of fresh popcorn, or serve with Turkey Jambalaya (page 318).

Cooking spray

1 large egg white

1 tablespoon plus 2 teaspoons Cajun Seasoning (page 30)

2 cups (290 g) unsalted dry-roasted peanuts

1. Preheat the oven to 350°F (180°C). Coat a large rimmed baking sheet with cooking spray.

2. Whisk the egg white and seasoning in a medium bowl. Add the peanuts and toss to coat.

3. Spread the peanuts in a single layer on the baking sheet. Bake for 8 minutes, then stir. Bake for an additional 8 minutes, until the peanuts are dry and toasted.

4. Remove from the oven and cool completely. Enjoy immediately or store in an airtight container in a cool, dark place for up to 3 months.

Serving Size ¼ cup (36 g); Calories 216; Protein 9 g; Carbs 8 g; Dietary Fiber 3 g; Added Sugars 0 g; Total Fat 18 g; Sat Fat 3 g; Omega-3s 10 mg; Sodium 13 mg; Potassium 243 mg

CURRY-ROASTED CASHEWS

Makes 4 servings

Add these nuts to your next bowl of air-popped popcorn or mix them into trail mix. Coated with cumin, curry, and chili powder, they're a natural fit for any Mediterranean salad or grain bowl.

1 tablespoon peanut or extra virgin olive oil

1 cup (135 g) whole unsalted cashews

½ teaspoon chili powder

½ teaspoon ground cumin

½ teaspoon Curry Powder (page 32)

¼ teaspoon red pepper flakes

¼ teaspoon kosher salt

¼ teaspoon freshly ground black pepper

1. Heat the oil in a medium skillet over medium-high heat. Add the cashews and stir well. Add the chili powder, cumin, curry powder, and red pepper flakes and stir to coat the cashews. Reduce the heat to medium-low and sauté until the spices are fragrant and nuts are toasted, about 3 minutes. Season with the salt and pepper.

2. Cool completely. Store in an airtight container in a cool, dark place for up to 1 month, in the refrigerator for up to 3 months, or in the freezer for up to 1 year.

Serving Size ¼ cup (34 g); Calories 228; Protein 5 g; Carbs 12 g; Dietary Fiber 1 g; Added Sugars 0 g; Total Fat 19 g; Sat Fat 4 g; Omega-3s 60 mg; Sodium 63 mg; Potassium 205 mg

MOROCCAN-SPICED ALMONDS

Makes 16 servings

Making almonds and other nuts part of your daily snacking routine is one of the best habits you can form to promote heart health and reduce the risk of type 2 diabetes. An ounce of almonds (30 grams, 23 nuts) provides protein, fiber, and half of the vitamin E we need every day.

1 large egg white

2 tablespoons honey

3 tablespoons Moroccan-Style Seasoning (page 35)

4 cups (570 g) unsalted almonds

1. Preheat the oven to 325°F (165°C). Line a large rimmed baking sheet with parchment paper.

2. Whisk the egg white in a medium bowl until foamy; add the honey and seasoning and whisk to combine. Add the almonds and toss well to coat. Spread the almonds in a single layer on the baking sheet, separating them as much as possible with a fork. Bake for 15 minutes. Stir and return to the oven for about 20 minutes, until the coating is dry. Remove from the oven and let cool completely.

3. Store in an airtight container in a cool, dark place for up to 3 months or in the freezer for up to 1 year.

Serving Size ¼ cup (37 g); Calories 224; Protein 9 g; Carbs 10 g; Dietary Fiber 4 g; Added Sugars 2 g; Total Fat 18 g; Sat Fat 1 g; Omega-3s 0 mg; Sodium 6 mg; Potassium 8 mg

PUMPKIN SPICE PECANS

Makes 12 servings

We couldn't resist putting a pumpkin spice–flavored snack in this recipe collection. We're confident you'll love these delicious morsels as a snack, as a crunchy addition to your morning oatmeal, or as a topping for the Pumpkin-Pear Mousse (page 360).

Cooking spray

3 cups (325 g) pecan halves

2 tablespoons real maple syrup

1 tablespoon honey

1 teaspoon pumpkin pie spice

¼ teaspoon kosher salt

1. Preheat the oven to 350°F (180°C). Line a large rimmed baking sheet with parchment paper. Coat the parchment paper with cooking spray.

2. Place the pecans in a medium bowl. Drizzle the syrup and honey over the pecans and toss well to coat. Sprinkle in about half of the pumpkin pie spice, toss well, and then slowly sprinkle in the rest while stirring and tossing the pecans. Spread the pecans in a single layer on the baking sheet, using a rubber spatula. Drizzle any syrup mixture left in the bowl over the pecans. Bake for 14 to 15 minutes, until the pecans are dry and dark brown.

3. Remove from the oven, sprinkle with the salt, and set aside to cool. Enjoy immediately or store in an airtight container at room temperature for up to 2 weeks.

Serving Size ¼ cup (27 g); Calories 202; Protein 3 g; Carbs 8 g; Dietary Fiber 3 g; Added Sugars 3 g; Total Fat 20 g; Sat Fat 2 g; Omega-3s 270 mg; Sodium 16 mg; Potassium 120 mg

SAVORY ROASTED MIXED NUTS

Makes 12 servings

Roasting nuts intensifies their unique flavors and develops their color. The savory coating on these nuts creates some unexpected bursts of heat and sweet. Use them as a crunchy topping for salads or a satisfying snack. Put them out at your next gathering and watch them disappear!

1 tablespoon peanut or extra virgin olive oil

1 tablespoon real maple syrup

1 teaspoon dried rosemary, crushed

1 teaspoon ground thyme

½ teaspoon ground cayenne

½ teaspoon ground sage

¼ teaspoon kosher salt

3 cups (425 g) unsalted mixed nuts

1. Preheat the oven to 275°F (135°C). Line a large rimmed baking sheet with parchment paper.

2. Combine the oil, syrup, rosemary, thyme, cayenne, sage, and salt in a medium bowl. Add the mixed nuts and toss well to coat. Spread the nuts in a single layer on the baking sheet. Bake for 10 minutes. Stir, then bake for another 8 to 10 minutes, until the nuts are toasted and fragrant.

3. Let cool for 10 minutes before serving. Store in an airtight container in a cool, dry place or in the refrigerator for up to 1 month or in the freezer for up to 1 year.

Serving Size ¼ cup (35 g); Calories 231; Protein 7 g; Carbs 9 g; Dietary Fiber 3 g; Added Sugars 1 g; Total Fat 20 g; Sat Fat 3 g; Omega-3s 230 mg; Sodium 18 mg; Potassium 223 mg

SMOKY ROASTED EDAMAME

Makes 6 servings

When roasted and spiced, edamame (green soybeans) can become an addictive snack. They are easy to make if you start with frozen shelled edamame. They're great on their own, but we also love them in Five-Spice Seasoned Popcorn (page 344).

One 16-ounce (454 g) bag frozen shelled edamame (green soybeans)

2 tablespoons freshly grated Parmesan

2 teaspoons Smoky Workaday Seasoning (page 37)

1 tablespoon extra virgin olive oil

Freshly ground black pepper

1. Preheat the oven to 375°F (190°C). Line a large rimmed baking sheet with parchment paper.

2. Rinse the edamame in a fine-mesh strainer under cold water until thawed, then drain well. Spread the edamame on one half of a kitchen towel, fold the other half over, and gently pat and roll them with your palms to remove as much moisture as possible. Let rest on the towel for a few minutes, then transfer to a medium bowl.

3. Whisk together the Parmesan and seasoning in a small bowl. Drizzle the edamame with the oil and toss to coat. Sprinkle with the Parmesan blend, add a few grinds of black pepper, and toss again.

4. Spread the edamame in a single layer on the baking sheet and roast for 30 minutes, stirring halfway through, until the outer shell is puffy with spots of dark to golden brown. Serve. Store in an airtight container in a cool, dry place for up to 2 months.

Serving Size 3 oz (76 g); Calories 136; Protein 9 g; Carbs 7 g; Dietary Fiber 4 g; Added Sugars 0 g; Total Fat 9 g; Sat Fat 2 g; Omega-3s 350 mg; Sodium 127 mg; Potassium 333 mg

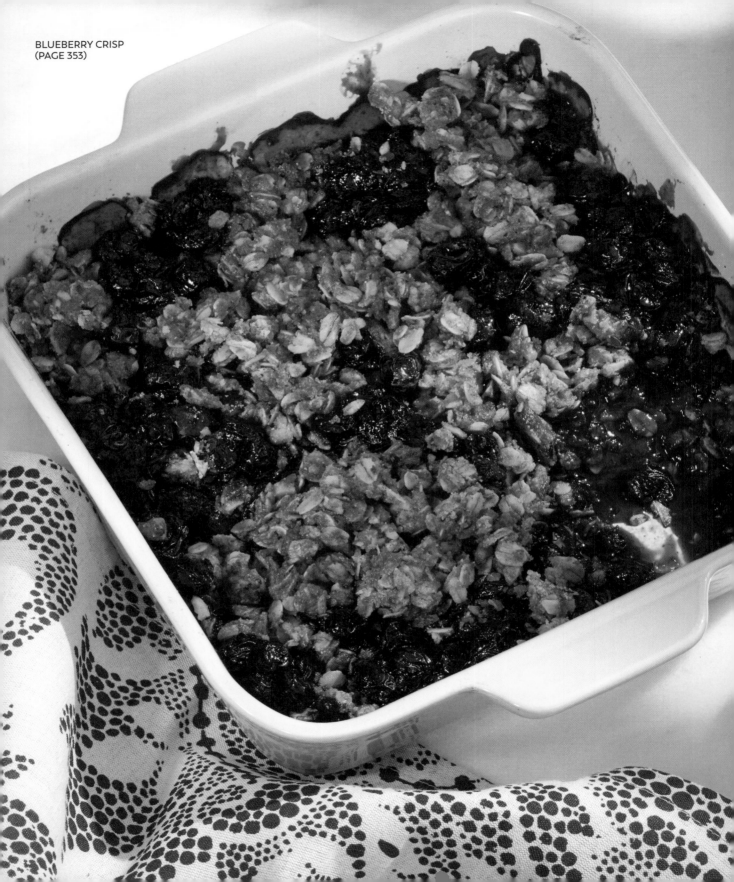

BLUEBERRY CRISP
(PAGE 353)

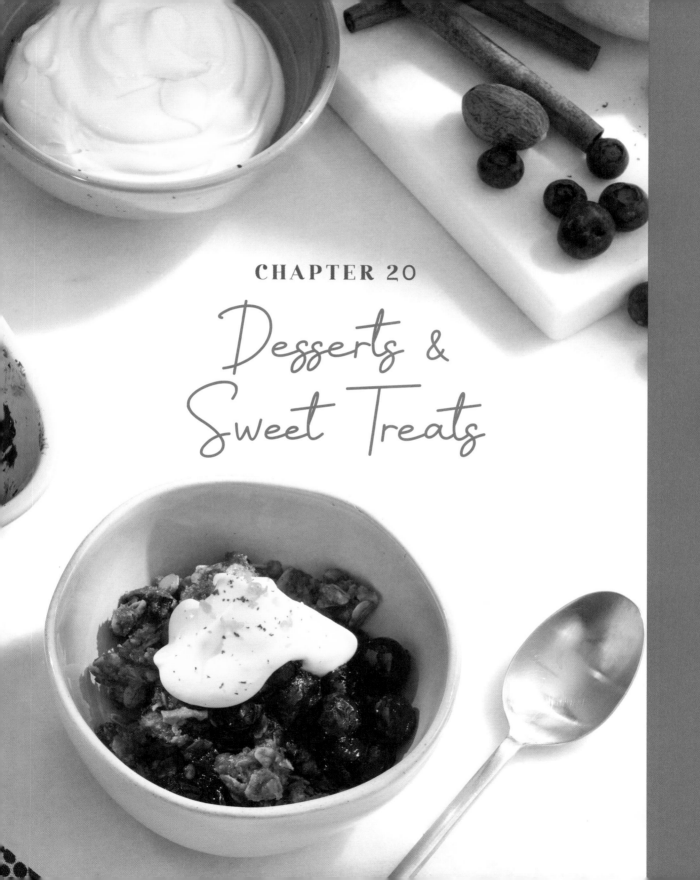

CHAPTER 20

Desserts & Sweet Treats

Desserts & Sweet Treats

Fruit Desserts

Berries with Cannoli Cream 351

Apple-Cinnamon Galette
with Gingerbread Crust. 352

Blueberry Crisp 353

Cranberry-Pear Crisp. 353

Strawberries with
Almond-Oat Crumble 354

Wine-Poached Pears 354

Bars, Cakes & Cookies

À la Heart Olive Oil Brownies 355

Almond-Orange Cake 355

Apple Walnut Date Coffee Cake. 356

Carrot Cake with Pecans 357

Chewy Molasses Cookies 357

Dark Chocolate Cranberry
Oatmeal Cookies with Walnuts 358

Pumpkin Spice Ginger Bars 358

Strawberry-Rhubarb Bars 359

Puddings & Mousses

Cherry-Farro Pudding Parfaits 359

Chocolate-Coconut Mousse. 360

Pumpkin-Pear Mousse. 360

Dessert Sauces & Toppings

Crème Fraîche 361

Citrus Curd 361

Spiced Ginger Cream 362

Other Sweet Treats

Blueberry Ginger Yogurt Bark
with Almonds. 362

Chocolate Cranberry
Almond Clusters 362

Pumpkin Apple Cranberry
Granola Bites. 363

There's definitely a place for dessert in healthful eating patterns. Remember, a health-promoting eating pattern isn't focused on single nutrients or single foods; it's focused on the overall pattern of foods you eat most of the time. Though we don't suggest indulging in sweets at the end of every meal, we want you to eat and enjoy dessert without regret. Life is too short for guilt; instead, focus on positive emotions to motivate you to make the best choices possible as much as you can.

We focused our recipe development efforts for this chapter on helping you find new ways to enjoy fruits, vegetables, whole grains, chocolate, nuts, dairy products, and even wine in lightly sweetened ways. Some recipes include granulated sugar. Some include heavy whipping cream. And, yes, a few even include butter. We worked to find a balance between using the very best ingredients for health with the very best ingredients for great flavor and enjoyment. We also focus on portion sizes, keeping them smaller than what you may be used to.

Since many of us love something creamy on top of crisps, cakes, and galettes, we also included a section with dessert toppings. Some of these are sweet like Orange Curd (page 361) while others like the Crème Fraîche (page 361) are tangy, providing a flavor counterbalance to the natural sweetness of many fruit desserts like our beautiful Blueberry Crisp (page 353). Spiced Ginger Cream (page 362) is the creamy topping most likely to get used in our homes. Amy loves it on Wine-Poached Pears (page 354) and Apple Walnut Date Coffee Cake (page 356) while Linda uses it to top Almond-Orange Cake (page 355) when she's entertaining family and friends.

You don't have to give up desserts and sweet treats, but we do hope you'll use these recipes as inspiration for making your dessert choices more intentional as you continue on your journey to the best health possible!

BERRIES WITH CANNOLI CREAM
Makes 4 servings

Cannoli are traditional Sicilian pastries, once made only for special holidays and festivals. Our version omits the tube-shaped fried pastry dough but still delivers the delicious cannoli cream. We nestle this heavenly creamy filling in fresh berries, topped with dark chocolate shavings and sprinkled with chopped pistachios.

- 2 cups (245 g) raspberries, sliced strawberries, or blueberries
- 1 teaspoon granulated sugar
- 1½ cups (370 g) reduced-fat ricotta
- ⅓ cup (40 g) confectioners' sugar
- 1 teaspoon pure vanilla extract
- 2 teaspoons grated orange zest
- 0.5 ounces (14 g) dark chocolate (72% or greater), grated
- ¼ cup (30 g) chopped pistachios

1. Toss the berries with the granulated sugar in a medium bowl.

2. Whip the ricotta in a blender, food processor, or with a handheld mixer until fluffy, 3 to 5 minutes. Add the confectioners' sugar and vanilla and whip until smooth and light, yet firm, 1 minute. Fold in the orange zest.

3. Divide the berries and any juices among 4 individual dessert dishes or stemmed coupes. Dollop the cannoli cream on top and sprinkle with the chocolate and pistachios.

Per Serving: Calories 270; Protein 13 g; Carbs 27 g; Dietary Fiber 5 g; Added Sugars 11 g; Total Fat 13 g; Sat Fat 6 g; Omega-3s 60 mg; Sodium 94 mg; Potassium 313 mg

APPLE-CINNAMON GALETTE WITH GINGERBREAD CRUST

Makes 8 servings

Galettes are a more casual way to make a pie. Instead of using a pie plate, the crust is laid flat on a baking sheet, the filling is piled in the middle, and the crust is folded up and around the filling without fully covering it. If making a pie intimidates you, try this galette, then top this yummy galette with Spiced Ginger Cream (page 362).

Gingerbread Crust

1⅓ cups (150 g) whole wheat pastry flour, plus more for dusting

1 teaspoon ground ginger

½ teaspoon ground allspice

⅛ teaspoon kosher salt

⅓ cup (80 ml) canola or peanut oil

2 tablespoons milk

1 large egg, lightly beaten, for brushing

Filling

1.5 pounds (680 g) apples, peeled, cored, and thinly sliced

1 tablespoon fresh lemon juice

4 tablespoons (50 g) sugar

1 tablespoon cornstarch

1 teaspoon ground cinnamon

½ teaspoon ground nutmeg

2 tablespoons cold unsalted butter or plant-based spread, cut into small pieces

1. Whisk together the flour, ginger, allspice, and salt in a medium bowl. Make a well in the center and add the oil and milk. Use a fork to stir until a soft dough forms. Dust your hands with flour and shape the dough into a ball, then flatten into a 5-inch (13 cm) circle. Wrap securely in wax paper, then plastic wrap. Chill for 20 minutes in the refrigerator.

2. Adjust an oven rack to the middle position. Preheat the oven to 375°F (190°C). Line a large rimmed baking sheet with parchment paper. Cut a separate 15-inch (38 cm) square of parchment to roll out the crust; cut a 13-inch (33 cm) square sheet of foil to protect the crust from overbrowning. Fold the foil in half and cut a 7-inch (18 cm) diameter semicircle from the center of the fold. When the foil is opened, the center

(a full circle) should be missing. (This allows the filling to be fully exposed while the foil covers the crust.)

3. Place the apples in a large bowl and sprinkle with lemon juice. Whisk together 3 tablespoons of the sugar, the cornstarch, cinnamon, and nutmeg in a small bowl. Sprinkle over the apples and mix to combine. Set the fruit aside as you roll out the crust.

4. Remove the dough from the refrigerator. Dust the 15-inch (38 cm) parchment square with flour, then roll out the dough to a 13-inch (33 cm) circle. Transfer the crust, still on the parchment, to the baking sheet.

5. Arrange the apples in the center of the dough, leaving a 2-inch (5 cm) border. The fruit can be layered in a circular design (pinwheel), mounded in the middle, or shingled (start at one edge and form even rows of apple slices, overlapping slices by one-third as you create a new row). Dot the filling with the butter.

6. Fold the crust over the filling in soft folds or pleats in 2-inch (5 cm) segments, allowing the center to remain uncovered. Brush the top and sides of the crust with the beaten egg and sprinkle with the remaining 1 tablespoon sugar. Trim away any excess parchment paper that hangs over the rim of the baking sheet.

7. Bake for 40 minutes. Place the foil over the galette to protect the crust from overbrowning, and bake for 20 minutes, until the crust is golden brown and the fruit is hot and bubbling. For a darker brown crust, remove the foil and bake for 10 minutes.

8. Let cool on the baking sheet for 10 minutes, then slide the galette, still on the parchment, onto a wire rack. Let cool for about 30 minutes to allow the filling to thicken. Slide a thin, long metal spatula under the galette to separate it from the parchment. Cut into eight pieces and serve. Store in an airtight container in the refrigerator for up to 2 days or on the counter covered with an overturned bowl for up to 2 days.

Per Serving: Calories 264; Protein 3 g; Carbs 34 g; Dietary Fiber 5 g; Added Sugars 6 g; Total Fat 13 g; Sat Fat 3 g; Omega-3s 900 mg; Sodium 45 mg; Potassium 103 mg

BLUEBERRY CRISP

Makes 6 servings

Regardless of the season, blueberries are available fresh or frozen, making this crisp practical to whip up most any night! Serve with a dollop of Crème Fraîche.

Filling

4 cups (590 g) blueberries

2 tablespoons granulated sugar

2 teaspoons cornstarch

½ teaspoon ground cinnamon

¼ teaspoon ground nutmeg

2 tablespoons fresh lemon juice

Topping

⅓ cup (75 g) butter or plant-based spread, softened

¼ cup (40 g) packed brown sugar

1 cup (90 g) quick-cooking rolled oats

⅓ cup (30 g) whole wheat pastry flour

3 tablespoons toasted flaxseed meal or chopped walnuts

½ teaspoon ground cardamom

½ teaspoon ground cinnamon

¾ cup (180 g) Buttermilk Crème Fraîche (page 361) for serving

1. Adjust an oven rack to the lower-third position. Preheat the oven to 375°F (190°C).

2. To make the filling, stir together the blueberries, granulated sugar, cornstarch, cinnamon, and nutmeg in a medium bowl. Transfer to a 9-inch (23 cm) square baking dish. Sprinkle with the lemon juice.

3. To make the topping, combine the butter and brown sugar in a medium bowl. Use a handheld mixer to beat until fluffy. Add the oats, flour, flaxseed meal, cardamom, and cinnamon. Use a fork to mix until the topping is crumbly and comes together in small clumps. Sprinkle the topping over the berries.

4. Bake for 30 to 35 minutes, until the topping is golden brown and the fruit is bubbling around the edges. Transfer the baking dish to a wire rack and let cool slightly, about 15 minutes. Serve warm with a dollop of crème fraîche. Store covered in the refrigerator for up to 3 days.

Per Serving: Calories 357; Protein 5 g; Carbs 43 g; Dietary Fiber 5 g; Added Sugars 10 g; Total Fat 20 g; Sat Fat 11 g; Omega-3s 120 mg; Sodium 108 mg; Potassium 218 mg

CRANBERRY-PEAR CRISP

Makes 6 servings

This juicy crisp is a wonderful option for fall and winter, when pears are readily available in stores. Cranberries and pears complement one another well, and the spices in the topping make this crisp very fragrant. Top this not-too-sweet crisp with Spiced Ginger Cream (page 362) or Sour Cream Crème Fraîche.

Filling

6 Bartlett or Bosc pears, peeled, cored, sliced ¾ inch (2 cm) thick, then halved

1½ cups (150 g) fresh or frozen cranberries

2 tablespoons granulated sugar

¾ teaspoon ground ginger

2 teaspoons cornstarch

1 tablespoon fresh lemon juice

Topping

⅓ cup (75 g) butter or plant-based spread, softened

¼ cup (40 g) packed brown sugar

1 cup (90 g) quick-cooking rolled oats

⅓ cup (30 g) almond flour

¼ cup (25 g) chopped slivered almonds

½ teaspoon ground cardamom

½ teaspoon ground cinnamon

¾ cup (160 g) Sour Cream Crème Fraîche (page 361) for serving

1. Adjust an oven rack to the lower-third position. Preheat the oven to 375°F (190°C).

2. Combine the pears, cranberries, granulated sugar, ginger, and cornstarch in a medium bowl. Toss well to combine. Pour the mixture into a 9-inch (23 cm) square baking dish. Sprinkle with the lemon juice. Combine the butter and brown sugar in a medium bowl. Use a handheld mixer to beat until fluffy. Add the oats, almond flour, almonds, cardamom, and cinnamon. Use a fork to mix until the topping is crumbly and comes together in small clumps. Sprinkle evenly over the filling.

3. Bake for 30 to 35 minutes, until the topping is golden brown and the fruit is bubbling around the edges. Transfer the baking dish to a wire rack and let cool slightly, about 15 minutes. Serve warm with a dollop of crème fraîche. Store covered in the refrigerator for up to 3 days.

Per Serving: Calories 440; Protein 7 g; Carbs 55 g; Dietary Fiber 9 g; Added Sugars 10 g; Total Fat 24 g; Sat Fat 11 g; Omega-3s 80 mg; Sodium 95 mg; Potassium 400 mg

STRAWBERRIES WITH ALMOND-OAT CRUMBLE

Makes 6 servings

Lovers of strawberry shortcake will go for this deconstructed version of the classic dessert. Serve topped with Crème Fraîche.

Almond-Oat Crumble

2 tablespoons extra virgin olive oil

2 tablespoons real maple syrup or honey

1 teaspoon pure vanilla extract

¼ teaspoon ground cardamom

¼ teaspoon kosher salt

1 cup (90) old-fashioned rolled oats

½ cup (45 g) slivered almonds, chopped

Strawberries

3 pints (865 g) strawberries, stems removed, diced

1 tablespoon sugar

1 teaspoon lemon zest

¼ cup plus 2 tablespoons (165 g) Sour Cream Crème Fraîche (page 361)

Mint sprigs, optional

1. Preheat the oven to 350°F (180°C). Line a large rimmed baking sheet with parchment paper.

2. Combine the oil, maple syrup, vanilla, cardamom, and salt in a small bowl. Add the oats and almonds and stir to coat.

3. Spread the mixture on the baking sheet. Bake for 7 minutes. Stir, then bake for 6 to 7 minutes, until the crumble starts to turn dark brown in spots. Let cool to room temperature.

4. Combine the strawberries, sugar, and lemon zest in a large bowl. Divide the strawberry mixture among six dessert bowls or plates. Top each portion of strawberries with the crumble, and finish with 1 tablespoon of crème fraîche. Garnish with mint, if desired.

Per Serving: Calories 292; Protein 5 g; Carbs 31 g; Dietary Fiber 5 g; Added Sugars 6 g; Total Fat 18 g; Sat Fat 6 g; Omega-3s 160 mg; Sodium 41 mg; Potassium 378 mg

WINE-POACHED PEARS

Makes 4 servings

Zinfandel works great for this recipe; its classic strawberry jam flavors complement the flavor of the pears so well.

2 Bosc pears, halved, cored (see Tip)

One 750 ml bottle Zinfandel

2 tablespoons honey

2 cinnamon sticks

One ½ × 2-inch (13 mm × 5 cm) strip orange peel

4 whole cloves

½ cup (60 g) Spiced Ginger Cream (page 362)

1. Combine the pears, wine, honey, cinnamon, orange peel, and cloves in a medium saucepan. Bring to a boil over high heat, then reduce the heat to medium-low and gently simmer until the pears can be easily pierced with a knife and are a pale red color, 15 to 20 minutes.

2. Use a slotted spoon to remove the pears from the poaching liquid. Serve at room temperature, cored side up, topped with spiced ginger cream.

TIP: *The poaching liquid is essentially mulled wine. Enjoy it as a festive warm cocktail served in a coffee or tea mug. Add a splash of Grand Marnier or Cointreau to enhance the orange flavor, if desired.*

NOTE: *A melon baller works well for removing the pear cores. You can leave the stem on for a more natural look.*

Per Serving: Calories 130; Protein 1 g; Carbs 18 g; Dietary Fiber 3 g; Added Sugars 5 g; Total Fat 6 g; Sat Fat 3 g; Omega-3s 20 mg; Sodium 5 mg; Potassium 115 mg

À LA HEART OLIVE OIL BROWNIES

Makes 16 brownies

If you love a brownie with a moist, fudgy middle, this is the recipe for you! For a more intense chocolate flavor, choose chocolate chips or chunks with a higher cacao percentage, which will provide more bitterness and intense chocolate flavor. If you prefer a sweeter brownie, use semi-sweet chocolate chips or chunks.

Cooking spray
½ cup (170 g) honey
½ cup (120 ml) extra virgin olive oil
½ cup (100 g) sugar
2 large eggs
¾ cup (90 g) whole wheat pastry flour
¼ cup (20 g) unsweetened cocoa powder
1 teaspoon instant espresso powder (see Tip)
1 teaspoon pure vanilla extract
½ teaspoon baking powder
¼ teaspoon kosher salt
½ cup (85 g) chocolate chips or chunks (62 to 72% cacao)
½ cup (60 g) chopped walnuts

1. Preheat the oven to 350°F (180°C). Line the bottom and two sides of a 9-inch (23 cm) square baking pan with parchment paper.

2. Combine the honey, oil, sugar, and eggs in a large bowl. Use a whisk or handheld mixer to mix until creamy and lightly golden in color. Add the flour, cocoa powder, espresso powder, vanilla, baking powder, and salt. Stir to incorporate.

3. Stir in the chocolate chips and walnuts. Pour the batter into the baking pan and spread evenly.

4. Bake for 30 minutes; the top will look dull (not shiny) and will have many holes. Transfer to a wire

rack and cool for 10 to 15 minutes in the pan before cutting into 16 bars. Serve immediately or store in an airtight container at room temperature for up to 1 week or in the freezer for up to 2 months.

TIP: *If you don't have instant espresso powder, you can grind ground dark roast coffee to a very fine powder with a coffee grinder or a mortar and pestle.*

Serving Size 1 brownie; Calories 203; Protein 3 g; Carbs 23 g; Dietary Fiber 2 g; Added Sugars 17 g; Total Fat 12 g; Sat Fat 3 g; Omega-3s 410 mg; Sodium 20 mg; Potassium 73 mg

ALMOND-ORANGE CAKE

Makes one 8-inch (20 cm) round cake

This delicate, moist, single layer cake is made from ground blanched almonds or almond flour. Scents of almond and orange will fill the air as it bakes. You can serve this cake the day you make it, but if you let it sit overnight, the flavors blend beautifully. Serve with a dollop of Crème Fraîche (page 361) or Spiced Ginger Cream (page 362), or a simple dusting of confectioners' sugar.

½ cup (115 g) unsalted butter, softened, plus more for greasing the pan
1¼ cups (120 g) almond flour or ground almonds, plus more for the pan
½ cup (60 g) whole wheat pastry flour
1 teaspoon baking powder
¼ teaspoon salt
½ cup (100 g) light brown sugar
1 tablespoon grated orange zest
1 teaspoon pure vanilla extract
3 large eggs, separated
¼ teaspoon cream of tartar
¼ cup (60 ml) fresh orange juice

1. Preheat the oven to 350°F (180°C). Line the bottom of an 8-inch (20 cm) round cake pan with parchment paper; lightly butter the parchment. Dust the pan with ground almonds; shake out any excess.

2. Whisk together the almond flour, pastry flour, baking powder, and salt in a medium bowl. Combine the butter and sugar in a large bowl. Use a handheld mixer to beat the butter and sugar until light and fluffy. Beat in the orange zest and vanilla. Add the egg yolks, one at a time, beating well after each addition.

3. In a medium bowl, with clean beaters, beat the egg whites with the cream of tartar to form soft peaks.

4. Add the flour mixture to the butter mixture. Beat for 10 seconds, then add the orange juice and beat until well blended.

5. Use a rubber spatula to gently fold the beaten egg whites into the batter. Spoon the batter into the pan. Bake for 35 minutes or until the cake is lightly golden and a toothpick inserted in the center comes out clean.

6. Transfer to a wire rack to cool for 30 minutes. Run a sharp knife around the sides of the cake to loosen it from the edge of the pan. Place a 9-inch (23 cm) plate over the top of the cake, then turn the plate and pan upside down to move the cake to the plate.

7. Remove the parchment paper from the cake. Turn the cake right side up. Let the cake cool completely. Cut into 8 pieces and serve. Store in an airtight container for 1 or 2 days or in the freezer for up to 3 months.

VARIATIONS: *Almond-Lemon Cake*

Replace the orange zest and juice with lemon zest and juice.

Gluten-Free Almond-Orange Cake

Replace the whole wheat pastry flour with ½ cup (55 g) coconut flour. Use 4 eggs instead of 3.

Serving Size 1 piece; Calories 298; Protein 6 g; Carbs 22 g; Dietary Fiber 3 g; Added Sugars 13 g; Total Fat 21 g; Sat Fat 8 g; Omega-3s 210 mg; Sodium 48 mg; Potassium 143 mg

APPLE WALNUT DATE COFFEE CAKE
Makes one 8-inch (20 cm) square cake

This cake is a perfect fall dessert. Serve with a dollop of Spiced Ginger Cream (page 362) and a cup of chai or coffee.

> 1 cup (200 g) packed light brown sugar
> ¼ cup (60 g) salted butter, softened
> ¼ cup (60 ml) extra virgin olive oil
> 2 large eggs
> ½ cup (120 ml) cold brewed coffee
> ½ teaspoon pure vanilla extract
> 2 cups (240 g) whole wheat pastry flour
> 1 teaspoon baking soda
> 1 teaspoon ground cinnamon
> ½ teaspoon ground cloves
> ½ teaspoon kosher salt
> 2 cups (250 g) chopped apples
> 1 cup (160 g) chopped pitted dates
> 1 cup (115 g) chopped walnuts

1. Preheat the oven to 350°F (180°C). Line the bottom and two sides of an 8-inch (20 cm) square baking dish with parchment paper.

2. Combine the sugar, butter, oil, and eggs in a large bowl. Beat with a handheld mixer until light, fluffy, and lightly golden. Add the coffee and vanilla and beat for 10 to 15 seconds. Use a rubber spatula to scrape down the sides of the bowl. Beat in the flour, baking soda, cinnamon, cloves, and salt. Stir in the apples, dates, and walnuts. Use a large spoon or spatula to stir until all the dry ingredients have been incorporated. Spread the batter in the pan.

3. Bake for 45 to 50 minutes, until a toothpick inserted into the center of the cake comes out clean.

4. Cool the cake in the pan for 30 minutes, to room temperature. Cut into 9 pieces and serve. Store covered at room temperature for up to 3 days, in the refrigerator for up to 7 days, or in the freezer for up to 2 months. Thaw at room temperature.

Serving Size 1 piece; Calories 340; Protein 6 g; Carbs 48 g; Dietary Fiber 5 g; Added Sugars 16 g; Total Fat 16 g; Sat Fat 4 g; Omega-3s 950 mg; Sodium 245 mg; Potassium 270 mg

CARROT CAKE WITH PECANS

Makes one 9 × 13-inch (23 × 33 cm) cake

Topping each piece of this moist, tender cake with a dollop of Crème Fraîche (page 361) provides a similar tang to a cream cheese frosting, with fewer calories and less saturated fat.

- Cooking spray
- 1½ cups (300 g) sugar
- ½ cup (120 ml) extra virgin olive oil
- ½ cup (115 g) butter or plant-based spread, softened
- 2 large eggs
- 3 cups (170 g) grated carrots (about 3 to 6 carrots)
- One 8-ounce (227 g) can crushed pineapple in 100% pineapple juice
- ½ cup (55 g) chopped pecans
- 1 teaspoon pure vanilla extract
- 1½ cups (190 g) all-purpose flour
- ½ cup (60 g) whole wheat pastry flour
- 2 teaspoons baking soda
- 2 teaspoons ground cinnamon

1. Preheat the oven to 325°F (165°C). Spray a 9 × 13-inch (23 × 33 cm) pan with cooking spray.

2. Combine the sugar, oil, and butter in large bowl. Beat with a handheld mixer until light, fluffy, and lightly golden, 2 to 3 minutes. Add the eggs and beat for 30 seconds to fully incorporate. Stir in the carrots, pineapple, pecans, and vanilla.

3. Whisk together the all-purpose flour, pastry flour, baking soda, and cinnamon in a medium bowl. Stir into the batter until incorporated. Spread the batter in the pan.

4. Bake for 60 minutes, until a toothpick inserted into the center comes out clean. Let cool in the pan for 20 to 30 minutes before cutting in a 4 × 6 pattern (each piece will be about 2 inches/5 cm square). Serve warm or at room temperature.

Serving Size 1 piece; Calories 195; Protein 2 g; Carbs 23 g; Dietary Fiber 1 g; Added Sugars 12 g; Total Fat 11 g; Sat Fat 3 g; Omega-3s 80 mg; Sodium 145 mg; Potassium 32 mg

CHEWY MOLASSES COOKIES

Makes 40 cookies

These deeply molasses-flavored cookies are crunchy on the outside and chewy on the inside—the perfect afternoon pick-me-up treat for those who love the sweet, smoky, and spicy flavor of molasses.

- 2½ cups (300 g) whole wheat pastry flour
- 1½ teaspoons ground cinnamon
- 1 teaspoon baking soda
- ½ teaspoon ground allspice
- ½ teaspoon ground ginger
- ¼ teaspoon kosher salt
- ⅔ cup (160 ml) light or dark molasses
- ½ cup (115 g) unsalted butter, melted
- 1 large egg, beaten
- 2 tablespoons fresh lemon juice
- ¼ cup (50 g) sugar

1. Combine the flour, cinnamon, baking soda, allspice, ginger, and salt in a medium bowl. Whisk together the molasses, butter, egg, and lemon juice in a large bowl, then add the flour mixture. Use a large spoon to mix well, creating a soft dough. Cover the dough or wrap in plastic wrap and chill in the refrigerator for 1 hour.

2. Adjust an oven rack to the middle position. Preheat the oven to 350°F (180°C). Line two baking sheets with parchment paper.

3. Place the sugar in a shallow bowl. Scoop out 1 tablespoon dough for each cookie. Roll it into a ball between your palms, then roll in the sugar and place on the baking sheet. Repeat for the remaining dough, placing the balls about 2 inches (5 cm) apart.

4. Bake one pan of cookies at a time for about 10 minutes, until the cookies are firm and the edges are set.

5. Remove from the oven and let rest for 2 minutes on the parchment before moving the cookies onto a wire rack to cool completely. Bake and cool the second pan of cookies. Store in an airtight container at room temperature for up to 3 days or in the freezer for up to 3 months.

Serving Size 1 cookie; Calories 71; Protein 1 g; Carbs 11 g; Dietary Fiber 1 g; Added Sugars 5 g; Total Fat 2 g; Sat Fat 1 g; Omega-3s 40 mg; Sodium 40 mg; Potassium 82 mg

DARK CHOCOLATE CRANBERRY OATMEAL COOKIES WITH WALNUTS

Makes 18 cookies

This simple cookie recipe includes a number of ingredients that not only taste great but may also provide some health benefits, including dark chocolate, cranberries, and walnuts. Have a cookie with a glass of milk for a nutrient-rich, feel-good snack!

4 tablespoons unsalted butter, softened

¼ cup (60 ml) peanut oil

½ cup (50 g) brown sugar

1 large egg

1½ teaspoons pure vanilla extract

1½ cups (140 g) old-fashioned rolled oats

¾ cup (90 g) whole wheat pastry flour

1 teaspoon ground cinnamon

½ teaspoon baking soda

¼ teaspoon kosher salt

½ cup (85 g) dark chocolate chips

½ cup (65 g) sweetened dried cranberries

½ cup (60 g) chopped English walnuts

1. Preheat the oven to 350°F (180°C). Line two baking sheets with parchment paper.

2. Combine the butter, oil, and sugar in a medium bowl. Beat with a handheld mixer until light and fluffy, 2 to 3 minutes. Add the egg and vanilla and beat until smooth, 1 minute.

3. Stir in the oats, pastry flour, cinnamon, baking soda, and salt until combined. Add the chocolate chips, cranberries, and walnuts, and stir to form a sticky dough.

4. Use two spoons to scoop out about a tablespoon of dough for each cookie, placing 9 balls of dough on each baking sheet.

5. If you can place both sheets on one oven rack, bake the cookies for 11 to 13 minutes, until the cookies start to turn light brown around the edges. If you need to place the sheets on separate racks, switch and rotate them after 6 minutes, and then bake for an additional 5 to 7 minutes. Remove from the oven and place cookies on a wire cooling rack to cool for a few minutes before enjoying a warm-from-the-oven treat. Store in an airtight container at room temperature for up to 1 week. (But we doubt they'll last that long . . .)

Serving Size 1 cookie; Calories 168; Protein 3 g; Carbs 18 g; Dietary Fiber 2 g; Added Sugars 7 g; Total Fat 10 g; Sat Fat 4 g; Omega-3s 340 mg; Sodium 50 mg; Potassium 78 mg

PUMPKIN SPICE GINGER BARS

Makes 24 bars

There are quite a few pumpkin spice recipes in this book! That's because we adore the flavor combination, and we suspect you do, too. This recipe is a wonderful option when you need to bring a dessert to an office party, church potluck, or family gathering. The bars pair well with a cup of coffee or tea, but they also go well with a glass of milk for the kids.

One 15-ounce (425 g) can 100% pure pumpkin (not pumpkin pie mix)

1 cup (240 ml) peanut oil

1 cup (150 g) light brown sugar

3 large eggs

2 cups (240 g) whole wheat pastry flour

2 teaspoons baking powder

2 teaspoons pumpkin pie spice

1 teaspoon baking soda

1 cup (160 g) golden raisins

1 cup (115 g) chopped walnuts or pecans

½ cup (80 g) finely chopped crystallized ginger

1. Preheat the oven to 350°F (180°C). Spray a 10 × 15-inch (25.5 × 38 cm) baking pan with cooking spray.

2. Beat together the pumpkin, oil, sugar, and eggs in a large bowl until light and fluffy. Add the flour, baking powder, pumpkin pie spice, and baking soda and stir well to fully incorporate. Stir in the raisins, walnuts, and ginger. Spread the batter in the prepared pan.

3. Bake for 25 to 30 minutes, until a toothpick inserted into the center comes out clean. Let cool for 30 minutes, then cut in a 4 × 6 pattern to make 24 bars. Store wrapped individually in wax paper or

parchment paper in an airtight container at room temperature for up to 1 week, in the refrigerator for up to 2 weeks, or in the freezer for up to 3 months. Thaw at room temperature.

Serving Size 1 bar; Calories 221; Protein 3 g; Carbs 24 g; Dietary Fiber 8 g; Added Sugars 17 g; Total Fat 13 g; Sat Fat 2 g; Omega-3s 450 mg; Sodium 62 mg; Potassium 72 mg

STRAWBERRY-RHUBARB BARS

Makes 24 bars

This is Linda's go-to bar recipe to take to potlucks and gatherings. It looks lavish, cuts easily, is filled with tangy fruit flavor, and has just the right ratio of crust to filling. Many people have been known to hunt Linda down to get the recipe. And this recipe works just as well with frozen fruit. Freeze rhubarb in the summer so you can make these bars anytime!

Filling

4 cups (490 g) sliced rhubarb, in ¼-inch (6 mm) pieces

1 cup (145 g) sliced or quartered strawberries

¾ cup (150 g) granulated sugar

¼ cup (60 ml) water

2 tablespoons cornstarch

1 tablespoon fresh lemon juice

Crust

1½ cups (180 g) whole wheat pastry flour

¾ cup (150 g) brown sugar

½ cup (115 g) salted butter, melted

½ cup (45 g) old-fashioned rolled oats

½ cup (60 g) chopped walnuts or pecans

2 tablespoons extra virgin olive oil

½ teaspoon baking soda

1. Adjust an oven rack to the middle position. Preheat the oven to 350°F (180°C). Line the bottom of a 9 × 13-inch (23 × 33 cm) baking pan with parchment paper.

2. To make the filling, combine the rhubarb, strawberries, granulated sugar, water, cornstarch, and lemon juice in a large saucepan over medium heat. Stir constantly until it begins to simmer, about 4 minutes, then stir occasionally until thickened, 1 to 2 minutes. Remove from the heat.

3. To make the crust, combine the flour, brown sugar, butter, oats, walnuts, oil, and baking soda in a medium bowl. Use a fork to blend the mixture together until large and small crumbles form. Gently pat two-thirds of the mixture into the pan. Reserve the remaining mixture to use as the topping.

4. Spoon the filling over the crust, spreading it evenly. Sprinkle the remaining crust mixture over the top of the filling to create a crumb topping. Bake for 30 to 35 minutes, until the topping is puffed, delicately browned, and firm.

5. Place on a wire rack to cool completely to room temperature, about 2 hours. Cut in a 4 × 6 pattern to make 24 bars. Leave the bars in the pan until you're ready to serve. Store in an airtight container at room temperature for up to 2 days, in the refrigerator for up to 4 days, or in the freezer for up to 3 months.

Serving Size 1 bar; Calories 152; Protein 2 g; Carbs 22 g; Dietary Fiber 2 g; Added Sugars 12 g; Total Fat 7 g; Sat Fat 3 g; Omega-3s 250 mg; Sodium 56 mg; Potassium 96 mg

CHERRY-FARRO PUDDING PARFAITS

Makes 4 parfaits

This recipe is an easy way to get fruit, whole grains, and dairy into a single dessert that can be endlessly customized to meet everyone's preferences. Instead of using cherries, amaretto, and almond extract, you can use strawberries or blueberries macerated with limoncello, with lemon extract in the cream. You can also prepare the almond cream ahead of time (storing it covered in the refrigerator) and assemble the parfaits right before serving.

Macerated Cherries

3 cups (465 g) thawed frozen or pitted fresh cherries

2 tablespoons amaretto liqueur

1 teaspoon grated orange zest

Almond Cream

2 cups (480 ml) milk

1 large egg

¼ cup (50 g) sugar

1 tablespoon all-purpose flour

½ teaspoon almond extract

Topping

¼ cup (60 g) whipping cream

1 teaspoon sugar

¼ cup (25 g) slivered almonds

2 cups (340 g) Simply Cooked Farro
(page 226)

1. Place a glass or stainless-steel bowl in the freezer to chill thoroughly.

2. To make the macerated cherries, combine the cherries, liqueur, and orange zest in a small bowl.

3. To make the almond cream, whisk together the milk, egg, sugar, and flour in a medium saucepan until blended. Place over medium-high heat. Stir constantly until the mixture starts to bubble up and thicken, 6 to 8 minutes. Remove from the heat and stir in the almond extract. Refrigerate for 10 minutes to cool slightly.

4. To make the topping, use a whisk or handheld mixer to beat the whipping cream in the chilled bowl until soft peaks form. Gently stir in the sugar.

5. Divide the farro among four stemless wine glasses, half-pint glass jars, or glass dessert dishes. Spoon the almond cream over the farro, followed by the cherries. Top with whipped cream and almonds and serve.

Serving Size 1 parfait; Calories 450; Protein 14 g; Carbs 67 g; Dietary Fiber 7 g; Added Sugars 14 g; Total Fat 15 g; Sat Fat 5 g; Omega-3s 135 mg; Sodium 200 mg; Potassium 575 mg

CHOCOLATE-COCONUT MOUSSE

Makes 2 servings

Dark chocolate syrup and coconut extract provide rich flavor in this vegan mousse. Blending a banana with a ripe avocado creates a lovely, creamy consistency. For a texture contrast, top the mousse with chopped macadamia nuts or toasted coconut.

1 ripe banana

1 ripe avocado, halved, pitted, peeled, and cubed

¼ cup (60 ml) dark chocolate syrup

¼ teaspoon coconut or peppermint extract

Pinch of salt

Combine the banana, avocado, chocolate syrup, coconut extract, and salt in a blender or food processor. Blend until smooth. Divide between two small dessert bowls and serve.

Per Serving: Calories 265; Protein 3 g; Carbs 43 g; Dietary Fiber 7 g; Added Sugars 20 g; Total Fat 10 g; Sat Fat 1 g; Omega-3s 100 mg; Sodium 20 mg; Potassium 550 mg

PUMPKIN-PEAR MOUSSE

Makes 8 servings

This no-bake dessert offers all the flavors we love in a pumpkin pie with fewer calories and less saturated fat. You'll feel good knowing you're getting fruits and vegetables in every delicious bite! Serve topped with Pumpkin Spice Pecans (page 346) and Spiced Ginger Cream (page 362).

One 15-ounce can (425 g) pears in 100% juice, drained, juice reserved

One 15-ounce can (425 g) 100% pure pumpkin (not pumpkin pie mix)

¼ cup (85 g) honey

1 teaspoon pumpkin pie spice

Two 0.25-ounce (7 g) packets unflavored gelatin

1 cup (240 g) whipping cream

1 tablespoon sugar

¼ teaspoon pure vanilla extract

1. Puree the pears in a blender or food processor until smooth.

2. Whisk together the pureed pears, pumpkin, honey, and pumpkin pie spice in a medium bowl.

3. Place the reserved pear liquid in small glass bowl. Transfer 3 tablespoons to a second small glass bowl. Microwave the pear juice in the first bowl on HIGH for 45 seconds. Sprinkle the gelatin over the 3 tablespoons pear juice and stir well to partially dissolve it. Add the warm juice and stir again to fully dissolve the gelatin.

4. Add the gelatin mixture to the pear-pumpkin mixture. Whisk well to combine. Cover and refrigerate for 30 to 45 minutes to allow the gelatin to set.

5. Beat the whipping cream in a stand mixer or with a handheld mixer until soft peaks form. Add the sugar and vanilla and beat until firm peaks form.

6. Add the whipped cream to the pumpkin mixture; use the mixer to combine well. Refrigerate until you're ready to serve. To serve, divide among eight serving dishes. Store covered in the refrigerator for up to 4 days. Top with whipped cream, if desired, when you're ready to serve the mousse.

Per Serving: Calories 190; Protein 2 g; Carbs 23 g; Dietary Fiber 2 g; Added Sugars 10 g; Total Fat 11 g; Sat Fat 7 g; Omega-3s 40 mg; Sodium 14 mg; Potassium 87 mg

CRÈME FRAÎCHE

Crème fraiche is the French version of sour cream. Our buttermilk version is made by adding buttermilk to heavy whipping cream; our sour cream crème fraiche uses sour cream to achieve the same effect. Both versions have a tart flavor and a smooth, silky creaminess. A dollop of crème fraîche is a lovely finishing touch for fresh fruit and many fruit desserts, such as the Blueberry Crisp (page 353) and Cranberry-Pear Crisp (page 353), and is also delicious on our Strawberry Pancakes (page 135).

Buttermilk Crème Fraîche
Makes 1½ cups (360 g)

1 cup (240 ml) heavy whipping cream
½ cup (120 ml) cultured buttermilk

Sour Cream Crème Fraîche
Makes 2 cups (430 g)

1 cup (240 ml) heavy whipping cream
1 cup (190 g) cultured sour cream

1. Combine the whipping cream and buttermilk or sour cream in a medium glass bowl, glass jar with lid, or a 2-cup (480 ml) glass measuring cup. Stir, then loosely cover the top with plastic wrap. Let stand at room temperature until thickened to the consistency of softly whipped cream, about 12 hours.

2. Refrigerate for 4 to 6 hours before using. The crème fraîche will thicken and become tangier as it sits in the refrigerator. Store covered in the refrigerator for up to 2 weeks.

Buttermilk Crème Fraîche Serving Size 2 tablespoons; Calories 73; Protein 1 g; Carbs 1 g; Dietary Fiber 0 g; Added Sugars 0 g; Total Fat 7 g; Sat Fat 5 g; Omega-3s 30 mg; Sodium 25 mg; Potassium 35 mg

Sour Cream Crème Fraîche Serving Size 2 tablespoons; Calories 75; Protein 1 g; Carbs 1 g; Dietary Fiber 0 g; Added Sugars 0 g; Total Fat 8 g; Sat Fat 5 g; Omega-3s 30 mg; Sodium 8 mg; Potassium 29 mg

CITRUS CURD
Makes 1 cup (390 g)

This is a wonderful accompaniment on our Gingery Lemon Scones (page 97) and heightens the citrus flavors in our Almond-Orange or Almond-Lemon Cake (page 355).

Lemon Curd
⅔ cup (160 ml) fresh lemon juice
½ cup (100 g) sugar
2 large eggs, beaten
1 tablespoon butter or lemon-infused extra virgin olive oil
2 tablespoons grated lemon zest

Orange Curd
⅔ cup (160 ml) fresh orange juice
¼ cup (50 g) sugar
2 large eggs, beaten
1 tablespoon butter or blood orange–infused extra virgin olive oil
2 tablespoons grated orange zest

1. Heat the juice and sugar in a small saucepan over low heat. Stir continuously to dissolve the sugar, about 30 seconds. Slowly pour into the beaten eggs, whisking constantly. Whisk for another 30 seconds.

2. Whisk in the butter and zest. Cook over low heat, whisking slowly, until thickened, 2 to 4 minutes. Do not allow to simmer or boil.

3. Remove from the heat. Serve immediately, or store in an airtight container in the refrigerator for up to 2 weeks.

Lemon Curd Serving Size 2 tablespoons; Calories 84; Protein 2 g; Carbs 14 g; Dietary Fiber 0 g; Added Sugars 13 g; Total Fat 3 g; Sat Fat 1 g; Omega-3s 30 mg; Sodium 27 mg; Potassium 24 mg

Orange Curd Serving Size 2 tablespoons; Calories 89; Protein 2 g; Carbs 15 g; Dietary Fiber 0 g; Added Sugars 12 g; Total Fat 3 g; Sat Fat 1 g; Omega-3s 30 mg; Sodium 27 mg; Potassium 46 mg

SPICED GINGER CREAM

Makes 1 cup (120 g)

This whipped cream with sweet spices pairs with so many desserts, including Wine-Poached Pears (page 354), Almond-Orange Cake (page 355), and Apple Walnut Date Coffee Cake (page 356).

- ½ cup (120 ml) cold whipping cream
- 1 teaspoon confectioners' sugar
- ¼ teaspoon ground ginger
- ¼ teaspoon ground cinnamon
- ⅛ teaspoon ground nutmeg

1. Chill a medium glass or stainless-steel bowl and the beaters of a stand or handheld mixer in the freezer until very cold.

2. Pour the cream into the bowl. Whip with the mixer until soft peaks start to form. Add the sugar, ginger, cinnamon, and nutmeg. Beat until the cream holds soft peaks and the tops of the peaks gently fold down. Serve immediately or store in the refrigerator, loosely covered, for up to 8 hours.

Serving Size 2 tablespoons; Calories 24; Protein 0 g; Carbs 1 g; Dietary Fiber 0 g; Added Sugars 0 g; Total Fat 2 g; Sat Fat 1 g; Omega-3s 20 mg; Sodium 3 mg; Potassium 9 mg

BLUEBERRY GINGER YOGURT BARK WITH ALMONDS

Makes 12 to 15 pieces

A small amount of crystallized ginger adds a bit of bite to this good-for-you treat!

- 1 cup (230 g) plain Greek yogurt
- ½ cup (75 g) fresh blueberries
- ¼ cup (25 g) toasted slivered almonds
- 1 tablespoon chopped crystallized ginger
- 1 teaspoon grated lemon zest
- 1 teaspoon grated lime zest

1. Cut a piece of parchment paper to fit the bottom of a 9-inch (23 cm) pie plate or round cake pan.

2. Combine the yogurt, ¼ cup (40 g) of the blueberries, 2 tablespoons of the almonds, the ginger, lemon

zest, and lime zest in a medium bowl. Spoon the mixture into the pie plate. Use a rubber spatula or the back of the spoon to spread it evenly in a ¼-inch (6 mm) thick oval. Sprinkle the remaining blueberries and almonds over the top and press them into the yogurt.

3. Freeze for at least 4 hours, preferably overnight, to allow the bark to freeze solid. Use a knife to gently break the bark into 12 to 15 pieces of varying sizes. Store between wax paper layers in an airtight container in the freezer for up to 2 months.

Serving Size 2 to 3 pieces; Calories 69; Protein 6 g; Carbs 5 g; Dietary Fiber 1 g; Added Sugars 0 g; Total Fat 3 g; Sat Fat 1 g; Omega-3s 10 mg; Sodium 15 mg; Potassium 107 mg

CHOCOLATE CRANBERRY ALMOND CLUSTERS

Makes 12 clusters

This is a simple way to put together a sweet, satisfying chocolate treat. Adding a bit of orange zest may call up flavor memories of the chocolate oranges that appear in many homes during the Christmas holidays.

- 8 ounces (227 g) dark chocolate (55 to 65% cacao), cut into small chunks
- ½ cup (45 g) slivered almonds
- ½ cup (65 g) sweetened dried cranberries
- 1 teaspoon grated orange zest

1. Line a large flat baking sheet with parchment paper.

2. Place the chocolate in the top of a double boiler over medium-low heat. (If you don't have a double boiler, you can place a heatproof glass bowl on top of a saucepan filled with 1 inch/2.5 cm water. Make sure the bottom of the bowl does not touch the water.) Stir the chocolate frequently until melted, then stir in the almonds, cranberries, and orange zest.

3. Working quickly, drop the mixture by tablespoonfuls onto the parchment paper in a 4 × 3 pattern to create 12 clusters.

4. Place the baking sheet in the refrigerator for 45 to 60 minutes to allow the clusters to harden. Store between wax paper layers in an airtight container at room temperature for up to 1 week, in the refrigerator for up to 2 weeks, or in the freezer for up to 3 months.

Serving Size 1 cluster; Calories 149; Protein 2 g; Carbs 15 g; Dietary Fiber 2 g; Added Sugars 4 g; Total Fat 9 g; Sat Fat 4 g; Omega-3s 20 mg; Sodium 2 mg; Potassium 135 mg

PUMPKIN APPLE CRANBERRY GRANOLA BITES

Makes 24 bites

These bite-size energy balls travel well because they are baked as a finishing touch, making them firm and storable at room temperature. Although the flavors are reminiscent of fall, all the ingredients are readily available to make these crunchy, sweet-tart bites year-round.

- 2 cups (185 g) old-fashioned rolled oats, toasted
- ½ cup (45 g) chopped dried apples
- ½ cup (65 g) unsweetened dried cranberries, chopped
- ½ cup (55 g) coarsely chopped pecans
- ¼ cup (15 g) raw, unsalted, shelled pepitas (pumpkin seeds) or sunflower seeds
- 3 tablespoons ground flaxseed or hemp seeds
- 1 cup (245 g) canned 100% pure pumpkin (not pumpkin pie mix)
- ¼ cup (85 g) honey
- 2 tablespoons canola oil or extra virgin olive oil
- 1 tablespoon grated orange zest
- 1 teaspoon ground cinnamon
- 1 teaspoon ground ginger
- ½ teaspoon ground nutmeg
- ¼ teaspoon ground cloves
- ⅛ teaspoon kosher salt

1. Preheat the oven to 350°F (180°C). Line a large rimmed baking sheet with parchment paper.

2. Combine the oats, apples, cranberries, pecans, pepitas, and flaxseed in a large bowl. Whisk the pumpkin, honey, oil, orange zest, cinnamon, ginger, nutmeg, and cloves in a medium bowl. Pour the wet ingredients into the dry ingredients and mix well to combine. Form into twenty-four 1½-inch (4 cm) balls

and place them 1 inch (2.5 cm) apart on the baking sheet.

3. Bake for about 15 minutes, until the balls are firm and lightly browned. Transfer to a wire rack to cool. Store in an airtight container at room temperature for up to 5 days or in the freezer for up to 3 months.

Serving Size 2 bites; Calories 185; Protein 3 g; Carbs 27 g; Dietary Fiber 4 g; Added Sugars 9 g; Total Fat 8 g; Sat Fat 1 g; Omega-3s 660 mg; Sodium 13 mg; Potassium 126 mg

References

CHAPTER 1

Appel, L. J., T. J. Moore, E. Obarzanek, et al. (DASH Collaborative Research Group.) "A Clinical Trial of the Effects of Dietary Patterns on Blood Pressure." *New England Journal of Medicine* 336, no. 16 (1997): 1117–1124.

Chiu, S., N. Bergeron, P. T. Williams, et al. "Comparison of the DASH (Dietary Approaches to Stop Hypertension) Diet and a Higher-Fat DASH Diet on Blood Pressure and Lipids and Lipoproteins: A Randomized Controlled Trial." *American Journal of Clinical Nutrition* 103, no. 2 (2016): 341–347.

Delichatsios, H. K., and F. K. Welty. "Influence of the DASH Diet and Other Low-Fat, High-Carbohydrate Diets on Blood Pressure." *Current Atherosclerosis Reports* 7, no. 6 (2005): 446–454.

Estruch, R., E. Ros, J. Salas-Salvadó, et al. (PREDIMED Study Investigators). "Primary Prevention of Cardiovascular Disease with a Mediterranean Diet Supplemented with Extra-Virgin Olive Oil or Nuts." *New England Journal of Medicine* 378, no.25, e34 (2018).

Hu, F. B. "Are Refined Carbohydrates Worse Than Saturated Fat?" *American Journal of Clinical Nutrition* 91, no. 6 (2010):1541–1542.

Liu, X., M. C. Morris, K. Dhana, et al. "Mediterranean-DASH Intervention for Neurodegenerative Delay (MIND) Study: Rationale, Design and Baseline Characteristics of a Randomized Control Trial of the MIND Diet on Cognitive Decline." *Contemporary Clinical Trials* 102, no. 106270 (2021).

Morris, M. C., C. C. Tangney, Y. Wang, et al. (2015). "MIND Diet Slows Cognitive Decline with Aging." *Alzheimer's & Dementia: The Journal of the Alzheimer's Association*, 11, no. 9 (2015): 1015–1022.

National Institute on Aging. https://www.nia.nih.gov/health/what-do-we-know-about-diet-and-prevention-alzheimers-disease, accessed December 2, 2021.

Seven Countries Study, The. https://www.sevencountriesstudy.com, accessed December 1, 2021.

Simopoulos, A. P. "The Mediterranean Diets: What Is So Special About the Diet of Greece? The Scientific Evidence." *Journal of Nutrition*, 131, no. 11 Suppl (2001): 3065S–73S.

Trichopoulos, Dr. Dimitrios. Quote as shared by Greg Drescher of The Culinary Institute of America on stage at the college's Worlds of Healthy Flavors Leadership Retreats during many education sessions focused on strategies for increasing vegetable consumption in the United States.

World Health Organization Hypertension Facts Page. https://www.who.int/news-room/fact-sheets/detail/hypertension, accessed December 1, 2021.

CHAPTER 2

Bitok, E., and J. Sabaté. (2018). "Nuts and Cardiovascular Disease." *Progress in Cardiovascular Diseases* 61, no. 1 (2018): 33–37.

Blesso, C. N., and M. L. Fernandez. "Dietary Cholesterol, Serum Lipids, and Heart Disease: Are Eggs Working For or Against You?" *Nutrients* 10, no. 4 (2018): 426.

Burd, N. A., J. W. Beals, I. G. Martinez, et al. (2019). "Food-First Approach to Enhance the Regulation of Post-Exercise Skeletal Muscle Protein Synthesis and Remodeling." *Sports Medicine* (Auckland, NZ) 49, Suppl 1: 59–68.

Dehghan, M., A. Mente, S. Rangarajan, et al. "Association of Egg Intake with Blood Lipids, Cardiovascular Disease, and Mortality in 177,000 People in 50 Countries." *American Journal of Clinical Nutrition* 111, no. 4 (2020): 795–803.

Delgado, C., and J. X. Guinard. "Sensory Properties of Californian and Imported Extra Virgin Olive Oils." *Journal of Food Science* 76, no. 3 (2011): S170–S176.

DiNicolantonio, J. J., and J. H. O'Keefe. (2020). "The Importance of Marine Omega-3s for Brain Development and the Prevention and Treatment of Behavior, Mood, and Other Brain Disorders." *Nutrients* 12, no. 8 (2020): 2333.

Ditano-Vázquez, P., J. D. Torres-Peña, F. Galeano-Valle, et al. (2019). "The Fluid Aspect of the Mediterranean Diet in the Prevention and Management of Cardiovascular Disease and Diabetes: The Role of Polyphenol Content in Moderate Consumption of Wine and Olive Oil." *Nutrients* 11, no. 11(2019): 2833.

Duyff, Roberta L., John R. Mount, and Joshua B. Jones. "Sodium Reduction in Canned Beans After Draining, Rinsing." *Journal of Culinary Science & Technology* 9, no. 2 (2011): 106–112.

Ertl, P., W. Knaus, and W. Zollitsch. (2016). "An Approach to Including Protein Quality When Assessing the Net Contribution of Livestock to Human Food Supply." *Animal: An International Journal of Animal Bioscience* 10, no. 11 (2016): 1883–1889.

Food and Agriculture Organization of the United Nations. "Food Wastage: Key Facts and Figures." https://www.fao.org/news/story/en/item/196402/icode/, accessed December 7, 2021.

Frankel, E. N. (2010). "Chemistry of Extra Virgin Olive Oil: Adulteration, Oxidative Stability, and Antioxidants." *Journal of Agricultural and Food Chemistry* 58, no. 10 (2010): 5991–6006.

Geiker, N., M. L. Larsen., J. Dyerberg, et al. "Egg Consumption, Cardiovascular Diseases and Type 2 Diabetes." *European Journal of Clinical Nutrition* 72, no. 1 (2018): 44–56.

Goodrow, E. F., T. A. Wilson, S. C. Houde, et al. "Consumption of One Egg Per Day Increases Serum Lutein and Zeaxanthin Concentrations in Older Adults Without Altering Serum Lipid and Lipoprotein Cholesterol Concentrations." *Journal of Nutrition* 136, no. 10 (2006): 2519–2524.

Gorzynik-Debicka, M., P. Przychodzen, F. Cappello, et al. "Potential Health Benefits of Olive Oil and Plant Polyphenols." *International Journal of Molecular Sciences* 19, no. 3 (2018): 686.

Greenfield, H., D. McCullum, and R. B. Wills. "Sodium and Potassium Contents of Salts, Salt Substitutes, and Other Seasonings." *Medical Journal of Australia* 140, no. 8 (1984): 460–462.

Hansson, P., K. B. Holven, L. Øyri, et al. "Meals with Similar Fat Content from Different Dairy Products Induce Different Postprandial Triglyceride Responses in Healthy Adults: A Randomized Controlled Cross-Over Trial." *Journal of Nutrition* 149, no. 3 (2019): 422–431.

Harnack, L. J., M. E. Cogswell, J. M. Shikany, et al. "Sources of Sodium in US Adults From 3 Geographic Regions." *Circulation* 135, no. 19 (2017): 1775–1783.

Herreman, L., P. Nommensen, B. Pennings, and M.C. Laus. "Comprehensive Overview of the Quality of Plant- and Animal-Sourced Proteins Based on the Digestible Indispensable Amino Acid Score." *Food Science & Nutrition* 8, no. 10 (2020): 5379–5391.

Hoffman, R., and M. Gerber. "Food Processing and the Mediterranean Diet." *Nutrients* 7, no. 9 (2015): 7925–7964.

Huth, P. J., and K. M. Park. "Influence of Dairy Product and Milk Fat Consumption on Cardiovascular Disease Risk: A Review of the Evidence." *Advances in Nutrition* 3, no. 3 (2012): 266–285.

Kessler, David. *Fast Carbs, Slow Carbs: The Simple Truth About Food, Weight, and Disease*. New York: Harper Wave, 2020.

King, J. C., and J. L. Slavin. "White Potatoes, Human Health, and Dietary Guidance." *Advances in Nutrition* 4, no. 3 (2013): 393S–401S.

Lai, H. T., M. C. de Oliveira Otto, R. N. Lemaitre, et al. "Serial Circulating Omega 3 Polyunsaturated Fatty Acids and Healthy Ageing Among Older Adults in the Cardiovascular Health Study: Prospective Cohort Study." *BMJ* 363, k4067 (2018).

Li, Q., Y. Cui, R. Jin, et al. "Enjoyment of Spicy Flavor Enhances Central Salty-Taste Perception and Reduces Salt Intake and Blood Pressure." *Hypertension* 70, no. 6 (2017): 1291–1299.

Liu, G., M. Guasch-Ferré, Y. Hu, et al. "Nut Consumption in Relation to Cardiovascular Disease Incidence and Mortality Among Patients with Diabetes Mellitus." *Circulation Research* 124, no. 6 (2019): 920–929.

Marinangeli, C., and J. D. House. "Potential Impact of the Digestible Indispensable Amino Acid Score as a Measure of Protein Quality on Dietary Regulations and Health." *Nutrition Reviews* 75, no. 8 (2017): 658–667.

McGill, C. R., A. C. Kurilich, and J. Davignon. "The Role of Potatoes and Potato Components in Cardiometabolic Health: A Review. *Annals of Medicine* 45, no. 7 (2013): 467–473.

Moeller, S. M., P. F. Jacques, and J. B. Blumberg. "The Potential Role of Dietary Xanthophylls in Cataract and Age-Related Macular Degeneration." *Journal of the American College of Nutrition* 19, no. 5 Suppl (2000): 522S–527S.

Nestel, P. J., N. Mellett, S. Pally, et al. "Effects of Low-Fat Or Full-Fat Fermented and Non-Fermented Dairy Foods on Selected Cardiovascular Biomarkers in Overweight Adults." *British Journal of Nutrition* 110, no. 12 (2013): 2242–2249.

Nosworthy, M. G., G. Medina, A. J. Franczyk, et al. "Effect of Processing on the In Vitro and In Vivo Protein Quality of Beans (*Phaseolus vulgaris* and *Vicia Faba*)." *Nutrients* 10, no. 6 (2018): 671.

O'Connor, L. E., D. Paddon-Jones, A. J. Wright, and W. W. Campbell. "A Mediterranean-Style Eating Pattern with Lean, Unprocessed Red Meat Has Cardiometabolic Benefits for Adults Who Are Overweight Or Obese in a Randomized, Crossover, Controlled Feeding Trial." *American Journal of Clinical Nutrition* 108, no. 1 (2018): 33–40.

Pan, A., Q. Sun, J. E. Manson, et al. "Walnut consumption is associated with lower risk of type 2 diabetes in women." *Journal of Nutrition* 143, no. 4 (2013): 512–518.

Phillips S. M. "Current Concepts and Unresolved Questions in Dietary Protein Requirements and Supplements in Adults." *Frontiers in Nutrition* 4, no. 13 (2017).

Potato Glory Nutrition Information. https://www.potatoglory.com, accessed December 7, 2021.

ReFED. https://refed.org, accessed December 7, 2021.

Santangelo, C., R. Vari, B. Scazzocchio, et al. "Anti-Inflammatory Activity of Extra Virgin Olive Oil Polyphenols: Which Role in the Prevention and Treatment of Immune-Mediated Inflammatory Diseases?" *Endocrine, Metabolic & Immune Disorders Drug Targets* 18, no. 1 (2018): 36–50.

Shi, J., and M. Le Maguer. "Lycopene in tomatoes: chemical and physical properties affected by food processing." *Critical Reviews in Biotechnology* 20, no. 4 (2000): 293–334.

Sun, W., B. Frost, and J. Liu. "Oleuropein, unexpected benefits!" *Oncotarget* 8, no. 11 (2017): 17409.

U.S. Food and Drug Administration. https://www.fda.gov/consumers/consumer-updates/eating-too-much-salt-ways-cut-backgradually, accessed January 17, 2022.

Wallace, T. C., R. Bailey, J. B. Blumberg, et al. "Fruits, Vegetables, and Health: A Comprehensive Narrative, Umbrella Review of the Science and Recommendations for Enhanced Public Policy to Improve Intake." *Critical Reviews in Food Science and Nutrition* 60, no. 13 (2020): 2174–2211.

Yamaguchi, S., and K. Ninomiya. "Umami and Food Palatability." *Journal of Nutrition* 130, no. 4S Suppl (2000): 921S–6S.

SMOOTHIES

Mathai, J. K., Y. Liu, and H. H. Stein. "Values for Digestible Indispensable Amino Acid Scores (DIAAS) for Some Dairy and Plant Proteins May Better Describe Protein Quality Than Values Calculated Using the Concept for Protein Digestibility-Corrected Amino Acid Scores (PDCAAS)." *British Journal of Nutrition* 117, no. 4 (2017): 490–499.

Marinangeli, C., and J. D. House. "Potential Impact of the Digestible Indispensable Amino Acid Score as a Measure of Protein Quality on Dietary Regulations and Health." *Nutrition Reviews* 75, no. 8 (2017): 658–667.

U.S. Department of Agriculture, Agricultural Research Service. FoodData Central, 2019. fdc.nal.usda.gov.

MEDITERRANEAN BEANS & GREENS SMOOTHIE

Bi, H., Y. Gan, C. Yang, et al. "Breakfast Skipping and the Risk of Type 2 Diabetes: A Meta-Analysis of Observational Studies." *Public Health Nutrition* 18, no. 16 (2015): 3013–3019.

Kaplan, A., H. Zelicha, G. Tsaban, et al. "Protein Bioavailability of Wolffia Globosa Duckweed, A Novel Aquatic Plant—A Randomized Controlled Trial." *Clinical Nutrition* 38, no. 6 (2019): 2576–2582.

Ma, X., Q. Chen, Y. Pu, et al. "Skipping Breakfast Is Associated with Overweight and Obesity: A Systematic Review and Meta-Analysis." *Obesity Research & Clinical Practice* 14, no. 1 (2020): 1–8.

O'Neil, C. E., T. A. Nicklas, and V. L. Fulgoni III. "Nutrient Intake, Diet Quality, and Weight/Adiposity Parameters in Breakfast Patterns Compared with No Breakfast in Adults: National Health and Nutrition Examination Survey 2001–2008." *Journal of the Academy of Nutrition and Dietetics* 114, no. 12 Suppl (2014): S27–S43.

Rong, S., L. G. Snetselaar, G. Xu, et al. (2019). "Association of Skipping Breakfast with Cardiovascular and All-Cause Mortality." *Journal of the American College of Cardiology* 73, no. 16 (2019): 2025–2032.

Takagi, H., Y. Hari, K. Nakashima, et al., for ALICE (All-Literature Investigation of Cardiovascular Evidence) Group. "Meta-Analysis of Relation of Skipping Breakfast with Heart Disease." *American Journal of Cardiology* 124, no. 6 (2019): 978–986.

Tsaban, G., A. Yaskolka Meir, E. Rinott, et al. "The Effect of Green Mediterranean Diet on Cardiometabolic Risk; A Randomised Controlled Trial." *Heart* (British Cardiac Society) heartjnl-2020-317802 advance online publication (2020).

Tsaban, G., A. Yaskolka Meir, H. Zelicha, et al. "Diet-Induced Fasting Ghrelin Elevation Reflects the Recovery of Insulin Sensitivity and Visceral Adiposity Regression." *Journal of Clinical Endocrinology and Metabolism* dgab681 advance online publication (2021).

Yaskolka Meir, A., E. Rinott, G. Tsaban, et al. "Effect of Green-Mediterranean Diet on Intrahepatic Fat: The DIRECT PLUS Randomised Controlled Trial." *Gut* 70, no. 11 (2021): 2085–2095.

BEEF & MUSHROOM BURGERS

Myrdal Miller, A., K. Mills, T. Wong, et al. "Flavor-Enhancing Properties of Mushrooms in Meat-Based Dishes in Which Sodium Has Been Reduced and Meat Has Been Partially Substituted with Mushrooms." *Journal of Food Science* 79, no. 9 (2014): S1795–S1804.

PERFECT PASTA PREP

Ostmann, B. and J. Baker, *The Recipe Writer's Handbook*. New York: John Wiley & Sons, 2001.

TABLE 8: COOKING PULSES FROM DRY

Bean Institute, The. https://beaninstitute.com/cook-with-beans-overview/.

USA Pulses. https://www.usapulses.org/consumers/get-cooking.

SIMPLY ROASTED GARLIC

Ried, K., C. Toben, and P. Fakler. "Effect of Garlic on Serum Lipids: An Updated Meta-Analysis." *Nutrition Reviews* 71, no. 5 (2013): 282–299.

FOOD SAFETY & QUALITY GUIDELINES FOR COOKING BEEF, VEAL, LAMB & PORK

United States Department of Agriculture (USDA). Safe Minimum Cooking Temperatures Chart. https://www.foodsafety.gov/food-safety-charts/safe-minimum-cooking-temperature.

BLUEBERRY GINGER YOGURT BARK WITH ALMONDS

Koo, J. Y., Y. Jang, H. Cho, et al. (2007). Hydroxy-alpha-sanshool Activates TRPV1 and TRPA1 in Sensory Neurons. *European Journal of Neuroscience* 26, no. 5 (2007): 1139–1147.

Zhang Q. B., L. Zhao H. Y. Gao, et al. "The Enhancement of the Perception of Saltiness By Sichuan Pepper Oleoresin in a NaCl Model Solution." *Food Research International* 136, no. 109581 (October 2020). doi: 10.1016/j.foodres.2020.109581. Epub 2020 Jul 24. PMID: 32846612.

Acknowledgments

Linda Hachfeld would like to thank:

Matthew Lore and Peter Burri, *for believing in me . . .*

My grandmothers, Henrietta and Emma, for their warm, cozy kitchens that produced ten loaves of bread at a time and the best stick-to-your-ribs goulash, providing me with my first cup of milk-coffee (today's latte) at a time when children weren't allowed to drink coffee. *Thank you for showing me that the kitchen is the best place to be, people matter, it's OK to bend a few rules, and love is what makes life better.*

My mother, Betty Jane, and mother-in-law, Marcella, who spent copious amounts of time in large gardens and year-round in their kitchens, for welcoming me into the kitchen to bake to my heart's content and experiment with new recipes, and for deeming my cooking efforts worthy. *Thank you for your dedication, encouragement, and, by your example, teaching me that the kitchen is the heart of the home.*

My late husband, Gary, and my children, Ed and Alicia, for their unconditional love and support. *Thank you, dear ones, for your fortitude as we go through the wide and narrow spaces in life's hourglass together.*

My lifelong friends Barb Druar Schmidt, my rhubarb conspirator and bake-off opponent; Alice Blume Schoon, a whole foods and gardening extraordinaire; Ginny Bird, a fabulous listener who keeps me on my toes with her food-related questions; Nancy Fogelberg, Susan McPartland, and Nancy Wendt, WEB buddies who lean in and are gifted in finding the humor in most situations; Patrice Mosley Mc-Clafferty and the late Alice Griffiths, college chums who cooked, crammed, and celebrated dietetics milestones; Karen Holtmeier, my steadfast FNCE traveling companion, fellow nutrition entrepreneur, and confidante; and Mary McComb, faithful recipe tester and consummate assistant. *Thank you for your friendship, caring hearts, and sage advice.*

My instructors, the late Julia Rowe, Beth Zimmer, the late Aileen Eick, and Pat Splett, my home economics, culinary, nutrition and dietetics mentors years ago and friends ever since. *Thank you for introducing me to the science of nutrition and for instilling the joy to be had in the pursuit of excellence.*

There would have been no first edition of *Cooking à la Heart* without the stimulus of the NIH-funded community research grant written and led by principal investigator Henry Blackburn, MD, at the University of Minnesota, Division of Epidemiology in the School of Public Health. Mankato, the first of three communities, embraced the importance of lifestyle in reducing the risks to prevent heart disease and stroke. Once aware, residents repeatedly requested practical, affordable, and delicious recipes to make healthy meals at home. *Thank you, Dr. Blackburn and your outstanding team of researchers and colleagues, in establishing the Minnesota Heart Health Program, which, in turn, created the Mankato Heart Health Program and sister programs in the communities of Fargo/Moorhead and Bloomington.*

A dedicated team of community volunteers answered the call for a heart-health cookbook and together we orchestrated its development. Members included the late Betsy Eykyn (coauthor), Nadine Sugden, Shirley Durfee, and the late Marion Lutes. Harland Bloomer, art instructor and designer, contributed his expertise in designing a cookbook with lasting appeal that reached far beyond the heart health programs. *I can't thank my fellow cookbook steering committee colleagues and recipe testers enough for their generous three-year commitment to define and triple-taste-test more than 450 recipes.*

Through Appletree Press, a small independent publishing house, Cooking à la Heart *enjoyed a revised second and third edition, earning accolades from food editors and awards of distinction for publishing excellence. The first through third editions of* Cooking à la Heart *achieved over 100,000 book sales, making it a bestseller whose proceeds went back to the community to fund various health-promoting projects.*

Cooking à la Heart, the fourth edition, also required a dedicated team of professionals to whom I owe much and am humbled by their contributions.

Hannah Thompson, a capable, trained culinary chef and recent graduate in dietetics, delightfully joined me (although too briefly) at the beginning of this undertaking. Her contributions were impactful, as she helped define dishes that speak to today's home chefs. *Hannah, someday, you will generate your own unique and successful cookbook; I wish you greatness as you explore more opportunities in the field of food, nutrition, and dietetics.*

Amy Myrdal Miller, my fearless and remarkable coauthor who said "Yes!" over the phone to someone she had never met, when invited to join me on rewriting *Cooking à la Heart.* You do not know my joy in discovering you, a fellow small business owner and nutrition entrepreneur. The skills of starting, growing, and tending a business are, no doubt, the same skills needed to develop this book. *Thank you for your willingness to step up to the challenge, for the fine work you've done, and for weaving your unique style and voice throughout the book. Your enthusiasm is persuasive, and I congratulate you on the completion of your first book.*

The Experiment editors Olivia Peluso, Hannah Matuszak, Zach Pace, Suzanne Fass, and Valerie Saint-Rossy. *Thank you for reading every word written, guiding it and when needed, making it better.* Beth Bugler, creative director; Sarah Hone, photographer; Melissa Mileto, food stylist; and the studio, OMS Photo, for shaping and transforming a massive amount of information into an appealing and lasting presentation that identifies and makes *Cooking à la Heart* unique. *Thank you for addressing the one request heard over and over: "Please add food photos." With all my heart, I appreciate and thank you for bringing our recipes to life. By showcasing their vibrant color, freshness, and the promise of fantastic flavor, you encourage our readers to look forward to cooking à la heart with joy in their kitchens.*

From Amy

I first need to thank my sweet, kind, generous, loving husband, Scott Miller, for his support and encouragement in all I do. He was an eager and honest taste tester throughout the recipe development process and an empathetic partner during the angst of multiple rounds of edits.

I owe much of my kitchen confidence and competence to my mom, Rosemarie Myrdal, who encouraged me to start cooking shortly after I was diagnosed with type 1 diabetes when I was seven. She knew my being able to cook would contribute immensely to my diabetes self-management skills and success.

My passion for farming and how food is produced comes from my dad, John Myrdal, who would start every supper table conversation with a review of the weather, how the crops and cattle were doing, what crop prices looked like, and what additional hard work would be needed to financially sustain the farm for another day, week, month, or year. My respect for the men and women who grow and produce food for the rest of us stems from the lessons my dad taught me through his words, work ethic, and actions.

Throughout my career, I have been blessed with bosses and mentors who encouraged me to pursue projects that fed my interest in the food and culinary world. Dr. James Rippe gave me the opportunity to collaborate with him on two books early in my career when I worked at the Rippe Lifestyle Institute, a clinical research firm that focused on improving cardiovascular health through diet and lifestyle changes. Dr. Lorelei DiSogra hired me to work for her at Dole Food Company, where her leadership in motivating people to eat more fruits and vegetables led me to pursue opportunities in this area. Greg Drescher gave me the opportunity to work for The Culinary Institute of America, where I got to learn about food cultures from around the world. Chefs John Ash, Iliana de la Vega, Joyce Goldstein, and Suvir Saran were especially generous when sharing their knowledge with me.

My cookbook collection wouldn't be nearly as complete without the many gifts presented by Roberta Klugman, who also spearheaded my nomination for Les Dames d'Escoffier International. Roberta has also given me numerous opportunities to learn about and appreciate extra virgin olive oil, offering oils from top California producers as well as invitations to olive sensory courses, orchard and mill tours, and tasting events.

And, of course, there are my many mentors who have soothed my spirit, boosted my ego, and coached me through chaos since the early days of my career, including Sue Borra, Carol Berg Sloan, Catharine Powers, Mary Kimbrough, Mary Christ-Erwin, and Barb Pyper.

My best friend Dana Zartner has been one of my most enthusiastic cheerleaders during so many seminal moments of my career, but especially while working on this book. I'm very blessed; Dana is among a large group of friends and family members who in ways great and small have supported me throughout my career and the writing of this book.

Speaking of this book, I must thank our editor Olivia Peluso for her soothing, joyful spirit and thoughtfulness with edits and queries. Her work pushed Linda and me to refine our messaging in subtle yet impactful ways.

Finally, I am very grateful Linda Hachfeld invited me to collaborate with her on this project. I admire her wit and wisdom, appreciate her sense of humor, and am honored by her friendship and faith in me.

Index

NOTE: Page numbers in *italics* refer to photos.

A

Adobo Seasoning, 30
Ahi Burgers with Wasabi-Ginger Slaw, 177
À la Heart Caesar Dressing, 47
À la Heart Classic Pizza Dough, 194
À la Heart House Dressing, *40*, 47
À la Heart Mexican-Inspired Mac & Cheese,
    206–7
À la Heart Olive Oil Brownies, 355
À la Heart Rice & Beans Bowl, 242
À la Heart Velouté Sauce, 52
Alfredo Sauce, 52–53
allspice, 271
almonds
    Almond-Crusted Chicken Strips, 303
    Almond-Orange Cake, 355–56
    Blueberry Ginger Yogurt Bark with
        Almonds, 362
    Chicken-Almond Stir-Fry with Carrots,
        Snow Peas & Plums, 304–5
    Chocolate Cranberry Almond Clusters,
        362–63
    Cranberry-Almond Coffee Cake, 98–99
    Crispy Almond Chicken Bowl, 310
    Moroccan-Spiced Almonds, 346
    Roasted Almond-Crusted Snapper, 291
    Strawberries with Almond-Oat Crumble,
        354
    Vegetable-Almond Rice with Parmesan, 233
Angel Hair Pasta with Tomatoes & Basil, 207
apples
    Apple-Cinnamon Compote, 128
    Apple-Cinnamon Galette with Gingerbread
        Crust, 352
    Apple-Cinnamon Pancakes, 128
    Apple Dutch Baby, 129
    Apple-Walnut Bread, 100–101
    Apple Walnut Date Coffee Cake, 356
    Arugula, Apple & Fennel Salad with
        Gorgonzola, 146
    Honey-Ginger Chicken & Apples, 312
    Pumpkin Apple Cranberry Granola Bites,
        363
    Roasted Sweet Potatoes & Ginger-Spiced
        Apples, 273
    Simply Roasted Root Vegetables with
        Apples, *252*, 261
    Spinach Salad with Honeycrisp Apples &
        Cheddar, 148
apricots
    Apricot & Sesame Roasted Carrots, 266
    Apricot-Chickpea Smoothie, 138, *138*
    Barley with Stone Fruit, 130
    Nutty Apricot Cottage Cheese Bread, 104
    Turkey & Squash Couscous with Apricots &
        Peanuts, 318–19
artichoke hearts
    Artichoke & Onions with Lemon & Thyme,
        263
    Chicken with Artichokes & Capers, 309–10

Italian Pasta Salad, 210
arugula
    Arugula, Apple & Fennel Salad with
        Gorgonzola, 146
    Pan-Seared White Fish, Arugula & Roasted
        Tomato Salad, 166
asparagus
    Asparagus with Sesame & Ginger, 263–64
    Crab, Asparagus & Avocado Salad, 163
    Creamy Asparagus Soup, 74–75
    Pasta Primavera, 211
Autumn Wild Rice & Chicken Bowls, 159
avocados
    Avocado Lemon Dill Aïoli, 43, *288*
    Avocado Lime Cilantro Aïoli, 44
    Avocado Salsa, 61
    Crab, Asparagus & Avocado Salad, 163
    Kefir, Spinach & Avocado Smoothie, 139, *139*
    Sausage, Egg & Avocado Breakfast
        Sandwiches, *116*, 124

B

bacon, Canadian, 242–43
Baked Beans with Maple Syrup, 242
Baked Beans with Pomegranate & Canadian
    Bacon, 242–43
Baked Ricotta, 341
Balsamic Vinaigrette, 170
bananas
    Banana Nut Bread, 101
    Banana Oat Blueberry Breakfast Bars,
        129–30
    Mixed Fruit with Yogurt-Cardamom
        Dressing, 144
barley
    Barley with Stone Fruit, 130
    Greek-Flavor Beef & Barley Bowls, 326–27
    Roasted Mushroom–Barley Pilaf, 223
    Simply Cooked Barley, 223
basil
    Angel Hair Pasta with Tomatoes & Basil,
        207
    Basil Pesto, 45
    Lemon-Basil Dressing, 152
    Tomato-Basil Soup, 83
beans
    À la Heart Caesar Dressing, 47
    À la Heart Mexican-Inspired Mac & Cheese,
        206–7
    À la Heart Rice & Beans Bowl, 242
    Baked Beans with Maple Syrup, 242
    Baked Beans with Pomegranate & Canadian
        Bacon, 242–43
    Bean & Baby Kale Frittata, 119
    Chicken & Bean Burritos, 186–87
    Chicken Chili Verde, 85–86
    Cooking À la Heart Salad, 168–69
    Four-Bean Salad, 169
    Mexican Black Bean Soup, 76–77
    Mexican-Inspired Egg & Veggie Skillet,
        122–23
    Midwestern Beef, Bean & Beer Chili, 87

Parmesan-Garlic Bean Dip, *336*, 342
Potato Salad with Red Wine Vinaigrette, 154,
    154–55
Quinoa & Black Bean Medley, 228
Red Beans & Rice, 243
Refried Beans, 243–44
Rotisserie Chicken & Farro Soup with
    Cannellini Beans, 82
Salade Niçoise, 166–67
Salmon & White Bean Bowl with Lime &
    Dill, 244
Simply Cooked Black Beans, 241
Simply Cooked White Beans, 241
Simply Roasted Green Beans, 258
Southwestern Beef & Bean Burgers, 180–81
Spicy Black Bean Chili, 244–45
White Bean Salad with Lemon & Rosemary,
    245
Béchamel, 53
beef
    Beef & Lentil Salad Bowls, 160
    Beef & Mushroom Burgers, 178
    Beef & Mushroom Taco Filling, 183
    Beef & Vegetable Kabobs, 324
    Beef & Vegetable Stir-Fry, 324–25
    Classic Beef Stroganoff, 325
    Easy Weeknight Ground Beef Stroganoff,
        325
    French-Style Beef Stew, 326
    Gorgonzola & Beef Piadine with Arugula
        Salad, 196–97
    grass-fed, 23
    Greek-Flavor Beef & Barley Bowls, 326–27
    Italian-Inspired Beef & Farro Bowls, *320*, 327
    Midwestern Beef, Bean & Beer Chili, 87
    Quebec City Shepherd's Pie (Pâté Chinois),
        328
    Sheet Pan Tri-Tip Roast, 328–29
    Smoked Tri-Tip, 329
    Southwestern Beef & Bean Burgers, 180–81
    Spaghetti with Meat Sauce, 215–16
    Spanish-Style Beef & Brown Rice Bowls, 330
    Spicy Shredded Beef Street Tacos, *174*, 186
    Super Savory Sloppy Joes, 181
    Swedish Meatballs, 330
beef bones, 69–70
Beef Stock, 69–70
beer
    Beer Breadsticks with Fennel, 106–7
    Midwestern Beef, Bean & Beer Chili, 87
beets
    Borscht, 73–74
    Citrus-Roasted Beets, 264
    Citrusy Golden Beet Salad, 148
berries
    Berries with Cannoli Cream, 351
    Berry-Turmeric Smoothie, 138, *138*
    Mixed Berry Compote, 134
    See also specific berries
blueberries
    Banana Oat Blueberry Breakfast Bars,
        129–30

blueberries (continued)
  Blueberry Crisp, *348*, 353
  Blueberry Ginger Yogurt Bark with
    Almonds, 362
  Blueberry Muffins, 94
  Blueberry Oat Flax Scones, 96–97
  Lemon-Blueberry Bread, 102–3
  Watermelon, Grapefruit & Blueberry Salad,
    145
Blue Cheese Vinaigrette, 48
bok choy
  Beef & Vegetable Stir-Fry, 324–25
  Simply Stir-Fried Vegetables, 262
  Very Veggie Miso Soup, 84
Borscht, 73–74
Bouquet Garni, 30
bran cereal, 94–95
bread
  Garlic & Herb Bread Crumbs, 33
  Parmesan-Herb Croutons, 172–73
  Very Veggie Grilled Cheese Sandwiches,
    182–83
bread crumbs
  Potato-Turnip Gratin, *278*, 278–79
  Savory Nut Crumb Topping, 36
Breaded Chicken Tenders with Herbs, 304
broccoli
  Beef & Vegetable Stir-Fry, 324–25
  Broccoli & Corn Salad, 149
  Broccoli with Coriander & Tomatoes, 264
  Cooking À la Heart Salad, 168–69
  Sheet Pan Chicken, Broccoli & Red Peppers,
    316
  Simply Stir-Fried Vegetables, 262
Broccoli Slaw, 149
Broiled Halibut with Pesto, 284
Brown Bag Popcorn with Herb Seasonings,
  344
Brown Rice with Pine Nuts & Roasted
  Butternut Squash, 230
Brussels sprouts, 265
bulgur
  Bulgur & Tomato Salad with Mint, 224–25
  Bulgur Breakfast Porridge with Sausage, 120
  Bulgur Sauté with Pomegranate &
    Pistachios, 224
  Bulgur-Stuffed Peppers, 275
  Bulgur-Tomato Salad with Tuna & Mint, 160
  Simply Cooked Bulgur, 224
  Tabbouleh, 225
  Turkish-Inspired Bulgur–Sweet Potato
    Patties, 225–26
Buttermilk Rolls, 107

C
cabbage
  Borscht, 73–74
  Napa Cabbage Slaw, 153
  Radish & Cabbage Slaw, 154
  Simply Stewed Cabbage, 257
  Southeast Asian–Style Shrimp & Napa
    Cabbage Salad with Rice Noodles, 167
  Tangy Sautéed Red Cabbage, 265
Cajun Seasoning, 30
Cajun-Spiced Peanuts, 345
capers, 309–10
Caramelized Garlic Sauce, 53
caraway seeds, 331
cardamom
  Cardamom & Orange Roasted Carrots, 266

  Lemon Cardamom Chickpea Muffins, *90*, 95
  Yogurt-Cardamom Dressing, 52
carrots
  Apricot & Sesame Roasted Carrots, 266
  Cardamom & Orange Roasted Carrots, 266
  Carrot & Fig Oats with Pistachios, 130
  Carrot & Pineapple Couscous Salad, 146
  Carrot Bran Muffins, 94–95
  Carrot Cake with Pecans, 357
  Chicken-Almond Stir-Fry with Carrots,
    Snow Peas & Plums, 304–5
  Citrus-Glazed Carrots, 265–66
  Curiously Compatible Cucumbers & Carrots,
    268–69
  Fennel & Pear Roasted Carrots, 266–67
  Herb-Roasted Turkey Breast with
    Vegetables, *40*, 317–18
  Italian Pasta Salad, 210
  Maple & Herb Roasted Carrots, 267
  Marinated Vegetable Salad, 152–53
  Pork Banh Mi Burgers, 180
  Simply Roasted Carrots, 257
  Simply Roasted Root Vegetables with
    Apples, *252*, 261
  Simply Steamed Vegetable Medley, 262
  Simply Stir-Fried Vegetables, 262
  Spicy North African-Style Carrot Dip, *337*,
    343
cashews
  Chicken Teriyaki with Soba Noodles &
    Cashews, 308
  Creamy Curry-Cashew Dip, 342
  Curry-Roasted Cashews, 346
catfish, 290–91
cauliflower
  Cauliflower & Kalamata Olive Salad, 150
  Cauliflower & Spinach Salad with Sesame-
    Orange Dressing, *143*, 147
  Cauliflower-Walnut Casserole, 276–77
  Indian-Spiced Cauliflower & Tomato Soup,
    76
  Sesame Chicken & Vegetable Foil Packs,
    315–16
  Simply Roasted Cauliflower, 258
  Simply Steamed Vegetable Medley, 262
  Spicy Cauliflower Stir-Fry, 267–68
celery, 152–53
Chana Dal, 248
Cheddar-Pepper Popovers, 120
cheese
  À la Heart Mexican-Inspired Mac & Cheese,
    206–7
  Alfredo Sauce, 52–53
  Arugula, Apple & Fennel Salad with
    Gorgonzola, 146
  Baked Ricotta, 341
  Bean & Baby Kale Frittata, 119
  Blue Cheese Vinaigrette, 48
  Cheddar-Pepper Popovers, 120
  Cheesy Mushroom Manicotti, 207–8
  Cherry Tomato Caprese Salad, 150
  Chicken Waldorf Tomato Blossoms with
    Feta & Dill, 162
  Creamy Feta & Mint Dressing, 49
  Creamy Spinach Lasagna, 208–9
  French Onion Soup, 75–76
  Garlic & Rosemary Egg Bites with Gruyère,
    121
  Gorgonzola & Beef Piadine with Arugula
    Salad, 196–97

  Greek-Inspired Baked Chickpeas with
    Tomatoes & Feta, *236*, 246–47
  Lentil & Mixed Greens Salad with Goat
    Cheese, 170–71
  Margherita Pizza, 197
  Nutty Apricot Cottage Cheese Bread, 104
  Orzo with Peas & Parmesan, 210
  Parmesan-Garlic Bean Dip, *336*, 342
  Parmesan-Herb Croutons, 172–73
  Peach Caprese Salad with Burrata, *140*, 144
  Penne with Spicy North African-Style Carrot
    Sauce & Goat Cheese, 211
  Potato-Cheddar Breakfast Casserole, 123
  Potato-Turnip Gratin, *278*, 278–79
  Roasted Vegetable Lasagna, 213–14
  Spaghetti Squash Sauté with Black Olives
    & Feta, 272
  Spinach Salad with Honeycrisp Apples &
    Cheddar, 148
  Tomato-Topped Veggie-Egg Bake, 127–28
  Vegetable-Almond Rice with Parmesan, 233
  Very Veggie Grilled Cheese Sandwiches,
    182–83
  Very Veggie Pizza, 200–201, *201*
cherries
  Cherry-Farro Pudding Parfaits, 359–60
  Persian-Inspired Rice Pilaf with Cherries &
    Pistachios, 232
Cherry Tomato Caprese Salad, 150
Chewy Molasses Cookies, 357
chia seeds, 136
chicken
  Almond-Crusted Chicken Strips, 303
  Autumn Wild Rice & Chicken Bowls, 159
  Breaded Chicken Tenders with Herbs, 304
  Chicken-Almond Stir-Fry with Carrots,
    Snow Peas & Plums, 304–5
  Chicken & Bean Burritos, 186–87
  Chicken & Chanterelles, 305
  Chicken & Wild Rice Salad with Grapes &
    Candied Pecans, 162
  Chicken Caesar Salad, 161
  Chicken Chili Verde, 85–86
  Chicken Enchiladas, 306
  Chicken Fried Rice, 306–7
  Chicken Lentil Spinach Bowls, 161
  Chicken-Pesto Pizza, 196
  Chicken Stock, 70
  Chicken Tandoori Skewers, 307–8
  Chicken Teriyaki with Soba Noodles &
    Cashews, 308
  Chicken Tikka Masala, 309
  Chicken Waldorf Tomato Blossoms with
    Feta & Dill, 162
  Chicken with Artichokes & Capers, 309–10
  Cilantro-Lime Chicken & Corn Salad, 163
  Classic Chicken Soup, 74
  Crispy Almond Chicken Bowl, 310
  Crispy Chicken Nuggets, 310
  Curry-Glazed Chicken, 311
  Habanero Chicken Wings, 311
  Have a Plant Curried Chicken Salad, 164
  Honey-Ginger Chicken & Apples, 312
  Lemon Chicken with Smoked Paprika, 312
  Moroccan-Inspired Chicken & Couscous,
    313
  Mulligatawny Soup, 78
  Roast Chicken with Lemon & Thyme, 313–14
  Rosemary-Citrus Chicken, 314
  Rosemary-Garlic Chicken Wings, 315

Rotisserie Chicken & Farro Soup with Cannellini Beans, 82
Sesame Chicken & Vegetable Foil Packs, 315–16
Sheet Pan Chicken, Broccoli & Red Peppers, 316
Singapore-Inspired Chicken Rice Noodles, 214–15
Zesty Chicken Bites, 316–17
See also sausage
chickpeas
Apricot-Chickpea Smoothie, 138, *138*
Chickpea Burgers, 178–79
Classic Hummus, 245–46
Cooking À la Heart Salad, 168–69
Crunchy Italian-Flavored Chickpeas, 172
Eastern Mediterranean Bowls with Hummus & Tabbouleh, 246
East Indian–Inspired Lentil & Chickpea Dal Bowl, 248
Four-Bean Salad, 169
Greek-Inspired Baked Chickpeas with Tomatoes & Feta, *236*, 246–47
Lemon Cardamom Chickpea Muffins, *90*, 95
Wild Rice & Chickpea Salad, 171
chiles
Habanero Spice Rub, 33
Hot Curried Egg Bites, 121–22
Jalapeño-Peach Barbecue Sauce, 56
Midwestern Beef, Bean & Beer Chili, 87
Roasted Poblano Soup, 81
Simply Roasted Peppers, 259
Singapore-Inspired Chicken Rice Noodles, 214–15
Thai-Inspired Shrimp Soup, 82–83
chili powder
Oven-Roasted Seasoned Popcorn, 344–45
Taco Seasoning, 38, *38*
Chimichurri, 54
Chinese Five Spice Blend, 31
chipotles in adobo
Chipotle Aïoli, 44
Raspberry-Chipotle Sauce, 57
chives, 108–9
chocolate, dark
Chocolate Cranberry Almond Clusters, 362–63
Dark Chocolate Cranberry Oatmeal Cookies with Walnuts, 358
Chocolate-Coconut Mousse, 360
Chocolate Energy Bars, 131
chocolate syrup, dark, 360
cilantro
Avocado Lime Cilantro Aïoli, 44
Cilantro-Lime Chicken & Corn Salad, 163
Cilantro-Lime Vinaigrette, 170–71
Cilantro-Mint Pesto, 46
Cilantro Pesto, 46
Creamy Cilantro Coleslaw, 151, *174*
Lamb Chops with Cilantro-Mint Pesto, 333–34
cinnamon
Apple-Cinnamon Compote, 128
Apple-Cinnamon Galette with Gingerbread Crust, 352
Apple-Cinnamon Pancakes, 128
Cinnamon & Ginger Granola, 131
Cinnamon-Honey Dressing, 148
Cinnamon Spice Mix, 31
Roasted Potatoes with Cinnamon, 270

Cioppino, 86
Citrus, Spinach & Mushroom Salad, 147
Citrus Curd, 361
Citrus-Glazed Carrots, 265–66
Citrus-Mint Dressing, 144–45
Citrus-Mint Salad with Ginger-Lime Vinaigrette, 143
Citrus-Roasted Beets, 264
Citrusy Golden Beet Salad, 148
Citrusy Walnut Gremolata, 63
citrus zest/juice, 144–45
clams
Clams in Chorizo Tomato Saffron Sauce, 284–85
Hearty Clam Chowder, 88
Classic Beef Stroganoff, 325
Classic Chicken Soup, 74
Classic Hummus, 245–46
cocoa powder
À la Heart Olive Oil Brownies, 355
Chocolate Energy Bars, 131
coconut/coconut milk/coconut extract
Chocolate-Coconut Mousse, 360
Coconut Fish Curry, 285
Mango-Coconut Overnight Oats with Macadamia Nuts, 133
Mussels in Coconut-Lemongrass Broth, 290
Coffee & Fennel Rub, 31
coleslaw mix, 155
Cooking À la Heart Salad, 168–69
coriander, 264
corn
À la Heart Mexican-Inspired Mac & Cheese, 206–7
Broccoli & Corn Salad, 149
Cilantro-Lime Chicken & Corn Salad, 163
Italian-Seasoned Corn Muffins, 95–96
Mexican-Inspired Egg & Veggie Skillet, 122–23
Smoked Salmon & Corn Chowder, 88–89
Smoky Workaday Sweet Corn & Pepper Sauté, 268
Southwest Corn Bread, 105
Tomato-Corn Salsa, 62–63
cornmeal
Italian-Seasoned Corn Muffins, 95–96
Southwest Corn Bread, 105
couscous
Carrot & Pineapple Couscous Salad, 146
Couscous with Vegetables & Pine Nuts, *204*, 206
Moroccan-Inspired Chicken & Couscous, 313
Simply Steamed Couscous, 205
crab
Crab, Asparagus & Avocado Salad, 163
Mini Crab Cakes, *288*, 289
Seafood Trio Rolls, 294
Wild Crab Salad, 168
cranberries
Chocolate Cranberry Almond Clusters, 362–63
Cranberry-Almond Coffee Cake, 98–99
Cranberry-Orange Bread, 101–2
Cranberry-Pear Crisp, 353–54
Cranberry Sauce with Lime & Crystallized Ginger, 54
Dark Chocolate Cranberry Oatmeal Cookies with Walnuts, 358
Fresh Cranberry Citrus Pear Relish, *40*, 64

Pumpkin Apple Cranberry Granola Bites, 363
cream, whipping
Crème Fraîche, 361
Light-Hearted Clotted Cream, 98
Spiced Ginger Cream, *348*, 362
Creamy Asparagus Soup, 74–75
Creamy Cilantro Coleslaw, 151, *174*
Creamy Cucumber-Dill Salad, 151
Creamy Cucumber Dressing, 48
Creamy Curry-Cashew Dip, 342
Creamy Dijon Dressing, 48, 168
Creamy Dill Dressing, 49
Creamy Eggplant with Tomatoes, 277
Creamy Feta & Mint Dressing, 49
Creamy Spinach Lasagna, 208–9
Crème Fraîche, 361
Crispy Almond Chicken Bowl, 310
Crispy Cajun Corn Chips, 339
Crispy Chicken Nuggets, 310
Crispy Fish Sticks, 286
Crispy Tofu Bites, 250–51
Crispy Tofu with Lentils & Mixed Greens, 169
Crunchy Italian-Flavored Chickpeas, 172
cucumbers
Creamy Cucumber-Dill Salad, 151
Creamy Cucumber Dressing, 48
Cucumber & Tomato Salad, 152
Cucumber-Dill Sauce, 54–55
Cucumber-Grape Gazpacho, 72
Cucumber Mint Yogurt Sauce, 189
Cucumber Raita, 63–64
Cucumber-Shrimp Soup, 72
Curiously Compatible Cucumbers & Carrots, 268–69
Dilly Cucumber Salad, 152
Fish Roast with Cucumber-Dill Sauce, *280*, 286
Marinated Vegetable Salad, 152–53
Mediterranean Oats with Cucumbers & Olives, 122
Tzatziki, 60
cumin
Cumin, Sage & Turmeric Seasoning, 32
Cumin-Garlic Tortilla Chips, *336–37*, 340
Curiously Compatible Cucumbers & Carrots, 268–69
curry powder
Coconut Fish Curry, 285
Creamy Curry-Cashew Dip, 342
Curried Peach Soup, 73
Curried Rice–Stuffed Tomatoes, 276
Curry-Glazed Chicken, 311
Curry Powder, 32
Curry-Roasted Cashews, 346
Have a Plant Curried Chicken Salad, 164
Hot Curried Egg Bites, 121–22

D
Dark Chocolate Cranberry Oatmeal Cookies with Walnuts, 358
Dashi Broth, 70
dates
Apple Walnut Date Coffee Cake, 356
Chocolate Energy Bars, 131
Diamond Crystal Kosher Salt, 13
dill
Avocado Lemon Dill Aïoli, 43, *288*
Chicken Waldorf Tomato Blossoms with Feta & Dill, 162

dill (continued)
Creamy Cucumber-Dill Salad, 151
Creamy Dill Dressing, 49
Cucumber-Dill Sauce, 54–55
Dill Vinaigrette, 49
Dilly Cucumber Salad, 152
Fish Roast with Cucumber-Dill Sauce, *280*, 286
Salmon & White Bean Bowl with Lime & Dill, 244
Smoked Salmon Flatbread with Dill, 200

E
Eastern Mediterranean Bowls with Hummus & Tabbouleh, 246
East Indian–Inspired Lentil & Chickpea Dal Bowl, 248
East Indian–Inspired Spice Blend, 32
Easy Weeknight Ground Beef Stroganoff, 325
edamame
Edamame-Pea Pesto Spread, 342
Scallops en Papillote with Shallots, Edamame & Bell Pepper, 293–94
Smoky Roasted Edamame, 347
Very Veggie Miso Soup, 84
eggplants
Creamy Eggplant with Tomatoes, 277
Mediterranean Rice Bake with Eggplant and Tomatoes, 231
Vegetarian Shepherd's Pie, 279
eggs
Bean & Baby Kale Frittata, 119
Garlic & Rosemary Egg Bites with Gruyère, 121
Hot Curried Egg Bites, 121–22
Make-Ahead Layered Salad with Eggs, 165
Mexican-Inspired Egg & Veggie Skillet, 122–23
Potato-Cheddar Breakfast Casserole, 123
Quinoa-Veggie Egg Bites, 123–24
Salade Niçoise, 166–67
Sausage, Egg & Avocado Breakfast Sandwiches, *116*, 124
Shiitake & Spinach Quiche with Rosemary & Sage, 125, *126*
Spinach Scramble Pita Pockets, 127
Tomato-Topped Veggie-Egg Bake, 127–28
English muffins, *116*, 124

F
Fajita Vegetables, 273
farro
Cherry-Farro Pudding Parfaits, 359–60
Farro With Roasted Grapes, 226–27
Italian-Inspired Beef & Farro Bowls, *320*, 327
Rotisserie Chicken & Farro Soup with Cannellini Beans, 82
Simply Cooked Farro, 226
fennel
Arugula, Apple & Fennel Salad with Gorgonzola, 146
Beer Breadsticks with Fennel, 106–7
Coffee & Fennel Rub, 31
Fennel & Pear Roasted Carrots, 266–67
Lentil-Fennel Lasagna, 249–50
White Fish with Fennel & Leeks, 299, *300*
figs, 130
fish
Cioppino, 86
Crispy Fish Sticks, 286

Fish Broth, 71
Fish Roast with Cucumber-Dill Sauce, *280*, 286
Fish Tacos, *39*, 184
Nordic Fish Soup, 78–79
Pan-Seared White Fish, Arugula & Roasted Tomato Salad, 166
Sheet Pan Fish & Vegetable Bake, 295
Summer Lake Bake, 299
White Fish with Fennel & Leeks, 299, *300*
See also specific types of fish
flaxseed
Blueberry Oat Flax Scones, 96–97
Super Seeds Protein Power Bars, 136
flour, whole wheat
Hearty Wheat Buns, 110–11
Honey Whole Wheat Bread, 111
Honey Whole Wheat Potato Pizza Dough, 194–95
Honey Whole Wheat Waffles, 132
Whole Wheat French Baguette, 114
Whole Wheat–Herb Pizza Dough, 195
Four-Bean Salad, 169
Four-Grain Sunflower Seed Bread, 108
Fragrant Warm Spiced Lentils, 247
French Onion Soup, 75–76
French-Style Beef Stew, 326
Fresh Chive–Yogurt Buns, 108–9
Fresh Cranberry Citrus Pear Relish, *40*, 64
Fresh Herb & Honey Batter Bread, 102
Fresh Salmon Burgers, 179–80

G
garlic
Caramelized Garlic Sauce, 53
Cumin-Garlic Tortilla Chips, *336–37*, 340
Garlic & Herb Bread Crumbs, 33
Garlic & Rosemary Egg Bites with Gruyère, 121
Garlicky Lemon Dressing, 150
Garlicky Wild Rice & Mushroom-Stuffed Acorn Squash, 274–75
Garlic-Lime Vinaigrette, 147
Garlic-Tomato Confit, 64
Ginger-Garlic Sauce, 214–15
Gingery Mackerel with Lemon & Garlic, 287
Parmesan-Garlic Bean Dip, *336*, 342
Roasted Garlic Aïoli, 45
Rosemary-Garlic Chicken Wings, 315
Simply Roasted Garlic, 258
Skordalia, 59
ginger
Apple-Cinnamon Galette with Gingerbread Crust, 352
Asparagus with Sesame & Ginger, 263–64
Blueberry Ginger Yogurt Bark with Almonds, 362
Cinnamon & Ginger Granola, 131
Citrus-Mint Salad with Ginger-Lime Vinaigrette, 143
Cranberry Sauce with Lime & Crystallized Ginger, 54
Ginger-Apple Cider Dressing, 148
Ginger-Garlic Sauce, 214–15
Ginger Lentil & Brown Rice Bake, 249
Ginger Lentils, 249
Ginger-Pear Compote, 132
Gingery Lemon Scones, 97–98
Gingery Mackerel with Lemon & Garlic, 287

Honey-Ginger Chicken & Apples, 312
Honey-Ginger Dressing, 50
Millet Morning Cakes with Ginger-Pear Compote, 134
Pumpkin Spice Ginger Bars, 358–59
Roasted Sweet Potatoes & Ginger-Spiced Apples, 273
Smoke & Pepper Ginger Rub, 37
Spiced Ginger Cream, *348*, 362
Wasabi-Ginger Coleslaw, 155
Gorgonzola & Beef Piadine with Arugula Salad, 196–97
grapefruit
Citrus-Mint Salad with Ginger-Lime Vinaigrette, 143
Citrus-Roasted Beets, 264
Citrusy Golden Beet Salad, 148
Pear & Grapefruit Toss with Citrus-Mint Dressing, 144–45
Tropical Fruit Salsa, 63
Watermelon, Grapefruit & Blueberry Salad, 145
grapes
Chicken & Wild Rice Salad with Grapes & Candied Pecans, 162
Cucumber-Grape Gazpacho, 72
Farro With Roasted Grapes, 226–27
Mixed Fruit with Yogurt-Cardamom Dressing, 144
grass-fed beef, 23
Greek-Flavor Beef & Barley Bowls, 326–27
Greek-Inspired Baked Chickpeas with Tomatoes & Feta, *236*, 246–47
Greek Orzo Salad with Spinach & Tomatoes, 209
greens, mixed
Crispy Tofu with Lentils & Mixed Greens, 169
Lentil & Mixed Greens Salad with Goat Cheese, 170–71
Make-Ahead Layered Salad with Eggs, 165
Wild Crab Salad, 168

H
Habanero Chicken Wings, 311
Habanero Spice Rub, 33
halibut, 284
Harvest Crescents, 109–10, *115*
Have a Plant Curried Chicken Salad, 164
Have a Plant Movement, 19, 164
Hearty Clam Chowder, 88
Hearty Wheat Buns, 110–11
hemp seeds, 136
Herb Blend for Beef, 34
Herb Blend for Pork, 34
Herb Blend for Poultry, 34
Herbed Red Wine Vinaigrette, 50
Herb-Infused Vinegar, 50
Herb-Roasted Turkey Breast with Vegetables, *40*, 317–18
Homestyle Barbecue Sauce, 55
honey
Cinnamon-Honey Dressing, 148
Fresh Herb & Honey Batter Bread, 102
Honey Balsamic Onion Jam, 64–65
Honey-Ginger Chicken & Apples, 312
Honey-Ginger Dressing, 50
Honey Lemon Dijon Dressing, 146
Honey Mustard Sauce, 55

Honey Whole Wheat Bread, 111
Honey Whole Wheat Potato Pizza Dough,
194–95
Honey Whole Wheat Waffles, 132
Roasted Salmon with Honey Walnut Lemon
Sauce, 292
Horseradish-Dijon Aïoli, 44
Hot Curried Egg Bites, 121–22
Hot Mango Chutney, 65

I

Icelanders in America Cereal, 133
Indian-Spiced Cauliflower & Tomato Soup, 76
Italian-Inspired Beef & Farro Bowls, *320*, 327
Italian Pasta Salad, 210
Italian-Seasoned Corn Muffins, 95–96
Italian Seasoning, 34

J

Jalapeño-Peach Barbecue Sauce, 56
Jamaican Jerk Rub, 35

K

kale
Bean & Baby Kale Frittata, 119
Kale Chips, 340
Kefir, Spinach & Avocado Smoothie, 139, *139*

L

lamb
Lamb & Rice-Stuffed Bell Peppers, 334
Lamb Chops with Cilantro-Mint Pesto,
333–34
Seared Lamb Pita Pockets with Cucumber
Mint Yogurt Sauce, 189
South African Lamb Pie (Bobotie), 334–35
leeks
Portobello-Pesto Pizza with Leeks, *190*, 198
Potato-Leek Soup, 79
White Fish with Fennel & Leeks, 299, *300*
lemongrass, 290
lemons/lemon juice
Artichoke & Onions with Lemon & Thyme,
263
Avocado Lemon Dill Aïoli, 43, *288*
Citrusy Walnut Gremolata, 63
Fresh Cranberry Citrus Pear Relish, *40*, 64
Garlicky Lemon Dressing, 150
Gingery Lemon Scones, 97–98
Gingery Mackerel with Lemon & Garlic, 287
Honey Lemon Dijon Dressing, 146
Lemon-Basil Dressing, 152
Lemon-Blueberry Bread, 102–3
Lemon Cardamom Chickpea Muffins, *90*, 95
Lemon Chicken with Smoked Paprika, 312
Lemon Curd, 361
Lemon-Herb Dressing, 149
Lemon Vinaigrette, 170
Pineapple Salsa with Tomato & Lemon, 62
Roast Chicken with Lemon & Thyme, 313–14
Roasted Salmon with Honey Walnut Lemon
Sauce, 292
Rosemary-Citrus Chicken, 314
White Bean Salad with Lemon & Rosemary,
245
lentils
Beef & Lentil Salad Bowls, 160
Chicken Lentil Spinach Bowls, 161
Crispy Tofu with Lentils & Mixed Greens,
169
East Indian–Inspired Lentil & Chickpea Dal
Bowl, 248

Fragrant Warm Spiced Lentils, 247
Ginger Lentil & Brown Rice Bake, 249
Ginger Lentils, 249
Lentil & Brown Rice Salad with Thyme, 170
Lentil & Mixed Greens Salad with Goat
Cheese, 170–71
Lentil Caprese Salad, 170
Lentil-Fennel Lasagna, 249–50
Red Lentil & Vegetable Soup, 79–80
Simply Cooked Lentils, 247
lettuce
Chicken Caesar Salad, 161
Mixed Greens & Mushroom Salad, 153
Pork Lettuce Wraps, 187
Wedge Salad, 155
Light-Hearted Clotted Cream, 98
limes/lime juice
Avocado Lime Cilantro Aïoli, 44
Cilantro-Lime Chicken & Corn Salad, 163
Cilantro-Lime Vinaigrette, 170–71
Citrus-Mint Salad with Ginger-Lime
Vinaigrette, 143
Citrusy Walnut Gremolata, 63
Cranberry Sauce with Lime & Crystallized
Ginger, 54
Garlic-Lime Vinaigrette, 147
Lime & Thyme Vinaigrette, 50–51
Oven-Roasted Seasoned Popcorn, 344–45
Peanut-Lime Dressing, 167
Salmon & White Bean Bowl with Lime &
Dill, 244
Sesame-Lime Dressing, 154

M

macadamia nuts, 133
Make-Ahead Layered Salad with Eggs, 165
mangos
Hot Mango Chutney, 65
Mango, Spinach & Shrimp Salad, *156–57*, 165
Mango-Coconut Overnight Oats with
Macadamia Nuts, 133
Mango Tofu Soy Milk Smoothie, 139, *139*
maple syrup
Baked Beans with Maple Syrup, 242
Maple & Herb Roasted Carrots, 267
Maple-Roasted Brussels Sprouts, 265
Maple-Yogurt Dressing, 149
Margherita Pizza, 197
Marinated Vegetable Salad, 152–53
Mediterranean Oats with Cucumbers &
Olives, 122
Mediterranean Rice Bake with Eggplant and
Tomatoes, 231
Mediterranean Tilapia en Papillote, 287
Mexican Black Bean Soup, 76–77
Mexican-Inspired Egg & Veggie Skillet, 122–23
Midwestern Beef, Bean & Beer Chili, 87
millet
Icelanders in America Cereal, 133
Millet Curry Cakes with Tomato-Corn Salsa,
218, 227–28
Millet Morning Cakes with Ginger-Pear
Compote, 134
Simply Cooked Millet, 227
Mini Crab Cakes, *288*, 289
mint
Bulgur & Tomato Salad with Mint, 224–25
Bulgur-Tomato Salad with Tuna & Mint, 160
Cilantro-Mint Pesto, 46

Citrus-Mint Salad with Ginger-Lime
Vinaigrette, 143
Creamy Feta & Mint Dressing, 49
Cucumber Mint Yogurt Sauce, 189
Lamb Chops with Cilantro-Mint Pesto,
333–34
Pear & Grapefruit Toss with Citrus-Mint
Dressing, 144–45
Strawberry, Pineapple & Mint Salad, 145
Mirepoix Soupe, 77
miso
Miso-Glazed Scallops, 289
Very Veggie Miso Soup, 84
Mixed Berry Compote, 134
Mixed Fruit with Yogurt-Cardamom Dressing,
144
Mixed Greens & Mushroom Salad, 153
Mock Risotto with Zucchini, 231
molasses
Chewy Molasses Cookies, 357
Molasses Brown Bread, 103
Moroccan-Inspired Chicken & Couscous, 313
Moroccan-Spiced Almonds, 346
Moroccan-Style Seasoning, 35
Mulligatawny Soup, 78
mushrooms
Beef & Mushroom Burgers, 178
Beef & Mushroom Taco Filling, 183
Beef & Vegetable Kabobs, 324
Cheesy Mushroom Manicotti, 207–8
Chicken & Chanterelles, 305
Citrus, Spinach & Mushroom Salad, 147
Classic Beef Stroganoff, 325
Easy Weeknight Ground Beef Stroganoff,
325
Garlicky Wild Rice & Mushroom-Stuffed
Acorn Squash, 274–75
Mixed Greens & Mushroom Salad, 153
Mushroom & Spinach–Stuffed Tomatoes,
275–76
Pasta Primavera, 211
Portobello-Pesto Pizza with Leeks, *190*, 198
Portobello Street Tacos, 184–85
Roasted Mushroom–Barley Pilaf, 223
Sheet Pan Fish & Vegetable Bake, 295
Shiitake & Spinach Quiche with Rosemary
& Sage, 125, *126*
Shrimp & Vegetable Pasta Bake, 214
Simply Steamed Vegetable Medley, 262
Smoky Roasted Mushrooms, 269
Tomato-Topped Veggie-Egg Bake, 127–28
Vegetable Fried Rice, 233–34
Wild Rice with Mushrooms, Tarragon &
Pine Nuts, 234
Mussels in Coconut-Lemongrass Broth, 290
mustard
Creamy Dijon Dressing, 48, 168
Honey Lemon Dijon Dressing, 146
Honey Mustard Sauce, 55
Horseradish-Dijon Aïoli, 44

N

Napa Cabbage Slaw, 153
nectarines, 62
noodles
À la Heart Mexican-Inspired Mac & Cheese,
206–7
Angel Hair Pasta with Tomatoes & Basil,
207
Cheesy Mushroom Manicotti, 207–8

noodles (*continued*)

    Chicken Teriyaki with Soba Noodles & Cashews, 308

    Creamy Spinach Lasagna, 208–9

    Greek Orzo Salad with Spinach & Tomatoes, 209

    Italian Pasta Salad, 210

    Lentil-Fennel Lasagna, 249–50

    Orzo with Peas & Parmesan, 210

    Pasta Primavera, 211

    Penne with Spicy North African-Style Carrot Sauce & Goat Cheese, 211

    Rice Noodles with Snow Peas & Shrimp, 212

    Roasted Red Pepper Fettuccine, *202*, 212–13

    Roasted Vegetable Lasagna, 213–14

    Shrimp & Vegetable Pasta Bake, 214

    Singapore-Inspired Chicken Rice Noodles, 214–15

    Southeast Asian–Style Shrimp & Napa Cabbage Salad with Rice Noodles, 167

    Spaghetti with Meat Sauce, 215–16

    Stir-Fried Vegetable & Farfalle Bowl, 216

    Summer Vegetable Pasta Toss, 217, *217*

Nordic Fish Soup, 78–79

nuts

    Savory Nut Crumb Topping, 36

    Savory Roasted Mixed Nuts, 347

    See also specific nuts

Nutty Apricot Cottage Cheese Bread, 104

O

oats, rolled

    Banana Oat Blueberry Breakfast Bars, 129–30

    Blueberry Oat Flax Scones, 96–97

    Carrot & Fig Oats with Pistachios, 130

    Cinnamon & Ginger Granola, 131

    Dark Chocolate Cranberry Oatmeal Cookies with Walnuts, 358

    Mango-Coconut Overnight Oats with Macadamia Nuts, 133

    Mediterranean Oats with Cucumbers & Olives, 122

    Pecan-Oat Muffins, 96

    Pumpkin Apple Cranberry Granola Bites, 363

    Pumpkin Spice Oats with Pecans, 135

    Strawberries with Almond-Oat Crumble, 354

olive oil, 355

olives

    Cauliflower & Kalamata Olive Salad, 150

    Mediterranean Oats with Cucumbers & Olives, 122

    Red Potato & Onion Roast with Cherry Tomatoes & Kalamata Olives, 269–70

    Spaghetti Squash Sauté with Black Olives & Feta, 272

onions

    Artichoke & Onions with Lemon & Thyme, 263

    French Onion Soup, 75–76

    Honey Balsamic Onion Jam, 64–65

    Red Potato & Onion Roast with Cherry Tomatoes & Kalamata Olives, 269–70

    Simply Quick-Pickled Red Onions, 259

oranges/orange juice

    Almond-Orange Cake, 355–56

    Cardamom & Orange Roasted Carrots, 266

    Cauliflower & Spinach Salad with Sesame-Orange Dressing, *143*, 147

    Citrus, Spinach & Mushroom Salad, 147

    Citrus-Glazed Carrots, 265–66

    Citrus-Mint Salad with Ginger-Lime Vinaigrette, 143

    Citrus-Roasted Beets, 264

    Citrusy Golden Beet Salad, 148

    Citrusy Walnut Gremolata, 63

    Cranberry-Orange Bread, 101–2

    Fresh Cranberry Citrus Pear Relish, *40*, 64

    Mixed Fruit with Yogurt-Cardamom Dressing, 144

    Orange Curd, 361

    Rosemary-Citrus Chicken, 314

Orzo with Peas & Parmesan, 210

Oven-Roasted Seasoned Popcorn, 344–45

P

Pan-Seared Crispy Catfish, 290–91

Pan-Seared White Fish, Arugula & Roasted Tomato Salad, 166

papayas, 63

paprika, smoked

    Lemon Chicken with Smoked Paprika, 312

    Smoke & Pepper Ginger Rub, 37

    Smoky Workaday Seasoning, 37

Parmesan-Garlic Bean Dip, *336*, 342

Parmesan-Herb Croutons, 172–73

parsley, 63

parsnips, *252*, 261

Pasta Primavera, 211

peaches

    Barley with Stone Fruit, 130

    Curried Peach Soup, 73

    Jalapeño-Peach Barbecue Sauce, 56

    Peach Caprese Salad with Burrata, *140*, 144

    Stone Fruit Salsa, 62

peanut butter

    Peanut-Lime Dressing, 167

    Peanut Sauce, 56

    West African–Inspired Sweet Potato & Peanut Stew, *66*, 85

peanuts

    Cajun-Spiced Peanuts, 345

    Turkey & Squash Couscous with Apricots & Peanuts, 318–19

pears

    Cranberry-Pear Crisp, 353–54

    Fennel & Pear Roasted Carrots, 266–67

    Fresh Cranberry Citrus Pear Relish, *40*, 64

    Ginger-Pear Compote, 132

    Millet Morning Cakes with Ginger-Pear Compote, 134

    Mixed Fruit with Yogurt-Cardamom Dressing, 144

    Pear & Grapefruit Toss with Citrus-Mint Dressing, 144–45

    Prosciutto & Pear Piadine with Balsamic Drizzle, 198–99

    Pumpkin-Pear Mousse, 360–61

    Wine-Poached Pears, 354–55

peas

    Chicken-Almond Stir-Fry with Carrots, Snow Peas & Plums, 304–5

    Edamame-Pea Pesto Spread, 342

    Nordic Fish Soup, 78–79

    Orzo with Peas & Parmesan, 210

    Pasta Primavera, 211

    Rice Noodles with Snow Peas & Shrimp, 212

    Shrimp & Vegetable Pasta Bake, 214

    Vegetable Fried Rice, 233–34

pecans

    Carrot Cake with Pecans, 357

    Chicken & Wild Rice Salad with Grapes & Candied Pecans, 162

    Nutty Apricot Cottage Cheese Bread, 104

    Pecan-Oat Muffins, 96

    Pumpkin Spice Oats with Pecans, 135

    Pumpkin Spice Pecans, 346–47

    Smoky Pecan Bits, 173

    Spicy Candied Pecans, 173

    Zucchini-Nut Bread, 106

Penne with Spicy North African-Style Carrot Sauce & Goat Cheese, 211

pepitas (pumpkin seeds)

    Pumpkin Spice Pepita Bread, 104–5

    Super Seeds Protein Power Bars, 136

pepper, black

    Cheddar-Pepper Popovers, 120

    Smoke & Pepper Ginger Rub, 37

peppers, bell

    Beef & Vegetable Kabobs, 324

    Bulgur-Stuffed Peppers, 275

    Fajita Vegetables, 273

    Lamb & Rice-Stuffed Bell Peppers, 334

    Pico de Gallo, 61

    Roasted Red Pepper Fettuccine, *202*, 212–13

    Sausage & Roasted Red Pepper Breakfast Pizza, 199

    Scallops en Papillote with Shallots, Edamame & Bell Pepper, 293–94

    Sheet Pan Chicken, Broccoli & Red Peppers, 316

    Simply Roasted Peppers, 259

    Smoky Workaday Sweet Corn & Pepper Sauté, 268

    Sweet & Tangy Red Pepper Sauce, 60

Persian Fresh Herb Mix, 35

Persian-Inspired Rice Pilaf with Cherries & Pistachios, 232

pesto

    Broiled Halibut with Pesto, 284

    Chicken-Pesto Pizza, 196

    Pork Chops with Pesto, 331

Pico de Gallo, 61

pineapple

    Carrot & Pineapple Couscous Salad, 146

    Pineapple Salsa with Tomato & Lemon, 62

    Strawberry, Pineapple & Mint Salad, 145

    Sweet & Sour Sauce, 60

pine nuts

    Brown Rice with Pine Nuts & Roasted Butternut Squash, 230

    Couscous with Vegetables & Pine Nuts, *204*, 206

    Wild Rice with Mushrooms, Tarragon & Pine Nuts, 234

pistachios

    Bulgur Sauté with Pomegranate & Pistachios, 224

    Carrot & Fig Oats with Pistachios, 130

    Persian-Inspired Rice Pilaf with Cherries & Pistachios, 232

    Turkey Tenderloins with Spinach Pesto & Pistachios, 319

pita pockets

    Seared Lamb Pita Pockets with Cucumber Mint Yogurt Sauce, 189

Southwest Pita Chips, 340–41
Spinach Scramble Pita Pockets, 127
plums
Chicken-Almond Stir-Fry with Carrots, Snow Peas & Plums, 304–5
Plum Sauce, 57
pomegranates/pomegranate juice
Baked Beans with Pomegranate & Canadian Bacon, 242–43
Bulgur Sauté with Pomegranate & Pistachios, 224
popcorn
Brown Bag Popcorn with Herb Seasonings, 344
Oven-Roasted Seasoned Popcorn, 344–45
pork
Pork Banh Mi Burgers, 180
Pork Chops with Caraway Rice, 331
Pork Chops with Pesto, 331
Pork Fried Rice, 332
Pork Lettuce Wraps, 187
Simply Cooked Pork Tenderloin, 332–33
Smoky Workaday Pork Tenderloin, 333
Spicy Sage Breakfast Sausage, 124–25
Swedish Meatballs, 330
Tomatillo-Pork Stew, 89
Tuscan-Inspired Pork, 333
See also sausage
Portobello-Pesto Pizza with Leeks, 190, 198
Portobello Street Tacos, 184–85
potatoes
Borscht, 73–74
Hearty Clam Chowder, 88
Herb-Roasted Turkey Breast with Vegetables, 40, 317–18
Honey Whole Wheat Potato Pizza Dough, 194–95
Potato-Cheddar Breakfast Casserole, 123
Potato Dinner Rolls, 112
Potato-Leek Soup, 79
Potato Salad with Red Wine Vinaigrette, 154, 154–55
Potato-Turnip Gratin, 278, 278–79
Quebec City Shepherd's Pie (Pâté Chinois), 328
Red Potato & Onion Roast with Cherry Tomatoes & Kalamata Olives, 269–70
Roasted Potatoes with Cinnamon, 270
Rosemary Mashed Potatoes, 270
Salade Niçoise, 166–67
Sesame Chicken & Vegetable Foil Packs, 315–16
Simply Roasted Potatoes, 260
Simply Smashed Potatoes, 260
Simply Spanish-Style Mashed Potatoes, 259–60
Smoked Salmon & Corn Chowder, 88–89
Turkey-Vegetable Soup, 84
Vegetarian Shepherd's Pie, 279
See also sweet potatoes
Prosciutto & Pear Piadine with Balsamic Drizzle, 198–99
prunes, 130
Pumpernickel Bread, 113
pumpkin
Pumpkin Apple Cranberry Granola Bites, 363
Pumpkin Butter, 135
Pumpkin-Pear Mousse, 360–61
Pumpkin Spice Ginger Bars, 358–59

Pumpkin Spice Oats with Pecans, 135
Pumpkin Spice Pepita Bread, 104–5
Roasted Butternut Bisque, 80–81
Pumpkin Spice Pecans, 346–47

Q
Quebec City Shepherd's Pie (Pâté Chinois), 328
Quick-Pickled Vegetables, 274
quinoa
Quinoa & Black Bean Medley, 228
Quinoa-Veggie Egg Bites, 123–24
Simply Cooked Quinoa, 228

R
Radish & Cabbage Slaw, 154
raisins, 109–10, 115
Raspberry-Chipotle Sauce, 57
Red Beans & Rice, 243
Red Lentil & Vegetable Soup, 79–80
Red Potato & Onion Roast with Cherry Tomatoes & Kalamata Olives, 269–70
Refried Beans, 243–44
rhubarb
Rhubarbecue Sauce, 58
Rhubarb-Strawberry Coffee Cake, 99–100
Strawberry-Rhubarb Bars, 359
rice, brown
À la Heart Rice & Beans Bowl, 242
Brown Rice with Pine Nuts & Roasted Butternut Squash, 230
Chicken Fried Rice, 306–7
Cooking À la Heart Salad, 168–69
Curried Rice–Stuffed Tomatoes, 276
Ginger Lentil & Brown Rice Bake, 249
Lamb & Race-Stuffed Bell Peppers, 334
Lentil & Brown Rice Salad with Thyme, 170
Mediterranean Rice Bake with Eggplant and Tomatoes, 231
Mock Risotto with Zucchini, 231
Persian-Inspired Rice Pilaf with Cherries & Pistachios, 232
Pork Chops with Caraway Rice, 331
Pork Fried Rice, 332
Red Beans & Rice, 243
Shrimp Fried Rice, 296–97
Shrimp Jambalaya, 297
Simply Cooked Brown Rice, 230
Spanish-Style Beef & Brown Rice Bowls, 330
Thai-Inspired Shrimp Soup, 82–83
Tofu Fried Rice, 232
Tomato-Topped Veggie-Egg Bake, 127–28
Vegetable-Almond Rice with Parmesan, 233
Vegetable Fried Rice, 233–34
rice, wild
Autumn Wild Rice & Chicken Bowls, 159
Chicken & Wild Rice Salad with Grapes & Candied Pecans, 162
Garlicky Wild Rice & Mushroom-Stuffed Acorn Squash, 274–75
Simply Cooked Wild Rice, 234
Wild Rice & Chickpea Salad, 171
Wild Rice with Mushrooms, Tarragon & Pine Nuts, 234
Wild Rice with Sausage & Sage, 235
Rice Noodles with Snow Peas & Shrimp, 212
Roast Chicken with Lemon & Thyme, 313–14
Roasted Acorn Squash with Allspice & Sage, 271
Roasted Almond-Crusted Snapper, 291
Roasted Balsamic-Glazed Salmon, 291–92
Roasted Butternut Bisque, 80–81

Roasted Garlic Aïoli, 45
Roasted Mushroom–Barley Pilaf, 223
Roasted Poblano Soup, 81
Roasted Potatoes with Cinnamon, 270
Roasted Red Pepper Fettuccine, 202, 212–13
Roasted Salmon with Honey Walnut Lemon Sauce, 292
Roasted Sweet Potatoes & Ginger-Spiced Apples, 273
Roasted Vegetable Lasagna, 213–14
Romesco Sauce, 58
rosemary
Garlic & Rosemary Egg Bites with Gruyère, 121
Rosemary-Cider Vinaigrette, 169
Rosemary-Citrus Chicken, 314
Rosemary-Garlic Chicken Wings, 315
Rosemary Mashed Potatoes, 270
Rosemary-Sage Gremolata, 63
Shiitake & Spinach Quiche with Rosemary & Sage, 125, 126
White Bean Salad with Lemon & Rosemary, 245
Rotisserie Chicken & Farro Soup with Cannellini Beans, 82
Rustic Herb Seasoning, 36

S
saffron threads, 284–85
sage
Cumin, Sage & Turmeric Seasoning, 32
Roasted Acorn Squash with Allspice & Sage, 271
Rosemary-Sage Gremolata, 63
Shiitake & Spinach Quiche with Rosemary & Sage, 125, 126
Spicy Sage Breakfast Sausage, 124–25
Wild Rice with Sausage & Sage, 235
Salade Niçoise, 166–67
salmon
Fresh Salmon Burgers, 179–80
Roasted Balsamic-Glazed Salmon, 291–92
Roasted Salmon with Honey Walnut Lemon Sauce, 292
Salmon & White Bean Bowl with Lime & Dill, 244
Salmon Spring Rolls, 188, 188–89
Simply Broiled Salmon, 298
Smoked Salmon & Corn Chowder, 88–89
Smoked Salmon Flatbread with Dill, 200
Smoky Seared Salmon for One, 298
Salmon Rub, 36
sardines, 166–67
sausage
Bulgur Breakfast Porridge with Sausage, 120
Clams in Chorizo Tomato Saffron Sauce, 284–85
Sausage, Egg & Avocado Breakfast Sandwiches, 116, 124
Sausage & Roasted Red Pepper Breakfast Pizza, 199
Turkey Jambalaya, 318
Wild Rice with Sausage & Sage, 235
See also chicken; pork
Sautéed Shrimp & Scallops, 292–93
Savory Nut Crumb Topping, 36
Savory Roasted Mixed Nuts, 347
Savory Sorghum Porridge, 229
Savory Sweet Potato Fries, 272

scallops
  Miso-Glazed Scallops, 289
  Sautéed Shrimp & Scallops, 292–93
  Scallops en Papillote with Shallots,
    Edamame & Bell Pepper, 293–94
Seafood Seasoning, 37
Seafood Trio Rolls, 294
Seared Lamb Pita Pockets with Cucumber
  Mint Yogurt Sauce, 189
sea salt, 13
Sesame Chicken & Vegetable Foil Packs, 315–16
sesame seeds/sesame oil
  Apricot & Sesame Roasted Carrots, 266
  Asparagus with Sesame & Ginger, 263–64
  Cauliflower & Spinach Salad with Sesame-
    Orange Dressing, *143*, 147
  Sesame-Lime Dressing, 154
  Sesame Shrimp en Papillote, 294–95
  Sweet & Sour Sesame Dressing, 51
shallots, 293–94
Sheet Pan Chicken, Broccoli & Red Peppers,
  316
Sheet Pan Fish & Vegetable Bake, 295
Sheet Pan Tri-Tip Roast, 328–29
Shiitake & Spinach Quiche with Rosemary &
  Sage, 125, *126*
shrimp
  Cioppino, 86
  Cucumber-Shrimp Soup, 72
  Mango, Spinach & Shrimp Salad, *156–57*, 165
  Rice Noodles with Snow Peas & Shrimp, 212
  Sautéed Shrimp & Scallops, 292–93
  Seafood Trio Rolls, 294
  Sesame Shrimp en Papillote, 294–95
  Shrimp & Vegetable Pasta Bake, 214
  Shrimp Curry, 296
  Shrimp Fried Rice, 296–97
  Shrimp Jambalaya, 297
  Shrimp Stock, 71
  Shrimp Tacos, 185
  Southeast Asian–Style Shrimp & Napa
    Cabbage Salad with Rice Noodles, 167
  Thai-Inspired Shrimp Soup, 82–83
Simply Broiled Salmon, 298
Simply Cooked Barley, 223
Simply Cooked Black Beans, 241
Simply Cooked Brown Rice, 230
Simply Cooked Bulgur, 224
Simply Cooked Farro, 226
Simply Cooked Fresh Tomato Sauce, 59
Simply Cooked Lentils, 247
Simply Cooked Millet, 227
Simply Cooked Pork Tenderloin, 332–33
Simply Cooked Quinoa, 228
Simply Cooked Sorghum, 229
Simply Cooked White Beans, 241
Simply Cooked Wild Rice, 234
Simply Quick-Pickled Red Onions, 259
Simply Roasted Butternut Squash, 257
Simply Roasted Carrots, 257
Simply Roasted Cauliflower, 258
Simply Roasted Garlic, 258
Simply Roasted Green Beans, 258
Simply Roasted Peppers, 259
Simply Roasted Potatoes, 260
Simply Roasted Root Vegetables with Apples,
  252, 261
Simply Sautéed Zucchini, 262–63
Simply Slow-Roasted Tomatoes, 260–61

Simply Smashed Potatoes, 260
Simply Spanish-Style Mashed Potatoes,
  259–60
Simply Steamed Couscous, 205
Simply Steamed Vegetable Medley, 262
Simply Stewed Cabbage, 257
Simply Stir-Fried Vegetables, 262
Singapore-Inspired Chicken Rice Noodles,
  214–15
Skordalia, 59
Smoke & Pepper Ginger Rub, 37
Smoked Salmon & Corn Chowder, 88–89
Smoked Salmon Flatbread with Dill, 200
Smoked Tri-Tip, 329
Smoky Pecan Bits, 173
Smoky Roasted Edamame, 347
Smoky Roasted Mushrooms, 269
Smoky Seared Salmon for One, 298
Smoky Workaday Pork Tenderloin, 333
Smoky Workaday Seasoning, 37
Smoky Workaday Sweet Corn & Pepper Sauté,
  268
snapper, 291
sole, 294
sorghum
  Savory Sorghum Porridge, 229
  Simply Cooked Sorghum, 229
South African Lamb Pie (Bobotie), 334–35
Southeast Asian–Style Shrimp & Napa
  Cabbage Salad with Rice Noodles, 167
Southwest Corn Bread, 105
Southwestern Beef & Bean Burgers, 180–81
Southwest Pita Chips, 340–41
Southwest Seasoning, 37
soy milk, 139, *139*
Spaghetti Squash Sauté with Black Olives &
  Feta, 272
Spaghetti with Meat Sauce, 215–16
Spanish-Style Beef & Brown Rice Bowls, 330
Spiced Ginger Cream, *348*, 362
Spicy Black Bean Chili, 244–45
Spicy Candied Pecans, 173
Spicy Cauliflower Stir-Fry, 267–68
Spicy North African-Style Carrot Dip, *337*, 343
Spicy Roasted Squash with Tuscan-Style
  Glaze, 271
Spicy Sage Breakfast Sausage, 124–25
Spicy Shredded Beef Street Tacos, *174*, 186
spinach
  Cauliflower & Spinach Salad with Sesame-
    Orange Dressing, *143*, 147
  Chicken Lentil Spinach Bowls, 161
  Citrus, Spinach & Mushroom Salad, 147
  Creamy Spinach Lasagna, 208–9
  Greek Orzo Salad with Spinach & Tomatoes,
    209
  Hot Curried Egg Bites, 121–22
  Kefir, Spinach & Avocado Smoothie, 139, *139*
  Mango, Spinach & Shrimp Salad, *156–57*, 165
  Mushroom & Spinach–Stuffed Tomatoes,
    275–76
  Quinoa-Veggie Egg Bites, 123–24
  Roasted Vegetable Lasagna, 213–14
  Shiitake & Spinach Quiche with Rosemary
    & Sage, 125, *126*
  Spinach-Lentil Dal, 248
  Spinach Pesto, 46–47
  Spinach Salad with Honeycrisp Apples &
    Cheddar, 148

Spinach Scramble Pita Pockets, 127
Turkey Tenderloins with Spinach Pesto &
  Pistachios, 319
Very Veggie Grilled Cheese Sandwiches,
  182–83
Very Veggie Pizza, 200–201, *201*
squash
  Brown Rice with Pine Nuts & Roasted
    Butternut Squash, 230
  Garlicky Wild Rice & Mushroom-Stuffed
    Acorn Squash, 274–75
  Red Lentil & Vegetable Soup, 79–80
  Roasted Acorn Squash with Allspice &
    Sage, 271
  Roasted Butternut Bisque, 80–81
  Simply Roasted Butternut Squash, 257
  Spaghetti Squash Sauté with Black Olives
    & Feta, 272
  Spicy Roasted Squash with Tuscan-Style
    Glaze, 271
  Turkey & Squash Couscous with Apricots &
    Peanuts, 318–19
Stir-Fried Vegetable & Farfalle Bowl, 216
Stone Fruit Salsa, 62
strawberries
  Rhubarb-Strawberry Coffee Cake, 99–100
  Strawberries with Almond-Oat Crumble,
    354
  Strawberry, Pineapple & Mint Salad, 145
  Strawberry Pancakes, 135–36
  Strawberry-Rhubarb Bars, 359
  Strawberry Salsa, 62
Summer Lake Bake, 299
Summer Vegetable Pasta Toss, 217, *217*
sunflower seeds, 108
Super Savory Sloppy Joes, 181
Super Seeds Protein Power Bars, 136
Super Smoothie Secrets, 137
sustainability, 24–25
Swedish Meatballs, 330
Sweet & Sour Sauce, 60
Sweet & Sour Sesame Dressing, 51
Sweet & Tangy Red Pepper Sauce, 60
sweet potatoes
  Harvest Crescents, 109–10, *115*
  Roasted Sweet Potatoes & Ginger-Spiced
    Apples, 273
  Savory Sweet Potato Fries, 272
  Turkish-Inspired Bulgur–Sweet Potato
    Patties, 225–26
  West African–Inspired Sweet Potato &
    Peanut Stew, *66*, 85

T
Tabbouleh, 225
Taco Seasoning, 38, *38*
tahini, sesame
  Classic Hummus, 245–46
  Eastern Mediterranean Bowls with
    Hummus & Tabbouleh, 246
Tangy Sautéed Red Cabbage, 265
tarragon
  Tarragon & Thyme Vinaigrette, 51
  Wild Rice with Mushrooms, Tarragon &
    Pine Nuts, 234
Thai-Inspired Shrimp Soup, 82–83
thyme
  Artichoke & Onions with Lemon & Thyme,
    263
  Lentil & Brown Rice Salad with Thyme, 170

Lime & Thyme Vinaigrette, 50–51
Roast Chicken with Lemon & Thyme, 313–14
Tarragon & Thyme Vinaigrette, 51
tilapia
    Coconut Fish Curry, 285
    Mediterranean Tilapia en Papillote, 287
tofu
    Crispy Tofu Bites, 250–51
    Crispy Tofu with Lentils & Mixed Greens, 169
    Mango Tofu Soy Milk Smoothie, 139, *139*
    Tofu Fried Rice, 232
    Tofu Italiano Bake, 251
    Tofu Sloppy Joes, 182
    Zoodle Tofu Bowls, 171–72
Tofu Seasoning, 38
Tomatillo-Pork Stew, 89
tomatoes
    Angel Hair Pasta with Tomatoes & Basil, 207
    Broccoli with Coriander & Tomatoes, 264
    Bulgur & Tomato Salad with Mint, 224–25
    Bulgur-Tomato Salad with Tuna & Mint, 160
    Cherry Tomato Caprese Salad, 150
    Chicken Waldorf Tomato Blossoms with Feta & Dill, 162
    Clams in Chorizo Tomato Saffron Sauce, 284–85
    Creamy Eggplant with Tomatoes, 277
    Cucumber & Tomato Salad, 152
    Curried Rice–Stuffed Tomatoes, 276
    Garlic-Tomato Confit, 64
    Greek-Inspired Baked Chickpeas with Tomatoes & Feta, *236*, 246–47
    Greek Orzo Salad with Spinach & Tomatoes, 209
    Indian-Spiced Cauliflower & Tomato Soup, 76
    Lentil Caprese Salad, 170
    Margherita Pizza, 197
    Mediterranean Rice Bake with Eggplant and Tomatoes, 231
    Mexican-Inspired Egg & Veggie Skillet, 122–23
    Mushroom & Spinach–Stuffed Tomatoes, 275–76
    Pan-Seared White Fish, Arugula & Roasted Tomato Salad, 166
    Pasta Primavera, 211
    Pico de Gallo, 61
    Pineapple Salsa with Tomato & Lemon, 62
    Red Lentil & Vegetable Soup, 79–80
    Red Potato & Onion Roast with Cherry Tomatoes & Kalamata Olives, 269–70
    Romesco Sauce, 58
    Sheet Pan Fish & Vegetable Bake, 295
    Simply Cooked Fresh Tomato Sauce, 59
    Simply Slow-Roasted Tomatoes, 260–61
    Spaghetti with Meat Sauce, 215–16
    Tomato-Basil Soup, 83
    Tomato-Corn Salsa, 62–63
    Tomato Jam, 343
    Tomato-Topped Veggie-Egg Bake, 127–28
    Very Veggie Pizza, 200–201, *201*
tomato sauce, 55
tortillas
    Chicken & Bean Burritos, 186–87
    Chicken Enchiladas, 306
    Crispy Cajun Corn Chips, 339

Cumin-Garlic Tortilla Chips, *336–37*, 340
Fish Tacos, *39*, 184
Portobello Street Tacos, 184–85
Shrimp Tacos, 185
Spicy Shredded Beef Street Tacos, *174*, 186
Tropical Fruit Salsa, 63
tuna
    Ahi Burgers with Wasabi-Ginger Slaw, 177
    Bulgur-Tomato Salad with Tuna & Mint, 160
    Salade Niçoise, 166–67
turkey
    Herb-Roasted Turkey Breast with Vegetables, *40*, 317–18
    Turkey & Squash Couscous with Apricots & Peanuts, 318–19
    Turkey Jambalaya, 318
    Turkey Tenderloins with Spinach Pesto & Pistachios, 319
    Turkey-Vegetable Soup, 84
Turkish-Inspired Bulgur–Sweet Potato Patties, 225–26
turmeric
    Berry-Turmeric Smoothie, 138, *138*
    Cumin, Sage & Turmeric Seasoning, 32
turnips
    Potato-Turnip Gratin, *278*, 278–79
    Simply Roasted Root Vegetables with Apples, *252*, 261
Tuscan-Inspired Pork, 333
Tzatziki, 60

V
Vegetable-Almond Rice with Parmesan, 233
Vegetable Broth, 72
Vegetable Fried Rice, 233–34
vegetables
    Quick-Pickled Vegetables, 274
    Stir-Fried Vegetable & Farfalle Bowl, 216
    See also specific vegetables
Vegetarian Shepherd's Pie, 279
Very Veggie Grilled Cheese Sandwiches, 182–83
Very Veggie Miso Soup, 84
Very Veggie Pizza, 200–201, *201*
vinegar
    Balsamic Vinaigrette, 170
    Blue Cheese Vinaigrette, 48
    Cilantro-Lime Vinaigrette, 170–71
    Dill Vinaigrette, 49
    Ginger-Apple Cider Dressing, 148
    Herbed Red Wine Vinaigrette, 50
    Herb-Infused Vinegar, 50
    Honey Balsamic Onion Jam, 64–65
    Lemon Vinaigrette, 170
    Lime & Thyme Vinaigrette, 50–51
    Potato Salad with Red Wine Vinaigrette, 154, *154–55*
    Prosciutto & Pear Piadine with Balsamic Drizzle, 198–99
    Roasted Balsamic-Glazed Salmon, 291–92
    Rosemary-Cider Vinaigrette, 169
    Tarragon & Thyme Vinaigrette, 51

W
walnuts
    Apple-Walnut Bread, 100–101
    Apple Walnut Date Coffee Cake, 356
    Banana Nut Bread, 101
    Cauliflower-Walnut Casserole, 276–77
    Chocolate Energy Bars, 131
    Citrusy Walnut Gremolata, 63
    Dark Chocolate Cranberry Oatmeal Cookies with Walnuts, 358
    Roasted Salmon with Honey Walnut Lemon Sauce, 292
    Zucchini-Nut Bread, 106
Wasabi-Ginger Coleslaw, 155
Watermelon, Grapefruit & Blueberry Salad, 145
Wedge Salad, 155
West African–Inspired Sweet Potato & Peanut Stew, *66*, 85
White Bean Salad with Lemon & Rosemary, 245
White Fish with Fennel & Leeks, 299, *300*
Whole Wheat French Baguette, 114
Whole Wheat–Herb Pizza Dough, 195
Wild Crab Salad, 168
Wild Rice & Chickpea Salad, 171
Wild Rice with Mushrooms, Tarragon & Pine Nuts, 234
Wild Rice with Sausage & Sage, 235
Wine-Poached Pears, 354–55
Wonton Crisps, 341

Y
yogurt, Greek
    Blueberry Ginger Yogurt Bark with Almonds, 362
    Cucumber Mint Yogurt Sauce, 189
    Fresh Chive–Yogurt Buns, 108–9
    Maple-Yogurt Dressing, 149
    Mixed Fruit with Yogurt-Cardamom Dressing, 144
    Tzatziki, 60
    Yogurt-Cardamom Dressing, 52

Z
Zesty Chicken Bites, 316–17
Zoodle Tofu Bowls, 171–72
zucchini
    Couscous with Vegetables & Pine Nuts, *204*, 206
    Italian Pasta Salad, 210
    Mock Risotto with Zucchini, 231
    Roasted Vegetable Lasagna, 213–14
    Simply Sautéed Zucchini, 262–63
    Summer Vegetable Pasta Toss, 217, *217*
    Zoodle Tofu Bowls, 171–72
    Zucchini-Nut Bread, 106

About the Authors

LINDA HACHFELD, MPH, RDN, served as the first community registered dietitian nutritionist in the Minnesota Heart Health Program, one of three NIH-funded community trials (Stanford, Minnesota, and Pawtucket) to reduce heart disease and stroke risk-factors through community-wide health-promotion efforts. Linda was tasked with developing healthy-eating strategies through grocery stores (Shop Smart), restaurants (Dining à la Heart), and in homes (Eat Smart) through recipe development, cooking demonstrations, and public speaking.

Afterward, as a nutrition entrepreneur, she founded and ran an independent publishing company, Appletree Press, focused on producing practical culinary health books written by nutrition experts that inspire and encourage healthful eating to reduce the risk of heart disease, diabetes, and obesity. As an avid volunteer, she spearheaded community and state efforts under the umbrellas of the American Heart Association, addressing women's issues and heart disease (Go Red Program), and the National Cancer Society (Nutrition Puts the Bite on Cancer), helping individuals choose and prepare health-promoting foods.

Linda received awards of excellence and recognition in the fields of dietetics, publishing, community leadership, and a variety of health initiatives from her state public health department, the Academy of Nutrition & Dietetics, the YWCA, Women Executives in Business, the Independent Book Publishers Association (recipient of the prestigious Benjamin Franklin Award of Excellence), the Midwest Independent Publishers Association (Distinguished Service Award), the Small Business Administration (Small Business Advocate of the Year Award for Women in Business), and she was honored as the outstanding alumna from the FCS department at her alma mater and with a certificate of commendation for community health promotion from the Governor of Minnesota, where she was cited for her dedication, enthusiasm, and inspiration.

Linda received her bachelor of science degree in dietetics from Minnesota State University, Mankato.

She earned a credential of advance studies in health services administration and a master of public health from the University of Minnesota, with an emphasis on nutrition administration. Linda has earned certificates in community partnerships from the Department of Health and Human Services and in publishing specialties for technical books from the University of Chicago.

Apart from her love of lifelong learning and the ongoing (re)search for the best molasses or ginger cookie, Linda's passions include a fondness for Scottish terriers, rescuing painted turtles on the byways of Minnesota, and championing her two adult children, Ed and Alicia, in their ongoing personal and professional pursuits.

AMY MYRDAL MILLER, MS, RDN, FAND, is an award-winning dietitian, farmer's daughter, public speaker, author, and president of Farmer's Daughter Consulting, Inc., an agriculture, food, and culinary communications firm. Amy's career highlights include working for Dole Food Company, the California Walnut Board and Commission, and The Culinary Institute of America. Today Amy works with a variety of clients across the food system, including seed companies, food startups, grower cooperatives, commodity boards, national brands, nonprofits, campus dining operations, and restaurants. Amy earned her undergraduate degree from the University of California, Davis and her master's degree from Tufts University Friedman School of Nutrition Science and Policy. She has been a member of the Academy of Nutrition and Dietetics since 1991 and a member of Les Dames d'Escoffier International since 2010. A farmer's daughter from North Dakota, she has been cooking since age seven, when she was diagnosed with type 1 diabetes. Today, Amy and her husband Scott live in Carmichael, California, where backyard gardening, cooking together, and wine tasting bring them great joy.